Essentials of Clinical Nutrition in Healthcare

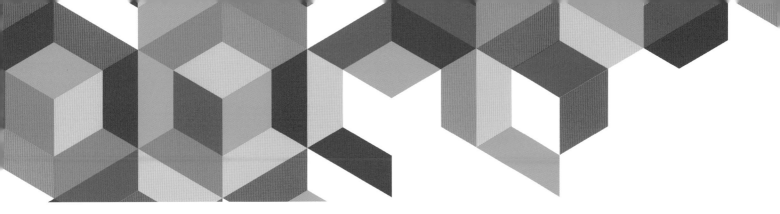

Essentials of Clinical Nutrition in Healthcare

Beth Frates, MD, FACLM, DipABLM
President of the American College of Lifestyle Medicine
Assistant Professor, Part Time
Department of Physical Medicine and Rehabilitation
Harvard Medical School
Spaulding Rehabilitation Hospital
Director of Lifestyle Medicine and Wellness
Department of Surgery
Massachusetts General Hospital
Boston, Massachusetts

Marie-France Hivert, MD, MMSc
Associate Professor, Department of Population Medicine
Director, Curricular Theme Nutrition and Lifestyle Medicine
Harvard Medical School
Division of Chronic Disease Research Across the Lifecourse (CoRAL)
Harvard Pilgrim Health Care Institute
Endocrinologist, Diabetes Unit
Massachusetts General Hospital
Boston, Massachusetts

Christopher P. Duggan, MD, MPH
Samuel Meltzer Professor of Pediatrics in the Field of Gastroenterology
Director, Division of Nutrition
Harvard Medical School
Director, Center for Nutrition
Division of Gastroenterology, Hepatology and Nutrition
Boston Children's Hospital
Professor, Departments of Nutrition and Global Health and Population
Harvard TH Chan School of Public Health
Boston, Massachusetts

McGraw Hill

Essentials of Clinical Nutrition in Healthcare

1 2 3 4 5 6 7 8 9   DSS   29 28 27 26 25 24

ISBN 978-1-264-58188-7
MHID 1-264-58188-2

The editors were Victor Lopez and Christina M. Thomas.
The production supervisor was Catherine Saggese.
Project management was provided by Karan Rana, MPS Limited.

Library of Congress Cataloging-in-Publication Data

Names: Frates, Elizabeth Pegg, 1967- author. | Hivert, Marie-France, author. |
    Duggan, Christopher (Christopher P.), author.
Title: Essentials of clinical nutrition in healthcare / Elizabeth Frates, Marie-France Hivert,
    Christopher Duggan.
Description: New York : McGraw Hill, [2024] | Includes bibliographical references and index.
Identifiers: LCCN 2023042982 (print) | LCCN 2023042983 (ebook) |
    ISBN 9781264581887 (paperback) | ISBN 9781264583379 (ebook)
Subjects: MESH: Nutrition Therapy | Nutritional Physiological Phenomena
Classification: LCC RM216 (print) | LCC RM216 (ebook) | NLM WB 400 |
    DDC 615.8/54—dc23/eng/20231107
LC record available at https://lccn.loc.gov/2023042982
LC ebook record available at https://lccn.loc.gov/2023042983

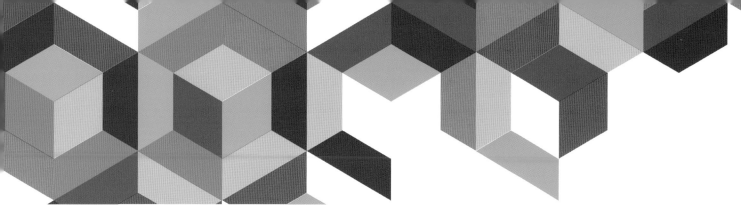

Contents

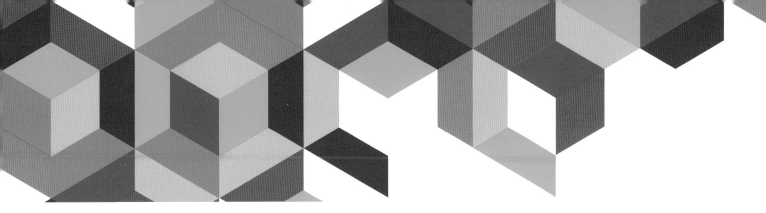

Student Reviewers

Andre Dempsey
Harvard Medical School
Class of 2024

Alaina Bever, PhD
Harvard Medical School
Class of 2026

Allison Fialkowski, MD
Clinical Fellow in Pediatrics
Harvard Medical School

Jake Cantrell
Harvard School of Dental Medicine
Class of 2025

Becca Clem
Harvard School of Dental Medicine
Class of 2025

Tashuana Holms
Harvard School of Dental Medicine
Class of 2025

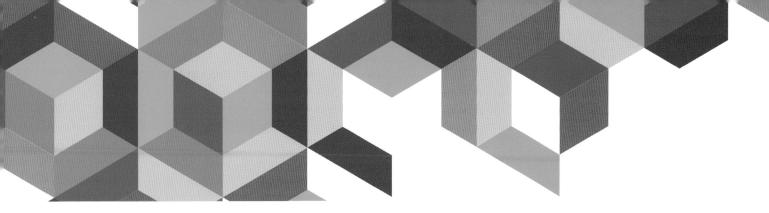

Contributors

Sondos Alghamdi, BDS, MMSc, FRCDC
Instructor, Department of Pediatric Dentistry and
    Orthodontics
King Khalid University, College of Dentistry, Saudi Arabia
Lecturer, Department of Oral Health Policy and
    Epidemiology
Harvard School of Dental Medicine
Boston, Massachusetts

Katelyn Ariagno, MPH, RD, LDN, CNSC
Senior Clinical Nutrition Specialist
Division of Gastroenterology, Hepatology and Nutrition
Boston Children's Hospital
Boston, Massachusetts

S. Bryn Austin, ScD
Professor
Department of Social and Behavioral Sciences
Harvard T.H. Chan School of Public Health
Division of Adolescent/Young Adult Medicine, Boston
    Children's Hospital
Department of Pediatrics, Harvard Medical School
Boston, Massachusetts

Robert Bandsma, MD, PhD
Staff Gastroenterologist, Nutritionist, Division of
    Gastroenterology, Hepatology and Nutrition,
    The Hospital for Sick Children
Associate Professor, Departments of Paediatrics and
    Nutritional Sciences, University of Toronto
Toronto, Ontario, Canada

Mandy B. Belfort, MD MPH
Associate Professor of Pediatrics, Harvard Medical School
Attending Neonatologist
Brigham and Women's Hospital
Department of Pediatrics
Division of Newborn Medicine
Boston, Massachusetts

Gerard T. Berry, MD
Division of Genetics and Genomics
Boston Children's Hospital
Professor of Pediatrics
Harvard Medical School
Boston, Massachusetts

Alaina Bever, PhD
MD Candidate
Department of Epidemiology, Harvard TH Chan School
    of Public Health
Harvard-MIT Division of Health Sciences and Technology,
    Harvard Medical School
Boston, Massachusetts

Lea Borgi, MD, MMSc
Associate Physician, Renal Division, Brigham and
    Women's Hospital
Instructor in Medicine, Harvard Medical School
Boston, Massachusetts

Cora C. Breuner, MD, MPH, FAAP
Professor
Department of Pediatrics
Adolescent Medicine Division
Adjunct Professor
Orthopedics and Sports Medicine
Seattle Childrens Hospital
University of Washington
Seattle, Washington

Nigel Brockton, PhD
Vice President, Research
American Institute for Cancer Research
Arlington, Virginia
Associate Professor (Adjunct)
Department of Community Health Sciences
University of Calgary
Calgary, Alberta

W. Scott Butsch, MD, MSc, FTOS
Director of Obesity Medicine
Bariatric and Metabolic Institute
Department of Surgery
Department of Internal Medicine and Geriatrics
Cleveland Clinic
Cleveland, Ohio

Andrew T. Chan, MD, MPH
Daniel K. Podolsky Professor of Medicine
Clinical and Translational Epidemiology Unit
Division of Gastroenterology
Massachusetts General Hospital and Harvard Medical School
Boston, Massachusetts

Denis Chang, MD
Attending Physician
Division of Gastroenterology, Hepatology, and Nutrition
Boston Children's Hospital
Boston, Massachusetts

Ariana Cerro, RD, LDN, CNSC
Clinical Nutrition Specialist
Center for Nutrition, Boston Children's Hospital
Division of Gastroenterology, Hepatology, and Nutrition
Boston, Massachusetts

Caitlin Colling, MD
Instructor of Medicine, Harvard Medical School
Assistant in Medicine, Massachusetts General Hospital
Co-Director, Inpatient Diabetes Management Service
Department of Medicine, Division of Endocrinology,
    Diabetes & Metabolism
Boston, Massachusetts

Amy Comander, MD, DipABLM
Instructor in Medicine, Harvard Medical School
Director of Lifestyle Medicine,
Massachusetts General Cancer Center
Medical Director, Mass General Cancer Center at Waltham
Director of Breast Oncology, Massachusetts General Cancer
    Center at Waltham and at Newton-Wellesley Hospital
Waltham, Massachusetts

Melanie V. Connolly, MSc, RD, LDN, CNSC
Clinical Nutrition Specialist
Center for Nutrition
Boston Children's Hospital
Boston, Massachusetts

McGreggor Crowley, MD
Instructor in Pediatrics
Harvard Medical School
Attending Physician
Center for Nutrition, Boston Children's Hospital
Division of Gastroenterology, Hepatology, and Nutrition
Boston, Massachusetts

Helen Delichatsios, MD, SM, DipABLM
Assistant Professor of Medicine
Harvard Medical School
Primary Care Physician, MGH Beacon Hill
Boston, Massachusetts

Ashley C. Draviam, MS, RD, LDN, CSO
Senior Clinical Dietitian
Mass General Cancer Center
Boston, Massachusetts

David Eisenberg, MD
Director of Culinary Nutrition
Adjunct Associate Professor
Department of Nutrition
Harvard T.H. Chan School of Public Health
Boston, Massachusetts

Jessica Fanzo, PhD
Professor of Climate
Director of the Food for Humanity Initiative
Columbia Climate School
Columbia University
New York, New York

Lauren G. Fiechtner, MD
Assistant Professor of Pediatrics
Division of Pediatric Gastroenterology and Nutrition,
    Mass General Hospital for Children
Department of Pediatrics, Harvard Medical School
Boston, Massachusetts

Mary Flanagan, MB, BCh, BAO, BPharm
Clinical Gastroenterology Fellow
Division of Gastroenterology, Hepatology and Nutrition,
    The Hospital for Sick Children
Toronto, Ontario, Canada

Beth Frates, MD, FACLM, DipABLM
President of the American College of Lifestyle Medicine
Assistant Professor, Part Time
Department of Physical Medicine and Rehabilitation
Harvard Medical School
Spaulding Rehabilitation Hospital
Director of Lifestyle Medicine and Wellness
Department of Surgery
Massachusetts General Hospital
Boston, Massachusetts

Christopher D. Golden PhD, MPH
Associate Professor of Nutrition and Planetary Health
Department of Nutrition, Harvard TH Chan School
    of Public Health
Boston, Massachusetts

Connor Hatfield, BSc
California Polytechnic State University-San Luis Obispo
San Luis Obispo, California
Incoming DO-MPH Student
Touro University California
Vallejo, California

Michelle Hauser, MD, MS, MPA, FACP, FACLM, DipABLM
Clinical Associate Professor, Medicine (Surgery), General
    Surgery and, by courtesy, Primary Care and Population
    Health
Stanford University School of Medicine
Stanford, California
Obesity Medicine, Medical Service
Veterans Affairs Palo Alto Health Care System
Palo Alto, California

Catherine Hayes, DMD, SM, DMSc
Chair, Department of Oral Health Policy and Epidemiology
DPH Program Director
Harvard School of Dental Medicine
Boston, Massachusetts

Awab Ali Ibrahim, MD
Instructor in Pediatrics, Harvard Medical School
Attending Physician
Division of Pediatric Gastroenterology and Nutrition,
    Mass General Hospital for Children
Boston, Massachusetts

Jamieson D. Johnson, MSS, CLMC, CITC, CPWC, CEP
Lifestyle Medicine Coach
Institute of Lifestyle Medicine
Topsham, Maine

Allison Kimball, MD
Assistant Professor of Medicine, Harvard Medical School
Assistant Physician, Massachusetts General Hospital
Department of Medicine, Division of Endocrinology,
    Diabetes & Metabolism
Boston, Massachusetts

Kevin C. Klatt, PhD, RD
Associate Research Scientist
Nutritional Sciences & Toxicology
University of California Berkeley
Berkeley, California

Andrée LeRoy, MD, FAAPMR, DipABLM
Assistant Professor
Harvard Medical School
Spaulding Rehabilitation Hospital
Massachusetts General Hospital
Boston, Massachusetts

Julia V. Loewenthal, MD
Associate Physician
Division of Aging, Department of Medicine
Brigham and Women's Hospital
Instructor in Medicine, Harvard Medical School
Boston, Massachusetts

John D. Matthews, MD, MSc
Benson-Henry Institute for Mind Body Medicine
Massachusetts General Hospital
Assistant Professor of Psychiatry, Harvard Medical School
Boston, Massachusetts

Kathy McManus, MS, RD, LDN
Director
Department of Nutrition
Brigham and Women's Hospital
Boston, Massachusetts

Nilesh M. Mehta, MD, FASPEN
Professor of Anaesthesia
Harvard Medical School
Chair, Critical Care Nutrition & Metabolism
Vice Chair for Quality & Outcomes
Department of Anesthesiology, Critical Care and Pain Medicine
Associate Medical Director
Division of Critical Care Medicine
Boston Children's Hospital
Boston, Massachusetts

Jordi Merino, PhD
Associate Professor
Diabetes Unit and Center for Genomic Medicine,
    Massachusetts General Hospital
Boston, Massachusetts
Program in Medical and Population Genetics, Broad Institute
Cambridge, Massachusetts
Department of Medicine, Harvard Medical School
Boston, Massachusetts
Novo Nordisk Foundation Center for Basic Metabolic
    Research, Faculty of Health and Medical Sciences,
    University of Copenhagen
Copenhagen, Denmark

Jad Mitri, MD
Resident Physician
Department of Medicine, St Elizabeth's Medical Center
Boston, Massachusetts

Kris M. Mogensen, MS, RD-AP, LDN, CNSC
Team Leader Dietitian Specialist
Department of Nutrition
Brigham and Women's Hospital
Boston, Massachusetts

Uma Naidoo, MD
Director of Nutritional and Metabolic Psychiatry,
    Massachusetts General Hospital
Instructor in Psychiatry, Harvard Medical School
Boston, Massachusetts

Stacey L. Nelson, MS, RDN
Manager, Clinical Nutrition
Department of Nutrition Services/Department of
    Obstetrics & Gynecology
Massachusetts General Hospital
Boston, Massachusetts

Khristopher Nicholas, PhD
Yerby Postdoctoral Fellow
Harvard T.H. Chan School of Public Health
Boston, Massachusetts

Nancy Oliveira, MS, RD, LDN, CDCES
Manager
Nutrition and Wellness Service
Brigham and Women's Hospital
Boston, Massachusetts

Simone Passarelli, PhD
Post-doctoral Fellow
Department of Nutrition, Harvard TH Chan School
    of Public Health
Boston, Massachusetts

Chetan P. Phadke, BPhT, DRPT, PhD
Research Manager, Providence Care Centre
Adjunct Professor, School of Rehabilitation Therapy
Queen's University
Kingston, Ontario, Canada

Aleksandra Pikula, MD, DipABPN, DipABLM
Associate Professor of Medicine (Neurology),
    University of Toronto
Clinician Investigator, Krembil Brain Institute
Stroke Staff, University Health Network/Toronto
    Western Hospital
Toronto, Ontario, Canada

Daniel J. Pomerantz, MD
Research Fellow in Pediatrics
Division of Genetics and Metabolism, Boston
    Children's Hospital
Department of Pediatrics, Harvard Medical School
Boston, Massachusetts

Amanda Raffoul, PhD
Instructor in Pediatrics
Division of Adolescent/Young Adult Medicine, Boston
    Children's Hospital
Department of Pediatrics, Harvard Medical School
Boston, Massachusetts

Shirly (Shalu) Ramchandani, MD
Bariatric Medicine, St Elizabeth's Medical Center
Benson Henry Institute Mind Body Medicine, MGH
Boston, Massachusetts

Coral Rudie, MS, RD, LDN, CNSC
Senior Clinical Nutrition Specialist
Center for Nutrition
Boston Children's Hospital
Program Manager
Division of Nutrition
Harvard Medical School
Boston, Massachusetts

Sara Saliba, MD, RD, LDN
Resident Physician
Department of Internal Medicine
Cleveland Clinic
Cleveland, Ohio

Christopher R. Sudfeld, ScD
Associate Professor of Global Health and Nutrition
Departments of Global Health and Population and Nutrition
Harvard T.H. Chan School of Public Health
Boston, Massachusetts

Carol Sullivan, MS, RD, CSO, LDN
Senior Clinical Dietitian
Lead Nutritionist, Lifestyle Medicine Program, Massachusetts
    General Hospital Cancer Center
Mass General Cancer Center at Waltham
Waltham, Massachusetts

Karen M. Switkowski, PhD, MPH
Senior Research Scientist
Division of Chronic Disease Research Across the Lifecourse,
    Department of Population Medicine
Harvard Medical School and Harvard Pilgrim Health
    Care Institute
Boston, Massachusetts

Nadine Tassabehji, PhD, RDN, LDN
Assistant Professor
Course Director Craniofacial Biology
Department of Comprehensive Care
Tufts School of Dental Medicine
Division of Nutrition Interventions, Communication, and
    Behavior change
Friedman School of Nutrition Science and Policy
Boston, Massachusetts

Deirdre K. Tobias, ScD
Assistant Professor and Epidemiologist
Division of Preventive Medicine, Department of Medicine
Brigham and Women's Hospital and Harvard Medical School
Nutrition Department
Harvard T.H. Chan School of Public Health
Boston, Massachusetts

Armida Lefranc Torres, MD
Clinical Fellow in Medicine
Renal Division, Brigham and Women's Hospital
Boston, Massachusetts

Francine K Welty, MD, PhD
Associate Professor of Medicine, Harvard Medical School
Division of Cardiology, Beth Israel Deaconess Medical Center
Boston, Massachusetts

Walter Willett, MD, MPH, DrPH
Professor of Epidemiology and Nutrition
Harvard T.H. Chan School of Public Health
Boston, Massachusetts

Loren N. Winters, MSN, ANP-BC, OCN, DipABLM
Assistant Director of Lifestyle Medicine, Mass General
    Hospital Cancer Center
Assistant Director of Breast Cancer Survivorship, Mass
    General Cancer Center at Waltham
Waltham, Massachusetts

Allison J. Wu, MD, MPH
Assistant Professor of Pediatrics
Division of Gastroenterology, Hepatology, and Nutrition,
    Department of Pediatrics
Boston Children's Hospital, Harvard Medical School
Boston, Massachusetts

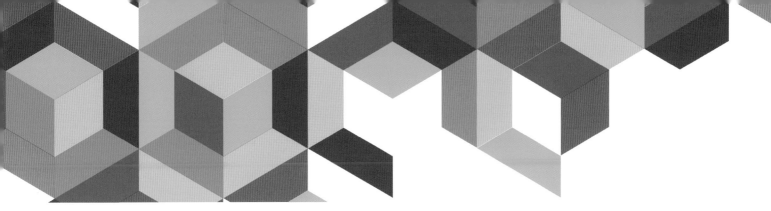

Preface

At a time when diet and lifestyle are among the most important factors in determining health and wellness, and when paradoxically instruction in these topics is scant in medical school and training afterwards, we are so pleased to publish the inaugural edition of *Essentials of Clinical Nutrition in Healthcare*. This book provides the essential facts in nutrition that every medical student and trainee needs to know before entering the wards, clinics, or practice. Many currently practicing providers will also find this book greatly informative, as historically few medical schools have been providing sufficient material and clinically applicable knowledge related to nutrition. Nutrition and lifestyle play such a critical role in the pathophysiology of many acute and chronic conditions that physicians treat each day. For example, diabetes and heart disease are greatly impacted by a person's eating patterns and other health behaviors, while susceptibility to infections, cancer, a wide variety of gastrointestinal diseases, and many others are impacted by diet and nutritional status. What food is healthy and why are questions patients routinely ask physicians, and physicians are expected to know the answers. This book prepares medical students, trainees, and lifelong learners to answer these questions.

The 32 chapters in this text are arranged in a progressive order. The first section covers nutrition in health, and includes chapters on biochemistry, metabolism, nutrition assessment, popular diets, and food system sustainability. The second section covers nutrition in disease, and includes chapters on several disease entities with strong nutritional etiologies, and/or for which nutritional management is core to treatment plans. The third section includes chapters with practical advice about how to counsel patients about nutrition and food.

Each chapter opens with learning objectives to help focus the reader. A clinical case is then presented to mimic a real-world clinical encounter, followed by clinically relevant questions emerging from the case. The questions are presented again at the end of the chapter, at which time the reader will have read the information necessary to answer the questions correctly. At the end of each chapter, there are key takeaways to remind the reader of the salient points.

Our expert authors have grounded this text in the latest research, and the book provides up-to-date evidence about how diet and nutritional status influence the development, progression, treatment, and prevention of many medical conditions. Each chapter addresses different conditions, and many chapters refer to information in different chapters. Readers can read the book from cover to cover, or they can select the topics most interesting to them and read based on their own interest. It will be important to read the whole book to understand the essentials of nutrition.

During clerkships and clinical practice, this nutrition text can serve as a reference for nutrition basics and counseling strategies that are effective for many medical conditions and as part of preventive practice. Unlike any other nutrition book currently available, this book also discusses how lifestyle medicine topics such as exercise, sleep, stress, and social connection interact with nutrition to impact a person's health.

In addition to our team of excellent authors, we are thankful to Coral Rudie, MS, RD, LDN, CNSC, who provided outstanding administrative and logistical support during the process of creating this textbook, as well as Michael Weitz and his colleagues at McGraw Hill for advice and help along the way to publication.

Beth Frates, MD, FACLM, DipABLM
Marie-France Hivert, MD, MMSc
Christopher P. Duggan, MD, MPH
Harvard Medical School
Boston, Massachusetts

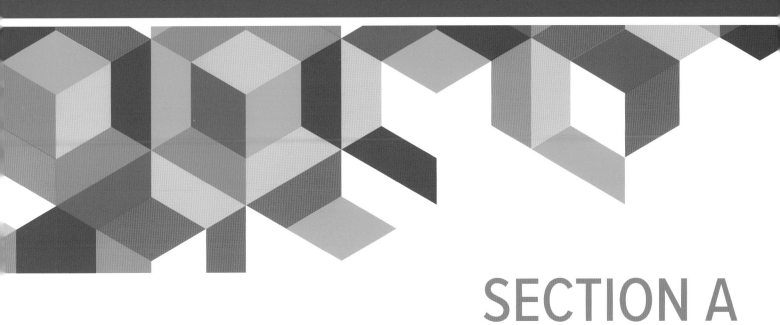

SECTION A

Nutrition and Metabolism in Health

Macronutrient Metabolism

Daniel J. Pomerantz, MD / Gerard T. Berry, MD

Chapter Outline

CASE STUDY

A 25-year-old otherwise healthy man with COVID-19 infection is admitted to the Intensive Care Unit for respiratory failure, dehydration, and inadequate nutrition. Along with requiring intubation for management of his respiratory failure, he has been unable to eat or drink anything for the past three days before presentation. Since he is expected to be intubated for a number of days due to his respiratory symptoms and is also too hemodynamically unstable to receive enteral nutrition at this time, the Intensive Care Unit has decided to start parental nutrition (i.e., intravenous nutrition).

1. The three critical macronutrients that are components of standard parenteral nutrition include all of the following except:
   A. Dextrose (carbohydrates)
   B. Vitamin A
   C. Amino acids
   D. Fatty acids

2. Starches, disaccharides, proteins, cholesterols, sphingolipids, and glycosaminoglycans are not included in parenteral nutrition. How does the body compensate for their absence?

3. The most important functions of macronutrient metabolism include:
   A. Energy production and storage
   B. Complex molecule formation and degradation for cellular development and signaling
   C. Macronutrient waste degradation and clearance
   D. A and B only
   E. A, B, and C

● WHAT ARE MACRONUTRIENTS AND WHY DO THEY MATTER?

Macronutrients are biochemical molecules for which life requires large amounts of regular consumption to support essential energy production and complex molecule formation. The five basic classes of macronutrients involved in human nutrition include sugars, fats, amino acids, nucleic acids, and water. These five macronutrients can be used in varying degrees and efficacy in energy production via the breakdown of these macronutrients, as well as complex molecule formation critical for energy storage and cellular functioning. Important complex molecules that can be formed from these macronutrients include polysaccharides such as starches, complex lipids including sphingolipids and cholesterols, amino acid formations such as proteins and glycosaminoglycans, and complex nucleic acid threads such as DNA and RNA. For each macronutrient and macromolecule class, the following sections will describe: (a) definition of specific macronutrient class, (b) important types of macronutrients and macromolecules within a specific class, (c) function of critical pathways in metabolism of macronutrients, and (d) health implications.

● CARBOHYDRATES

What Are Simple Carbohydrates and Monosaccharides?

Carbohydrates can be simply defined as biomolecules consisting of carbon, hydrogen, and oxygen, typically within a ratio of $C_xH_{2x}O_x$. These biomolecules form the basis of what we think of as sugars, also known as saccharides, which can be used in a diversity of different functions, depending on their size and molecular complexity. The complexity of saccharides is dependent upon glycosidic bonds between the carbon of one saccharide and the hydroxyl group of another saccharide. Monosaccharides are the least complex form of sugars as they cannot be decomposed into simpler sugars via the hydrolysis of glycosidic bonds. Classically, a monosaccharide has a carbohydrate structure that includes an aldehyde and a ketone with multiple hydroxyl groups added to each of the primary carbon groups. The typical structure of these monosaccharides is $H–(CHOH)_x(C=O)–(CHOH)_y–H$.[1,2]

What Are the Important Types of Monosaccharides?

The five most clinically significant forms of monosaccharides include three hexoses (i.e., six-carbon sugars, including glucose, fructose, and galactose), as well as two pentoses (i.e., five-carbon sugars, including ribose and deoxyribose).[1,2] Figure 1-1 shows the structural ring formations of these two sugar groups.

Glucose is a hexose with an aldehyde on its first carbon and is the most abundant monosaccharide macronutrient found in a number of plant-based food products. Galactose is a C-4 epimer of glucose, meaning that the hydroxyl group attached to the fourth carbon is positioned in the mirror image of glucose and can be found enriched in dairy products such as milk and cheese. Fructose is a hexose from which a ketone group is based on the second carbon, rather than an aldehyde group on the first carbon, and can be found enriched in fruits and vegetables. Collectively, these three hexoses are the primary carbohydrate-based macronutrients, from which humans accrue energy in the form of adenosine triphosphate (ATP).[1,2]

The most critical of these pathways includes glycolysis, a 10-step biochemical metabolic pathway that converts glucose into two pyruvate molecules. Pyruvate is a three-carbon macromolecule that can be readily metabolized into acetyl CoA and oxaloacetate via pyruvate dehydrogenase and pyruvate carboxylase respectively in order to fuel another 10-step biochemical pathway known as the citric acid cycle. The two pyruvate molecules formed from one glucose molecule can be converted into ATP, GTP, NADH, and $FADH_2$. The NADH and $FADH_2$ formed from the glycolysis and citric acid can be further formed into ATP in the mitochondria of cells via a process known as oxidative phosphorylation. Collectively through glycolysis, the citric acid cycle, and oxidative phosphorylation,

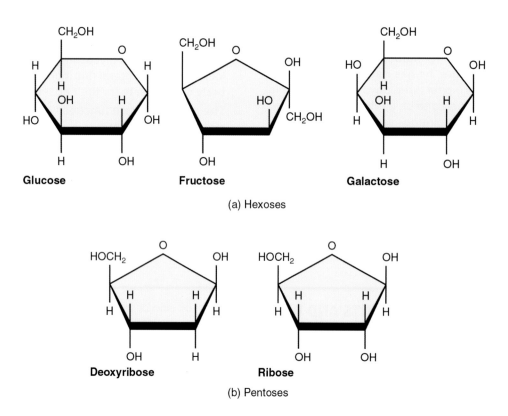

(a) Hexoses

Glucose   Fructose   Galactose

(b) Pentoses

Deoxyribose   Ribose

FIGURE 1-1 • Structures of important monosaccharides. (Copyright © 2022 The Consortium of Glycobiology Editors, La Jolla, California; published by Cold Spring Harbor Laboratory Press; doi:10.1101/glycobiology.4e.2. All rights reserved.[2])

one molecule of glucose can be metabolized to form 38 ATP molecules for energy.[1,2]

Fructose, which can be classically found in fruits, honeys, and vegetables such as corn, can form energy either by the conversion of fructose into glucose via a process known as gluconeogenesis, or through direct metabolism into pyruvate via fructolysis. Galactose cannot be directly converted into pyruvate like glucose or fructose can, but still can provide a source of ATP via conversion into glucose via a process known as the Leloir Pathway. The body also can regulate the uptake of glucose, fructose, and galactose via a number of monosaccharide transporters, including glucose transporters, galactose transporters, and fructose transporters in the gastrointestinal tract.[1-3]

Ribose and deoxyribose are five-carbon sugars that play a critical role in a number of cellular functions. Ribose plays a critical role in energy metabolism, as it is a core component of NADH, $FADH_2$, and NADPH. Ribose also is a building block of the signaling molecule cyclic adenosine monophosphate (cAMP). However, ribose and deoxyribose are most recognized as the sugar moiety that, through a process known as de novo nucleotide biosynthesis, form the nucleotides critical for the molecular coding of life: ribonucleic acid (RNA) and deoxyribonucleic acid (DNA). These pentoses can also be derived from glucose via an archaic metabolic pathway known as the pentose phosphate pathway, a pathway that can help fuel the production of nucleotides as well as the production of pyruvate and coenzymes such as NADH.[1-3]

These five aforementioned monosaccharides, along with hexoses such as mannose, and pentoses such as fucose, can also play a critical role in the glycosylation of proteins and lipids. The importance of these macronutrients in glycosylation will be discussed later in this chapter. These monosaccharides can also be converted into sugar alcohols, such as sorbitol, galactitol, and mannitol, which can be useful as artificial sweeteners, food preservatives, and medications.[1-4]

What Are Some of the Health Implications of These Monosaccharides?

Glucose levels are critical for energy homeostasis in human health and disease, providing a critical source of fuel for the brain, red blood cells, and renal medulla. Each gram of carbohydrate provides 4 kilocalories of energy.[1,5] High dietary intake of carbohydrates can lead to accumulation of the macronutrients throughout the body, such as through Non-Alcoholic Fatty Liver Disease (NAFLD). Hyperglycemia, or high blood sugars, classically defined as greater than 125 mg/dL in the fasting state or greater than 200 mg/dL in the fed state, can lead to excessive thirst and appetite, excessive urination to clear glucose, vomiting, confusion, cerebral edema, and coma.[1,5] While hyperglycemia can sometimes be secondary to excessive intravenous administration of glucose, more classically this is secondary to disorders of insulin. These include autoimmune reduction of insulin production (type 1 diabetes), metabolic cellular resistance to insulin (type 2 diabetes), and congenital disorders of insulin production (maturity-onset diabetes of youth [MODY]). Hypoglycemia, or low blood sugar levels, classically defined as less than 70 mg/dL in adults, can begin

to manifest with clinical symptoms such as hunger, fatigue, headache, and dizziness and can progress to more serious symptoms such as slurred speech, blurred vision, fainting, seizures, and coma. Classically, hypoglycemic episodes can occur in the context of secondary hyperinsulinism, such as through the administration of excess insulin for the treatment of disorders such as diabetes mellitus. Primary hyperinsulinism can also occur through the excess production of insulin from insulin-producing tumors, known as insulinomas, as well as congenital disorders of insulin function, known as congenital hyperinsulinism syndromes.[2]

Other disorders of monosaccharide metabolism include disorders of galactose, fructose, and ribose metabolism ranging from rare disorders such as classical galactosemia and hereditary fructose intolerance to very rare disorders affecting other enzymes in the Leloir Pathway, the Fructolysis Pathway, the Pentose Phosphate Pathway, and the Glycosylation Pathways. Collectively, these disorders lead to the accumulations of these non-glucose monosaccharides in organs such as the brain, eyes, and liver and can also lead to secondary disruptions in glucose levels as well, among other symptoms based upon the specific disorder.[1-5]

Disaccharides, Oligosaccharides, and Polysaccharides: Complex Sugars and Starches

What Are the Different Classes of Complex Sugars and Why Do We Have Them? Complex sugars are simply defined as two or more monosaccharides bound together by a glycolytic bond. The three main groups of these complex sugars include disaccharides (2 monosaccharides), oligosaccharides (3 to 10 monosaccharides), and polysaccharides (more than 10 monosaccharides). Globally, these complex sugars allow for improved storage of carbohydrates for utilization for energy production as well as structural macromolecule formation in human health and disease.[1,2,5]

What Are Some of the Important Types of Complex Sugar Macronutrients? While there are a number of types of disaccharides, the three most clinically significant types of disaccharides include maltose, lactose, and sucrose. Maltose is composed of one glucose molecule bound at its sixth carbon to the first carbon of a second glucose molecule. This molecule is classically found in foods such as grains and malts. Lactose is composed of one galactose molecule bound at its sixth carbon to the first carbon of a glucose molecule. This compound can be found in human milk as well as in dairy product such as milk and cheese, as well as whey products. Sucrose is composed of one glucose molecule bound at its sixth carbon to the second carbon of a fructose molecule (Figure 1-2). This compound is classically found in fruits, nectars, and honeys. Collectively, these disaccharides allow for readily storable forms of carbohydrates that can be converted into either more complex saccharides, or more bioavailable monosaccharides for energy utilization. These disaccharides can be readily digested in the human gut by enzymes known as disaccharidases, most significant among them including lactase, which metabolizes lactose, and sucrase-isomaltase, an enzyme that breaks down both sucrose and maltose.[2,5,6]

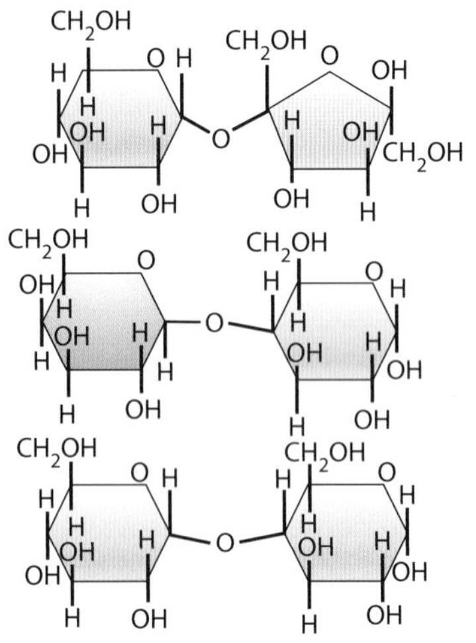

FIGURE 1-2 • Different types of disaccharides.[6]

Oligosaccharides can be divided into two main classes of function: dietary oligosaccharides and glycosylation structures. Dietary oligosaccharides include chains of 3 to 10 monosaccharides and disaccharides from foods such as fruits, vegetables, and dairy products enriched with compounds such as lactooligosaccharides, also known as human milk oligosaccharides (HMOs), fructooligosaccharides (FOS), and galactooligosaccharides (GOS). Notably, while these oligosaccharide groups cannot be absorbed directly by the human intestines, these oligosaccharides can be utilized as bacteria in the human gut to promote healthy gut ecology and facilitate their breakdown into monosaccharides and disaccharides, which can be absorbed by the gut via glucose transporters. Glycosylation structures of oligosaccharides will be discussed later in the chapter.[4]

Polysaccharides, carbohydrate complexes composed of more than 10 monosaccharides, can also be used in a diversity of functions in human health, including long-term carbohydrate storage for energy as well as structural macromolecule formations in food. Starches are plant-based polysaccharides composed of polyglucose molecules, known as amylose and amylopectin, for glucose energy storage and metabolism. Glycogens are animal-based polysaccharides composed of polyglucose molecules analogous to starch but with increased branching of polyglucose chains. Inulins are plant based, composed of polyfructose molecules also used in fructose energy metabolism. These molecules can be comprehensively broken down via salivary and pancreatic amylases as well as intestinal mucosal glucosidases into disaccharides and monosaccharides, which can be readily processed and transported into the bloodstream for either immediate energy utilization or via processing into human glycogen. Excess glucose molecules can be stored into glycogen via a metabolic pathway known as glycogenesis, by which large chains of glucoses can bind together for energy storage. These glycogen molecules are classically stored in the liver and muscles, but can also be found in the heart and brain as well. During periods of fasting, these stored macromolecules can be readily degraded into glucose

molecules via a process known as glycogenolysis. Thus, the formation and degradation of glycogen allows for appropriate storage and release of glucose for energy utilization during times of feeding and fasting, respectively. Celluloses (plant-based structural polysaccharides) and chitins (animal-based structural polysaccharides) are abundant in foods but hold limited to no nutritional value for humans.[1,2,5,6]

What Are the Health Implications of These Complex Carbohydrates? Metabolism of glycogen and starches focuses catabolism for energy production on carbohydrate metabolism, shunting away from lipid or other macromolecule classes for energy metabolism. Insulin plays a critical role in the regulation of the processes of glycogenolysis and glycogenesis, thus playing a critical role in energy homeostasis. Rare disorders of the biochemical pathways of glycogenolysis and glycogenesis, known as glycogen storage disorders, can lead to inappropriate storage and utilization of glycogen for energy production in cells enriched with glycogen, such as the liver and muscles. Complications range from episodic hypoglycemia, lactic acidosis, hepatomegaly, rhabdomyolysis, and elevated lipid levels, depending on the type of disease. Certain glucosidases enrich within the lysosomes of cells, leading to inappropriate storage of glycogen in the heart and brain cells to cause lysosomal glycogen storage diseases. Congenital deficiencies in disaccharidases such as lactase and sucrase-isomaltase can lead to inadequate absorption and metabolism of disaccharides in the diet and typically lead to chronic diarrhea in the neonatal period. Later-onset lactase deficiency occurs in people as the relative production of endogenous lactase is reduced and can manifest in gastrointestinal distress during the consumption of milk products.[1,2,5,6] Disorders of oligosaccharides are not a classically described entity. However, further research exploring the role of gut bacterial utilization of dietary oligosaccharides in neonatal disorders such as necrotizing enterocolitis, as well as gastrointestinal disorders of the microbiome such as infectious colitis, inflammatory bowel disease, and colon cancer, warrants further investigation.

● LIPIDS, FATTY ACIDS, AND CHOLESTEROLS

What Are Lipids and Why Are They Important?

Lipids, or fats, are a class of macromolecules of which non-polar polycarbon biomolecules are relatively insoluble in water, and are comprised predominantly of carbon and hydrogen chains. Different types of fats are dependent upon the types of added oxygen and nitrogen molecules in specific biochemically significant ways. These lipids can be broadly classified under the following groups: fatty acids and triglycerides, cholesterols and sterols, and complex lipids.[1,7,8]

Fatty acids are carboxylic acids (R-COOH) of varying lengths and saturation that are used for energy storage. While the smallest fatty acid is formic acid and the smallest multi-carbon fatty acid is acetic acid (Figure 1-3), carbon chains attached to the carboxylic acid group can range from

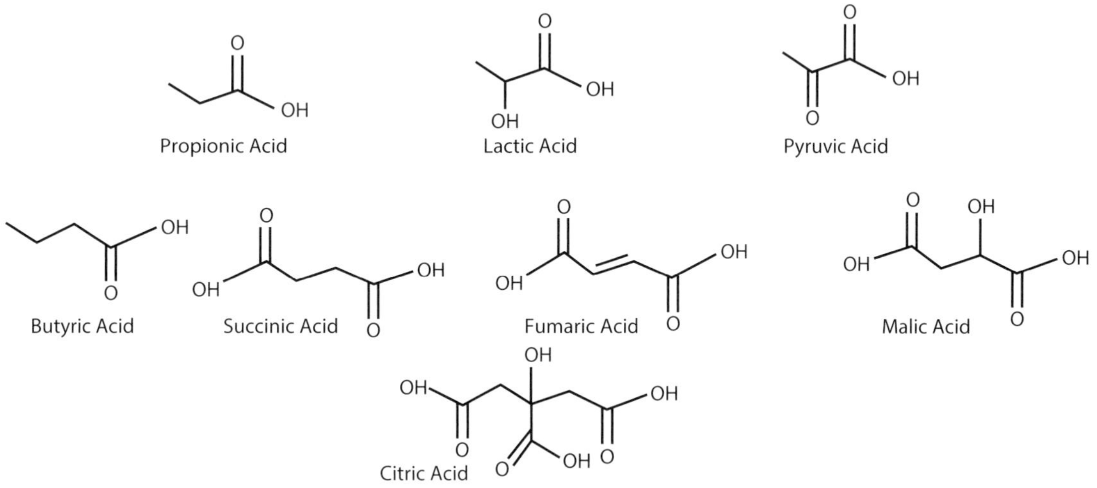
Propionic Acid
Lactic Acid
Pyruvic Acid
Butyric Acid
Succinic Acid
Fumaric Acid
Malic Acid
Citric Acid

FIGURE 1-3 • Examples of carboxylic acids. (Reproduced with permission from Yang ST (ed.). *Bioprocessing for value-added products from renewable resources: new technologies and applications*. Elsevier. 2007; 1-24.[9])

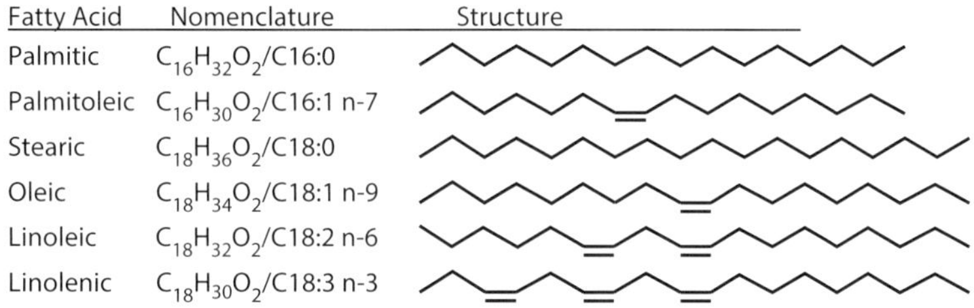
Fatty Acid
Nomenclature
Structure
Palmitic $C_{16}H_{32}O_2$/C16:0
Palmitoleic $C_{16}H_{30}O_2$/C16:1 n-7
Stearic $C_{18}H_{36}O_2$/C18:0
Oleic $C_{18}H_{34}O_2$/C18:1 n-9
Linoleic $C_{18}H_{32}O_2$/C18:2 n-6
Linolenic $C_{18}H_{30}O_2$/C18:3 n-3

FIGURE 1-4 • Examples of fatty acids. (Díez-Pascual AM, Rahdar A. Composites of vegetable oil-based polymers and carbon nanomaterials. *Macromol.* 2021;1(4):276-292.[10])

small (0–5 carbons), medium (6–12 carbons), long (13–21 carbons), and very long (22 or more carbons) fatty acids (Figures 1-3 and 1-4). These chains can also be saturated, meaning that the carbon bonds are entirely without double bonds, or unsaturated, meaning that the carbon chains have one or more double bonds between the carbons. This saturation component increases the energy storage of each fatty acid structure. Classically, these fatty acids are stored further into more complex energy units known as triglycerides. Triglycerides are simply three fatty acid groups esterified to glycerol for long-term fatty acid storage.[1,7,8]

Fundamentally, these fatty acids and triglycerides provide for another form of energy for which the body can utilize, particularly during times of fasting when glycogen stores are reduced or depleted. Fatty acids and triglycerides can be absorbed from dietary sources such as meats, nuts, and certain highly fat-enriched vegetables like avocados. Enzymes such as gastric and pancreatic lipases help break down triglycerides into fatty acids, which can bind to bile produced in the biliary tract and liver to form micelles. These micelles and free triglycerides can be further processed into lipid transport molecules known as chylomicrons that are absorbed into the bloodstream by the small intestines via specific transporter proteins. The pathways of lipogenesis (the endogenous formation of lipid groups) and fatty acid oxidation (the breakdown of fatty acids for energy production) can regulate the catabolism and anabolism of fatty acid groups into acetyl CoA to feed into energy production in the citric acid cycle, as discussed earlier in this chapter. Further regulation of longer-chain fatty acids can be performed by via carnitine transporters, which regulate trafficking of long-chain fatty acids into the mitochondria for utilization in fatty acid oxidation.[3,5,7,8]

Sterols and cholesterols are a distinct class of lipid groups comprised in multi-carbon ring structures of $C_{17}H_{28}O$. These molecules not only form the basis behind distinctive classes of lipid-based energy storage units akin to fatty acid, but can also be molecules that can regulate a diversity of signaling pathways ranging from hormonal regulation of reproduction, electrolyte concentration regulation, and cortisol regulation glycemic control and growth. While the basic mechanisms of dietary absorption of cholesterols are quite similar to those of dietary fatty acid processing, endogenous synthesis of cholesterol and steroid groups plays a significant role in human nutrition. Other types of complex lipids, such as phospholipids, prenols, sphingolipids, and glycolipids will be discussed below.[3,5,7,8]

What Are the Health Implications of Lipid Macronutrients?

Lipids play an integral role in long-term energy storage and dynamics to complement carbohydrate metabolism. Lipids provide as much as 9 kilocalories per gram of energy, more than double that of carbohydrates. Malabsorption of fat (steatorrhea) or diets lacking in fat can lead to nutritional and energy storage deficiencies such as severe acute malnutrition. Lipid storage regulates weight and adiposity and may play a role in insulin regulation of carbohydrate metabolism. Hypercholesterolemia can manifest in hyperlipidemia, which can manifest in disease and obstruction of coronary arteries. Cholesterol synthesis can also play a critical role in essential steroid synthetic pathways as well as lipid storage.[1,3,5,7,8]

While the balance of these metabolic pathways and dietary consumption of fat and carbohydrates may present later in life via chronic, cardiometabolic diseases (see Chapters 17–20), there are also inborn errors of metabolism that can present in the neonatal period, infancy, and even early adulthood with disruptions in lipid metabolism. Disorders of fatty acid oxidation metabolism range from disorders of medium-chain metabolism (medium-chain acyl CoA dehydrogenase deficiency) to long- and very-long-chain metabolism (very-long-chain acyl CoA dehydrogenase deficiency, carnitine palmitoyltransferase type 1 and 2 deficiencies, carnitine acylcarnitine translocase deficiency, long-chain 3 hydroxyacyl-CoA dehydrogenase deficiency, mitochondrial trifunctional protein deficiency). Early-onset hypercholesterolemia may be secondary to deficiencies in chylomicron transporter proteins. Other enzymatic deficiencies can lead to disruptions in steroid production, which can lead to inappropriate regulation of electrolytes and sexual characteristics as well as glycemic control and growth.[3,7,8]

AMINO ACIDS AND PROTEINS

What Are Amino Acids and Proteins and Why Are They Important Macronutrients?

Amino acids are organic compounds composed of a carboxylic acid functional group and an amino group. While there are dozens of amino acids that exist in the nature, the most clinically significant amino acids are the alpha amino acids, which form small chains known as peptides and larger complex chains called proteins. Proteins from dietary sources, such as meats, dairy products, nuts, and certain vegetables can be broken down by enzymes known as proteases in the stomach into peptides and amino acids for absorption in the small intestine via specific amino acid transporters. Amino acids can be divided into two main classes: essential amino acids and non-essential amino acids. Essential amino acids are not made by the human body and thus a dietary source is required to produce proteins. These include leucine, isoleucine, valine, phenylalanine, histidine, lysine, tryptophan, and threonine. Non-essential amino acids are 11 amino acids made endogenously by the human body via distinctive amino acid synthesis pathways and do not require dietary consumption. These amino acids are alanine, serine, asparagine, aspartate, glutamate, cysteine, tyrosine, glutamine, arginine, proline, and glycine.[1,3,5,8,11] Common structures of amino acids are noted in Figure 1-5.

The large number of synthetic and degradative pathways for amino acids is beyond the scope of this chapter.

The synthesis of peptides and proteins as complex amino acid chains is a tightly regulated highly complicated process that broadly involves two critical steps: the transcription of DNA into RNA transcripts and the translation of RNA into amino acid chains that form peptides and proteins. Briefly, the human genome is comprised of ~3.2 billion DNA nucleotides that form nucleotide base pairs across 24 pairs of DNA storage units known as chromosomes. These chromosomes provide the packaging for thousands of "recipes" for proteins known as genes. These genes can be selectively opened up for the "transcription" into new copies of a specific type of RNA, known as mRNA, through an enzyme known as RNA polymerase. These mRNA "transcripts" are trafficked to macromolecular machines known as ribosomes, where they bind with tRNA transcripts that have been bound to specific amino acids, allowing for the "translation" of mRNA transcripts into amino acid sequences known as peptides. These peptides can be further processed into proteins, which can provide a diversity of functions in human biology, including energy production, cellular growth, and structure formation (Figure 1-6).[1,3,5,8,11]

What Are the Health Implications of Amino Acids and Proteins?

Proteins provide 4 kilocalories per gram, equivalent to that of carbohydrates, but less than that of lipids. However, due to the critical nature of proteins as structural building blocks, inappropriate utilization of proteins for energy consumptions can lead to significant nutritional deficiency states. Protein malnutrition can present with sarcopenia (low muscle mass and function) as well as low blood concentrations of the "visceral" proteins albumin and prealbumin. Hypoalbuminemia in increased protein consumption in the general population may be associated with lipid and carbohydrate consumption, which can undergird growth and muscle buildup. Less commonly, people who present with inborn errors of amino acid metabolism may lead to toxic accumulations of amino acids and amino acid by-products, including ammonia. Classes of such disorders include urea cycle disorders, branched chain aminoacidopathies (maple syrup urine disease), phenylketonuria, tyrosinemia, non-ketotic hyperglycinemia, and organic acidurias like propionic acidemia, methylmalonic acidemia, and glutaric acidemia. Specific strategies in the regulation of these disorders include limiting the dietary exposure to non-essential amino acids that the body can already synthesize and closely regulating the essential amino acids that these patients have difficulty metabolizing to levels that are sufficient for adequate growth through childhood and beyond.[1,3,5,8,11]

NUCLEIC ACIDS, WATER, AND OTHER COMPLEX MOLECULES

What Other Types of Macronutrients Are There and What Are Their Functions?

Other important classes of macronutrients and molecules derived from macronutrients are less important for energy production but are rather for structural and other functions

Alanine	Ala	A	$-CH_3$
Arginine	Arg	R	$-CH_2-CH_2-CH_2-NH-\overset{\underset{\|}{NH}}{C}-NH_2$
Asparagine	Asn	N	$-CH_2-\overset{\underset{\|}{O}}{C}-NH_2$
Asparate	Asp	D	$-CH_2-\overset{\underset{\|}{O}}{C}-OH$
Cysteine	Cys	C	$-CH_2-SH$
Glutamate	Glu	E	$-CH_2-CH_2-\overset{\underset{\|}{O}}{C}-OH$
Glutamine	Gln	Q	$-CH_2-CH_2-\overset{\underset{\|}{O}}{C}-NH_2$
Glycine	Gly	G	$-H$
*Histidine	His	H	$-CH_2$ (imidazole ring)
*Isoleucine	Ile	I	$-\overset{\underset{\|}{CH_3}}{C}-CH_2-CH_3$

*Leucine	Leu	L	$-CH_2-\overset{\underset{\|}{CH_3}}{CH}-CH_3$
*Lysine	Lys	K	$-CH_2-CH_2-CH_2-CH_2-NH_2$
*Methionine	Met	M	$-CH_2-CH_2-S-CH_3$
*Phenylalanine	Phe	F	$-CH_2$ (phenyl ring)
Proline	Pro	P	(pyrrolidine ring)
Serine	Ser	S	$-CH_2-OH$
*Threonine	Thr	T	$-\overset{\underset{\|}{OH}}{CH}-CH_3$
*Tryptophan	Trp	W	$-H_2C$ (indole ring)
*Tyrosine	Tyr	Y	$-CH_2$ (phenol ring) $-OH$
*Valine	Val	V	$-\overset{\underset{\|}{CH_3}}{CH}-CH_3$

FIGURE 1-5 • Amino acid structures and types. (Reproduced with permission from Maloy S, Hughes K (eds.). *Brenner's Encyclopedia of Genetics*. Academic Press; 2013: Chapter 13, Amino Acids.)

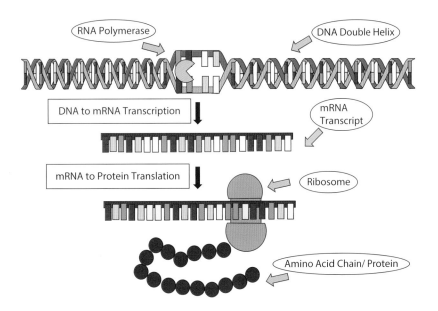

FIGURE 1-6 • DNA transcription and RNA translation into proteins.[12]

of cells in human physiology. Nucleic acids are biomolecules composed of a five-carbon sugar (deoxyribose or ribose), a phosphate group, and a nitrogenous base. As detailed above, nucleic acids such as DNA and RNA play an integral role in the storage of information, rather than energy, specifically as it relates to the formation of proteins (Figure 1-7). Classically these nucleic acids are derived from five types of nitrogenous

bases; the purines adenine and guanine; along with the pyrimidines cytosine, thymine, and uracil. While the first three nitrogenous bases are found in both DNA and RNA, thymine is exclusively found in DNA, while uracil is found exclusively in RNA. Nucleic acids are particularly enriched in diets with high cellular and protein content, particularly meats, fish, mushrooms, and legumes. Digestion and absorption are facilitated

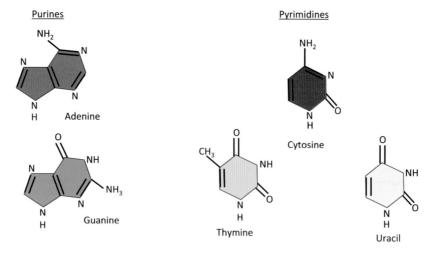

FIGURE 1-7 • Nucleic acid types.[13]

by pepsin in the stomach and brush border enzymes such as nucleotidases and phosphatases in the intestine, which allows for the three components of nitrogenous bases, pentoses, and phosphate groups to be transported into the bloodstream via intestinal transporters. These nucleotides can be endogenously synthesized and degraded via processes such as the pentose phosphate pathway as well as other purine and pyrimidine de novo and salvage synthesis and other degradation pathways.[1,3,5,8,13]

Water is a ubiquitous polar inorganic compound with two hydrogens and one oxygen with the unique capacity to act as a solvent as both an H^+ and OH^-, providing features of both acids and bases, depending on the context. Water's unique properties as a solvent allow for it to help facilitate a number of critical reactions to facilitate building and utilizing many of the macronutrients and complex molecules derived from these macronutrients critical in human functions. There is a diversity of mechanisms by which water can be absorbed and utilized as a macronutrient, most notably via osmosis of water across cellular domains and the utilization of proteins such as aquaporins to transport water throughout the digestive system, including intestinal cells, into the bloodstream for use by other cell types.[1,5]

While not classically defined as macronutrients, there are several large biomolecules found in the diet that are composed of smaller macronutrients from which these macronutrients can be utilized. Examples of such complex molecules include glycoproteins, glycosaminoglycans, glycolipids, and sphingolipids, all of which can classified by the fact that they are composed of two or more macronutrient classes. Glycoproteins are proteins with oligosaccharides covalently linked to asparagine (N-linked glycosylation) and serine/threonine/tyrosine (O-linked glycosylation). Complex chains of mannose-, glucose-, galactose-, and fructose-derived oligosaccharides can be used in N- and O-linked glycosylation of proteins and lipids, which can play a critical role in cell adhesion and cell recognition. The process by which these oligosaccharides are formed

in humans is a highly complex multi-enzymatic process across multiple cellular domains, including the cytosol, endoplasmic reticulum, and Golgi bodies, details of which are beyond the scope of this chapter. Importantly, glycoproteins in the diet provide an enriched source of carbohydrates and amino acids that need to be adequately digested via many of the stomach and intestinal enzymes and transporters previously described.[4]

Glycosaminoglycans (GAGs) are polysaccharides composed of disaccharides based in one amino sugar and either a uronic sugar or galactose. GAGs are derived and degraded via a number of complex enzymatic pathways. Examples of important GAGs include heparan sulfate, keratan sulfate, and dermatan sulfate and can be found throughout cell types and nutritional sources and play a critical role in structural scaffolding and cell signaling. Similar to glycoproteins, the dietary GAGs provide an enriched source of carbohydrates and amino acids that need to be adequately digested via many of the stomach and intestinal enzymes and transporters previously described.[3-5]

Finally, sphingolipids and glycosphingolipids are sphingosine-based lipids with or without fatty acid and/or oligosaccharide groups attached via covalent bonds. The base of these molecules is derived from a sphingoid base such as sphingosine, can become increasingly more complex with either fatty acid groups added in isolation, known as ceramides, or with other biomolecules and macronutrient components such as phosphatidylcholines (sphingomyelins), monosaccharides (cerebrosides), oligosaccharides, and amino sugars (gangliosides and globosides). Other important glycolipids include glycophosphatidylinositols. Globally, their functions are diverse and critical for intracellular diversity, cell adhesion and cell signaling, and disruptions in the processing and clearance of these molecules can lead to complex inborn errors of metabolism. However, as these molecules can be found throughout a diverse array of dietary sources, particularly lipid-rich animal-based foods, it is important to recognize that these macronutrient sources can be broken down for utilization via many of the processes described throughout this chapter.[3-5]

THREE TAKE-HOME POINTS

1. Human nutrition requires five key classes of simple macronutrients for functioning and metabolism: carbohydrates, fats, proteins, nucleic acids, and water

2. The formation of complex molecules critical for cellular function, such as starches, cholesterols, sphingolipids, proteins, glycosaminoglycans, and DNA, requires the metabolism of the four groups of simple macronutrients as key building blocks.

3. While all classes of macronutrients (except water) can be theoretically metabolized for energy production, the two most important for normal energy production use carbohydrate and fat metabolism, whereas amino acids and nucleic acids are important for the formation of critical structural macronutrients. Macronutrient by-product buildup also requires biochemical and cellular pathways for clearance to ensure adequate homeostasis of energy production and complex molecule formation.

CASE STUDY ANSWERS

1. **B**; Carbohydrates (i.e., anhydrous dextrose), fats (i.e., fatty acids), and protein (i.e., amino acids) are all macronutrients. Vitamin A is a micronutrient.

2. Starches, disaccharides, proteins, cholesterols, sphingolipids, and glycosaminoglycans are complex building blocks that can be formed by endogenous metabolic pathways using dextrose, fats, and amino acids provided in parenteral nutrition.

3. **E**; Energy production and storage, complex molecule formation and degradation for cellular development and signaling, and macronutrient waste degradation and clearance are all important functions.

REFERENCES

1. Lanham-New SA, Hill TR, Gallagher AM, Vorster HH. (Eds.). *Introduction to Human Nutrition.* John Wiley & Sons; 2019.

2. Aryal S. *Carbohydrates—Monosaccharides, Disaccharides and Polysaccharides.* Microbe Notes; 2022, June 21. https://microbenotes.com/carbohydrates/.

3. Fernandes J, Saudubray JM, Van den Berghe G, Walter JH. (Eds.) *Inborn Metabolic Diseases: Diagnosis and Treatment.* Springer Science & Business Media; 2006.

4. Seeberger PH. Monosaccharide Diversity. In: Varki A, Cummings RD, Esko JD, et al., editors. *Essentials of Glycobiology [internet].* 4th edition. Cold Spring Harbor Laboratory Press; 2022. Chapter 2. Available from: https://www.ncbi.nlm.nih.gov/books/NBK579981/; doi: 10.1101/glycobiology.4e.2.

5. Boyer SW, Barclay LJ, Burrage LC. Inherited metabolic disorders: aspects of chronic nutrition management. *Nutr Clin Prac.* 2015;30(4):502-510.

6. Helminstine A. *Disaccharide Examples—What Is a Disaccharide?* Science Notes; 2021 September 6. https://sciencenotes.org/disaccharide-examples-what-is-a-disaccharide/.

7. Wenk MR. The emerging field of lipidomics. *Nat Rev Drug Discov.* 2005 July;4(7):594-610.

8. Begum RM. *A Textbook of Foods, Nutrition & Dietetics.* Sterling Publishers Pvt. Ltd.; 2008.

9. Yang ST (Ed.). *Bioprocessing for Value-Added Products From Renewable Resources: New Technologies and Applications.* Elsevier; 2011.

10. Díez-Pascual AM, Rahdar A. Composites of vegetable oil-based polymers and carbon nanomaterials. *Macromol.* 2021; 1(4):276-292.

11. The Albert Team. *Amino Acid Study Guide; Structure and Function* (2022, March 1). The Albert Team. https://www.albert.io/blog/amino-acid-study-guide-structure-and-function/.

12. Clancy S, Brown W. Translation: DNA to mRNA. *Nature Education*; 2008.

13. Life of Plants Blog (2011, March), *Nucleic Acids, Life of Plants Blog.* http://lifeofplant.blogspot.com/2011/03/nucleic-acids.html.

Micronutrient Metabolism

Ariana Cerro, RD, LDN, CNSC / McGreggor Crowley, MD

Chapter Outline

CASE STUDY

Luisa is a 12-year-old girl with no prior medical or surgical history who was referred to a pediatric gastroenterology clinic for 6 years of selective eating and severe anxiety at mealtimes. She expresses long-standing and significant sensory aversions to many foods, including meats, fruits, and vegetables, and she reports no concerns about her body image. A 3-day dietary recall reveals that Luisa's meals consist entirely of cupcakes, mixed nuts (pistachios, walnuts, and cashews), French fries, and soy milk. Food insecurity screening is negative. She does not take any medications, nutritional supplements, or multivitamins. Despite her severe dietary limitations, Luisa's height, weight, and body mass index have been consistently normal. Her exam is notable for pallor, lateral gaze impairment, and involuntary "piano-playing" finger movements when her arms are outstretched. Several regions of confluent ecchymosis are observed on her extremities. Based on her history and clinical presentation, Luisa is diagnosed with avoidant restrictive food intake disorder (ARFID), and a comprehensive assessment of micronutrient status is performed.

1. **What micronutrient deficiencies best explain Luisa's pallor and neurological exam findings? (More than one answer may be selected.)**
   A. Vitamin A
   B. Vitamin B1
   C. Vitamin B12
   D. Vitamin C

2. **How are Luisa's micronutrient deficiencies best assessed? (More than one answer may be selected.)**
   A. Cross-sectional imaging of brain and spine
   B. Serum testing
   C. Assessment of inflammatory markers
   D. Esophagogastroduodenoscopy (EGD)

● INTRODUCTION

Micronutrients are organic molecules and ions necessary for appropriate growth, homeostasis, anabolism and catabolism, energy production, repair of oxidative stress, response to inflammation, cell signaling, gene expression, and reproduction. Though some micronutrients can be synthesized by the human body, many essential micronutrients must be obtained from dietary sources.[1] Micronutrients can be divided further by their chemical structure into trace elements, water-soluble vitamins, and fat-soluble vitamins.

The small intestine is the primary site of absorption for most micronutrients obtained from the diet, though some absorption of copper, iodine, fluoride, and molybdenum occurs in the stomach.[2] Non-dietary-derived vitamin K and biotin (B7) synthesized by gut flora may be absorbed in the large intestine.[3,4]

The question of which micronutrients to assess for a patient presents a challenge for the clinician for many reasons. Although a patient's signs and symptoms may help predict which deficiency is complicit, deficiencies for many micronutrients have similar presentations. For example, inadequate intake of iron, folate, B12, or vitamin A may lead to forms of anemia. In addition, clinically apparent symptoms may only be apparent with severe deficiency, so biochemical monitoring is critically important. Patients with one micronutrient deficiency may also be deficient in other micronutrients, leading to complex presentations.

Considerable care should be used when obtaining and interpreting serum micronutrient concentrations. First, low circulating plasma concentrations of many essential trace elements make assessment of their nutritional status challenging and potentially unreliable. Additionally, circulating levels of many micronutrients may be influenced by recent dietary intake, leading to artificially normal concentrations even in the setting of deficiency; to diminish the impact of recent dietary intake, micronutrient labs may be drawn only after fasting. Because several micronutrients are either positive or negative acute phase reactants, meaning that their serum concentrations are influenced in part by a patient's inflammatory status, these micronutrients should be assessed simultaneously along with C-reactive protein (CRP) and/or erythrocyte sedimentation rate (ESR). Finally, interpretation of resulting values presents diagnostic and interpretive complexity for even experienced clinicians and may be aided by consultation with either a registered dietitian or a nutrition-focused gastroenterologist.

Due to the large number of essential micronutrients, this chapter focuses on several archetypal examples, including iron, zinc, vitamin B12, and vitamin D, and describes their dietary sources, mechanisms of absorption, and the symptoms associated with deficiency and excess. These examples, combined with additional guidance provided in a series of concise tables throughout the chapter, may aid clinicians in the appropriate assessment of the full range of essential micronutrients for their patients.

● ESSENTIAL TRACE ELEMENTS

Chromium, copper, iodine, iron, manganese, molybdenum, selenium, and zinc comprise the group of essential trace elements for humans, while the designation of fluoride and molybdenum as trace elements has been debated. Unlike essential major elements like sodium, phosphorus, and calcium, which occur in relatively large amounts within the human body, essential trace elements are present in only minute amounts. Nonetheless, essential trace elements have important roles in establishing protein structure and serve as cofactors in numerous enzymatic reactions. Zinc, for example, is integral to the function of over 700 human proteins, many of which have roles in DNA transcription regulation.[5] These minerals originate within the soil and may enter the diet directly through plant sources, indirectly through animal sources, or through water. Table 2-1 highlights a laboratory-based assessment of these trace elements' nutritional status.

Iron

Iron, the most abundant trace element within the human body, is a necessary component of the oxygen transport proteins hemoglobin and myoglobin and is required for the mitochondrial oxidation/phosphorylation system.[15] There are two forms of dietary iron: non-heme and heme. Non-heme iron is derived from plant sources, such as cereal, legumes, fruits, and vegetables. Heme iron, contained within hemoglobin and myoglobin proteins, is derived from animal food sources such as meat, poultry, and fish and is more bioavailable (more easily absorbed) than non-heme iron.

Absorption of iron occurs in the duodenum and the proximal jejunum, followed by transfer across the duodenal mucosa into the blood where it can then be transported to tissues by the carrier, protein transferrin. Rates of absorption are indirectly proportional to the body's iron stores, and absorption is increased in patients with iron deficiency.[16] Absorption of iron is adversely affected by the presence of other food components, such as phytic acid (a non-digestible sugar commonly found in grains), polyphenols, calcium, and peptides that inhibit iron absorption. In contrast, vitamin C enhances iron absorption in a dose-dependent manner by preserving iron in its absorbable form.

Iron deficiency is commonly related to inadequate intake, but may also be caused by chronic inflammation, malabsorption, parasitic infection, fluoroquinolone use, pregnancy, blood loss from menstruation, gastrointestinal bleeding, chronic renal disease, and chronic liver disease.[17] Signs and symptoms of iron deficiency include microcytic anemia, pallor, weakness, tachycardia, increased risk of sepsis in pregnancy, restless legs, and decreased cognitive abilities. Iron overload is associated with hereditary disorders such as hemochromatosis, in addition to over-supplementation and chronic transfusions for treatments of hematological disorders, and may lead to zinc deficiency, cirrhosis, pancreatic failure, cardiac failure, and a characteristic bronze pigmentation of sun-exposed skin.

Hemoglobin, hematocrit, mean corpuscular hemoglobin concentration, and mean corpuscular volume may partially characterize iron nutrition status, but these are neither sensitive nor specific markers of iron deficiency. Serum ferritin and transferrin saturation may be more helpful when assessing iron nutrition status, though both ferritin and transferrin are acute phase reactants and their serum concentration may fluctuate in the setting of infection or inflammation. Interpretation of these markers of nutrition status may be aided by obtaining a concurrent CRP to assess for such inflammation. Table 2-2 illustrates expected serum labs in the setting of iron deficiency anemia, anemia of chronic disease, and iron overload. Note that iron deficiency anemia can coexist with anemia of chronic disease and that recent blood transfusions can lead to complex, sometimes confounding, patterns of serum labs.

Zinc

An essential trace element and the second most abundant micronutrient in the human body after iron, zinc is intracellularly ubiquitous. Zinc is involved in gene expression and many

TABLE 2-1 • Nutritional status tests for trace elements

Element	Test(s)	Comments	References
Chromium	Serum chromium	As chromium does not equilibrate within tissue pools, serum chromium may not fully reflect tissue stores.	6
Copper	1. Serum copper 2. Ceruloplasmin	Both serum copper and ceruloplasmin are positive acute phase reactants (APR) and may be elevated in the setting of inflammation. Both may be normal in the setting of mild to moderate copper deficiency.	7
Iodine	1. Urine iodine 2. Serum thyroxine 3. Serum thyroglobulin	Urine iodine may be influenced by recent dietary intake. TSH levels may be in normal range for older children and adults with marginal iodine deficiency.	8
Iron	Combination of serum iron, ferritin, transferrin saturation (TS), and total iron binding capacity (TIBC) with complete blood count (CBC)	Ferritin is a positive APR and may be elevated in the setting of inflammation. Iron is a negative APR.	9
Manganese	1. Whole blood manganese 2. Urine manganese	There is poor correlation between whole blood or urine manganese levels and dietary intake.	10
Molybdenum	1. Serum molybdenum 2. Urine molybdenum	Neither serum nor urine Mo levels accurately reflect Mo nutritional status. Serum Mo may be impacted by inflammation (especially hepatic inflammation) or recent dietary intake.	11
Selenium	1. Serum selenium 2. Erythrocyte selenium concentration 3. Glutathione peroxidase (GPX) activity	Serum Se may be influenced by recent dietary intake. GPX activity assay is not commonly available.	12
Zinc	1. Serum zinc 2. Serum alkaline phosphatase	Neither test is adequate for assessing zinc status. Serum zinc is a negative APR. Alkaline phosphatase is not a sensitive indicator of zinc stores.	13
Fluoride	1. Serum fluoride 2. Urine fluoride	Serum fluoride is a better indicator of body fluoride stores.	14

cellular processes that affect growth and development, such as differentiation, apoptosis, and proliferation. Zinc serves as a catalyst for many enzymatic reactions by providing structural stabilization of zinc finger proteins and plays an integral role in fertility, neurotransmission, neurodevelopmental, hormonal regulation, immune function, and skeletal growth.[18]

Zinc absorption occurs throughout the small intestine with major absorption sites in the duodenum and jejunum. In zinc-replete diets, between 17% and 50% of enteral zinc is absorbed by healthy individuals in a process regulated by body zinc homeostasis, bioavailability, and bioaccessibility, while in zinc-deficient diets, absorption rates exceeding 90% have been observed. It is important to note that co-ingestion of calcium or iron can negatively affect zinc absorption, perhaps by worsening phytate-mediated chelation or through competitive inhibition of transport proteins. Following absorption, zinc binds to albumin or α-2-macroglubin and is then excreted into the serum to be delivered to its primary storage sites in skeletal muscles and bones, with only a small amount of zinc (<0.1%) remaining in the plasma.[19] Excess zinc can be excreted via both urine and feces.

Zinc deficiency impacts more than 2 billion people worldwide and is a leading cause of death globally for children under the age of 5.[20] Inadequate intake, poor bioavailability from dominant diet sources, and poverty may predispose to deficiency. Vegans and vegetarians, the elderly, those with

TABLE 2-2 • Expected changes in laboratory studies influenced by iron nutrition status

Disease state	Hemoglobin	Hematocrit	MCV	MCHC	Serum iron	TIBC	Ferritin	Transferrin	Transferrin saturation
Iron Deficiency Anemia	Low	Low	Low	Low	Low	High	Low	High	Low
Anemia of Chronic Disease	Low	Low	Low or Normal	Low	Low	Low	High	Low	Low
Iron Overload	High	High	High or Normal	High	High	Low	High	Low	High

MCV, mean corpuscular volume; MCHC, mean corpuscular hemoglobin concentration; TIBC, total iron binding capacity

conditions leading to poor absorption such as celiac disease, and those with conditions associated with increased gastrointestinal losses, such as inflammatory bowel disease or diarrhea, are also at high risk for deficiency.

Signs and symptoms of deficiency include alopecia, rash, immunodeficiency, irritability, diarrhea, oral ulcers, and poor linear growth. Zinc toxicity may manifest as irritability, tremor, sideroblastic anemia, and sensorimotor neuropathy, and is most commonly linked to over-supplementation or environmental exposure.

Though serum zinc concentration is the most widely used biomarker for assessing nutritional status, multiple conditions may impact circulating zinc concentrations. Like iron, zinc is a negative acute phase reactant, and serum concentrations can decrease in the setting of inflammation. Additionally, hypoalbuminemia may also lead to artificially low serum zinc concentrations, while fasting may increase concentrations.[13] Obtaining a CRP and albumin along with plasma zinc concentration may help improve interpretation of zinc nutritional status.

WATER-SOLUBLE VITAMINS

There are nine essential water-soluble vitamins that humans are unable to synthesize, including vitamin C and the B vitamins: folate (B1), riboflavin (B2), niacin (B3), pantothenic acid (B5), pyridoxine (B6), biotin (B7), folate (B9), and cobalamin (B12). Due to their water-soluble nature, most of these vitamins cannot be stored in large amounts within the human body and deficits can develop rapidly in the setting of inadequate intake or inflammation. Water-soluble vitamins are derived from a wide variety of plant, fungal, and animal sources and have important roles as cofactors in glycolysis, fatty acid metabolism, DNA and RNA synthesis, and protection against reactive oxygen species. Table 2-3 highlights laboratory-based assessment of these water-soluble vitamins' nutritional status.

Vitamin B12

Vitamin B12, also known as cobalamin, is a structurally complex, water-soluble molecule that integrates a single atom of the trace element cobalt (Co) within its center. Though

TABLE 2-3 • Nutritional status tests for water-soluble vitamins			
Vitamin	Test(s)	Comments	References
B1 Thiamin	1. Whole blood thiamin 2. Transketolase enzymatic activity	Transketolase activity testing may have limited availability. Serum thiamin is not reflective of thiamin nutritional status. Not an Acute Phase Reactant (APR).	21
B2 Riboflavin	Pre- and post-supplementation erythrocyte glutathione reductase activity coefficient (EGRAC)	Spot urine riboflavin assays are influenced by recent dietary intake but 24-hour assays may be used if EGRAC cannot be tested. Not an APR.	22
B3 Niacin	First morning void or 24-hour urine niacin metabolites	Niacin metabolites in urine include N-methylnicotinamide and N-methyl-6-pyridone-3-carboxamide. Serum niacin does not reflect total body niacin stores. Not an APR.	23
B5 Pantothenic Acid	Urine pantothenic acid level	Very rarely assessed and of limited clinical utility. Not an APR.	24
B6 Pyridoxine	1. Plasma pyridoxal-5-phosphate (PLP) 2. Erythrocyte aspartic acid transaminase (AST) and alanine transaminase (ALT) activity	Plasma PLP may be influenced by inflammation, hypophosphatasia, and hypoalbuminemia. Erythrocyte AST and ALT are not influenced by these factors but assays may not be widely available. Possible negative APR.	25
B7 Biotin	1. Leukocyte holocarboxylases 2. Urine 3-hydroxyisovaleric acid	Urine biotin does not identify deficiency. Urine 3-hydroxyisovaleric acid testing has lower sensitivity than leukocyte holocarboxylase assays, which have limited availability. Not an APR.	26
B9 Folate	1. Red blood cell folate level 2. Serum folate level	RBC folate may be less influenced by recent dietary folate intake. Obtain with B12 due to overlap in deficiency symptoms. Not an APR.	27
B12 Cyanocobalamin	1. Serum B12 level 2. Urine or serum methylmalonic acid (MMA)	MMA may be both more sensitive and specific for B12 deficiency compared to serum B12 assay. Obtain with folate due to overlap in deficiency symptoms. Not an APR.	28
Vitamin C	1. Serum ascorbic acid level 2. Leukocyte ascorbic acid concentration	Though both serum and leukocyte AA correlate with dietary intake, leukocyte AA is a more sensitive indicator of tissue stores. Negative APR.	29
Choline	Serum choline	Serum choline has limited use in assessing choline nutritional status. Unknown if APR.	30

vitamin B12 exists in many dietary-derived forms, including methyl, deoxyadenosyl-, and hydroxy-cobalamin, it is the chemically stable cyanocobalamin form that is commonly found in commercial B12 supplements. Most dietary forms of B12, including cyanocobalamin, can be converted intracellularly into adenosylcobalamin or methylcobalamin, bioactive forms that are cofactors for three classes of enzyme families. Adenosylcobalamin is an integral cofactor in the breakdown of amino acids via conversion of L-methylmalonyl-CoA to succinyl-CoA, while the methylcobalamin within methionine synthase is required for purine and pyrimidine synthesis in a reaction that also relies on folate (B9).[31]

B12 absorption is complex. First, B12 bound to food proteins must be separated from these proteins by hydrochloric acid produced by gastric parietal cells. Freed cobalamin then binds to haptocorrin, also known as R-factor, a salivary gland–produced protein that protects cobalamin from degradation in the stomach's acidic environment. In the duodenum, haptocorrin-bound B12 is cleaved by proteases, and free cobalamin is then bound to the intrinsic factor, a protein produced by gastric parietal cells. In the distal ileum, the intrinsic factor-cobalamin complex can be absorbed via endocytosis in the presence of calcium. B12 is secreted in bile and reabsorbed through enterohepatic circulation, which also requires intrinsic factor. Excess vitamin B12 can be excreted via feces. Bioavailability of vitamin B12 is affected by the gastrointestinal absorption of each individual.[32]

Deficiency of B12 is caused by inadequate dietary provision or malabsorption and may take several years to manifest after depletion of body stores. Since B12 is found only in animal food sources, those who follow strict vegetarian and vegan diets are at higher risk for developing a deficiency. The elderly are also at risk for vitamin B12 deficiency due to increased incidence of the development of autoantibodies against gastric parietal cells that secrete intrinsic factor in addition to age-related reduction of hydrochloric acid secretion.[32] Patients who have undergone ileal or gastric resection are also at higher risk for deficiency. Medications such as proton pump inhibitors, metformin, nitrous oxide anesthesia, some antiepileptic drugs, cholestyramine, and colchicine can also negatively impact B12 absorption or metabolism. Deficiency manifests as megaloblastic anemia, paresthesia, discoordination, and possibly irreversible dementia and disorientation. Toxicity has not been well documented. The majority of the body's B12 stores are intracellular; thus, serum B12 levels may not adequately reflect nutritional status or deficiency. To aid interpretation of B12 nutritional status, serum methylmalonic acid, and homocysteine levels should be obtained along with serum B12; serum concentrations of methyl malonic acid and homocysteine increase in true B12 deficiency as they cannot be converted to succinyl Co-A or methionine, respectively.[28]

Fat-Soluble Vitamins

Vitamins A, D, E, and K are termed *fat-soluble* due to their molecular structure; dissolvability within organic solvents; and absorption, transportation, and storage pathways that are similar to fats. Like the water-soluble vitamins, each of the fat-soluble vitamins is considered essential, though some endogenous vitamin D may be synthesized in human skin upon UV light exposure and some absorbed vitamin K may have colonic flora origins.[33,34] Table 2-4 highlights a laboratory-based assessment of these fat-soluble vitamins' nutritional status.

Vitamin D

Vitamin D is vital in the development, growth, and maintenance of bones throughout the human life cycle. Vitamin D also plays an important role in calcium homeostasis through regulating intestinal calcium absorption and parathyroid hormone-mediated bone mineralization, maintaining vascular integrity, regulating aspects of glucose metabolism, and impacting growth and differentiation of numerous immunomodulatory cells.

There are three primary sources of vitamin D: dietary-derived vitamin D2 (ergocalciferol), dietary-derived vitamin D3 (cholecalciferol), and endogenously produced cholecalciferol generated in epithelial tissue upon ultraviolet B ray exposure. After emulsification and integration into mixed micelles, more than 50% of ingested vitamin D is then absorbed primarily in the proximal small intestine via passive diffusion, putative vitamin D–specific membrane transporters, and cholesterol transporters, with bioavailability influenced by co-ingestion

TABLE 2-4 • Nutritional status tests for fat-soluble vitamins			
Vitamin	**Test(s)**	**Comments**	**References**
Vitamin A	1. Retinol binding protein (RBP) concentration 2. Serum retinol level	RBP is a negative acute phase reactant (APR) and may also be depressed in malnutrition/protein deficiency states.	35
Vitamin D	1-25-OHD	25-OHD in obese patients is inversely correlated with percentage body fat content and may not accurately reflect vitamin D body stores. Possible negative APR.	36
Vitamin E	1. Serum tocopherol level 2. Tocopherol:Total lipid ratio	Levels of vitamin E/tocopherols fluctuate with plasma lipid concentrations. Ratio is especially important in settings of pathologically elevated lipids.	37
Vitamin K	1. aPTT and PTT 2. Proteins induced in vitamin K absence or antagonism-factor II (PIVKA-II)	Consider evaluating aPTT/PTT pre- and post–vitamin K supplementation to determine therapy efficacy.	38

TABLE 2-5 • Luisa's micronutrient labs

Lab	Value	Normal range
C-reactive Protein	0.05 mg/L	<1 mg/L
HCT	31%	35%–44%
MCV	105 fL	78–90 fL
Vitamin B12	88 pg/mL	200–900 pg/mL
Homocysteine	66 μmol/L	5–15 μmol/L
Methylmalonic Acid	0.9 μmol/L	0.07–0.27 μmol/L
Vitamin C	7 μmol/L	23–114 μmol/L
25-OH Vitamin D	12 ng/mL	30–70 ng/mL
Folate/Vitamin B9	14 ng/mL	2.7–17 ng/mL
Transferrin Saturation	17%	15%–50%
Prothrombin Time	12 s	11–13.5 s
INR	1.1	0.8–1.1

of fatty acids. After uptake by enterocytes, vitamin D is then secreted within chylomicrons into the lymphatic circulation, then sequestered in adipocytes until hydroxylation in the liver and kidneys converts it to bioactive forms. Excess absorbed vitamin D is almost entirely excreted through bile into feces.

Vitamin D deficiency is widespread due to dietary insufficiency and inadequate environmental exposure, along with malabsorption, inflammation, chronic liver disease, chronic renal disease, exclusive breastfeeding, obesity, short bowel syndrome, medication side effects, and bariatric surgery all increase the risk of deficiency.[39] Signs of deficiency like rickets and osteomalacia are typically associated with aberrant osteogenesis and calcium absorption. Excess vitamin D secondary to over-supplementation or (less commonly) granuloma-forming disorders may eventually lead to confusion, dehydration, diarrhea, irritability, and emesis.[39] Biochemical assessment of vitamin D can be achieved by serum 25-hydroxy vitamin D levels. There is considerable controversy, however, regarding target serum 25-hydroxy vitamin D levels, the need for vitamin D supplementation, and health-related consequences of marginal (near-normal) vitamin D nutritional status.[40]

THREE TAKE-HOME POINTS

1. Micronutrients, including trace elements, water-soluble vitamins, and fat-soluble vitamins, are essential for a multitude of day-to-day cellular functions. These micronutrients must be acquired exogenously from the diet.

2. Micronutrient deficiencies may have important health consequences that can be addressed through repletion and dietary changes.

3. Since micronutrient levels are dependent upon recent ingestion and inflammation and may not reflect true nutritional status or body stores, care should be used when assessing a patient's micronutrient status.

CASE STUDY ANSWERS

1. **B, D**; Deficiencies in B12 can explain Luisa's pallor and neurological exam findings; deficiencies in vitamin C may contribute to her ecchymosis. Luisa, a 12-year-old girl with ARFID and a constellation of neurological findings, is at considerable risk for multiple micronutrient deficiencies due to her limited dietary intake. Her diet consists predominantly of carbohydrates and is likely calorie-sufficient, as evidenced by her normal height, weight, and BMI. The soy milk and mixed nuts that she consumes are relatively good dietary sources of protein, iron, zinc, vitamin A, vitamin E, and vitamin K, provided she eats a sufficient quantity, and the iodinated salt on the nuts and her French fries makes iodine deficiency less likely. Though the enriched flour found in her cupcakes and other processed baked goods provides her with many B vitamins, she has no apparent dietary source of vitamin B12. She is also at risk for vitamin C and vitamin D deficiencies.

2. **B, C**; Luisa's micronutrient deficiencies are best assessed through serum testing combined with assessment of inflammatory markers. Based on this assessment, a complete blood count and comprehensive micronutrient panel were obtained along with a CRP, and the results from her testing are displayed in Table 2-5. Luisa's normal CRP indicates low likelihood of systemic inflammation and allows for appropriate interpretation of the remainder of her micronutrient panel. Her hematocrit is low and her mean corpuscular volume is elevated, revealing a megaloblastic anemia that is consistent with B12 deficiency. Further supporting Luisa's B12 deficiency is low serum B12 in combination with elevated serum homocysteine and methyl malonic acid. Serum vitamin C is deficient, however, and symptomatic hypovitaminosis C (also known as scurvy) may help explain her ecchymosis. Luisa also has a vitamin D deficiency. Luisa has a normal folate, her transferrin saturation is normal, indicating normal iron stores, and the normal prothrombin time and international normalized ratio (INR) likely reflect normal vitamin K stores.

REFERENCES

1. Said HM. Intestinal absorption of water-soluble vitamins in health and disease. *Bioche J.* 2011;437:357-372. Preprint at: https://doi.org/10.1042/bj20110326.

2. Goff JP. Invited review: mineral absorption mechanisms, mineral interactions that affect acid-base and antioxidant status, and diet considerations to improve mineral status. *J Dairy Sci.* 2018;101:2763-2813.

3. Said HM. Cell and molecular aspects of human intestinal biotin absorption. *J Nutr.* 2009;139:158-162.

4. Karl JP, Meydani M, Barnett JB, et al. Fecal concentrations of bacterially derived vitamin K forms are associated with gut microbiota composition but not plasma or fecal cytokine concentrations in healthy adults. *Am J Clin Nutr.* 2017;106:1052-1061.

5. Vilas CK, Emery LE, Denchi EL, Miller KM. Caught with one's zinc fingers in the genome integrity cookie jar. *Trends Genet.* 2018;34:313-325.

6. Anderson RA, Polansky MM, Bryden NA. Stability and absorption of chromium and absorption of chromium histidinate complexes by humans. *Biol Trace Elem Res.* 2004;101:211-218.

7. Bost M, Houdart S, Oberli M, Kalonji E, Huneau JF, Margaritis I. Dietary copper and human health: current evidence and unresolved issues. *J Trace Elem Med Biol.* 2016;35:107-115.

8. Zimmermann MB, Aeberli I, Andersson M, et al. Thyroglobulin is a sensitive measure of both deficient and excess iodine intakes in children and indicates no adverse effects on thyroid function in the UIC range of 100–299 μg/L: A UNICEF/ICCIDD Study Group Report. *J Clin Endocrin Metab.* 2013;98:1271-1280. Preprint at https://doi.org/10.1210/jc.2012-3952.

9. Terri D, Johnson-Wimbley DYG. Diagnosis and management of iron deficiency anemia in the 21st century. *Therap Adv Gastroenterol.* 2011;4:177-184.

10. Santos D, Batoreu C, Mateus L, Marreilha Dos Santos AP, Aschner M. Manganese in human parenteral nutrition: considerations for toxicity and biomonitoring. *Neurotoxicology.* 2014;43:36-45.

11. Institute of Medicine (US); Panel on Micronutrients. Molybdenum. In: *Dietary Reference Intakes for Vitamin A, Vitamin K, Arsenic, Boron, Chromium, Copper, Iodine, Iron, Manganese, Molybdenum, Nickel, Silicon, Vanadium, and Zinc:* National Academies Press; 2001.

12. Combs GF Jr. Biomarkers of selenium status. *Nutrients.* 2015;7:2209-2236. Preprint at https://doi.org/10.3390/nu7042209.

13. Wieringa FT, Dijkhuizen MA, Fiorentino M, Laillou A, Berger J. Determination of zinc status in humans: which indicator should we use? *Nutrients.* 2015;7:3252-3263.

14. Rango T, Vengosh A, Jeuland M, Whitford GM, Tekle-Haimanot R. Biomarkers of chronic fluoride exposure in groundwater in a highly exposed population. *Sci Total Environ.* 2017;596-597:1-11. Preprint at https://doi.org/10.1016/j.scitotenv.2017.04.021.

15. *Annual Review of Nutrition.* 23, 2003. Preprint at https://doi.org/10.1146/nutr.2003.23. issue-1.

16. Hallberg L, Hultén L, Gramatkovski E. Iron absorption from the whole diet in men: how effective is the regulation of iron absorption? *Am J Clin Nutr.* 1997;66:347-356.

17. Abbaspour N, Hurrell R, Kelishadi R. Review on iron and its importance for human health. *J Res Med Sci.* 2014;19:164-174.

18. Chasapis CT, Ntoupa PSA, Spiliopoulou CA, Stefanidou ME. Recent aspects of the effects of zinc on human health. *Arch Toxicol.* 2020;94:1443-1460. Preprint at https://doi.org/10.1007/s00204-020-02702-9.

19. Smith KT, Failla ML, Cousins RJ. Identification of albumin as the plasma carrier for zinc absorption by perfused rat intestine. *Biochem J.* 1979;184:627-633. Preprint at https://doi.org/10.1042/bj1840627.

20. Walker CLF, Fischer Walker CL, Ezzati M, Black RE. Global and regional child mortality and burden of disease attributable to zinc deficiency. *Eur J Clin Nutr.* 2009;63:591-597. Preprint at https://doi.org/10.1038/ejcn.2008.9.

21. Whitfield KC, Bourassa MW, Adamolekun B, et al. Thiamine deficiency disorders: diagnosis, prevalence, and a roadmap for global control programs. *Ann N Y Acad Sci.* 2018;1430:3-43. Preprint at https://doi.org/10.1111/nyas.13919.

22. Institute of Medicine (US) Standing Committee on the Scientific Evaluation of Dietary Reference Intakes and its Panel on Folate, Other B Vitamins, and Choline. *Dietary Reference Intakes for Thiamin, Riboflavin, Niacin, Vitamin B, Folate, Vitamin B, Pantothenic Acid, Biotin, and Choline.* National Academies Press; 2012.

23. Soldi LR, Maltos AL, da Cunha DF, Portari GV. Correlation between first morning single void and 24-hour urines: the reliability to quantify niacin status. *Med Sci Monit Basic Res.* 2018; 24:206-209.

24. Kathman JV, Kies C. Pantothenic acid status of free living adolescent and young adults. *Nutr. Res.* 1984;4:245-250.

25. Ueland PM, Ulvik A, Rios-Avila L, Midttun Ø, Gregory JF. Direct and functional biomarkers of vitamin B6 status. *Annu Rev Nutr.* 2015;35:33-70.

26. Eng WK, Giraud D, Schlegel VL, Wang D, Lee BH, Zempleni J. Identification and assessment of markers of biotin status in healthy adults. *Br J Nutr.* 2013;110:321-329.

27. Bailey LB, Stover PJ, McNulty H, et al. Biomarkers of nutrition for development—Folate review. *J Nutr.* 2015;145:1636S-1680S.

28. Vashi P, Edwin P, Popiel B, Lammersfeld C, Gupta D. Methylmalonic acid and homocysteine as indicators of vitamin B-12 deficiency in cancer. *PLoS One.* 2016;11(1):e0147843.

29. Mitmesser SH, Ye Q, Evans M, Combs M. Determination of plasma and leukocyte vitamin C concentrations in a randomized, double-blind, placebo-controlled trial with Ester-C. *SpringerPlus.* 2016;5:1161. Preprint at https://doi.org/10.1186/s40064-016-2605-7.

30. Wallace TC, Blusztajn JK, Caudill MA, et al. Choline: the underconsumed and underappreciated essential nutrient. *Nutr Today.* 2018;53:240-253.

31. Calderón-Ospina CA, Nava-Mesa MO. B Vitamins in the nervous system: current knowledge of the biochemical modes of action and synergies of thiamine, pyridoxine, and cobalamin. *CNS Neurosci Ther.* 2020;26:5-13.

32. Sobczyńska-Malefora A, Delvin E, McCaddon A, Ahmadi KR, Harrington DJ. Vitamin B status in health and disease: a critical review. diagnosis of deficiency and insufficiency – clinical and laboratory pitfalls. *Crit Rev Clin Lab Sci.* 2021;58:399-429.

33. Wedad Z, Mostafa RAH. Vitamin D and the skin: focus on a complex relationship: a review. *J Adv Res.* 2015;6:793-804.

34. Cooke G, Behan J, Costello M. Newly identified vitamin K-producing bacteria isolated from the neonatal faecal flora. *Microb Ecol Health Dis.* 2006;18. Preprint at https://doi.org/10.3402/mehd.v18i3-4.7681.

35. Larson LM, Namaste SM, Williams AM, et al. Adjusting retinol-binding protein concentrations for inflammation: biomarkers reflecting inflammation and nutritional determinants of anemia (BRINDA) project. *Am J Clin Nutr.* 2017;106:390S-401S.

36. Pilz S, Zittermann A, Trummer C, et al. Vitamin D testing and treatment: a narrative review of current evidence. *Endocr Connect.* 2019;8:R27-R43.

37. Waniek S, di Giuseppe R, Esatbeyoglu T, et al. Vitamin E (α- and γ-Tocopherol) levels in the community: distribution, clinical and biochemical correlates, and association with dietary patterns. *Nutrients.* 2017;10:3.

38. Dituri F, Buonocore G, Pietravalle A, et al. PIVKA-II plasma levels as markers of subclinical vitamin K deficiency in term infants. *J Matern Fetal Neonatal Med.* 2012;25:1660-1663.

39. Marcinowska-Suchowierska E, Kupisz-Urbańska M, Łukaszkiewicz J, Płudowski P, Jones G. Vitamin D toxicity–A clinical perspective. *Front Endocrin.* 2018;9:550. Preprint at https://doi.org/10.3389/fendo.2018.00550.

40. Cummings SR, Rosen C. VITAL findings—A decisive verdict on vitamin D supplementation. *N Engl J Med.* 2022;387:368-370.

Nutritional Assessment

Melanie V. Connolly, MSc, RD, LDN, CNSC / Nancy Oliveira, MS, RD, LDN, CDCES

Chapter Outline

I. Case Studies
II. Introduction
III. Nutrition Screening
IV. Nutrition Assessment
   a. Dietary History
   b. Physical Assessment
   c. Anthropometrics
   d. Biochemical Data

V. Nutrient Requirements
   a. Energy
   b. Protein
   c. Fluid
VI. Take-Home Points
VII. Case study answers
VIII. References

CASE STUDY 1

A 68-year-old male presents to the Emergency Department with progressive abdominal pain, steatorrhea, fatigue, and weight loss of 30 pounds in the past 6 months. He denies nausea or vomiting. Blood pressure is 100/72 mm Hg. He has a medical history of hypertension and cardiovascular disease (s/p myocardial infarction 10 years ago) and is taking clopidogrel 75 mg (antiplatelet), aspirin 75 mg (NSAID), lisinopril 5 mg (angiotensin-converting enzyme inhibitor), and atorvastatin 10 mg (HMG-CoA reductase inhibitor). There is no history of gastrointestinal surgeries. Despite weight loss, his body mass index (BMI) is 32 kg/m². Bloodwork shows hemoglobin 12.9 g/dL, hematocrit 37.9%, and MCV 80 fL. Albumin is 3.5 mg/dL and AST/ALT are 50 and 62 U/L, respectively. Electrolytes including blood urea nitrogen and creatinine are normal.

1. **What additional nutrition screening questions might you ask the patient?**
   A. What are your usual stooling patterns?

   B. Do you have any food allergies or food intolerances?
   C. Have there been any changes in your access to food?
   D. Both A and B
   E. All of the above

2. **What further nutritional bloodwork will you order?**
   A. Anemia panel (ferritin, TIBC)
   B. B vitamins (folate, B6, B12)
   C. Vitamin D
   D. All of the above

3. **What is the differential diagnosis?**
   A. Foodborne illness
   B. Celiac disease
   C. Inflammatory bowel disease (ulcerative colitis, Crohn's disease)
   D. Both B and C
   E. All of the above

CASE STUDY 2

AJ is a 9-year-old girl with autism who presents for a well-child visit. She appears well hydrated with adequate fat and muscle stores; oral cavity exam is unremarkable. She complains of dry eyes and will be seeing an ophthalmologist next week. AJ's parents describe her as a "picky eater"; it has always been a struggle to find foods that she will eat. AJ's anthropometrics are as follows:

One year ago: Weight 30 kg, weight-for-age percentile = 80th, weight for age Z-score 0.84
Height: 124.5 cm, height-for-age percentile = 30th, height for age Z-score −0.53
BMI: 19.4 kg/m², BMI-for-age percentile = 91st, BMI for age Z-score 1.36
Today: Weight 30.5 kg, weight-for-age percentile = 61st, weight for age Z-score 0.27
Height: 129 cm, height-for-age percentile = 26th, height for age Z-score −0.64
BMI: 18.3 kg/m², BMI-for-age percentile = 79th, BMI for age Z-score 0.80

1. **How would you classify AJ's current nutritional status based on the anthropometric data provided?**
   A. Well nourished
   B. Mild protein-energy malnutrition
   C. Moderate protein-energy malnutrition
   D. We have insufficient data to classify AJ's nutritional status

2. **Based on the physical exam information provided, what biochemical data would you obtain?**
   A. Albumin and prealbumin
   B. Retinol
   C. Riboflavin
   D. Sodium and potassium

3. **If you were to review a 24-hour recall for AJ, which of the following findings would be most concerning?**
   A. Most grains are not whole
   B. Protein intake mostly coming from dairy and plant sources
   C. Extremely limited intake of fruits and vegetables, may have one serving once a week
   D. Her "picky" eating pattern

INTRODUCTION

Poor nutritional status increases the risk of health-related complications and poorer disease outcomes, whether patients are in acute care, sub-acute care, long-term care, or outpatient settings. Malnutrition can occur with both overnutrition (obesity) and undernutrition.[1] The prevalence of malnutrition in independently living older adults is less than 10% but in acute care settings and nursing homes is estimated to be as high as 30% to 50%.[2] In hospitalized children, estimates of undernutrition range from 6% to 51%,[3] and globally, 45% of all deaths of children under age 5 are attributable to malnutrition.[4] Obese hospitalized patients are also at risk of underfeeding and poor clinical outcomes.[5] Obesity itself is a costly epidemic that increases the risk of cardiovascular disease, type 2 diabetes, several types of cancer, and early death.[6] Identification of those individuals at increased nutrition risk is the cornerstone of nutrition assessment.

NUTRITION SCREENING

A nutrition screening includes a checklist of factors that increase the risk of nutritional problems and morbidities that can lead to a prolonged hospital stay or vulnerability to infections. It quickly identifies patients who would benefit from a more extensive nutrition assessment by a registered dietitian. Malnutrition in adults is often present prior to a hospitalization, so screenings can be performed not only during an inpatient hospitalization but in various settings: emergency or urgent care units, long-term care, behavioral care, ambulatory clinics, and rehabilitation units.[7] The Joint Commission, the accrediting body of healthcare organizations, requires that nutrition screenings be completed within 24 hours of an inpatient admission, or at the first visit at a primary care office or ambulatory clinic.[8] Early screening for nutrition risk and malnutrition can lead to interventions that potentially decrease hospitalization lengths of stay and lower the cost of care.[9]

Nutrition screenings are not typically completed by a registered dietitian but by a nurse or other healthcare provider, which may then trigger a referral for a registered dietitian assessment.[8,9] There are various simple validated screening tools used for adults in acute care, ambulatory, and long-term care settings, such as the Malnutrition Screening Tool[1] or the Mini Nutritional Assessment-Short Form.[10] Validated pediatric nutrition screening tools include the Pediatric Nutrition Screening Tool (PNST).[11] Table 3-1 includes examples of screening criteria for both adults and pediatrics.

NUTRITION ASSESSMENT

A comprehensive nutrition assessment is typically performed by a registered dietitian after a nutrition screening is completed. This includes assessing the patient's dietary history, a physical assessment, anthropometrics, biochemical data, and nutrient requirements.

A commonly used validated assessment tool is the one-page Subjective Global Assessment (SGA), which focuses on five areas: decreased nutrient intake, weight changes, symptoms that affect oral intake (nausea, vomiting, dental problems, dysphagia), functional capacity and fatigue, and metabolic demand.[12] It also includes a physical assessment, followed by a rating system (well nourished, mild/moderately malnourished, and severely malnourished with wasting).

TABLE 3-1 • Examples of screening criteria that may prompt a more in-depth nutrition assessment
• Adults with a body mass index (BMI) of < 18.5 kg/m^2 (underweight) or ≥ 40 kg/m^2 (severe obesity), or unintentional weight changes, either increased or decreased.
• Changes in appetite, dietary intake, or eating behaviors.
• Changes in oral health that decrease food intake: difficulty chewing or swallowing due to poor dentition or dysphagia, mouth or throat pain, taste changes, infants with difficulty latching/sucking.
• Having undergone major surgeries that interfere with digestion, nutrient metabolism, or the ability to drink or eat.
• Changes in bowel habits such as constipation or diarrhea.
• Having one or more food allergies or intolerances. Common allergens in the United States are milk, eggs, wheat, peanuts, tree nuts, soy, fish, shellfish, and sesame.
• Infants requiring high calorie or specialized formulas.
• Poor wound healing caused by inadequate nutrition before or during the healing process.
• Use of herbal supplements and "megadoses" of vitamins and minerals that potentially cause harmful metabolic effects and even organ damage. It is an unregulated industry, but The National Center for Complementary and Integrative Health (NCCIH) provides evidence-based research on some supplements (refer to Chapter 7, "Herbs and Dietary Supplements").
• Food insecurity that is associated with financial constraints, housing instability, lack of transportation, limited access to full-service grocery stores, race/ethnicity, or physical disability.
• Decreased mobility due to physical disability or extreme fatigue that makes meal preparation or transportation to purchase food difficult.
• A relevant family health history, especially immediate relatives (parent or sibling), with chronic diseases that increase the risk of disease development.

Adapted from Charney P, Malone A. *Pocket Guide to Nutrition Assessment.* 4th ed. Chicago, Illinois: Academy of Nutrition and Dietetics; 2022; Kaiser MJ, Bauer JM, Ramsch C, et al. Validation of the Mini Nutritional Assessment Short-Form (MNA®-SF): a practical tool for identification of nutritional status. *J Nutr Health Aging.* 2009;13:782; Duerksen DR, Laporte M, Jeejeebhoy K. Evaluation of nutrition status using the Subjective Global Assessment: malnutrition, cachexia, and sarcopenia. *Nutr Clin Pract.* 2021;36(5):942-956.

TABLE 3-2 • Diagnosis and classification of undernutrition: Pediatrics (< 18 years of age)			
Primary indicator	**Mild malnutrition**	**Moderate malnutrition**	**Severe malnutrition**
Weight-for-height Z-score or BMI-for-age Z-score[a]	−1 to −1.9	−2 to −2.9	−3 or lower
Length/height-for-age Z-score[b]	No data	−2 to −2.9	−3 or lower
Mid-upper arm circumference	Z-score −1 to −1.9	Z-score −2 to −2.9 or ≥ 115 to < 125 mm	Z-score −3 or lower or < 115 mm
Weight gain velocity (< 2 years of age)	$< 75\%$ of norm for expected weight gain	$< 50\%$ of the norm for expected weight gain	$< 25\%$ of the norm for expected weight gain
Weight loss (2–20 years of age)	5% usual body weight	7.5% usual body weight	10% usual body weight
Deceleration in weight-for-length/height Z-score	Decline of 1 Z-score	Decline of 2 Z-scores	Decline of 3 Z-scores
Inadequate nutrient intake	51%–75% estimated energy/protein needs	26%–50% estimated energy/protein needs	$\leq 25\%$ estimated energy/protein needs

[a]Low weight-for-height Z-score or BMI Z-score indicates wasting.
[b]Low height-for-age Z-score indicates stunting.
Adapted from references 13 and 14.

Each of the areas commonly included in a nutrition assessment is discussed below.

Dietary History

Several methods can be used to obtain information on an individual's eating patterns. All of them have the goal of identifying deficits or excesses in macro- or micronutrient intake, gaps in intake (e.g., omission of entire food groups or prolonged periods of eating only specific foods, known as "food jags"), or irregular eating patterns (e.g., binge eating). Cutoffs for suboptimal dietary intake can also be used in the classification of undernutrition in pediatrics and adults (Tables 3-2 and 3-3).

The commonly used 24-hour dietary recall involves the clinician asking the individual to recall all food and beverages consumed in the past 24 hours. As with any assessment of dietary intake, the clinician should confirm types and quantities of foods consumed, preparation methods, all beverages and snacks, and timing of food intake.[16] The 24-hour recall does not provide valid data on long-term dietary intake; however, it provides a quick snapshot of current intake, with minimal cognitive burden for the responder. Another useful tool is the prospectively collected 3-day or 7-day food diary, where the patient or caregiver records, in real time, all foods and beverages consumed on predetermined days including both a weekday and weekend day to capture variability throughout the

TABLE 3-3 • Diagnosis and classification of undernutrition: Adults (≥ 18 years of age)		
Clinical characteristic[a]	Moderate protein-energy malnutrition	Severe protein-energy malnutrition
Energy intake	Acute illness or injury Chronic illness Environmental/social circumstances	< 75% estimated energy requirement for > 7 days < 75% estimated energy requirement for ≥ 1 month < 75% estimated energy requirement for ≥ 3 months	≤ 50% estimated energy requirement for ≥ 5 days < 75% estimated energy requirement for ≥ 1 month ≤ 50% estimated energy requirement for ≥ 1 month
Interpretation of weight loss (as a percentage compared to usual body weight)	Acute illness or injury Chronic illness or environmental/social circumstances	1-2% in 1 week 5% in 1 month 7.5% in 3 months 5% in 1 month 7.5% in 3 months 10% in 6 months 20% in 1 year	>2% in 1 week 5% in 1 month 7.5% in 3 months 5% in 1 month >7.5% in 3 months 10% in 6 months >20% in 1 year
Loss of subcutaneous body fat	Mild	Acute illness: Moderate Chronic illness or environmental/social circumstances: Severe	
Loss of muscle mass	Mild	Acute illness: Moderate Chronic illness or environmental/social circumstances: Severe	
Fluid accumulation	Mild	Acute illness: Moderate to severe Chronic illness or environmental/social circumstances: Severe	
Reduced grip strength	N/A	Measurably reduced	

[a]At least two of the six characteristics is recommended in order to make a diagnosis of malnutrition. Modified with permission from Marsha Schofield, Ainsley Malone, Gordon Jensen, et al. Academy of Nutrition and Dietetics and American Society for Parenteral and Enteral Nutrition. *J Parenter Enteral Nutr.* 2012;36(3):259-364.

Modified with permission from Schofield M, Malone A, Jensen G, et al. Academy of Nutrition and Dietetics and American Society for Parenteral and Enteral Nutrition. *J Parenter Enteral Nutr.* 2012;36(3):259-364.[15]

week. The 3-day or 7-day food diary can also be combined with a "symptom diary"; for example, for an individual with clinical signs/symptoms which are thought to be related to food intolerance (rash, diarrhea, etc.). The individual records all foods/beverages consumed, including the times of day at which they are consumed and simultaneously records their symptoms, which can aid diagnosis of food allergies or intolerances.

A food frequency questionnaire is commonly used in research settings but not often in clinical practice, as it is a lengthy survey that relies on patient memory of historical dietary intake but provides valid measures of long-term intake.

Whether included in a clinician's review of dietary or medication history, it is also important to confirm whether an individual takes a multivitamin or any other vitamin/mineral or herbal supplements, including megadoses.

Physical Assessment

Nutrition-focused physical assessment is a key component in nutrition assessment of both the adult and pediatric patient. A thorough, systems-based assessment of key body parts is critical and can diagnose or confirm muscle wasting, subcutaneous fat loss, overhydration (edema) or dehydration, and micronutrient deficiencies (Table 3-4). Assessment of blood pressure and pulse should be included for the patient with an eating disorder, as bradycardia and orthostatic hypotension

are common findings in anorexia nervosa.[16] Fever, hypothermia, or tachycardia could indicate an inflammatory response that could impact nutritional requirements and interpretation of biochemical data.[15] It is not uncommon for a diagnosis of micronutrient deficiency to be made after skin, eye, or nail manifestations to lead the practitioner to explore further biochemical testing or confirmation by dietary/medical data. A physical exam can confirm or deny the presence of malnutrition diagnosed by an inaccurate length or height. Similarly, a documented weight may indicate overweight or obesity, but a thorough physical exam may reveal edema or external hardware, for example, and thus an artificially inflated weight.

Anthropometrics

Pediatric. The importance of obtaining accurate anthropometric measurements cannot be overstated. Inaccurate measurements can result in an incorrect or missed diagnosis of malnutrition. For pediatrics, weight, recumbent length (< 2 years), standing height (2–20 years), and head circumference (< 2 years) should be obtained.[3] For children older than 2 years on whom an accurate standing height is not feasible (for example, a nonambulatory child or one with contractures), proxy height measures such as a knee height, tibia length, or arm span can be obtained.[3,17] We refer the reader elsewhere for methods of obtaining pediatric anthropometrics.[20,21]

TABLE 3-4 • Clinical signs and symptoms of malnutrition in adult and pediatric patients	
Body part	**Sign/symptom of malnutrition**
Dorsal hand	When tip of forefinger touching tip of thumb, depressed area indicates malnutrition (muscle loss)
Triceps/biceps	With arm bent, very little skin/fat to pinch on underside of arm (fat loss)
Temporalis muscle	Hollowing, depression (muscle loss)
Clavicle and acromion regions	Protruding, prominent bones (muscle loss); lack of rounded curves at arm/shoulder/neck (muscle loss)
Ribs and iliac crest	Ribs and iliac crest apparent (fat loss)
Hand grip strength	A proxy for functional status, reduced handgrip strength reflects poor muscle function and reduced nutritional status. Adult: No universally accepted cut-off points; proposed cut-offs < 30 kg men and < 20 kg women Pediatric: Use device-dependent reference ranges
Hair	Thin, sparse, patchy (iron, zinc, biotin, protein deficiency); depigmentation (protein-energy malnutrition, Mn, Se, Cu deficiency); easily plucked, dull (malnutrition, essential fatty acid deficiency)
Nails	Spoon-shaped, concave (koilonychia) (iron or protein deficiency); brittle, flaky, weak (Mg deficiency), severe malnutrition (vitamin A or selenium toxicity); transverse lines (protein deficiency)
Skin	Acanthosis nigricans (insulin resistance, obesity); eczema (riboflavin or zinc deficiency); abnormal dryness (vitamin A or essential fatty acid deficiency); seborrheic dermatitis (deficiency of biotin, vitamin A, vitamin B6, zinc, riboflavin, essential fatty acids; vitamin A toxicity); petechiae (purple or red spots on the skin) (vitamin C or vitamin K deficiency associated with abnormal bleeding under the skin)
Extremities	Bilateral pitting edema in legs (protein-energy deficiency, vitamin C deficiency); thin or no muscle definition on gastrocnemius (calf) (muscle loss)
Eyes	Pale conjunctivae (deficiency of vitamin B6, vitamin B12, folate, iron, copper); night blindness, dry membrane, white/gray spots on conjunctivae (Bitot's spots) (vitamin A deficiency); photophobia and burning, itching (riboflavin); periorbital depressions, dark circles, loose skin, hollow look (fat loss)
Mouth	Redness, swelling, or fissures at corners of mouth (angular stomatitis or cheilitis) (deficiency of riboflavin, niacin, iron, vitamin B6, vitamin B12); soreness or burning of lips or mouth (riboflavin deficiency); swollen beefy-red tongue (folate, vitamin B12, or niacin deficiency); hypogeusia or dysgeusia (zinc deficiency); red, retracted, swollen, or bleeding gums (deficiency of vitamin C, folate, niacin, zinc, or severe vitamin D)

Adapted from references 13 and 17–19.

For all children under age 20 years, anthropometric measurements are plotted on growth charts. For infants under the age of 2 years, weight-for-age, length-for-age, head circumference-for-age, and weight-for-length are plotted on sex-specific WHO growth charts.[21] For children ages 2–20 years, weight-for-age, height-for-age, and BMI-for-age are plotted on sex-specific CDC growth charts.[22] BMI percentiles are used in the diagnosis of pediatric overweight/obesity (Table 3-5). A child's growth should be tracked over time and compared to both established norms and

to a child's own curve. For example, a child who is "following their own curve" at the 3rd percentile weight-for-age may be less concerning than a child who crosses more than two percentile curves over a period of time. Growth charts are available for specific conditions including prematurity[24] and Down syndrome.[25]

In the same manner, Z-scores may also be used to track a child's weight-for-age, length/height-for-age, head circumference-for-age, and weight-for-length or BMI-for-age over time. Changes in weight-for-length or BMI Z-score can be helpful in the assessment of the effectiveness of a nutrition intervention. Z-scores are also used in the classification of malnutrition, as outlined in Table 3-2. Refer to Chapter 13 (Severe Malnutrition and Refeeding Syndrome) for more information on severe acute malnutrition. All growth charts noted above and Z-scores can be obtained by inputting patient data in peditools.org.

Weight gain velocity is another useful tool in the assessment of the nutritional status of a child less than 2 years of age.[13] Using a child's weight from two different dates, weight gain velocity can be calculated for a specified timeframe and compared to published norms for gender and weight-for-age percentile. A child with a suboptimal weight gain velocity is at risk for growth failure; indeed, a slow weight gain velocity can be diagnostic of malnutrition in children less than 2 years of age (Table 3-2).

TABLE 3-5 • Diagnosis and classification of overnutrition		
	Overweight	**Obese**
Adult	BMI 25.0 to 29.9 kg/m²	Class I: 30.0 to 34.9 kg/m² Class II: 35.0 to 39.9 kg/m² Class III: ≥ 40.0 kg/m²
Pediatrics	BMI-for-age 85–94th percentile or weight-for-length or BMI-for-age Z-score > 2 to ≤ 3	BMI-for-age ≥ 95th percentile or weight-for-length or BMI-for-age Z-score > 3

Adapted from references 6, 14, and 23.

Mid-upper arm circumference (MUAC) is a relatively simple bedside measure of body composition that has been suggested as a proxy for weight or even lean body mass.[3,17] MUAC is recommended in the assessment of nutritional status of children ages 6–60 months, particularly those in whom accurate weight and length measurements are challenging; for example, the critically ill child who cannot be moved, or a child with fluid shifts or edema.[3,13] Published MUAC Z-scores exist for tracking serial measurements,[21] as well as defined Z-score cutoffs for the classification of malnutrition (Table 3-2).[13] Triceps skinfold measurement (TSF) reflects body fat stores and can be an adjunct to other markers of nutritional status, although it requires clinician training and specific equipment (calipers). Published TSF reference data (percentiles and Z-scores) are available for ages 3 months to 5 years.[21] Although not routinely used in clinical practice, arm muscle area (AMA) and arm fat area can be calculated from MUAC and TSF measurements.[17]

Adult. Body mass index (BMI) and clinical signs of malnutrition such as muscle loss, subcutaneous fat loss, and fluid status (Tables 3-3 and 3-4) can be used to assess for underweight in adults. BMI (Table 3-5), waist circumference, and waist-hip ratio may be used to assess for obesity and excess visceral fat. Sarcopenia (decreased skeletal muscle and fat-free mass) and sarcopenic obesity (decreased fat-free mass with increased fat mass) are conditions plaguing older adults that increase the risk of injury, disability, and mortality but that require not only body composition measures but an in-depth assessment of muscular strength and performance.[6] Refer to Chapter 17 (Overweight and Obesity) for more information on obesity.

Height and weight measurements are used to calculate BMI. There are specific guidelines on how to obtain accurate height measurements, such as having the patient remove shoes and stand with heels close together touching a wall. For patients with contractures or who cannot stand, the arm span method is used in which the patient extends one arm straight to the side, at a 90-degree angle from the torso. The length from the tip of the longest finger to the jugular notch is measured and multiplied by two.

When measuring weight, calculating the average of two to three measurements may be needed to increase accuracy, as well as comparison of past-recorded weights with a current weight. Reported weights from the patient, family members, or caregivers may not be reliable. Electronic and balance beam scales are the most accurate types and should be calibrated periodically. Shoes and heavy clothing/accessories should be removed. For heavier or immobile patients, a lift or bed scale may be used.

BMI is an inexpensive screening tool for weight categories (underweight, healthy weight, overweight, obesity) that may be associated with health problems. It is calculated from height and weight measurements: weight (kilograms) ÷ height (meters squared). Research has shown that BMI correlates well on a population level with "gold-standard" direct measures of fat mass and fat-free mass such as underwater weighing (hydrostatic weighing) and dual X-ray absorptiometry (DXA).[26]

The association of BMI and body fat percentage can differ, however, among populations and ethnicities.[27] Relying solely on BMI without other important clinical or anthropometric variables may not be an accurate tool to diagnose weight-related diseases.

BMI does not measure location of fat (e.g., abdominal or visceral fat associated with greater health risks) or muscle and bone mass. In addition, age, sex, race, and ethnicity can affect BMI. For example, women tend to carry more body fat and less muscle mass than men, and highly trained athletes may have a higher BMI due to greater muscle mass but carry little body fat. Older adults tend to carry more body fat than young adults, and differences in body composition have been reported among some ethnic groups (e.g., individuals of South Asian ancestry tend to develop insulin resistance at a lower BMI than non–South Asians).[26]

International studies show that certain populations have higher rates of obesity but do not have a high prevalence of metabolic diseases such as diabetes, and vice versa.[28] Therefore, a BMI measurement might be used with other measures such as waist-hip ratio, historical weight changes (progressive gain or loss), and biochemical assessment to help assess health risk.

Waist circumference is a simple tool to measure excess abdominal or visceral fat, which is associated with metabolic syndrome, type 2 diabetes, high blood pressure, and heart disease. A waist measurement taken just above the belly button of > 35 inches (89 cm) for women and > 40 inches (102 cm) for men indicates increased risk.

Waist-hip ratio (WHR) is also an estimate of abdominal fat. It is calculated by measuring circumferences of both the waist and hip (at the widest diameter of the buttocks), and then dividing the waist by the hip measurement. It is a good predictor of disease risk and early mortality. The World Health Organization defines abdominal obesity in men as WHR > 0.90 and in women > 0.85.[29] Skinfold thickness using special calipers can estimate total body fat by measuring the thickness of subcutaneous fat at various sites of the body. However, the method is prone to variable readings, both within and between observers, due to even slight differences in the location of measurement, how much of the skin is pinched, and the position of the calipers. The presence of edema can also affect the reading.

Other methods of body composition include bioelectrical impedance analysis (BIA) and dual-energy X-ray absorptiometry (DXA). These instruments can screen for sarcopenia and sarcopenic obesity, measuring both fat-free mass and fat mass.[6] BIA uses low-level electrical currents passing through the body, but results are affected by hydration status and are generated by protected algorithms. DXA is the preferred method for assessing bone density but can also estimate body composition. Its use of radiation limits its application in children and pregnant adults.

Biochemical Data

Biochemical indices comprise an important part of a thorough nutrition assessment. Abnormalities in a patient's basic chemistry panel (BUN, creatinine, Cl, CO_2, glucose, Na, K,

Ca, Mg, P) can lead the clinician to further diagnostic testing or referral to a registered dietitian. For example, abnormalities in blood glucose warrant further workup, including testing for diabetes; abnormalities in potassium or magnesium may indicate GI losses and potential malabsorption of micronutrients; and a finding of low serum levels of one micronutrient warrants investigation into the possibility of poor status of other micronutrients and, in pediatrics, the potential for poor growth. Historically, visceral protein markers (albumin, prealbumin, transferrin, retinol binding protein) were used in nutrition assessment, particularly prealbumin, with its shorter half-life of around 2 days, compared with albumin's 20-day half-life. Given the role of visceral proteins in the acute phase response and their highly variable serum levels in conditions such as inflammation, infection, trauma, and liver disease, the use of visceral protein markers is not recommended for the assessment of nutritional status nor for assessing the adequacy of protein provision.[5] When conducting a nutrition assessment, including the assessment of malnutrition, it is now considered imperative to determine whether or not inflammation is present, as described elsewhere.[3,15]

Whereas an exhaustive discussion of nutritional biochemical indices is beyond the scope of this chapter, Table 3-6 outlines the more common nutritional labs. Please also see Chapter 2 (Micronutrient Metabolism).

TABLE 3-6 • Common nutrition laboratory markers and their nutritional significance		
Common nutrition laboratory markers	**Normal serum reference range (both adult and pediatric unless otherwise specified)**	**Nutritional importance**
Sodium (Na) Potassium (K)	Na: 136–145 mEq/L K: 3.5–5.0 mEq/L (may be higher in neonates and premature infants)	• Serum Na not reflective of dietary sodium intake. • Serum Na may be falsely low with hyperglycemia. • Causes of low K: excessive urinary or gastrointestinal losses (chronic diarrhea, vomiting, potassium-wasting diuretics, laxatives), Cushing syndrome, refeeding syndrome. • Causes of high K: drugs that impair renal potassium excretion, acute kidney injury, chronic kidney disease. • Excess dietary K intake will not result in hyperkalemia unless underlying renal dysfunction is present.
Magnesium (Mg) Phosphorus (P)	Mg: 1.5–2.4 mEq/L P: 3.0–4.5 mg/dL (higher in infants and young children)	• Causes of high P: advanced kidney disease, hypoparathyroidism. • Causes of low P: undernutrition, refeeding syndrome, alcoholism, diabetic ketoacidosis. Chronic causes: hyperparathyroidism, diarrhea, diuretic use. • Causes of low Mg: alcoholism, chronic diarrhea, chronic use of diuretics or proton pump inhibitors. • Hypermagnesemia rare but seen in patients with kidney failure who are given magnesium-containing medications (e.g., antacids).
Calcium (Ca)	9.0–10.5 mg/dL	• Serum level tightly controlled, not reflective of dietary calcium intake. • Ionized calcium trends may be useful to assess adequacy of calcium provision in patients receiving nutrition support.
Lipid Panel: Total cholesterol Low-density lipoprotein (LDL) High-density lipoprotein (HDL) Triglycerides	Total cholesterol: 125–200 mg/dL LDL: < 100 mg/dL if no risk factors, LDL < 70 mg/dL in high-risk patients (hx of CHD, previous heart attack, stroke, T2DM) HDL: ≥ 40 mg/dL in men and ≥ 50 mg/dL in women Triglycerides: < 150 mg/dL	• Hypertriglyceridemia increases risk of pancreatitis, fatty liver disease, and heart disease. • With parenteral nutrition, check triglycerides at baseline and weekly thereafter.
Hemoglobin A1c (HbA1c)	Normal: <5.7% Prediabetes: 5.7%–6.4% Diabetes: ≥ 6.5% Less stringent goal of < 8% appropriate for patients with lower life expectancy or when harms of treatment are greater than benefits	• Testing should begin at age 35 years for adults, and earlier if diabetes risk factors are present. • Iron deficiency anemia and vitamin B12 and folate deficiency can falsely increase HbA1c in adults with or without diabetes due to decreased red blood cell turnover.

(Continued)

TABLE 3-6 · Common nutrition laboratory markers and their nutritional significance *(Continued)*		
Common nutrition laboratory markers	Normal serum reference range (both adult and pediatric unless otherwise specified)	Nutritional importance
Assessment of iron status: Hemoglobin (Hgb) Hematocrit (HCT) Mean corpuscular volume (MCV) Ferritin Total iron blood count (TIBC) Iron (Fe) Transferrin saturation (TSat) % reticulocyte count	Hgb: males 14–17 g/dL, females 12–16 g/dL HCT: males 41%–51%, females 36%–47% MCV: 80–100 fL Ferritin: adult males 12–300 ng/mL, adult females 10–150 ng/mL, < 1 mo–5 mo 50–200 ng/mL 6 mo–15 y: 7–142 ng/mL TIBC: 250–400 mcg/dL Iron: adult males 50–150 mcg/dL, adult females 35–145 mcg/dL Transferrin saturation: 20%–50 %	• Hgb low in late-stage iron deficiency anemia but is not sensitive to early deficiency states. • Hgb sensitive to hydration status and may appear normal in dehydration even if iron deficiency anemia is present. • MCV low in iron deficiency anemia and high in megaloblastic anemia (vitamin B12 or folate deficiency). • Ferritin is a positive acute-phase reactant that is low in early stages of iron deficiency without inflammation, but high in presence of inflammation, thus not useful in assessment of anemia during inflammation. • TIBC increases in iron deficiency. • Anemia of chronic disease (AOCD): Iron and transferrin are low to normal; ferritin is normal to elevated.
C-reactive protein (CRP)	< 0.8 mg/dL	• CRP is a positive acute phase reactant. Monitor serial measurements to track stress response; effectiveness of nutrition interventions (e.g., nutrition support) may be lessened during inflammation. • If CRP elevated, serum micronutrient levels may be falsely elevated or depressed due to inflammation.
Albumin (Alb) Prealbumin (PA)	Alb: 3.5–5 g/dL PA: 18–45 mg/dL	• Negative acute phase reactants; not reliable indicators of nutritional status in the presence of inflammation, trauma, edema, infections, and liver disease. • If normal CRP, low Alb and PA levels potentially indicative of inadequate dietary intake or poor nutritional status. • Zinc deficiency lowers PA levels.
25-OH Vitamin D Vitamin A (retinol) Vitamin C (ascorbic acid) Zinc	25-OH Vitamin D: 30–100 ng/mL (85–160 nmol/L) Retinol: 20–100 mcg/dL Vitamin C: 1–12 years: 0.2–2.3 mg/dL ≥ 13 years: 0.2–2.0 mg/dL Zinc: 0.7–1.2 mg/L (11-18 mmol/L)	• Check serum levels if concern for malnutrition, inadequate intake, or malabsorption, only after confirmation of no inflammation (e.g., normal CRP). • Serum zinc generally not sensitive indicator of zinc status but may confirm suspected deficiency in setting of clinical signs and if no inflammation.
Vitamin B1 (thiamine) Vitamin B6 (pyridoxine) Vitamin B9 (folate) Vitamin B12 (cobalamin)	Vitamin B1: 2.5–7.5 mcg/dL Vitamin B6: 5–50 mcg/L Vitamin B9: >140 mcg/L Vitamin B12: 200–800 pg/mL	• Vitamin B1, B6, and B9 deficiencies commonly seen with excess alcohol use that interferes with absorption and metabolism. • Vitamin B9 levels may decrease in pregnancy or lactation due to increased demand, and with malabsorption (e.g., celiac disease, intestinal surgeries). • Vitamin B12 deficiency occurs with vegans who do not eat animal products, pernicious anemia causing lack of intrinsic factor needed to absorb B12, and medications that decrease stomach acid (e.g., proton pump inhibitors) needed to metabolize B12.

Adapted from references 15, 16, 30, and 31.

● NUTRIENT REQUIREMENTS

Energy

In order to guide energy provision and minimize the risk of over- or underfeeding, the clinician should measure or estimate a patient's energy expenditure. A precise method to measure a patient's resting energy expenditure (REE) is by using indirect calorimetry (IC), which measures oxygen consumption and carbon dioxide production. IC is the preferred method to determine a patient's energy needs;[5,13] however, since many practitioners do not have routine access to IC, estimation equations are routinely used in clinical practice. Published equations estimating REE for adults include the Mifflin-St. Jeor and Penn State equations,[32] and in pediatrics, the Schofield and FAO/WHO/UNU equations.[13] Since REE estimation equations do not account for energy requirements for wound healing, trauma, or growth, among others, "stress factors" are commonly applied when using an REE equation; for example, a stress factor of REE x1.1 may be sufficient for an adult surgery patient,[33] whereas x1.3-1.8 might be used for an adult burn patient[33] or x1.5-2.0 for a child with growth failure.[34]

For healthy, active adults and children, many clinicians use the Dietary Reference Intakes (DRIs) for energy, known as the Estimated Energy Requirements (EERs).[35] These equations include factors for various physical activity levels for all ages, consideration of growth for children, and separate equations for individuals at higher BMIs.[35] We refer the reader elsewhere for equations estimating energy expenditure for individuals with conditions such as cerebral palsy, Down syndrome, myelomeningocele, and Prader-Willi syndrome.[36] Table 3-7 describes common clinical scenarios where various energy estimation equations may be used.

It is important to consider an individual's clinical status when choosing an energy equation; for example, the use of the EER equation may vastly overestimate energy expenditure if applied to a patient who is intubated/sedated/ventilated in a critical care setting, and can thus result in overfeeding. Despite their convenience, equations provide an estimation only. Ongoing nutrition assessment of weight trends, wound healing, muscle and fat mass, respiratory status, and biochemical data is imperative; it is not uncommon for nutrition clinicians to identify patients ultimately requiring more or less energy than was calculated by prediction equations. For patients receiving nutrition support or for those in whom fine-tuning of nutritional needs is needed, referral to a registered dietitian is crucial.

Protein

Table 3-7 outlines protein requirements for a variety of conditions and life stages. In many cases, a patient will meet their dietary protein needs by consuming the RDA, although many individuals regularly consume more than the RDA. In clinical scenarios including critical illness, wound healing, burns, and hemodialysis, protein requirements may be higher than

TABLE 3-7 • Selection of energy/protein estimation equations in various clinical scenarios		
	Energy	Protein
Adult		
Healthy, active	DRI equation for EER; or Mifflin-St. Jeor (REE) × activity factor	RDA: 0.8 g/kg
Overweight or obese, not critically ill[a]	Mifflin-St. Jeor (REE) using actual weight × DRI PAL	1.0–1.3 g/kg actual body weight
Not obese, critically ill	Mifflin-St. Jeor or Penn State (REE) × stress factor 25–30 kcal/kg	1.2–2 g/kg
Obese, critically ill[a]	11–14 kcal/kg actual body weight (BMI 30–50) 22–25 kcal/kg ideal body weight (using Hamwi) (BMI> 50)	2.0 g/kg ideal body weight (BMI 30–39) 2.0–2.5 g/kg ideal body weight (BMI ≥ 40)
Pediatric		
Critical illness (> 1 mo to < 18 years), not obese	Indirect calorimetry; Schofield or FAO/WHO/UNU equations without stress factor	1.5–3 g/kg
Critical illness (> 1 mo to < 18 years), obese	Indirect calorimetry; Schofield or FAO/WHO/UNU equations without stress factor	1.5–3 g/kg using ideal body weight
Healthy, active	EER equation	RDA/AI: 0–6 mos: 2.2 g/kg 7–12 mos: 1.2 g/kg 1–3 years: 1.05 g/kg 4–13 years: 0.95 g/kg 14–18 years: 0.85 g/kg
Overweight, not critically ill (ages 3–18 years)[a]	EER TEE equation for boys/girls with overweight (weight maintenance)	RDA/AI (see "Healthy, active")
Catch-up growth	Schofield or FAO/WHO/UNU using actual weight × 1.5–2.0	0–6 mos: 2.2 g/kg 6–12 mos: 1.6 g/kg 1–3 years: 1.2 g/kg 4–6 years: 1.1 g/kg 7–10 years: 1.0 g/kg 11–14 years: 1.0 g/kg 15–18 years: 0.9 g/kg

[a]The use of dry body weight is imperative for energy, protein, and fluid equations. For obese individuals, the use of actual body weight is recommended, unless otherwise specified.
Adapted from references 5, 13, 32, 34, 35, 37, and 38.

the RDA. In less-common situations such as adults with pre-dialysis renal disease, protein requirements may be slightly less than the RDA.[37] Referral to a registered dietitian is recommended to ensure appropriate protein provision in these scenarios.

Fluid

Table 3-8 outlines maintenance fluid needs across the life span. An individual may require more fluids if there are excessive insensible losses (drooling, sweating, large wounds), persistent fevers, vomiting/diarrhea, or other GI losses such as fistulas or ostomies.[39] Fluid intake may be restricted in heart failure, renal failure, edema, or ascites. Fluids from all sources, including liquids consumed orally, through parenteral or enteral nutrition support, and water consumed with medications, should be included in the estimation of fluid intake. Monitoring

TABLE 3-8 • Daily fluid requirements	
Adult	**Pediatric**
1 mL per kcal consumed OR 25–35 mL/kg; see reference[39] for discussion of adjusted equations for individuals > 65 years of age or use of obesity-adjusted weight	≤ 10 kg: 100 mL/kg 11–20 kg: 1,000 mL + 50 mL/kg for every kg above 10 kg > 20 kg: 1,500 mL + 20 mL/kg for every kg above 20 kg

Adapted from references 39 and 40.

biochemical (Table 3-6) and clinical signs will be helpful in the assessment of hydration.

We refer the reader to Chapter 2 (Micronutrient Metabolism) for the DRIs for micronutrients.

TAKE-HOME POINTS

1. When to refer to a registered dietitian
   - Nutritional intake is suboptimal to maintain weight or attain pediatric age-appropriate growth.
   - Critical conditions (e.g., burns, wound care, pressure ulcers, failure to thrive, malnutrition) or any other medical condition that increases the risk of micro- and macronutrient deficiencies.
   - Need for nutrition support (enteral or parenteral nutrition).
   - Patient requires in-depth nutrition education for chronic diseases or autoimmune conditions (e.g., high blood pressure, diabetes, inflammatory

   bowel disease, celiac disease, kidney disease, food allergies or sensitivities).
   - Disordered eating patterns including anorexia nervosa, bulimia nervosa, binge eating disorder, or avoidant restrictive food intake disorder (ARFID).
2. A complete nutrition assessment includes interpretation of accurate anthropometric measurements, a nutrition-focused physical exam, and review of dietary and biochemical data.
3. For patients receiving nutrition support, or those with a changing clinical status, ongoing assessment of macro- and micronutrients needs is imperative in optimizing nutrition status.

CASE STUDY ANSWERS

CASE 1: ADULT

1. *D.* Changes in weight and bowel habits suggest a gastrointestinal problem, so a screening should include asking about noticeable food intolerances or difficulty digesting meals. Although decreased food access could lead to weight loss, it would not be the primary cause of the other symptoms mentioned.
2. *D.* The patient's microcytic anemia suggests investigating iron deficiency anemia, and deficiencies in certain B vitamins can lead to anemia. Vitamin D is absorbed in the small intestine, so this deficiency is common in intestinal diseases.
3. *D.* Food-borne illness tends to cause acute, not progressive chronic abdominal pain, and typically

does not cause significant weight loss. Crohn's and celiac disease can cause all of the patient's reported symptoms.

The patient has celiac disease. A few reasons may cause a delayed or missed diagnosis. It is believed that celiac disease typically occurs in younger adults; however, about one-third of new patients diagnosed are 65 and older. This patient is also obese with a normal albumin, which may prevent further investigation into vitamin and mineral deficiencies, which are commonly seen in newly diagnosed celiac disease. Further antibody testing and an upper endoscopy with small bowel biopsy would confirm the diagnosis.

CASE 2: PEDIATRIC

1. *A.* Based on one data point (today's anthropometrics), AJ classifies as well nourished without malnutrition per WHO criteria (Table 3-2). It is worth noting that AJ's BMI Z-score dropped from 1.36 to 0.8 over the past year; this decline of 0.56 is less than the unintentional drop of > 1.0 Z-score which would have classified AJ with mild protein-energy malnutrition. Despite the fact that AJ presents well nourished, this drop in BMIZ warrants further investigation with AJ's parents, as ongoing BMIZ decline could result in a diagnosis of malnutrition at AJ's next well-child visit. AJ's BMI was at the 91st percentile 1 year ago, indicating an overweight status, and it's possible this reduced weight gain velocity and resultant change in BMI was intentional.

2. *B.* Dry eye could be a symptom of xerophthalmia related to retinol deficiency, and it would be prudent to check a serum retinol (vitamin A) and CRP (to reduce the inappropriate interpretation of artificially low micronutrient levels in the setting of inflammation). Vitamin A deficiency has been identified in children with autism and restricted dietary intake. In light of AJ's limited dietary variety, it may also be worth checking iron studies, vitamin C, 25-OH vitamin D, thiamine (B1), vitamin B12, folate, and zinc.

3. *C.* Avoidance of entire food groups is considered a dietary red flag. Individuals with limited dietary variety who do not take a daily multivitamin are at risk for micronutrient deficiencies. AJ's extremely limited intake of fruits and vegetables puts her at risk for deficiencies in vitamins A and C in particular.

REFERENCES

1. Mueller C, Compher C, Ellen DM; American Society for Parenteral and Enteral Nutrition (A.S.P.E.N.) Board of Directors. A.S.P.E.N. clinical guidelines: nutrition screening, assessment, and intervention in adults. *J Parenter Enteral Nutr.* 2011;35(1):16-24.

2. O'Keeffe M, Kelly M, O'Herlihy E, et al. Potentially modifiable determinants of malnutrition in older adults: a systematic review. *Clin Nutr.* 2019;38(6):2477-2498.

3. Mehta NM, Corkins MR, Lyman B, et al. Defining pediatric malnutrition: a paradigm shift toward etiology-related definitions. *J Parenter Enteral Nutr.* 2013;37(4):460-481.

4. World Health Organization. Malnutrition. https://www.who.int/news-room/fact-sheets/detail/malnutrition. Updated June 9, 2021. Accessed March 6, 2023.

5. McClave SA, Taylor BE, Martindale RG, et al. Guidelines for the provision and assessment of nutrition support therapy in the adult critically ill patient: Society of Critical Care Medicine (SCCM) and American Society of Parenteral and Enteral Nutrition (A.S.P.E.N.). *J Parenter Enteral Nutr.* 2016;40(2):159-211.

6. Holmes CJ, Racette SB. The utility of body composition assessment in nutrition and clinical practice: an overview of current methodology. *Nutrients.* 2021;13(8):2493.

7. Charney P, Malone A. *Pocket Guide to Nutrition Assessment.* 4th ed. Chicago, IL: *Academy of Nutrition and Dietetics;* 2022.

8. Patel V, Romano M, Corkins MR, et al. Nutrition screening and assessment in hospitalized patients: a survey of current practice in the United States. *Nutr Clin Pract.* 2014;29(4):483-490.

9. Freijer K, van Puffelen E, Joosten KF, Hulst JM, Koopmanschap MA. The costs of disease related malnutrition in hospitalized children. *Clin Nutr ESPEN.* 2018;23:228-233.

10. Kaiser MJ, Bauer JM, Ramsch C, et al. Validation of the Mini Nutritional Assessment Short-Form (MNA®-SF): a practical tool for identification of nutritional status. *J Nutr Health Aging.* 2009;13:782.

11. White M, Lawson L, Ramsey R, et al. Simple nutrition screening tool for pediatric inpatients. *J Parenter Enteral Nutr.* 2016;40(3):392-398.

12. Duerksen DR, Laporte M, Jeejeebhoy K. Evaluation of nutrition status using the subjective global assessment: malnutrition, cachexia, and sarcopenia. *Nutr Clin Pract.* 2021;36(5):942-956.

13. Becker P, Carney LN, Corkins MR, et al. Consensus statement of the Academy of Nutrition and Dietetics/American Society for Parenteral and Enteral Nutrition: indicators recommended for the identification and documentation of pediatric malnutrition (undernutrition). *Nutr Clin Pract.* 2015;30(1):147-161.

14. World Health Organization. *Guideline: Assessing and Managing Children at Primary Health-Care Facilities to Prevent Overweight and Obesity in the Context of the Double Burden of Malnutrition: Updates for the Integrated Management of Childhood Illness (IMCI).* Geneva: World Health Organization; 2017. Accessed January 25, 2023. Available at: https://www.ncbi.nlm.nih.gov/books/NBK487900/table/fm.s1.t1/.

15. White JV, Guenter P, Jensen G, Malone A, Schofield M; Academy Malnutrition Work Group; A.S.P.E.N. Malnutrition Task Force; A.S.P.E.N. Board of Directors. Consensus statement: Academy of Nutrition and Dietetics and American Society for Parenteral and Enteral Nutrition: characteristics recommended for the identification and documentation of adult malnutrition (undernutrition). *J Parenter Enteral Nutr.* 2012;36(3):275-283.

16. Raymond JL, Morrow K, eds. *Krause and Mahan's Food & The Nutrition Care Process.* St. Louis, MO: Elsevier; 2021.

17. Corkins KG, Teague EE. Pediatric nutrition assessment: anthropometrics to zinc. *Nutr Clin Pract.* 2017;32(1):40-51.

18. Mordarski B, Wolff J, eds. *Pediatric Nutrition Focused Physical Exam Pocket Guide.* Chicago, IL: Academy of Nutrition and Dietetics; 2015.

19. Cruz-Jentoft AJ, Baeyens JP, Bauer JM, et al. Sarcopenia: European consensus on definition and diagnosis: report of the European working group on sarcopenia in older people. *Age Ageing.* 2010;39(4):412-423.

20. Abbott Nutrition Health Institute. Clinical demonstration series: Measuring infant weight; measuring infant length; measuring head circumference; measuring toddler weight; measuring toddler height. Updated September 25, 2020. Accessed October 23, 2022. Available at: https://anhi.org/resources/podcasts-and-videos/clinical-demonstration-modules.

21. World Health Organization. Child growth standards. Accessed October 23, 2022. Available at: https://www.who.int/tools/child-growth-standards.

22. Centers for Disease Control and Prevention. Clinical growth charts. Updated June 16, 2017. Accessed January 25, 2023. Available at: https://www.cdc.gov/growthcharts/clinical_charts.htm.

23. Barlow SE; Expert Committee. Expert committee recommendations regarding the prevention, assessment, and treatment of child and adolescent overweight and obesity: summary report. *Pediatrics.* 2007;120(supp l4):S164-S192.

24. Fenton TR, Kim JH. A systematic review and meta-analysis to revise the Fenton growth chart for preterm infants. *BMC Pediatr.* 2013:13-59.

25. Zemel BS, Pipan M, Stallings VA, et al. Growth charts for children with Down syndrome in the United States. *Pediatrics.* 2015;136(5):e1204-e1211.

26. Centers for Disease Control and Prevention. Body Mass Index: Considerations for practitioners. Available at: https://www.cdc.gov/obesity/downloads/bmiforpractitioners.pdf. Accessed May 28, 2022.

27. Akindele MO, Phillips JS, Igumbor EU. The relationship between body fat percentage and body mass index in overweight and obese individuals in an urban african setting. *J Public Health Afr.* 2016;7(1):515.

28. Lustig RH, Collier D, Kassotis C, et al. Obesity I: overview and molecular and biochemical mechanisms. *Biochem Pharmacol.* 2022 Mar 30:115012.

29. World Health Organization. *Waist Circumference and Waist-Hip Ratio: Report of a WHO Expert Consultation, Geneva, 8-11, December 2008.* Geneva: World Health Organization; 2011. Accessed October 24, 2022. Available at: https://www.who.int/publications/i/item/9789241501491.

30. Merck Manual, Professional Version. Table: Representative laboratory reference values: Blood, plasma, and serum. Updated December 2021. Accessed June 15, 2022. Available at: https://www.merckmanuals.com/professional/resources/normal-laboratory-values.

31. American Diabetes Association. Standards of medical care in diabetes-2022 abridged for primary care providers. *Clin Diabetes.* 2022;40(1):10-38.

32. Frankenfield D. Energy. In: Mueller CM, ed. *The ASPEN Adult Nutrition Support Core Curriculum,* 3rd ed. ASPEN;2017:27-40.

33. Mogensen KM, Robinson MK. Surgical Metabolism & Nutrition. In: Doherty GM. eds. *Current Diagnosis & Treatment: Surgery,* 15edn. McGraw Hill; 2020. Accessed July 27, 2022. Available at: https://accessmedicine.mhmedical.com/content.aspx?bookid=2859&sectionid=242154209.

34. Academy of Nutrition and Dietetics. *Pediatric Nutrition Care Manual.* Academy of Nutrition and Dietetics. Accessed July 28, 2022. Available at: www.nutritioncaremanual.org.

35. Institute of Medicine. *Dietary Reference Intakes for Energy, Carbohydrate, Fiber, Fat, Fatty acids, Cholesterol, Protein, and Amino Acids.* Washington, DC; The National Academies Press; 2005. Accessed January 25, 2023. Available at: https://nap.nationalacademies.org/catalog/10490/dietary-reference-intakes-for-energy-carbohydrate-fiber-fat-fatty-acids-cholesterol-protein-and-amino-acids.

36. Tougas L, Weston S. Developmental disabilities. In: Sonneville K, Duggan C, eds. *Manual of Pediatric Nutrition,* 5th ed. PMPH; 2014:303-315.

37. Academy of Nutrition and Dietetics. *Nutrition Care Manual.* Academy of Nutrition and Dietetics. Accessed July 25, 2022.

38. Mehta NM, Skillman HE, Irving SY, et al. Guidelines for the provision and assessment of nutrition support therapy in the pediatric critically ill patient: Society of Critical Care Medicine and American Society for Parenteral and Enteral Nutrition. *Pediatr Crit Care Med.* 2017;18(7):675-715.

39. Canada TW, Lord LM. Fluids, electrolytes, and acid-base disorders. In: Mueller CM, ed. *The ASPEN Adult Nutrition Support Core Curriculum.* 3rd ed. ASPEN; 2017:113-137.

40. Holliday MA, Segar WE. The maintenance need for water in parenteral fluid therapy. *Pediatrics.* 1957;19:823-832.

Food Insecurity

Awab Ali Ibrahim, MD / Lauren G. Fiechtner, MD

Chapter Outline

CASE STUDY

A 15-month-old boy with a past history of three hospitalizations for viral infections presents for evaluation of anemia. Point-of-care testing done by his primary care physician showed a Hgb of 6.7 His diet consists of human milk, minimal cow's milk, and some table foods. He stools twice per day with no blood or mucus in his stools. The patient lives with his mother and some relatives. The mother works full time in retail and is currently renting an apartment with no reported housing instability. The patient has normal vital signs, his weight is 13 kg, and his length is 75 cm. His weight for length is > 99%ile (Z = 3.78). His physical exam is otherwise normal. Lab work done is shown below.

White blood cell count	6.6 (6.0–17.5 K/µL)
Red blood cell count	4.93 (3.7–5.3 M/µL)
Hemoglobin	6.7 (10.5–13.5 g/dL)
Hematocrit	24.5 (33%–39%)
Mean corpuscular volume	59 (70–86 fL)
MCHC	23 (23–31 pg)
Platelet count	270 (150–450 K/µL)
Red cell distribution width	30 (11.5%–16%)
Iron	12 µg/dL (45–169 µg/dL)

Iron saturation	4% (14%–50%)
Total iron binding capacity	500 µg/dL (230–400 µg/dL)
Ferritin	6 µg/L (10–75 µg/L)
Folate	13.5 ng/mL (> 4.7 ng/mL)
Vitamin B12	413 pg/mL (> 231 pg/ml)
Stool guaiac	Negative

The patient was diagnosed with iron deficiency due to insufficient dietary intake. He was started on oral iron supplementation. A nutrition consult showed that the family would often run out of food and that the patient and parent would frequently skip meals.

1. How can you screen this patient for food insecurity? (select all that apply)
   A. USDA food security survey
   B. Hunger Vital Sign
   C. Ask the patient directly if they suffer from food insecurity
   D. This patient clearly does not have food insecurity, no further investigations needed

2. What is the association between weight and food insecurity?

3. What federal and local resources can you refer the family to for help with access to food?

WHAT IS FOOD INSECURITY VS. HUNGER?

The U.S. Department of Agriculture (USDA) defines food insecurity (FI) as the lack of consistent access to enough food for an active, healthy life.[1] This could be due to the unavailability of food and/or lacking the resources to access food. Hunger, in contrast, is an uncomfortable sensation or desire to consume food. FI and hunger are closely related since most people with FI will likely experience hunger; however, the concepts and terms of hunger and food insecurity should not be used interchangeably[2].

HOW COMMON IS FOOD INSECURITY?

The COVID-19 pandemic has led to a sharp increase in the prevalence of FI worldwide.[3] Nearly 30% of the people in the world (2.37 billion) did not have access to adequate food in 2020. Disturbingly, that is an increase of almost 320 million people in just 1 year.[4] With this rapid increase in food insecurity, the prevalence of malnutrition is also on the rise.[4] These are some statistics regarding the global burden of food insecurity: More than half of all undernourished people live in Asia (418 million), one-third in Africa (282 million and 1% of the population which is more double any other region), and a smaller portion (60 million) live in Latin America and the Caribbean.

Based on USDA data from 2020, it is estimated that the prevalence of FI in the United States is ~11% (13.8 million) of the total population.[5] There is a large variability in this prevalence depending on the household characteristics, with a higher prevalence of FI in ethnic under-represented groups (22% in Black non-Hispanic and 17% in Hispanic household).[5] Moreover, households with young children (15% have FI) and single-family households (28% of single mothers and 16% of single fathers have FI) are at higher risk of FI.

HOW DO WE IDENTIFY FOOD INSECURITY IN THE CLINICAL PRACTICE?

FI is associated with poor health outcomes at all age groups. The American Academy of Pediatrics (AAP) and the American Association of Retired Persons (AARP) have both recommended a FI screening in both pediatric and adult healthcare visits.[6,7] The gold standard for assessing FI is the USDA household food insecurity module.[8] This is comprehensive questionnaire that consist of 18 items. The length of this questionnaire makes it difficult to administer in a clinical setting. There are various shorter assessment tools developed with similar efficacy to the USDA questionnaire. The two-item Hunger Vital Sign[9] is the most commonly used health screening questionnaire, with 89%–97% sensitivity and 83%–84% specificity compared to the gold standard USDA questionnaire[10] (Table 4-1).

TABLE 4-1 • The hunger vital sign®	
The Hunger Vital Sign®	
"Within the past 12 months, we worried whether our food would run out before we got money to buy more."	• Often True • Sometimes True • Never True
"Within the past 12 months, the food we bought just didn't last and we didn't have enough money to get more."	• Often True • Sometimes True • Never True

Note: If the answer to either or both these questions is "often true" or "sometimes true," then the individual is at risk for food insecurity.

WHAT ARE THE HEALTH CONSEQUENCES OF FOOD INSECURITY?

FI is associated with lower-quality food (defined as lower fruit, vegetable, and dairy consumption) and suboptimal micronutrient content in adults unrelated to their socioeconomic status.[11] With children, the risk of FI and lower-quality food is not clear.[11] This is believed to be due to caregivers protecting their children by prioritizing the child's nutrition and skipping meals themselves. Analysis of National Health and Nutrition Examination Surveys (NHANES) suggests that micronutrient malnutrition is surprisingly common in the United States, with an estimated 31% of the population at risk of developing one or more micronutrient deficiencies.[9] Chapter 2 focuses on specific micronutrients and their deficiencies.

In the case of the 15-month-old above, the family's FI has likely resulted in lower intake of iron-rich food such as meat, leafy green vegetables, and some fish. Iron deficiency is the most common micronutrient deficiency worldwide.[10] Iron deficiency anemia has multiple effects, including delays in cognitive, motor, and psychological development.[12]

FI has many other physical and psychological effects (Table 4-2).

TABLE 4-2 • Physical and psychological effects of food insecurity	
Child	• Higher frequency of chronic illness • Delays in cognitive function • Obesity • Substance use
Parents	• Increased risk of depression • Substance use • Post-traumatic stress disorder • Parental Stress • Less responsive caregiver practices
Adults	• Substance use • Tobacco use • Obesity

WHAT ARE THE SYSTEMIC EFFECTS OF FOOD INSECURITY?

FI disproportionately affects racial and ethnic minority communities and people with lower socioeconomic status. The cause of these inequities is rooted in systemic racism and other policies including housing segregation that combine to limit access to healthy foods. Unfortunately, the physical and psychological effects of FI are interconnected and are passed down in families and generations. Figure 4-1 visualizes the vicious cycle of FI. Understanding this is crucial in the implementation of systemic and public health policies to help eradicate this problem.

RELATIONSHIP BETWEEN FOOD INSECURITY AND OBESITY

Most individuals with FI live in lower socioeconomic environments. Living in these lower socioeconomic states predisposes individuals to a suboptimal diet.[13] With limited financial resources, individuals have to purchase high-calorie foods with lower nutrient density to stretch their budgets.[14] These foods are generally "more filling" and protect individuals from experiencing hunger. High-calorie foods also predispose individuals to the development of obesity.[13-15]

Moreover, neighborhoods with lower incomes are more likely to have limited food outlets to purchase fresh produce (food deserts) as well as an increase in fast-food restaurants (food swamps).[14] There is mixed evidence on the correlation between food deserts and obesity rates.[15] Alternatively, food swamps with increased access to unhealthy foods have been found to be a better predictor of obesity rates than food deserts.[11] Understanding these concepts is important in managing and preventing obesity. Weight stigma is pervasive, including from their families and medical providers and often individuals are blamed for their weight status when environmental and structural racism factors are at play.

HOW DO WE END FOOD INSECURITY?

Food Banks and Pantries

Feeding America is a nationwide network of 200 food banks that provides food to 60,000 food pantries and meal programs throughout the United States. A food bank is a nonprofit organization that collects and distributes food to food pantries. Food pantries are where members of the community can reach out for food assistance. Food banks rely on both state and federal funding as well as philanthropy to purchase and distribute food. Many have national nutrition standards and distribute produce, lean meat, and dairy. Many food banks help families connect with food assistance programs such as the supplemental nutrition assistance program (SNAP); they can also play a role in antihunger advocacy and policy. The national network of food banks can be found on the Feeding American website.

Universal School Meals

The National School Lunch Program (NSLP) was established in 1946 to provide children with free or reduced-price meals. These school meals can account for over 50% of a child's calories and have also been linked to improved academic performance.[12] Providing meals at school can also reduce stress from families experiencing food insecurity. Unfortunately, not all children who qualify for free or reduced meals participate in this program. Cost and stigma are two of the biggest reasons for this.[16] Universal School Meals legislation, which has been passed in a growing number of states, ensures that all children would receive free school breakfast and lunch. The cost of this intervention is generally covered by the NSLP as well as the state.

Hunger-Fighting Organizations

For many people who struggle with FI, getting help can be a challenge. These challenges can occur due to various reasons, such as language barriers, transportation, and fear of stigma. Hunger-fighting organizations can play a pivotal role in getting people the help they need. Connecting patients with local hunger-fighting institutions can be a helpful tool to resolve FI. For example, in Massachusetts, Project Bread is a nonprofit organization that connects people and communities to reliable sources of food while advocating for policies that make food more accessible. The food source hotline provided by Project Bread helps connect patients (through 180 languages) with the reliable food sources and federal assistance programs they need.

Federal Food Assistance Programs

Subsidized food and food programs are one of the most effective ways to combat hunger and FI. These are funded by government programs rather than donations, making them more sustainable. Table 4-3 is a list of the most common food subsidy programs.

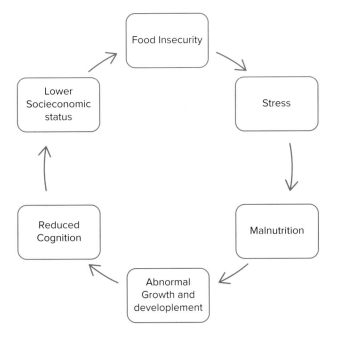

FIGURE 4-1 • The food insecurity cycle and how it can be passed down through generations (self-created).

TABLE 4-3 · Food subsidiary programs available in the United States

Program	About	Who qualifies (varies by state)	How to apply (Hunger-fighting organization can help connect patients)

Supplemental Nutritional Assistance Program (SNAP)	• Largest supplemental program administered by the USDA
	• Electronic Benefits Transfer (EBT) card provided
	  ○ Acts like a debit card
	  ○ Benefits loaded on card each month
	• EBT card can be used to buy food and drinks (not alcohol) as well as seeds and food producing plants
	• Cannot be used for ready-made meals
		• Gross income below 130% of poverty limit
		• Net income below 100% of poverty limit
			• SNAP local office, which can be located on the USDA website for SNAP

Woman, Infants, and Children (WIC)	• Provided by the USDA • Provides nutritional needs for woman and children • Some states might offer food lists or a phone app detailing foods that are available through the program	• Pregnant woman • Woman up to 6 months postpartum • Breastfeeding mothers up to infants first birthday • Children under 5 years old	• Local WIC office, which can be located on the USDA website for WIC
Senior Farmers Assistance Program (SFMNP)	• Provided by USDA • Low-income seniors receive coupons that can be used in participating locations • Benefits from $20–50 annually	• Seniors over 60 • Income less than 180% of poverty limit	• Local SFMNP office, which can be located on the USDA website for SFMNP
Commodity Supplemental Food Program (CSFP)	• USDA program • Low-income seniors receive monthly food packages	• Seniors over 60 • Income less than 130% of poverty limit	• Local CSFP office, which can be located on the USDA website for CSFP

THREE TAKE-HOME POINTS

1. Food insecurity is highly prevalent and should be considered in all clinical encounters.
2. The Hunger Vital Sign is a quick and efficient way of screening for food insecurity during clinical visits.
3. Patients who screen positive for food insecurity should be enrolled and referred to federal and other charitable food assistance programs.

CASE STUDY ANSWERS

1. **A, B;** The gold standard for screening food insecurity is the USDA food security survey tool; however, this is time intensive and difficult to implement during clinic visits. The Hunger Vital Sign® is a two-question questionnaire that screens for FI with good sensitivity and specificity.
2. Patients with FI are at an increased risk of developing obesity. FI patients often need to prioritize the purchase of high-calorie food with lower nutrient density to help stretch their budget and relieve hunger. Moreover, many people with FI will live in "food swamps," which have been linked to obesity.
3. The patient and his mother likely qualify for both WIC and SNAP based on the criteria in Table 4-1. To help patients sign up for these programs, you can refer them to hunger-fighting organizations or local social services that can connect them with appropriate resources. Referring the patient to a food bank can also be helpful to get immediate access to food. Food banks can also help connect patients with supplemental nutrition programs.

REFERENCES

1. U.S. Department of Agriculture. Definitions of Food Security, 2019. Available online at: https://www.ers.usda.gov/topics/food-nutrition-assistance/food-security-in-the-us/definitions-of-food-security.aspx Accessed 03/15/2022.

2. https://www.fao.org/hunger/en/ Accessed 05/01/2022

3. https://www.who.int/news/item/12-07-2021-un-report-pandemic-year-marked-by-spike-in-world-hunger Accessed 04/23/2022

4. https://www.fao.org/state-of-food-security-nutrition Accessed 05/03/2022

5. https://www.ers.usda.gov/topics/food-nutrition-assistance/food-security-in-the-u-s/key-statistics-graphics/.

6. Council on Community Pediatrics, Committee on Nutrition. Promoting food security for all children. *Pediatrics*. 2015;136(5): e1431-1438. Accessed 05/03/2022

7. Pooler J, Levin M, Hoffman V, Karva F, Lewin-Zwerdling A. *Implementing food security screening and referral for older patients in primary care: A resource guide and toolkit.* AARP Foundation and IMPAQ International; 2016.

8. Bickel G, Nord M, Price C, Hamilton W, Cook J. Guide to measuring household food security, revised 2000. U.S. Department of Agriculture, Food and Nutrition Service Alexandria VA. 2000.

9. Bird JK, Murphy RA, Ciappio ED, McBurney MI. Risk of deficiency in multiple concurrent micronutrients in children and adults in the United States. *Nutrients*. 2017;9(7):E655.

10. https://www.who.int/health-topics/anaemia#tab=tab_1 Accessed 05/03/2022

11. Hanson KL, Connor LM. Food insecurity and dietary quality in US adults and children: a systematic review. *Am J Clin Nutr*. 2014;100:684-692.

12. Cohen JFW, Hecht AA, McLoughlin GM, Turner L, Schwartz MB. Universal school meals and associations with student participation, attendance, academic performance, diet quality, food security, and body mass index: a systematic review. *Nutrients*. 2021 Mar 11;13(3):911.

13. Tester JM, Rosas LG, Leung CW. Food insecurity and pediatric obesity: a double whammy in the era of COVID-19. *Curr Obes Rep*. 2020 Dec;9(4):442-450.

14. Larson NI, Story MT, Nelson MC. Neighborhood environments: disparities in access to healthy foods in the U.S. *Am J Prev Med*. 2009 Jan;36(1):74-81.

15. Drewnowski A. The cost of US foods as related to their nutritive value. *Am J Clin Nutr*. 2010 Nov;92(5):1181-1188.

16. https://www.ers.usda.gov/webdocs/publications/44003/53570_eib143.pdf?v=8379.8 Accessed 05/04/2022.

chapter 5

Nutrition Through the Life Span

Julia V. Loewenthal, MD / Karen M. Switkowski, PhD, MPH / Allison J. Wu, MD, MPH

Chapter Outline

CASE STUDY

In family medicine clinic, a 65-year-old grandmother, 30-year-old mother, and her 6-month-old son present for their annual physical exams. They are awaiting a visit with the clinic's registered dietician, and they would value any dietary advice in the meantime.

1. **The mother tells you she adheres to a vegan diet and that she would like to continue to breastfeed for the next 6 months. She asks if this is okay and if she should make any changes to her existing diet.**
   A. What, if any, potential nutrient deficiencies might a lactating mother, who adheres to a vegan diet, be at risk for?
   B. She asks if she should change her diet to be pescatarian in anticipation of a future pregnancy. What are the benefits and other considerations to keep in mind when consuming fish and seafood during pregnancy?

2. **The mother is interested in starting her 6-month-old son, who has been healthy and exclusively breastfed, on solids.**
   A. What foods should she introduce first to the 6-month-old?
   B. What foods or beverages should she avoid giving him, and why?
   C. What, if any, supplements should an exclusively or partially breastfed infant receive from 0 to 6 months of age? What about from 6 to 12 months of age?

3. **The grandmother has osteoporosis as well as an upcoming hip surgery in the next few months.**
   A. What are some risk factors for osteoporosis in an older adult?
   B. In anticipation of her surgery, what, if any, specific diet and nutrition recommendations may be helpful for her?

INTRODUCTION

Each life stage is distinct and requires a healthy diet pattern to prevent disease and promote optimal health through the life span. Comprehensive patient care requires multidisciplinary support for nutritional health throughout the life span. The goal of this chapter is to outline the key elements and "clinical pearls" for each life stage. We will selectively cover key evidence that informs the Dietary Guidelines for Americans (DGAs), which is drawn from robust scientific reviews and the Dietary Guidelines Advisory Committee.

By the end of this chapter, readers will be able to describe (1) ideal nutrient needs, (2) important areas of consideration, and (3) health implications of inadequate nutrition or dietary

TABLE 5-1 • Summary of distinct nutritional needs, considerations, and implications for each life stage

	Ideal nutrient needs	Important areas of consideration	Health implications
Infancy and toddlerhood	• Human milk (preferred) and/or infant formula • Complementary foods beginning ~6 mos • <1,000 kcal/day	• Development of self-regulation • Repeated exposure to a variety of foods/flavors • Risk of deficiency in vitamin D, iron, and zinc • Avoidance of added sugars/sodium	• Brain development in the first 1,000 days • Early introduction of potential food allergens can help prevent allergy • Rapid weight gain in the first year may increase cardiometabolic risk later in life

Childhood and adolescence (F: female, M: male)	• 2–4 years (cals/day):
	  ○ F: 1,000–1,400
	  ○ M: 1,000–1,600
	• 5–8 years:
	  ○ F: 1,200–1,800
	  ○ M: 1,200–2,000
	• 9–13 years:
	  ○ F: 1,400–2,200
	  ○ M: 1,600–2,600
	• 14–18 years:
	  ○ F: 1,800–2,400
	  ○ M: 2,000–3,200
		• Avoidance of sugar-sweetened beverages
		• Lactose intolerance
			• Inadequate diets are associated with malnutrition (including overnutrition) and poor bone health

Adulthood (19–59 years old)	• Adult calorie level patterns range from 1,600 to 3,000 calories/day and include vegetables, fruits, grains, dairy, protein foods, and oils	• Reproductive age women • Menopause • Alcohol intake	• High prevalence of overweight and obesity in general population • Emergence of many chronic diseases (diabetes, cancer, hypertension, cardiovascular disease, etc.)
Pregnancy and lactation	• Additional 300–500 kcal required from the second trimester through lactation • Ensure adequate protein, folate, iron, calcium, iodine, choline, vitamin D, B vitamins, and omega-3s.	• Gestational weight gain • Alcohol and caffeine intake • Allergy prevention • Nutrient deficiencies and excess • Meeting nutrient needs with nausea and aversions	• Food safety (listeria, methylmercury • Gestational diabetes • Adequate intake of macro- and micronutrients to support fetal growth

Older adulthood (≥ 60 years old)	• Older adult caloric needs range from 1,600 to 2,800 calories/day (depending on sex and activity level)	• Eating to support a healthy aging trajectory
		• Oral health
			• Diet, chronic disease, and social factors may contribute to:
			  ○ Unintentional weight loss
			  ○ Sarcopenia
			  ○ Osteoporosis

deficits for the following life stages: infancy and toddlerhood, childhood and adolescence, adulthood (19–59 years old), pregnancy and lactation, and older adulthood (≥ 60 years old). We have outlined a summary for each life stage in Table 5-1 and provided relevant clinical pearls in Table 5-2.

INFANCY AND TODDLERHOOD

Ideal Nutrient Needs

Human milk is the preferred source of nutrients for infants during the first 6 months of life, with infant formula used as an alternative or supplement if necessary. Beginning at around 6 months, infants continue to meet their nutrient needs primarily through human milk or formula, with complementary foods increasingly added to the diet. Infants and toddlers have a very high ratio of nutrient-to-energy needs to support their rapid growth and development, but most need less than 1,000 kcal/day.[1] From 12 to 23 months, toddlers require between 700 and 1,000 kcal/day and their diet should include foods from a variety of different sources.

Important Areas of Consideration

Self-Regulation and Responsive Feeding From birth, infants show both hunger and satiety cues. Parents may be advised to learn to recognize and respond to these cues, offering food when an infant demonstrates hunger and not forcing or pressuring a child to drink or eat after showing signs of satiety. This will help infants learn to self-regulate their intake by responding to their own internal signals rather than external cues from their environment.

TABLE 5-2 • Clinical pearls

Clinical pearl	Section
A review of the infant or toddler's diet, including any restrictions, is important to identify potential deficiencies as supplemental sources may be required if the diet is inadequate.	III. Infancy and Toddlerhood-Important Areas of Consideration: Nutrients of Potential Concern
Formula is not typically indicated in infants after the age of 12 months. Among infants younger than 12 months, juice is not recommended. Among toddlers older than 12 months, guidelines suggest that 100% fruit juice consumption is limited to 4 oz per day or less.[1]	III. Infancy and Toddlerhood-Important Areas of Consideration: Complementary Feeding
Current guidelines recommend introduction of food allergens during complementary feeding. If an infant has an increased risk of peanut allergy, age-appropriate peanut containing foods should be introduced into the diet as early as 4–6 months of age.[1] If there are any additional concerns or doubts, caregivers are recommended to discuss complementary food introduction with their infant's healthcare provider.	III. Infancy and Toddlerhood-Important Areas of Consideration: Food Allergy
Eliminating SSB consumption in children and adolescents is considered "low-hanging fruit" in dietary education and counseling and can set the stage for healthy behaviors throughout the life course.	Childhood and Adolescence-Important Areas of Consideration: Sugar-Sweetened Beverages
When lactose intolerance is suspected in children, the initial approach is to recommend a lactose-exclusion diet and assess for resolution of symptoms. If confirmed, patients and families should be further counseled on alternative calcium and vitamin D sources, which are important for bone health.	Childhood and Adolescence-Important Areas of Consideration: Lactose Intolerance
Nutrient-dense foods include vegetables, fruits, whole grains, seafood, eggs, beans, peas, lentils, unsalted nuts and seeds, fat-free and low-fat dairy products, and lean meats and poultry, when prepared with no or little added sugars, saturated fat, and sodium.[1] Adolescents, who have increasing autonomy over their food preferences, require nutrition education from providers and role-modeling from caregivers to guide them to make healthy diet choices.	IV. Childhood and Adolescence-Health Implications: Risk of Dietary Inadequacy in Adolescence
In addition to regular weight-bearing physical activity, promoting a healthy dietary pattern, and specifically adequate dairy consumption and/or vitamin supplementation, will optimize peak bone mass accrual during adolescence.	IV. Childhood and Adolescence-Health Implications: Risk of Dietary Inadequacy in Adolescence
Clinician counseling to most U.S. adults generally should include increasing consumption of vegetables and reducing intake of processed food with added sugars, fat, and sodium. Other dietary recommendations should be individualized to patient characteristics and medical conditions.	Adulthood- Ideal Nutrient Needs-Daily Energy Requirements
Food sources that are rich in fiber include lentils, chickpeas, nuts, berries, popcorn, apples, pears, peaches, grapes, vegetables, avocados, seeds, oat and rice bran, oatmeal, barley, and rye. For some individuals, an easy way to consume a sizable serving of fiber is to eat a bowl of bran cereal each morning topped with fruits and nuts.	Adulthood- Ideal Nutrient Needs: Fiber
Vitamin D aids the absorption of calcium. If not sufficiently achieved through food or beverage sources, a supplement can support individuals. These nutrients are especially important among women 19–30 years old and during menopause, in addition to weight-bearing exercise, to optimize bone health.	Adulthood- Ideal Nutrient Needs: Calcium and Vitamin D
Absorption of iron from non-heme sources (mostly non-animal) is optimized by consuming them with vitamin C-rich foods, which is why iron pills are often recommended to be taken with 100% orange juice.	V. Adulthood- Important Areas of Consideration: Reproductive-Age Women*
Soy may have a beneficial or neutral effect on various health conditions, including menopausal symptoms, and it can be safely consumed several times a week. For the general adult population, soy may be a healthy alternative to red and processed meat.	V. Adulthood- Important Areas of Consideration: Menopause and soy
Calories from alcoholic and other beverages are often overlooked in consideration of an individual's total daily calories. A thorough dietary and social history includes assessment of alcoholic beverage intake.	V. Adulthood- Important Areas of Consideration: Alcoholic Beverages
Energy requirements increase after the first trimester of pregnancy, and increased energy needs should be met through intake of nutrient-dense foods including sources of protein.	VI. Pregnancy and Lactation- Ideal Nutrient Needs: Macronutrient and Energy Needs Throughout Pregnancy and Lactation

(Continued)

TABLE 5-2 • Clinical pearls *(Continued)*	
Clinical pearl	**Section**
While there is no clear evidence on benefits or harmful effects of caffeine intake during pregnancy, pregnant individuals are recommended to restrict their intake to < 300 mg/day, which is approximately one caffeinated drink per day (e.g., 12 oz commercial drip coffee ~250 mg of caffeine).	VI. Pregnancy and Lactation- Important Areas of Consideration: Caffeine
MyPlate for Older Adults, available on USDA MyPlate.gov website, is a helpful tool to use with older adults to guide meal composition.	VII. Older Adults- Ideal Nutrient Needs
Calcium carbonate is a readily available, cost-effective supplement that is best absorbed with meals. However, individuals taking proton pump inhibitors (PPIs) or H_2 blockers should take calcium citrate supplements instead. When >500 mg/d is taken from supplements the dose should be split into two administration times (e.g., morning and evening).	VII. Older Adults- Ideal Nutrient Needs: Calcium
Serum magnesium levels do not correlate well with total body magnesium stores as magnesium is primarily located intracellularly or within the bones.	VII. Older Adults- Ideal Nutrient Needs: Magnesium
For older adults with dental implants or dentures it is important to ask about denture fit or pain as this may contribute to difficulty eating.	VII. Older Adults- Important Areas of Consideration: Oral Health

Food and Flavor Exposure It is important that older infants receive a wide variety of foods, flavors, and textures during the complementary feeding period (see "Complementary Feeding" below). Caregivers should introduce and continue to offer a variety of foods, even if the infant does not accept them the first time. Infants innately dislike foods that taste bitter, an adaptive mechanism that helps to protect them from ingesting toxic substances but can also limit acceptance of foods such as vegetables. Repeated exposure to foods, especially those that are initially rejected, can promote their eventual acceptance by increasing familiarity and teaching infants that the food is safe to consume.[2] Parents may also increase comfort with different foods by modeling behavior, whereby their infant observes them eating and enjoying the food.

Nutrients of Potential Concern Infants receiving human milk, including those fed both human milk and formula, should be given a daily supplement containing at least 400 IU/day of vitamin D starting soon after birth. Vitamin D does not pass efficiently into human milk and even if the mother has sufficient vitamin D levels, the baby will not receive enough. If the mother has low levels of iron or vitamin B12, as may be the case with women following a vegetarian or vegan diet, breastfed infants might also need supplemental sources of these vitamins. Infant formula is generally fortified with vitamin D, iron, and B12, among other nutrients, and exclusively formula-fed babies do not need supplemental nutrients.

Older infants and toddlers should consume dietary sources of iron and zinc, such as meats, seafood, eggs, dairy products, and legumes. These minerals are extremely important for infant growth and development but are commonly not consumed at the necessary levels, especially in babies whose diet is mostly human milk, which will not meet infants' needs for iron and zinc after 6 months. Infant formulas sold in the United States are typically fortified with iron and sometimes with zinc. Infants and toddlers eating a diet that includes limited or no animal products may be at particular risk of iron and zinc deficiency and may benefit from supplementation or inclusion of additional iron and zinc-fortified foods in the diet.

Complementary Feeding Complementary feeding is defined as "the introduction of foods and liquids other than formula or human milk."[3] Infants should start receiving complementary foods at around 4 to 6 months of age. Individual readiness varies within this age range, but research supports waiting until at least 4 months of age but not past 6 months. The DGAs recommend introducing foods from all five of the "core" food groups, including fruits, vegetables, grains, protein foods, and dairy, early in complementary feeding. This will help ensure that the infant is getting adequate nutrients as well as exposure to a variety of foods. Potentially allergenic foods, including peanuts, tree nuts, eggs, fish, soy, wheat, shellfish, and cow's milk products (but not actual cow's milk), should be introduced along with other foods.[4] See "Health Implications-Food Allergy" for more information.

For the first 6 months of life, only human milk and/or formula are recommended liquids for infants. Infants may be offered up to 8 oz of water per day between 6 and 12 months, with amounts slowly increased after 12 months of age. While older infants may be offered dairy products made from cow's milk, such as yogurt and cheese, liquid cow's milk should be avoided until 12 months of age. After 12 months, children may be introduced to whole milk or unsweetened, fortified plant-based milks. Toddler formulas and "toddler milk" products are not necessary for children who consume a varied diet.

Food Safety Honey and unpasteurized foods may contain bacterial spores that cause botulism in young children.[5] As the immune system matures, children can safely eat some of these foods; for example, honey is safe after 12 months, although others may still present some risk.

Added Sugars and Sodium Infants are born with an innate preference for sweetness and will readily accept sweet-tasting foods and beverages. However, foods and beverages with added sugars are energy-dense, providing excessive calories and few nutrients. Foods and drinks with added sugars, including soda, juice drinks, sports drinks, sweet snacks, and desserts are not recommended for infants and toddlers because these energy-dense foods will supplant required nutrient-dense foods in the diet. Additionally, more exposure to sweets during early life might increase the innate preference for sweetness and could result in a preference for increasingly sweeter foods and beverages.

Infants given foods high in sodium may also learn to prefer salty foods, and high sodium intake in infancy and toddlerhood can establish a lifelong pattern of excess sodium intake[6] and associated impacts on blood pressure in older children and adults.[7] Guidelines suggest consumption of no more than 370 mg of sodium per day for infants younger than 12 months, and no more than 1,200 mg per day for toddlers 12 to 14 months.[1] Cured meats, fast food, snacks, and other processed foods are commonly high in sodium and often poor in essential nutrients.

Health Implications

Brain Development The "first 1,000 days," which is the period approximately from conception to age 2, is a critical time for brain development. Disturbances during this window of development may lead to lifelong consequences. Long-chain polyunsaturated fatty acids support the formation of neurons and membrane integrity and dietary sources such as fish and seafood are important to include in the diet of infants and toddlers. Iron and zinc are other key micronutrients supporting brain development, and foods rich in iron and zinc should be introduced during complementary feeding and maintained as a regular component of the infant and toddler diet to support the developing brain.

Food Allergy Estimates of the prevalence of a food allergy among U.S. children range from 5% to 8%,[8] with allergies to peanuts, eggs, and cow's milk most common in young children. Food allergy is an immune-mediated reaction to ingestion of a food with specific, reproducible signs and symptoms. Blood and skin-prick testing respond to the presence of IgE and will not detect food allergies that are not IgE-mediated. Thus, oral food challenges are the recommended method for clinical diagnosis of food allergy. Allergen-specific IgE (sIgE) to food allergens typically develops during the first 2 years of life and during the first year of life for milk allergy.

Reactions to food allergens can range from mild cutaneous or gastrointestinal symptoms to life-threatening anaphylaxis, and an individual can have variable reactions to the same food at different times. Food intolerances can cause similar symptoms in children but are not immune-mediated.[9] Food allergy can impact growth, nutritional status, and quality of life, even when reactions are mild.

Growth Infants and toddlers grow rapidly, including length/height growth as well as gains in adipose tissue and muscle mass. Growth patterns in the first year of life differ between breastfed and formula-fed infants, primarily due to differences in protein intake in the first months of life.[10] Rapid weight gain in infancy and early childhood is associated with higher subsequent risk of obesity and possibly with other cardio-metabolic risk factors.[11]

CHILDHOOD AND ADOLESCENCE

While growth rates are higher in early infancy than at any other life stage, childhood and adolescence are also critical periods of growth. Pubertal "growth spurts" occur in girls beginning in early puberty and are nearly completed by menarche. In boys, the pubertal growth spurt occurs towards the end of puberty, at an average age of 2 years older than in girls.[12] During childhood and adolescence, nutrient requirements vary with levels of physical activity as well as growth rate, body composition, and composition of new growth (i.e., fat mass, lean mass, etc.).

Ideal Nutrient Needs

Daily Energy Requirements While physical activity and individual growth requirements of children vary, the recommended ranges of total energy requirements in children and adolescents can be summarized as follows in Table 5-3.

In children older than 4 years of age, energy requirements based on body weight decrease progressively. The estimated daily energy requirement is about 40 kcal/kg/day at the end of adolescence. Intakes also depend on the energy density of the food offered; energy-dense foods have many calories per serving. For example, calories from ½ cup of raw carrots, a good source of vitamins and minerals, cannot be equated with the same number of calories from potato chips, which often are high in sodium and poor in essential vitamins and micronutrients.

Macronutrients As discussed in Section A, Chapter 1 ("Macronutrient Metabolism"), a regular dietary supply of protein is essential to optimal growth in children. However, excess protein intake of more than 4 g/kg/day in older children and adolescents may lead to elevated blood urea nitrogen, acidosis, and hyperammonemia, in addition to increased calcium losses in urine, and over the life span, may increase loss of renal mass.[13] Adolescents focused on muscle building and/or weight-lifting and consuming protein supplements should be cautioned to

TABLE 5-3 • Total calorie requirements (range in calories) per day in children and adolescents[a]

	Females	Males
Early Childhood (2–4 years old)	1,000–1,400	1,000–1,600
School-age Children (5–8 years old)	1,200–1,800	1,200–2,000
Early Adolescence (9–13 years old)	1,400–2,200	1,600–2,600
Later Adolescence (14–18 years old)	1,800–2,400	2,000–3,200

[a]Adapted from U.S. Department of Agriculture and U.S. Department of Health and Human Services. *Dietary Guidelines for Americans, 2020–2025.* DietaryGuidelines.gov. Published online 2020:164.

avoid excess protein intake given the long-term consequences on renal health over the life course.

With relation to intake of fat, children older than 2 years of age are recommended to switch to a diet with approximately 30% of total calories from total fat, with no more than 10% of calories from saturated fat.

Important Areas of Consideration

Sugar-Sweetened Beverages In the United States, many children and adolescents consume large quantities of sucrose and high-fructose corn syrup in soft drinks and other sugar-sweetened beverages (SSB), candy, syrups, sweetened cereals, and other processed food. As mentioned above, energy provided by such beverages displaces "room" for energy from nutritious complementary foods and beverages, leading to potential nutrient deficiencies. In addition, a systematic review and meta-analyses demonstrate that SSB consumption by young children is associated with weight gain and higher body mass index.[14]

Lactose Intolerance Lactose intolerance can result from lactase deficiency. This is the most common brush border disaccharidase deficiency and is a frequent etiology of diarrhea, abdominal pain, gassiness, and bloating, which becomes evident as early as childhood. Children as young as 2 years old may start developing symptoms of lactase deficiency. Lactose is abundant in many components of processed foods and in dairy products.

Health Implications

Risk of Dietary Inadequacy in Adolescence Diet quality has been demonstrated to worsen through childhood and into adolescence. An estimated 41% of children in the United States have overweight or obesity.[15] The goal for children and adolescents with overweight or obesity is to reduce the trajectory of weight gain while enabling normal growth and development. This can primarily be done by encouraging regular physical activity, choosing nutrient-dense foods and beverages, and reducing calories from sources that are not part of a healthy dietary pattern.

By late adolescence, average fruit and vegetable consumption is about half the recommended range of intake in the United States and many developed countries. Starchy vegetables, including white potatoes and corn, which are often fried or prepared with butter and salt, are more frequently consumed than other vegetable subgroups. Consumption of dairy among adolescents is typically below recommended intake levels. However, adolescents have increased needs of calcium and vitamin D to support the accrual of bone mass.

● ADULTHOOD (19–59 YEARS OLD)

In general, individuals enter adulthood with an already established dietary pattern, which is set during childhood and adolescence. Collaborative efforts, between the clinical care team and the patient, are necessary to support the adult patient in adopting dietary and behavioral changes that adhere to a healthy dietary pattern if not established earlier in life. This often requires the adult patient to deviate from their learned food and beverage preferences. In addition, these behaviors extend beyond the individual to large social networks and other family members. Especially among adults caring for children, role-modeling healthy dietary choices is crucial.[1]

Ideal Nutrient Needs

Daily Energy Requirements Generally, adult females require fewer total daily calories compared to adult males, and calorie needs decline throughout the lifespan during adulthood secondary to aging and changes in metabolism. Further, psychological, socioeconomic, cultural, and disease processes may contribute to changes in regulation of appetite and hunger in response to energy demands.[16] Additional influences on an individual's calorie needs include level of physical activity, body composition, medications, and medical history. Figure 5-1 is a summary table from the DGAs outlining the eight calorie levels that are suitable for most adults 19 to 59 years old. The table also includes daily and weekly amounts from food groups, subgroups, and components, including vegetables, fruits, grains, dairy, protein, and oils.

Among U.S. adults 19 to 59 years old, the average daily intake of fruits, vegetables, and dairy is lower than recommended intake ranges. The average daily intake of grains is close to or within the lower range of recommended intake for males and females. Males on average have a higher daily intake of protein exceeding the recommended intake range, while females have an average daily intake of protein in the lower end of the recommended intake range. Most adults exceed the recommended intake limits of added sugars, saturated fat, and sodium.

Fiber Most adults do not meet recommended intakes for dietary fiber, because fruits, vegetables, and whole grains are generally being underconsumed. Dietary fiber is important to reduce the risk of some cancers, cardiovascular disease, and diabetes.

Calcium and Vitamin D Bone mass is actively accumulating between ages 19 and 30 years. Foods adequate in calcium and vitamin D, such as dairy, including low-fat cow's milk, fortified soy alternatives, and seafood, are critical to promote bone health and prevent the onset of osteoporosis. These nutrients are further needed among women during the post-menopausal period, when rapid bone remodeling occurs.

Important Areas of Consideration

Reproductive-Age Women* Women of reproductive age require several nutrients, including folic acid, iodine, and iron. Folic acid and iodine are important nutrients for individuals capable of becoming pregnant, because often individuals are unaware of their pregnancy until weeks to months after conception. The U.S. Preventative Services Task Force (USPSTF) recommends

---

* We have used the term *women* to refer to persons who were biologically assigned female at birth.

Healthy U.S.-Style Dietary Pattern for Adults Ages 19 Through 59, With Daily or Weekly Amounts From Food Groups, Subgroups, and Components

CALORIE LEVEL OF PATTERN[a]	1,600	1,800	2,000	2,200	2,400	2,600	2,800	3,000
FOOD GROUP OR SUBGROUP[b]	Daily Amount of Food From Each Group (Vegetable and protein foods subgroup amounts are per week.)							
Vegetables (cup eq/day)	2	2 ½	2 ½	3	3	3 ½	3 ½	4
	Vegetable Subgroups in Weekly Amounts							
Dark-Green Vegetables (cup eq/wk)	1 ½	1 ½	1 ½	2	2	2 ½	2 ½	2 ½
Red & Orange Vegetables (cup eq/wk)	4	5 ½	5 ½	6	6	7	7	7 ½
Beans, Peas, Lentils (cup eq/wk)	1	1 ½	1 ½	2	2	2 ½	2 ½	3
Starchy Vegetables (cup eq/wk)	4	5	5	6	6	7	7	8
Other Vegetables (cup eq/wk)	3 ½	4	4	5	5	5 ½	5 ½	7
Fruits (cup eq/day)	1 ½	1 ½	2	2	2	2	2 ½	2 ½
Grains (ounce eq/day)	5	6	6	7	8	9	10	10
Whole Grains (ounce eq/day)	3	3	3	3 ½	4	4 ½	5	5
Refined Grains (ounce eq/day)	2	3	3	3 ½	4	4 ½	5	5
Dairy (cup eq/day)	3	3	3	3	3	3	3	3
Protein Foods (ounce eq/day)	5	5	5 ½	6	6 ½	6 ½	7	7
	Protein Foods Subgroups in Weekly Amounts							
Meats, Poultry, Eggs (ounce eq/wk)	23	23	26	28	31	31	33	33
Seafood (ounce eq/wk)	8	8	8	9	10	10	10	10
Nuts, Seeds, Soy Products (ounce eq/wk)	4	4	5	5	5	5	6	6
Oils (grams/day)	22	24	27	29	31	34	36	44
Limit on Calories for Other Uses (kcal/day)[c]	100	140	240	250	320	350	370	440
Limit on Calories for Other Uses (%/day)	6%	8%	12%	11%	13%	13%	13%	15%

[a] Calorie level ranges: Ages 19 through 30, Females: 1,800-2,400 calories; Males: 2,400-3,000 calories. Ages 31 through 59, Females: 1,600-2,200 calories; Males 2,200-3,000 calories. Energy levels are calculated based on median height and body weight for healthy body mass index (BMI) reference individuals. For adults, the reference man is 5 feet 10 inches tall and weighs 154 pounds. The reference woman is 5 feet 4 inches tall and weighs 126 pounds. Calorie needs vary based on many factors. The DRI Calculator for Healthcare Professionals, available at **nal.usda.gov/fnic/dri-calculator**, can be used to estimate calorie needs based on age, sex, height, weight, and activity level.

[b] Definitions for each food group and subgroup and quantity (i.e., cup or ounce equivalents) are provided in **Chapter 1** and are compiled in **Appendix 3**.

[c] All foods are assumed to be in nutrient-dense forms; lean or low-fat; and prepared with minimal added sugars, refined starches, saturated fat, or sodium. If all food choices to meet food group recommendations are in nutrient-dense forms, a small number of calories remain within the overall limit of the pattern (i.e., limit on calories for other uses). The number of calories depends on the total calorie level of the pattern and the amounts of food from each food group required to meet nutritional goals. Calories up to the specified limit can be used for added sugars, saturated fat, or alcohol, or to eat more than the recommended amount of food in a food group.

NOTE: The total dietary pattern should not exceed *Dietary Guidelines* limits for added sugars, saturated fat, and alcohol; be within the Acceptable Macronutrient Distribution Ranges for protein, carbohydrate, and total fats; and stay within calorie limits. Values are rounded. See **Appendix 3** for all calorie levels of the pattern.

FIGURE 5-1 • Healthy U.S.-style dietary pattern for adults ages 19 through 59, with daily or weekly amounts from food groups, subgroups, and components.
(Source: U.S. Department of Agriculture and U.S. Department of Health and Human Services. *Dietary Guidelines for Americans, 2020-2025.* 9th ed. December 2020; Chapter 4, Table 4-1. Available at DietaryGuidelines.gov.)

that all individuals who are planning or capable of pregnancy take a daily supplement of 400 to 800 micrograms of folic acid (see "Pregnancy and Lactation") to prevent neural tube defects during fetal development. In addition, iodine intake is important for fetal neurocognitive development. Iodine intake is generally adequate among those who regularly consume dairy products, eggs, seafood, or iodized table salt. For all individuals who menstruate, iron is a key nutrient. Heme iron, found in lean meats, poultry, and some seafood, is more readily absorbed than non-heme iron found in plants, such as beans and dark-green vegetables.

Menopause and Soy In the United States, menopause occurs at a median age of 51 years old. In lieu of and/or accompanying hormone replacement therapy, soy has been considered a popular alternative treatment for hot flashes and other menopausal symptoms, based on the notion that soy isoflavones provide an estrogen-like boost. Results from meta-analyses and reviews of the studies of soy and menopausal symptoms are conflicting, likely due to variation in the soy preparations used, quantities given, and duration of use.[17]

Limitation of Saturated Fats, Sodium, and Added Sugars As the prevalence of coronary heart disease increases with age, peaking in men between 50 and 59 years old and women 60 and 69 years old, limiting saturated fat intake is recommended. Examples of foods high in saturated fat and sodium include deli sandwiches, burgers, tacos, burritos, and hot dogs. Strategies to help lower intake of saturated fat include switching to lean meats and low-fat cheese or substituting beans in place of meats as the source of protein. When cooking, using olive oil instead of butter can also lower the intake of saturated fat.

In addition, reduced dietary intake of sodium is a modifiable risk factor that can help manage and prevent hypertension, which is a risk factor for cardiovascular disease and stroke. Most sodium comes from foods that have salt added during commercial processing, e.g., breads, canned soups, salad dressings, frozen pizzas and meals, and cold cuts, and from prepared foods outside the home, including fast food.

Last, many adults consume well above the recommended limits for added sugars, particularly from beverage sources, followed by desserts, snacks, candies, and sweetened beverage cereals. SSB including soda, sports drinks, energy drinks, fruit drinks, and sweetened coffees and teas supply over 40% of daily intake of added sugars. Of note, research on the health effects of artificial sweeteners is inconclusive, though beverages with artificial sweeteners may be a temporary replacement strategy to reduce intake of SSB in adults who are high consumers of SSB.

Alcoholic Beverages Roughly two-thirds of U.S. adults report consuming alcoholic beverages. Alcoholic beverages and their calories are considered discretionary. Alcoholic beverages, including mixed drinks, can contribute to added sugars and saturated fat intakes. Regular intake of alcoholic beverages can impede consumption of food group and nutrient needs while also contributing to excess calories. On days alcohol is consumed, intakes should be limited to one drink or less in a day for women and two drinks or less in a day for men. Alcohol in moderation has been associated with fewer cardiovascular events by helping to maintain higher HDL. However, excessive drinking is associated with liver damage and can increase risk of many cancers, among other health harms.

Health Implications

Overweight and Obesity In the United States, an estimated 42.5% of adults over 20 years old have obesity and an additional 31.1% of adults have overweight[18]. The notion that weight loss is achieved only if adults reduce the number of calories received from foods and beverages and increase calories expended from physical activity is an oversimplification. The complexity of this topic is beyond the scope of this chapter; for further detail, see Section B, Chapter 17, "Overweight and Obesity."

Other Chronic Diseases The life stage from 19 to 59 years old is most commonly when chronic diseases arise. For greater detail about the essential nutrition topics as they relate to specific chronic diseases, please refer to Section B.

⬤ PREGNANCY AND LACTATION

Pregnant individuals require an increased intake of macro- and micronutrients to support the physiologic adaptations of the mother to pregnancy as well as growth and development of the fetus. Nutrient needs change throughout the three trimesters of pregnancy and lactation.

Ideal Nutrient Needs

Macronutrient and Energy Needs Throughout Pregnancy and Lactation After the first trimester, pregnant women require additional energy to support growth of their own tissues (breast, uterus, adipose) as well as the synthesis of new tissue (fetus, placenta, amniotic fluid). The DGAs recommend an additional 340 kcal starting in the second trimester and an additional 452 kcal in the third trimester above typical (nonpregnant) requirements. Energy restriction during pregnancy may impair fetal growth and negatively impact birth weight. To meet the demands of milk production, the DGAs recommend an additional 330 calories per day above prepregnancy requirements in the first 6 months of lactation and an additional 400 calories per day at 6 months and beyond.[1]

Protein contributes to the synthesis of keratin and collagen as well as the function of enzymes, transport mechanisms, and hormones. Maternal protein metabolism adapts in early pregnancy to compensate for increased fetal demands, but increased protein intake is required in the second half to support additional protein synthesis. While higher protein intake (within the recommended 10%–25% range) may be associated with increased birth weight and reduced risk of SGA,[19] pregnant women should consume no more than 25% of total energy from protein.

Micronutrient Needs Throughout Pregnancy A higher intake of specific vitamins and minerals is recommended during pregnancy. Vitamins and minerals support cell proliferation and differentiation, production of hemoglobin and oxygen transport, and bone mineralization, all of which provide the basis of fetal growth. While many nutrient needs can be met with a balanced diet, a multivitamin formulated specifically for pregnancy can help ensure adequate intake of key micronutrients, and ideally should be started preconception.[18]

Folate: Folate occurs naturally in food and in the synthetic form folic acid. Folate acts as a coenzyme in one-carbon metabolism and plays a role in cell division and protein synthesis, which occur at a rapid rate in early pregnancy. Folate is essential for preventing neural tube defects and supporting fetal and placental growth and development. Recommended folate intake in pregnancy is 600 μg/day, and the American College of Obstetricians and Gynecologists (ACOG) recommends that women take a daily supplement containing 400 μg.[20] Supplementation should begin at least 1 month prior to becoming pregnant to ensure that levels are sufficient to support development of the neural tube, which occurs during the early stages of pregnancy when a woman might not know that she is pregnant. Women should continue to supplement with 400 μg/day through the first 12 weeks of pregnancy. Women with multiple pregnancies or severe vomiting during pregnancy are particularly at risk of folate deficiency, and higher-dose supplements may benefit women with pregestational diabetes.[21] However, excessive folic acid intake may be harmful to the mother and the fetus.

Iron: Iron supports the mother's increased blood volume, hemoglobin production, and oxygen transport. Iron is required for placental and fetal growth and brain development, and iron deficiency can have lasting and irreversible effects. Maternal transferrin delivers iron across the placenta to the fetus, which is entirely dependent on maternal iron during early gestation. If maternal iron levels are insufficient, iron will be preferentially transferred to the fetus, further depleting maternal stores.[22] Recommended iron intake in pregnancy is 27 mg/d and pregnant women should take a supplement containing iron to ensure that they are meeting their needs.[20] Pregnant women can eat foods rich in vitamin C, including citrus fruits and strawberries, broccoli, and peppers, along with iron-containing foods or supplements to enhance intestinal absorption of iron. Conversely, coffee and tea contain polyphenols that can interfere with iron absorption and should be consumed separately from iron-rich foods and iron supplements.

Calcium: Calcium is important to prevent bone loss and preeclampsia in the mother during pregnancy, and to support fetal development of bones and teeth. Pregnant adolescents (age 18 or younger) require 1,300 mg/d of calcium, while pregnant adults require 1,000 mg/d. Dietary sources of calcium include dairy products, leafy green vegetables, and sardines.

Iodine: Iodine maintains maternal thyroid function during pregnancy, supporting fetal brain development. The fetus relies on maternal thyroid hormones during early gestation, and maternal iodine deficiency and subsequent hypothyroidism can have lasting, nonreversible effects on fetal neurodevelopment. In the second half of gestation, adequate iodine is required for synthesis of fetal thyroid hormones (T3 and T4), which support development of the fetal brain and nervous system. Iodine needs increase by ~50% during pregnancy and ACOG recommends 220 μg/day.[20] Women who smoke tobacco, or have a short interpregnancy interval, vegan diet, or restricted food intake due to nausea/vomiting may all be susceptible to iodine deficiency.[18]

Choline: Choline is a precursor of key phospholipids and neurotransmitters and supports epigenetic programming of the fetal and placental genomes.[23] Adequate maternal choline intake before and during pregnancy facilitates healthy development of the placenta, potentially reducing maternal risk of placenta-related conditions such as preeclampsia. There is some evidence that lower periconceptual intake of choline and lower maternal blood levels of choline in mid-pregnancy are associated with increased risk of NTDs.[24] The Adequate Intakes (AIs) for choline are 450 mg/d for pregnancy and 550 mg/d for lactation, with a recommended upper limit (UL) of 3.5 g/d.[25] Many prenatal supplements do not include choline, and an estimated 90%–95% of pregnant women in the United States consume less than the AI.[26]

Vitamin D: There is a lack of consensus on the optimal 25(OH)D levels for pregnant women and the supplemental doses required to obtain sufficient plasma levels, yet a supplement containing at least 400 IU/day is generally recommended. Severe vitamin D deficiency during pregnancy can manifest in the mother as osteomalacia.

B-Complex Vitamins: Vitamin B1 (thiamine), B2 (riboflavin), B3 (niacin), B6 (pyridoxine), and B12 (cyanocobalamin) are involved as coenzymes in macronutrient metabolism. Along with folate, vitamin B12 supports methylation of RNA, DNA, proteins, neurotransmitters, and phospholipids, and maternal deficiency has been associated with risk of NTDs. Requirements increase during pregnancy, especially in the third trimester, due to increased maternal and fetal demand for both energy and protein.

Omega-3 Fatty Acids: Omega-3 fatty acids are a class of polyunsaturated fatty acids (PUFAs), which are essential membrane components. PUFAs are precursors of lipid mediators and are involved in regulating inflammation and gene expression. Omega-3 fatty acids include eicosapentaenoic acid (EPA), docosahexaenoic acid (DHA), and alpha-linolenic acid (ALA). DHA accumulates in the brain during fetal development and the first 2 years of life. Omega-3s are *essential* fatty acids; the body cannot synthesize them from scratch and must obtain them from foods. EPA and DHA are found mainly in fish. ALA is found in walnuts, flaxseeds, vegetable and flaxseed oils, leafy vegetables, and some fats from grass-fed animals. Omega-3 intake should be balanced with avoidance of methylmercury as both are found in seafood (see Health Implications: Food Safety during Pregnancy). Fish oils capsules may be a safe method of increasing omega-3 intake during pregnancy for women who do not consume seafood or have limited access to low-mercury varieties.

Important Areas of Consideration

Gestational Weight Gain Ranges for target gestational weight gain (GWG) are dependent on prepregnancy BMI, with more

TABLE 5-4 • Institute of medicine recommended ranges for gestational weight gain[a]	
Pre-pregnancy BMI category	Total recommended weight gain
Underweight (< 18.5 kg/m²)	20–40 lbs/12.5–18 kg
Normal weight (18.5–24.9 kg/m²)	25–35 lbs/11.5–16 kg
Overweight (25.0–29.9 kg/m²)	15–25 lbs/7–11.5 kg
Obesity (≥ 30.0 kg/m²)	11–20 lbs/5–9 kg

[a]Adapted from: Institute of Medicine and National Research Council. 2009. *Weight Gain During Pregnancy: Reexamining the Guidelines.* Washington, DC: The National Academies Press. https://doi.org/10.17226/12584.

weight gain recommended for individuals beginning pregnancy at a lower weight (Table 5-4). The Institute of Medicine (IOM) released their guidelines in 2009, though recent evidence has indicated that a single guideline for women in the "obese" category may not be appropriate and that risk of adverse outcomes such as gestational diabetes mellitus (GDM) and large for gestational age (LGA) would be best managed with guidance specific to each class of obesity. Additionally, the USPSTF recommends that clinicians offer counseling and behavioral interventions targeted towards a healthy lifestyle supporting healthy weight gain during pregnancy (often supported by additional health professionals), rather than simply offering recommended ranges for GWG with no accompanying behavioral support.[21]

Alcohol Heavy alcohol use or abuse during pregnancy, defined as having > 80 g or ≥ 8 standard drinks/day, is associated with fetal alcohol spectrum disorders (FASD). The effects of moderate alcohol use among pregnant women, defined as < 1 standard drink/day (or 0–6/week), are less clear. There are no definitive data to establish safe limits for alcohol intake during pregnancy, therefore, pregnant individuals are advised to avoid consumption of any alcohol.

Caffeine Caffeine is found in coffee, tea, chocolate, cocoa, cola, and some medications. Maternal caffeine clearance is reduced during pregnancy. The primary metabolite of caffeine is paraxanthine, which crosses the placenta and can promote maternal and fetal neural stimulation and potentially impact metabolic activities. High caffeine intake can result in placental and uterine vasoconstriction and increased fetal heart rate.

Potentially Allergenic Foods The eight primary food allergens in the United States are peanut, tree nut, wheat, soy, milk, egg, fish, and shellfish. Maternal diet during pregnancy and lactation does not appear to impact the development of food allergy in the offspring, and pregnant and lactating women do not need to avoid or restrict intake of potentially allergenic foods for purposes of preventing food allergy. However, allergens from the maternal diet can pass into human milk, and lactating women may need to eliminate certain foods from their diet if the baby shows signs of reacting to a component of the human milk.[9]

Nutrients with Potential Teratogenic Effects (Vitamin A) Vitamin A includes all dietary retinols, their metabolites, and the provitamin A carotenoids β-carotene, α-carotene, and β-cryptoxanthin. While liposoluble vitamin A contributes to regulating gene expression, cell differentiation, eye tissue development and vision, and immune system function, excessive doses can accumulate and are teratogenic. The safe upper limit is set at 3,000 µg/day (10,000 IU/day), and pregnant women should meet their vitamin A needs through dietary sources or supplements containing provitamin A carotenoids, generally β-carotene.[18]

Common Nutrient Deficiencies Among Pregnant Individuals Pregnant women can obtain most required nutrients from a balanced diet, yet are at risk of iron and vitamin D deficiencies and potentially others if the diet is limited. Nutrient deficiencies commonly occur together in resource-limited populations. An estimated 10%–25% of pregnant women in the United States are deficient in iron, with deficiency most common in the third trimester.[27] Pregnant women are often deficient in vitamin D, particularly during the winter.

Nausea and Food Aversions Nausea, vomiting, and food aversions are common particularly in early pregnancy and may make it difficult for pregnant women to meet their energy and nutrient needs. Women with aversions, nausea, and/or vomiting may reduce their intake of foods such as vegetables, meat, beans, and some fruits, increasing the risk of deficiencies in nutrients such as protein, iron, zinc, vitamin B12, and magnesium.[28] If fluid intake is limited or fluids are lost through vomiting, there is also a risk of dehydration.

Health Implications

Food Safety During Pregnancy Extra precautions around food safety are recommended during pregnancy. Pregnant women are recommended to consume cooked meats, poultry, seafood, and eggs; avoid raw sprouts and unpasteurized juices or milks; and avoid soft cheeses made from unpasteurized milk. It is safer for pregnant women to avoid foods from deli counters (deli meats, prepared eggs, or seafood salads, etc.). If consumed, deli meats and hot dogs should be heated to 165°F to kill *Listeria*, a bacteria that causes listeriosis. Listeriosis is often asymptomatic or very mild in adults (including pregnant women), but can cause harm to the fetus. Undercooked meats and poultry can also be a source of toxoplasmosis and salmonella bacteria, both of which can be harmful to the mother and fetus.

During pregnancy, avoiding consumption of fish high in methylmercury, including shark, king mackerel, tilefish, and swordfish, is recommended. While canned, light tuna is safe, albacore tuna is higher in mercury and intake should be limited to no more than one serving per week during pregnancy. It is safe for pregnant women to consume 8–12 oz per week of seafood, selecting a variety of types low in mercury.[1] The EPA provides a reference card with recommendations for safe fish and shellfish consumption.[29]

Health Conditions Impacting Pregnant Women Nutritional status can impact many of the health conditions commonly experienced by pregnant women. Gestational diabetes mellitus (GDM), defined as "any degree of glucose intolerance with onset or first recognition during pregnancy," is associated with excessive fetal growth and adiposity and increased risk of cesarean section. Glycemic control aiming to targeted pregnancy thresholds can be achieved with diet and physical activity in 70%–80% of GDM cases. Diets emphasizing low glycemic index foods and high fiber content may be helpful in improving glycemic control with no adverse effects.[30] Preeclampsia impacts up to 5% of pregnancies and is a leading cause of maternal and infant morbidity and mortality.[31]

Fetal Growth Optimal fetal growth requires a balance between sufficient macro- and micronutrients to meet fetal demands and avoid fetal overnutrition. The fetus requires glucose to meet energy requirements, and maternal energy restriction may impair fetal growth. Popular diets involving restriction of specific macronutrients, such as the Paleo or ketogenic diets, have been associated with low birth weight among other adverse effects related to micronutrient deficiencies. Micronutrients including folate and iron also support healthy fetal growth and deficiencies may contribute to preterm delivery and low birth weight. Conversely, fetal overnutrition, particularly in the context of excessive gestational weight gain and/or gestational diabetes, can promote fetal overgrowth and program adverse cardiometabolic trajectories over the life course of the offspring.

⬤ OLDER ADULTS

The older adult population, typically defined as 65 years and older, is heterogeneous and ranges from fit to frail. In general, body composition changes as an individual ages, resulting in loss of body weight and lean muscle mass along with increased body fat, reduced body water, and reduced bone density.[32] Nutritional needs are also altered as a result of aging physiology (e.g., reduced intestinal transit time), socioeconomic factors, the development of chronic disease, and medications.

Ideal Nutrient Needs

Dietary Reference Intakes (DRIs) include chronologic age categories of 51–70 years and > 70 years. Older adults' actual nutritional requirements may range widely depending on the individual. Overall, total energy requirements typically decline. Therefore, it is important to focus on nutrient-dense foods. Other important considerations for macro- and micronutrients as they relate to aging are highlighted below.

Protein Consuming adequate protein is a challenge for many older adults. Reduced appetite, poor oral health, low physical activity, functional impairment, financial hardship, and other factors contribute to the problem. Insufficient protein intake is related to poor wound healing, impaired immune function, skin fragility, and overall frailty.[33] Though there is no consensus, a protein intake of 0.80 g/kg body weight/day has been suggested for older adults.[34] More recent studies have suggested that a higher intake of 1–1.2 g/kg/day is protective of lean mass, maintains grip strength, and decreases risk of functional decline.[35]

Fiber Fiber helps manage body weight and chronic diseases, in addition to providing other benefits such as reducing constipation. Older adults typically consume less than recommended amounts.[36] Current recommendations for older adults range from 25 to 35 g/day.[34]

Fluid Intake Older adults have difficulty reaching recommended fluid intakes due to changes in physiology, especially reduced thirst and impaired renal function. Adequate intake is between 2.7 and 3.7 L daily for those over age 51.[37]

Micronutrients Recommended Dietary Allowances (RDAs) for vitamins and minerals are provided based on chronologic age groups 51–70 years and > 70 years.[38] Older adults have difficulty meeting the RDA for several micronutrients due to age-related physiologic changes.

Calcium: Approximately 10%–30% of calcium is absorbed from the diet, primarily from the duodenum and jejunum. Calcium absorption is reduced with aging due to vitamin D deficiency and reduced stomach acidity; high consumption of fiber and of sodium may impair calcium absorption. The RDA for people aged 51–70 years is 1,200 mg/d for women and 1,000 mg/d for men; for those 70 years of age and older the RDA is 1,200 mg/d.[39] Older adults have difficulty meeting these levels and older adults in the United States usually consume 580–735 mg/d (without supplements).[40]

Vitamin D: With aging, the skin is less efficient at synthesizing vitamin D and there is decreased production of the 1,25 hydroxylated form in the kidneys. Older adults typically consume less vitamin D in the diet and spend more time indoors, placing them at higher risk of deficiency. The IOM's recommendation for DRI for vitamin D in the context of bone health is 800–1,000 International units (IU).[39] Levels of serum 25(OH)-vitamin D3 may be measured to assess for deficiency, though is not recommended in asymptomatic individuals;[41] there is no consensus for cutoff levels for deficiency, but less than 20–30 ng/ml is considered to be insufficient.[42] Recent clinical trial data suggests that vitamin D supplementation does not lower risk of fractures in generally healthy midlife and older adults.[43] However, the benefit of vitamin D supplementation appears to be greater among institutionalized or hospitalized individuals.[44]

Vitamin B12: Vitamin B12 absorption is impacted by age-related changes in the gut, including a reduction in gastric acid, reduced intrinsic factor, and atrophic gastritis, which can be exacerbated by previous gastric surgery, small intestine bacterial overgrowth, and medication such as PPIs. Adults 51 years and older are suggested to consume at least 2.4 mg of vitamin B12 daily.[38]

Magnesium: Magnesium deficiency is one of the most common micronutrient deficiencies in older adults.[45] Older adults tend to consume lower amounts due to decreased total caloric intake. Magnesium absorption also decreases due to less intestinal absorption and increased excretion in the urine. The RDA for those aged 51 years and older is 420 mg/d for men and 320 mg/d for women.[38] There is no specific recommendation for magnesium supplements in otherwise healthy older adults.

Important Areas of Consideration

Diets That Support a Healthy Aging Trajectory Healthy aging has been defined multiple ways, but may be viewed as a multidimensional construct of five key health promotion domains focusing on promoting and optimizing: (1) health, preventing injury, and managing chronic conditions; (2) cognitive health; (3) physical health; (4) mental health; and (5) facilitating social engagement and resilience.[46] There are several dietary patterns that have been associated with "healthy aging," though definitions vary across studies. The Mediterranean Diet has been associated with a healthy aging trajectory,[47] lower incidence of cardiovascular disease and stroke,[48] reduced cognitive decline,[49] and reduced incident frailty.[50] The MIND Diet, a combination of Mediterranean and Dietary Approaches to Stop Hypertension (DASH) diets, has been shown to reduce cognitive decline.[51] For more information on some of these diets, refer to Section A, Chapter 6 ("Popular Diets") and Section B, Chapters 17–20 ("Overweight and Obesity," "Diabetes Mellitus," "Stroke and Hypertension," and "Cardiovascular Disease").

Oral Health Oral health is essential to older adults' ability to maintain a healthy diet and consume a variety of foods (see Section B, Chapter 15, "Oral Conditions"). The sense of smell tends to decline with age, leading to changes in taste and therefore appetite. In addition, medications and chronic disease may cause xerostomia, tooth loss, and difficulty with chewing and swallowing. Signs of malnutrition may first appear in the mouth, such as glossitis due to iron, vitamin B12, or folate deficiency.

Health Implications

Unintentional Weight Loss Undernutrition and subsequent unintentional weight loss are important considerations for both community-dwelling and institutionalized older adult populations. The etiology of unintentional weight loss is typically multifactorial and may include economic barriers, social isolation, oral health issues, dysphagia, medical illness (e.g., cancer), chronic diseases requiring dietary restriction, medications (e.g., cholinesterase inhibitors, SSRIs), functional disability interfering with meal preparation, poor appetite, depression, cognitive impairment, and others. Treatment should focus on addressing as many modifiable factors as possible. Ideally, older adults should obtain nutrition from food, but protein or energy supplements may be used in older adults at risk of malnutrition. Ideally, they should be given between meals and not before meals to maximize appetite for food. There are no FDA-approved appetite stimulants to promote weight gain in older adults and guidelines recommend avoiding use.[52]

Sarcopenia Sarcopenia is age-related loss of muscle mass associated with weakness, functional limitation, and disability.[53] Causes include decreased physical activity, inadequate protein intake, increased inflammatory cytokines, and other changes due to age-related physiology. Sarcopenia is one factor that may lead to development of the frailty syndrome,[54] leading to further declines in physical performance and functional status. Diets with higher protein intake may protect against this, as discussed in "Protein" in the older adults' section.

Osteoporosis Osteoporosis is an age-related condition characterized by reduced bone density and quality, predisposing the risk of fracture.[55] It is more common in older women but also prevalent in older men. There are many risk factors, including alcohol (> 2 drinks per day), lack of physical activity (weight bearing), and low body weight. Calcium and vitamin D status are important for both the prevention and management of osteoporosis (see "Calcium" and "Vitamin D" above for details). For older adults with osteoporosis who are unable to meet recommended dietary intakes of calcium and vitamin D, additional supplementation is recommended.

THREE TAKE-HOME POINTS

1. With each life stage, medical professionals must be aware of the distinct nutritional needs and what comprises a healthy dietary pattern.
2. There are rife opportunities for medical professionals to address "do not miss" nutritional issues, such as folate supplementation before and during pregnancy.
3. Nutrition is intertwined with health and disease, and nutrition through the life span has implications on short- and long-term health.

CASE STUDY ANSWERS

1A. Mothers following a vegetarian or vegan diet may have low levels of iron and vitamin B12, and possibly low DHA as well. As such, both the mother and her breastfed infant may need supplemental sources of these vitamins.

1B. For future pregnancies, a pescatarian diet may provide additional omega-3 fatty acids to support fetal brain development. However, omega-3 intake should be balanced with avoidance of methylmercury as both are found in seafood. A few examples of seafood that are lower in methylmercury include lobster, salmon, scallop, shrimp, and tilapia.

2A. Guidelines and evidence support introduction of all 5 of the "core" food groups, including fruits, vegetables, grains, protein foods, and dairy, early in complementary feeding. Dietary guidelines suggest introducing potentially allergenic foods, including peanut products, tree nuts, eggs, fish, soy, wheat, shellfish, and cow's milk products, along with other foods. If an infant has an increased risk of peanut allergy, age-appropriate peanut-containing foods should be introduced into the diet as early as 4–6 months of age. If there are any additional concerns or doubts, caregivers are recommended to discuss complementary food introduction with their infant's healthcare provider.

2B. Cow's milk, honey, fruit juice, or any beverages with added sugars are not recommended in infants younger than 1 year of age. Infants' digestive systems may not tolerate large quantities of cow's milk protein. Honey may contain bacterial spores that cause botulism in infants. Fruit juice and beverages with added sugars are not recommended in infants as they may supplant required nutrient-dense foods in the diet, and may increase the innate preference for sweetness, resulting in a preference for increasingly sweeter foods and beverages. Therefore, in addition to breastmilk and/or infant formula, water is recommended.

2C. Infants that are fed both formula and human milk, and those that are exclusively breastfed, should be receiving at least 400 IU/day of vitamin D. Infant formula is generally fortified with vitamin D, iron, and B12, among other nutrients, and exclusively formula-fed babies do not need additional supplemental nutrients. After 6 months, consider supplemental iron, zinc, B12, and DHA for infants and toddlers eating a diet that includes limited or no animal products.

3A. Risks factors for development of osteoporosis include aging, sex (more common in women than in men), alcohol consumption of > 2 drinks/day, lack of weight-bearing physical activity, and low body weight.

3B. Nutritional optimization prior to surgery, particularly in the elderly with sarcopenia, is important to reduce surgical complications and to promote swift healing and recovery. A protein intake of 0.8 g/kg/day, and in recent studies, up to 1–1.2 g/kg/day has been shown to protect lean mass, maintain grip strength, and decrease risk of functional decline.

REFERENCES

1. U.S. Department of Agriculture and U.S. Department of Health and Human Services. Dietary guidelines for Americans, 2020-2025. *DietaryGuidelines.gov.* Published online 2020:164.

2. Anzman-Frasca S, Ventura AK, Ehrenberg S, Myers KP. Promoting healthy food preferences from the start: a narrative review of food preference learning from the prenatal period through early childhood. *Obes Rev.* 2018;19(4):576-604.

3. Agostoni C, Decsi T, Fewtrell M, et al. Complementary feeding: a commentary by the ESPGHAN Committee on Nutrition. *J Pediatr Gastroenterol Nutr.* 2008;46(1):99-110.

4. Greer FR, Sicherer SH, Burks AW, American Academy of Pediatrics. Effects of early nutritional interventions on the development of atopic disease in infants and children: the role of maternal dietary restriction, breastfeeding, timing of introduction of complementary foods, and hydrolyzed formulas. *Pediatrics.* 2008; 121(1):183-191.

5. Prevention Botulism CDC. Published June 7, 2019. Accessed April 8, 2021. Available at: https://www.cdc.gov/botulism/prevention.html.

6. Mura Paroche M, Caton SJ, Vereijken CMJL, Weenen H, Houston-Price C. How infants and young children learn about food: a systematic review. *Front Psychol.* 2017;8:1046.

7. CDC. CDC VitalSigns—Reducing sodium in children's diets. Centers for Disease Control and Prevention. Published September 5, 2018. Accessed July 21, 2022. Available at: https://www.cdc.gov/vitalsigns/children-sodium/index.html.

8. Gupta RS, Springston EE, Warrier MR, et al. The prevalence, severity, and distribution of childhood food allergy in the United States. *Pediatrics.* 2011;128(1):e9-e17.

9. Boyce JA. Guidelines for the diagnosis and management of food allergy in the United States: Report of the NIAID-Sponsored Expert Panel. *J Allergy Clin Immunol.* 2010;126(6, Supplement):S1-S58.

10. Ren Q, Li K, Sun H, et al. The association of formula protein content and growth in early infancy: a systematic review and meta-analysis. *Nutrients.* 2022;14(11):2255.

11. Zheng M, Hesketh KD, Vuillermin P, et al. Determinants of rapid infant weight gain: a pooled analysis of seven cohorts. *Pediatr Obes.* 2022 Oct;17(10):e12928.

12. Styne D. Puberty. In: Gardner DG, Shoback D, eds. *Greenspan's Basic & Clinical Endocrinology*. 10th ed. McGraw-Hill Education; 2017. Accessed July 13, 2022. Available at: accessmedicine.mhmedical.com/content.aspx?aid=1144818197.

13. Diab LK, Haemer MA, Primak LE, Krebs NF. Normal childhood nutrition & its disorders. In: Bunik M, Hay WW, Levin MJ, Abzug MJ, eds. *Current Diagnosis & Treatment: Pediatrics*. 26th ed. McGraw-Hill Education; 2022. Accessed July 13, 2022; Available at: accessmedicine.mhmedical.com/content.aspx?aid=1190359669.

14. Nguyen M, Jarvis SE, Tinajero MG, et al. Sugar-sweetened beverage consumption and weight gain in children and adults: a systematic review and meta-analysis of prospective cohort studies and randomized controlled trials. *Am J Clin Nutr*. 2023;117(1):160-174.

15. Fryar CD, Carroll MD, Afful J. *Prevalence of Overweight, Obesity, and Severe Obesity Among Children and Adolescents Aged 2–19 Years: United States, 1963–1965 Through 2017–2018*. National Center for Health Statistics; 2020.

16. Sullivan DH, Johnson LE. Nutrition and obesity. In: Halter JB, Ouslander JG, Studenski S, et al., eds. *Hazzard's Geriatric Medicine and Gerontology*. 7ed. McGraw-Hill Education; 2017. Accessed July 20, 2022. Available at: accessmedicine.mhmedical.com/content.aspx?aid=1136588978.

17. Harvard TH. *Chan School of Public Health Straight Talk About Soy*. The Nutrition Source. Published 2018. Available at: https://www.hsph.harvard.edu/nutritionsource/soy/.

18. Jouanne M, Oddoux S, Noël A, Voisin-Chiret AS. Nutrient requirements during pregnancy and lactation. *Nutrients*. 2021;13(2):692.

19. Ota E, Hori H, Mori R, Tobe-Gai R, Farrar D. Antenatal dietary education and supplementation to increase energy and protein intake. *Cochrane Database Syst Rev*. 2015;(6):CD000032.

20. *Nutrition During Pregnancy*. Accessed July 22, 2022. Available at: https://www.acog.org/en/womens-health/faqs/nutrition-during-pregnancy.

21. Cantor AG, Jungbauer RM, McDonagh M, et al. Counseling and behavioral interventions for healthy weight and weight gain in pregnancy: evidence report and systematic review for the US Preventive Services Task Force. *JAMA*. 2021;325(20):2094-2109.

22. Lynch S, Pfeiffer CM, Georgieff MK, et al. Biomarkers of Nutrition for Development (BOND)-iron review. *J Nutr*. 2018;148(suppl_1):1001S-1067S.

23. Korsmo HW, Jiang X, Caudill MA. Choline: exploring the growing science on its benefits for moms and babies. *Nutrients*. 2019;11(8):E1823.

24. Shaw GM, Carmichael SL, Yang W, Selvin S, Schaffer DM. Periconceptional dietary intake of choline and betaine and neural tube defects in offspring. *Am J Epidemiol*. 2004;160(2):102-109.

25. Office of Dietary Supplements—Choline. Accessed July 22, 2022. Available at: https://ods.od.nih.gov/factsheets/Choline-HealthProfessional/.

26. Brunst KJ, Wright RO, DiGioia K, et al. Racial/ethnic and sociodemographic factors associated with micronutrient intakes and inadequacies among pregnant women in an urban US population. *Public Health Nutr*. 2014;17(9):1960-1970.

27. Micronutrient Inadequacies in the US Population: an Overview. Linus Pauling Institute. Published April 20, 2018. Accessed July 22, 2022. Available at: https://lpi.oregonstate.edu/mic/micronutrient-inadequacies/overview.

28. Crozier SR, Inskip HM, Godfrey KM, Cooper C, Robinson SM, SWS Study Group. Nausea and vomiting in early pregnancy: effects on food intake and diet quality. *Matern Child Nutr*. 2017;13(4):e12389.

29. US Environmental Protection Agency. EPA-FDA Advice about Eating Fish and Shellfish. Published July 30, 2015. Accessed May 11, 2023. Available at: https://www.epa.gov/fish-tech/epa-fda-advice-about-eating-fish-and-shellfish.

30. Mahajan A, Donovan LE, Vallee R, Yamamoto JM. Evidenced-based nutrition for gestational diabetes mellitus. *Curr Diab Rep*. 2019;19(10):94.

31. Poon LC, Shennan A, Hyett JA, et al. The International Federation of Gynecology and Obstetrics (FIGO) initiative on pre-eclampsia: a pragmatic guide for first-trimester screening and prevention. *Int J Gynecol Obstet*. 2019;145(S1):1-33.

32. Bernstein M. Nutritional needs of the older adult. *Phys Med Rehabil Clin N Am*. 2017;28(4):747-766.

33. Chernoff R. Protein and older adults. *J Am Coll Nutr*. 2004;23(6 Suppl):627S-630S.

34. Institute of Medicine. *Dietary Reference Intakes for Energy, Carbohydrate, Fiber, Fat, Fatty Acids, Cholesterol, Protein, and Amino Acids*. The National Academies Press; 2002. doi:10.17226/10490.

35. Bradlee ML, Mustafa J, Singer MR, Moore LL. High-protein foods and physical activity protect against age-related muscle loss and functional decline. *J Gerontol A Biol Sci Med Sci*. 2017;73(1):88-94.

36. Hoy, G.. Dietary fiber intake of the US population, what we eat in America, NHANES 2009-2010. Accessed July 22, 2022. Available at: https://www.ars.usda.gov/research/publications/publication/?seqNo115=309591.

37. Institute of Medicine, Food, and Nutrition Board. *Dietary Reference Intakes for Water, Potassium, Sodium, Chloride, and Sulfate*. The National Academies Press; 2004.

38. Institute of Medicine. *Dietary Reference Intakes: The Essential Guide to Nutrient Requirements*. The National Academies Press; 2006.

39. Institute of Medicine (US). Committee to review dietary reference intakes for vitamin D and calcium. In: Ross AC, Taylor CL, Yaktine AL, Del Valle HB, eds. *Dietary Reference Intakes for Calcium and Vitamin D*. The National Academies Press; 2011. Accessed July 22, 2022. Available at: http://www.ncbi.nlm.nih.gov/books/NBK56070/.

40. Ervin RB, Kennedy-Stephenson J. Mineral intakes of elderly adult supplement and non-supplement users in the third national health and nutrition examination survey. *J Nutr*. 2002;132(11):3422-3427.

41. Aung K, Htay T. USPSTF found insufficient evidence on benefits and harms of screening for vitamin D deficiency in asymptomatic adults. *Ann Intern Med*. 2021;174(9):JC100.

42. Holick MF, Binkley NC, Bischoff-Ferrari HA, et al. Evaluation, treatment, and prevention of vitamin D deficiency: an Endocrine Society clinical practice guideline. *J Clin Endocrinol Metab*. 2011;96(7):1911-1930.

43. LeBoff MS, Chou SH, Ratliff KA, et al. Supplemental Vitamin D and Incident Fractures in Midlife and Older Adults. *N Engl J Med*. 2022;387(4):299-309.

44. Iuliano S, Poon S, Robbins J, et al. Effect of dietary sources of calcium and protein on hip fractures and falls in older adults in residential care: cluster randomised controlled trial. *BMJ*. 2021;375:n2364.

45. ter Borg S, Verlaan S, Hemsworth J, et al. Micronutrient intakes and potential inadequacies of community-dwelling older adults: a systematic review. *Br J Nutr.* 2015;113(8):1195-1206.

46. Friedman SM, Mulhausen P, Cleveland ML, et al. Healthy aging: American Geriatrics Society White Paper Executive Summary. *J Am Geriatr Soc.* 2019;67(1):17-20.

47. Samieri C, Sun Q, Townsend MK, et al. The association between dietary patterns at midlife and health in aging: an observational study. *Ann Intern Med.* 2013;159(9):584-591.

48. Estruch R, Ros E, Salas-Salvadó J, et al. Primary prevention of cardiovascular disease with a mediterranean diet supplemented with extra-virgin olive oil or nuts. *N Engl J Med.* 2018;378(25):e34.

49. Valls-Pedret C, Sala-Vila A, Serra-Mir M, et al. Mediterranean diet and age-related cognitive decline: a randomized clinical trial. *JAMA Intern Med.* 2015;175(7):1094-1103.

50. Kojima G, Avgerinou C, Iliffe S, Walters K. Adherence to mediterranean diet reduces incident frailty risk: systematic review and meta-analysis. *J Am Geriatr Soc.* 2018;66(4):783-788.

51. Morris MC, Tangney CC, Wang Y, Sacks FM, Bennett DA, Aggarwal NT. MIND diet associated with reduced incidence of Alzheimer's disease. *Alzheimers Dement.* 2015;11(9):1007-1014.

52. American Geriatrics Society: Ten Things Clinicians and Patients Should Question. Published February 24, 2015. Accessed July 22, 2022. Available at: https://www.choosingwisely.org/societies/american-geriatrics-society/.

53. Kim JS, Wilson JM, Lee SR. Dietary implications on mechanisms of sarcopenia: roles of protein, amino acids and antioxidants. *J Nutr Biochem.* 2010;21(1):1-13.

54. Fried LP, Tangen CM, Walston J, et al. Frailty in older adults: evidence for a phenotype. *J Gerontol A Biol Sci Med Sci.* 2001;56(3):M146-M156.

55. Siris ES, Adler R, Bilezikian J, et al. The clinical diagnosis of osteoporosis: a position statement from the National Bone Health Alliance Working Group. *Osteoporos Int.* 2014;25(5):1439-1443.

chapter 6

Popular Diets

Kevin C. Klatt, PhD, RD / Deirdre K. Tobias, ScD

Chapter Outline

CASE STUDY

Mr. Macro is an 82-year-old man who presents with Alzheimer's disease. Mr. Macro lives with his daughter, Ms. Calor, and is cared for by his full-time nurse. Mr. Macro presents with significant memory impairment and has retained most functional abilities but exhibits feeding difficulties, requiring assisted feeding from his full-time nurse; Mr. Macro, however, does not currently require artificial nutrition. His BMI is 20.5 kg/m² and has remained stable at this weight for the past 6 months; 12 months ago, Mr. Macro developed an upper respiratory infection that resulted in 5.2% weight loss over a 1-month period. Now that Mr. Macro's weight remains stable, his daughter wants to discuss the potential of feeding Mr. Macro a ketogenic diet. His current dietary pattern reflects a low-variety, Western-style eating pattern, including oatmeal and fruit at breakfast, sandwiches with cold cuts at lunch, and soups for dinner, but is not a picky eater. Ms. Calor describes herself as very physically active and interested in wellness, and had seen a detailed post on social media noting that ketones are beneficial for brain function and may reverse or slow cognitive impairment.

Ms. Calor wants to discuss whether switching Mr. Macro to a ketogenic diet as an adjunctive therapy to his current pharmacotherapy (Donepezil).

1. **Which of the following would be potential concerns related to initiating a ketogenic diet for Mr. Macro? Select all that apply.**
   A. Unintentional weight loss
   B. Nutrient adequacy
   C. Lack of support
   D. Strict food preferences
   E. Adherence to a strict ketogenic regimen

2. **True or False: Mechanistic evidence supporting the beneficial effects of ketones in dementia is sufficient to support recommending a ketogenic diet to patients with Alzheimer's disease.**

3. In reviewing the literature, you find a pilot trial reporting positive effects of modified ketogenic diet without protein restriction in patients with Alzheimer's disease, as well as a small randomized controlled trial showing improvements in mild cognitive impairment in patients consuming a medium-chain triglyceride drink enriched in the ketogenic fatty acid, C8:0. However, you find no authoritative medical guidelines or systematic reviews that recommend or support an indication for implementing ketogenic diets or supplements in patients with cognitive impairments/dementia. How would you best facilitate patient-centered care and informed decision making? Select all that apply.
   A. Emphasize your enthusiasm for the diet and discuss your personal experience seeing other patients trial ketogenic diets.
   B. Explain that some limited data supports a beneficial effect of ketogenic diets and supplements in cognitive impairment, but there have not been

(Continued)

rigorous trials and thus, no major medical organizations recommend it.

C. Recommend referral to a registered dietitian for further discussion of considerations when implementing a ketogenic diet and/or use ketogenic supplements.

D. Note that other dietary patterns have similarly limited data for a potential benefit in

cognitive impairment, such as the MIND diet, a Mediterranean and DASH hybrid diet with an emphasis on hypothesized neuroprotective intakes of specific nutrients.

E. Dismiss the idea of pursuing a ketogenic diet because the data is poor and keto diets are hard to implement.

INTRODUCTION

Physicians may be approached by patients to discuss whether adopting a popular diet would be appropriate for them for improvement or maintenance of general health and wellness. Further, patients may be interested in starting a popular diet for the prevention or treatment of a specific health condition or disease. These patient interactions require the clinician to know the specific foods that the eating pattern promotes or restricts, validity of the health claims made by the diet's developers and proponents, and an understanding of your patient's motive(s) and expectations. The clinical evaluation also includes potential concerns for contraindications, safety, and efficacy. This chapter will provide an overview of these considerations, with the objective of improving competency in synthesizing and discussing pros and cons of popular diets with patients.

WHAT IS A POPULAR DIET?

A popular diet refers generally to any eating plan, dietary approach, or implementation tool trending among the public purported to promote human health. Popular diets can fall in relative accordance or in direct contradiction to national dietary guidelines, and range in durability from quick fads to long-lasting. The evidence underlying the claims of popular diets is widely variable. In this chapter, we will discuss types of popular diets, common health claims, approaches to assessing the safety and efficacy of such diets, and considerations for communicating with patients.

POPULAR DIETS THROUGHOUT HISTORY

Popular diets are seen throughout history, with therapeutics and rationale often reflecting the medical beliefs and values of the era. For example, Marcus Cato, the Roman senator and historian (234 B.C. to 149 B.C.), is documented as having promoted the medicinal value of cabbage over all other vegetables, claiming benefits for a variety of body systems and ailments.[1] A variant of this diet reappears in the 1950–1960s as a cabbage soup-based weight loss regimen. In the 1800s, Sylvester Graham, an Evangelical minister for whom the Graham cracker is named, promoted a vegetarian eating pattern rich in whole grains to promote general health, moral purity, and temperance; so-called "Grahamism" was further bolstered by John Harvey Kellogg,

MD, of the Kellogg family flaked cereals, who detailed benefits of the vegetarian dietary pattern in his 1923 book, *The Natural Diet of Man*. Prominent news and media platforms provided an outlet for a broader dissemination of popular diets. For example, in 1961, the physiologist Ancel Keys was featured on the cover of *Time* magazine for "Medicine: The Fat of the Land,"[2] launching a discussion of low-fat diets, obesity, and atherosclerosis into the forefront of the public domain. Over 50 years later, in 2014, *Time* depicted the reversal of public opinion for low-fat popular diets with its provocative cover title "Eat Butter." The second half of the 21st century saw an explosion of popular diets marketed largely through programs (e.g., Jenny Craig, WW) and lay books (e.g., Diet: Atkins, Zone, Ornish, Blood Type), most targeting general health and the emerging epidemic of overweight/obesity. With the advent of the Internet, social media, popular television shows, podcasts, blogs, and streaming services provide additional mediums for promoting and popularization of diets. The *U.S. News & World Report* publishes its expert opinion-based "Best Diets" annually, which provides a ranking and snapshot of the most common popular diets. Further, national statistics indicated in 2007–2008 that 14.3% of U.S. adults over age 20 years reported being "currently on any kind of diet to lose weight or for some other health-related reason," which increased to 17.1% of adults in 2015–2018.[3]

POPULAR DIETS AND YOUR PATIENT

There is an appreciation today that there is no one single optimal diet for all. This is recognized explicitly in the U.S. Dietary Guidelines for Americans, which offers guidance on how children and adults can meet nutrient needs through a variety of healthy dietary patterns, allowing for flexibility for Americans' vast cultural and personal preferences.[4] Nonetheless, popular diets for a variety of health claims persist, representing a multibillion dollar industry. Given the potential cost implications for your patient, it is also prudent not to assume that all popular diets are relatively harmless. However, scrutiny of a diet's health claims should be balanced with compassion and an understanding of your patient's health concerns or goals.

Types of Popular Diets

While the content and goals of popular diets vary across time and culture, they can be broadly grouped by common features of the intervention and/or health claims:

i. Restriction/elimination: A popular diet may be founded in a claim that a specific food, nutrient, or other food-related feature is a cause of illness or other negative health effects, and thus restricting intake below a certain threshold or eliminating it altogether is desirable. These are not the medically-indicated diets to treat allergies or intolerances, such as gluten-free diets for patients diagnosed with celiac disease (see Chapter 16). Rather, these diets are only purported to be a factor in general wellness or nonspecific symptoms, such as fatigue or bloating.

ii. Addition/supplementation: Popular diets may be founded in emphasizing an intake of specific foods or nutrients to enhance health (e.g., "superfoods"), often under the assumption that "more is better." While such foods often fit within a healthy dietary pattern, examples where evidence supports a leading role for the bioavailability and bioactivity of any one specific compound on clinical health benefits are rare, with the exception of clinical deficiency.

iii. Production and processing: For over a century, there have been advocates of "whole food diets" and other eating patterns with the shared objective of reducing or eliminating exposure to otherwise unregulated adulterations, contaminants, artificial ingredients, additives, colorings, texturizers, and/or other features of food production or processing.[4,5] Common diets today include "organic" and "non-GMO" diets. These popular diets may be agnostic to the foods that are consumed, so long as certain standards are met; however, lack of standardized definitions, food labeling, biologically meaningful thresholds of acceptable exposures, and verification measures may undermine these approaches.

iv. Mode and time restricted eating: Popular diets have long advocated for alterations in not only the types of foods consumed but also the manner in which the food is eaten. This includes food pairings, the order in which foods are eaten, the time of day that food is consumed, and fasting regimens. There are numerous combinations of these elements, including alternate-day fasting, fasting for 5 days then eating for 2 days (5:2 regimen), eating only between 10am and 5pm, and so forth. It is common for these diets to have no restrictions on food type or quantity during the allowed eating windows, and emphasis is instead on the benefits of food orders, aligning with the circadian rhythm, and/or independent benefits of fasting.

v. Dietary patterns: Dietary patterns refer to diets that provide comprehensive guidance on the totality of diet, including which foods/nutrients to consume more of and which to avoid, often with attention to maintaining balanced intake across the food groups. Some popular dietary patterns are inspired by ecological studies identifying countries or regions with lower prevalence of chronic diseases, longer life spans, etc. For example, the Mediterranean Diet is a popular dietary pattern based on the traditional foods, ingredients, and eating habits observed in countries around the Mediterranean, which historically maintained lower rates of cardiovascular disease, cancer, and other conditions than the United States and other Western European countries.[6]

Implementing Popular Diets

Implementation of a diet refers to the tools, education, and other methods that the patient uses to adopt and sustain a diet. Monetizing access to information and resources is common for proponents of popular diets. In addition to cost, popular diet implementation strategies also carry implications for patients' effort and time. Like the dietary goals themselves, the evidence to support any one implementation strategy as a means of long-term adherence is highly variable in quality and there does not appear to be any one approach that works best for all. Below are some common categories of options for adherence to a popular diet:

i. Patient education: The least invasive and intensive form of implementing a popular diet is educating the approach through diet books, recipes, online resources, and may be freely available or for a cost.

ii. Self-monitoring behaviors: Popular restrictive and addition diets typically require patients to be familiar with food labels and recipes and to closely monitor their daily intakes. This can be achieved through paper-based food journals and hand-counting of target nutrients. There are also countless smartphone apps and websites that provide tracking tools for patients to log foods and drinks and receive outputs of their nutrient intakes. These are increasingly sophisticated, allow patients to set and monitor diet goals in real time, capture foods and beverages with photos and food labels, and receive automated prompts about healthy eating and their adherence to input goals. Self-monitoring tools aimed at intake are frequently coupled with self-monitoring tools around body composition, physical activity levels, and metabolic outcomes, due to the increasing rise of electronic scales, wearable activity trackers, and automated continuous monitoring of metabolites (e.g., glucose). Increasingly, these tools interface across devices and platforms, aiming to shift intake in response to other outcome metrics.

iii. Food delivery: Many food delivery services cater to dietary needs and even accommodate or promote popular diets. The degree of food preparation or cooking can vary, and range from only dinners to provision of all meals/snacks and beverages, with varying levels of food preparation required. Quantity of food is often tailored to the individuals' nutritional needs and dietary preferences and goals.

iv. Behavior modification: Several notable popular diets are centered or accommodate in behavioral modification theories, focusing on individuals' behavior change rather than specific nutrient goals (e.g., Jenny Craig, WW). These programs vary and may include individualized interactive app-based resources, in-person group sessions, online 1:1 learning modules, and more. Behavior modification programs and platforms increasingly employ self-monitoring approaches and tools to promote adherence to a specific way of eating.

v. Precision and individualized nutrition: These implementation strategies are increasing in popularity, whereby the "no one diet fits all" approach leverages information provided by the patient to output a personalized eating plan.

Information is collected on health status, anthropometrics, taste preferences, biospecimen samples, and even genetics. Additional input from technology such as body weight scales, vital status and other wearables, glucose monitors, blood work services, symptom tracking, and more, are increasingly incorporated into algorithms of personalized nutrition. The types of recommended diets can follow many of the diet types described above.

Health Claims by Popular Diet Developers and Advocates

There are popular diets that claim to prevent or treat virtually any condition, symptom, or illness, in addition to those promoting overall wellness and healthy living. These include overweight/obesity, cardiometabolic disease, gastrointestinal symptoms and illnesses, hormonal regulation, reproductive health and sexual function, fatigue, and more. It should be emphasized that although there may be evidence supporting the rationale for diet's effects on one health outcome, there may be limited or no evidence for its role in other areas of health. This necessitates careful communication of the expected benefits with the patient. For example, ketogenic diets can be medically indicated in the management of refractory epilepsy with a sound evidence base, but have minimal research for their efficacy in other neurological conditions (e.g., Parkinson's disease).

Popular diet claims frequently lack consistent and reliable evidence (e.g., systematic reviews of high-quality prospective cohorts and randomized, controlled trials with disease endpoints). In the absence of such evidence, health claims might be inferred from biological plausibility, extrapolations from *in vitro* model systems and animal feeding experiments, and/or small short-term human interventions with surrogate endpoints instead of clinical outcomes. Surrogate outcomes are highly variable in prognostic value to inform conclusions about the longer-term clinical outcomes of interest. For example, advocates for consuming a gluten-free diet, regardless of celiac diagnosis, frequently claim that nonspecific symptoms and complaints like bloating, general malaise, mood, and more, occur from "leaky gut" syndrome, resulting from the impact of alpha gliadins, derived from the intestinal processing of gluten, on zonulin production. There are only *in vitro* and small human trials examining gluten-derived peptides on zonulin, a major regulator of intestinal permeability, and this is extrapolated to suggest there would then be detrimental effects to human health generally secondary to impaired barrier function of the gut.

A common rationale for diet-health relationships found throughout the popular diet landscape is that a diet, due to some bioactive component(s), impacts one or more mechanistic intermediates (e.g., inflammatory cytokines, circulating hormone levels, gut microbiota composition, cellular receptor), and thus, health and disease risk. Such theoretical mechanism of action-based claims would typically be viewed by medical researchers and evidence-based practitioners as preliminary hypotheses, owing to the lack of a causal relationship supported by clear mechanistic data, defined and plausible dose-response relationships, and measured clinical outcomes, but can be found cited in support of popular diets as being "evidence-based" throughout popular media. It should be emphasized that such mechanisms of action-based recommendations are not only scientifically lacking but exist in overabundance. Indeed, it is egregiously simple to identify at least one component of a food/dietary pattern involved in a metabolic pathway that has been hypothesized to be related to or disturbed in a disease process. For many foods/nutrients, their pleiotropic involvement across physiological systems allow for mechanisms of action-based recommendations with competing directionality. As in this chapter's case study, one may find the potential for ketogenic diets to be therapeutic in cognitive impairment compelling due to mechanistic data related to beta-hydroxybutyrate; however, one could readily hypothesize and cite similar potential detrimental effects of a ketogenic diet on cognitive impairment due to their high intakes of long-chain saturated fatty acids and lower intakes of plant-derived bioactives including fibers and phytochemicals. Such inconsistency and conflicting narratives underscore the low clinical utility of mechanism of action-based recommendations that provide much of the rationale for popular diets.

In instances where some supporting evidence from well-conducted controlled trials exists (e.g., macronutrient modified diets and weight loss), claims frequently overstate the magnitude of the benefit. For example, numerous popular diets and their associated media (e.g., books, blogs) claim rapid, significant weight loss and long-term weight-loss maintenance specific to following a macronutrient modified diet (e.g., low carb, low fat); however, systematic reviews of dozens of randomized controlled trials and authoritative medical guidelines for the management of overweight and obesity consistently demonstrate underwhelming weight loss after 12 months of following macronutrient modified diets, with minimal differences between different diets.[7] In other instances, there may be rigorous evidence with reliable and meaningful effects on certain intermediate outcomes that are extrapolated to draw inferences about longer-term efficacy or effectiveness on other related outcomes. For example, well-done intervention studies in patients with polycystic ovarian syndrome (PCOS) demonstrate that lower glycemic dietary patterns lead to significant improvement in metabolic factors (e.g., insulin, IGF-1). Although few of these studies evaluated PCOS-related ovulatory capacity and fecundity/fertility, these trials are regularly cited to support popular diets to improve cyclicity and live birth rates.[8] Many intermediate outcome markers are not validated to have prognostic capacity, yet are very commonly used to derive popular diet claims.

There are instances where well-conducted dietary intervention studies have measured clinically meaningful surrogates, event rates, and quality of life improvement, to inform dietary guidelines and clinical recommendations. However, skilled nutrition practitioners should be mindful of assessing a study's internal validity as well as the relevance or translation of its intervention and findings to your specific patient or patient population. Many nutrition interventions are challenging to conduct, limited by factors such as feasibility and cost to sustain change long term, inability to deliver interventions to participants in a blind manner, lack of placebo control group, and relatively low adherence. There are trade-offs made between generalizability to a broader population and the rigorous conducting of the trial. With regard to this chapter's case study, one might find pilot trial evidence suggesting a benefit for participants randomized to a ketogenic diet, but further interrogation of the study is required to determine the adherence to the ketogenic diet, what specific ketogenic diet composition was chosen, what behavioral interventions were utilized and/or foods provided to facilitate following the diet, what the baseline dietary pattern was of the group, and what dietary pattern the comparator group consumed. Popular diets proclaiming the *unique* benefits of ketogenic diet for cognitive impairment frequently fail to contextualize the effects relative to control groups (often a standard Western-style dietary pattern) and note the lack of head-to-head trials comparing ketogenic diets to other well-formulated diets associated with improved cognition (e.g., DASH, Mediterranean, MIND). Such factors need to be considered when determining the relevance of a proposed nutrition intervention to your specific patient or patient population and when making claims about the relative efficacy of one diet versus another.

Balancing Patient Motives, Safety, and Accurate Communication About Popular Diets

Assessing popular diets for your patient includes not only its safety and efficacy, but also the patient's motives, expectations, beliefs, and preferences. These interactions with patients also necessitate an appreciation for communicating about diet with sensitivity. Given the relative paucity of evidence to support many popular diet claims but high interest from patients in modifying diets (one of the few medical variables under their control) with the aim of potentially improving outcomes, it is imperative to facilitate patient-centered decision making that results from respecting patient autonomy and limiting practitioner biases, while as accurate and objective information as possible about efficacy and safety.

i. **Patient motives:** Practitioners must communicate sensitively and accurately about the risks and benefits of diets. Medicine has traditionally employed a deficit model of communication, assuming that providers hold knowledge that needs to be communicated to patients, who lack said knowledge. This approach is the subject of much critique due to its failure to facilitate patient-centered care and shared decision making. Indeed, many patients with interest in a popular diet pattern come with informed reasoning for wanting to pursue the diet, may have already begun investing in following the diet, and even perceive health improvements. The patient may prioritize psychosocial and/or cultural reasons for consuming a popular diet, regardless of the evidence base. Overall, practitioners should take care to address questions accurately and sensitively without being dismissive.

ii. **Safety:** Practitioners should readily consider acutely dangerous contraindications when considering popular diets. Serious contraindications commonly present because of additional medical indications; for example, patients with type 1 diabetes and acute porphyrias are strongly recommended to avoid low-carbohydrate diets, as well as popular diets that advocate fasting, due to the risk of hypoglycemia and attack onset, respectively. Such diets increase the chance of a metabolic crisis, the need for acute medical care, and can be life-threatening if not immediately addressed. Some popular diets also advocate for consumption of a variety of food products that present with foodborne illness risk (e.g., raw milk, home-brewed kombucha) that can prevent serious risks to immunocompromised patients, including patients having received transplants, pregnant persons, and individuals diagnosed with HIV/AIDs. Additional acute health threats from popular diets can include those that cause dramatic shifts in electrolytes (e.g., extreme weight-loss diets, prolonged fasting, excessive fluid intakes, homemade formulas).

Popular diets can be an acute threat to an individual's health when they are abjectly deficient in essential nutrients, especially protein-energy malnutrition (PEM) and water-soluble nutrients with shorter half-lives in the body. Many popular diets restricting a single food or macronutrient may result in intakes below the Dietary Reference Intakes (DRIs); however, most DRIs establish indicators of adequacy linked to physiological function in excess of the minimal requirement to prevent deficiency, resulting in lower intakes not necessarily presenting with an acute clinical manifestation. Some popular diets advocate for consumption of a single food or food group and likely increase the risk of PEM and micronutrient deficiencies. Thus, symptoms of acute deficiency states are important to monitor for in individuals pursuing popular diets but are unlikely to occur unless extremely restrictive patterns are pursued.

For most individuals in the general population and those with common chronic conditions, popular diets typically do not pose immediate, acute risks. However, popular diets may result in inadequate nutrient intakes (below the Estimated Average Requirement [EAR]), increased intakes of dietary factors linked to increased chronic disease risk (e.g., sodium) or eliminate factors that may be protective (e.g., fiber-rich plant foods and associated nutrients/bioactives), and may cause undue psychological harm. Depending on the popular diet and its inclusion guidelines, risks from the diet may be attenuated by prioritization of certain foods over others. For example, diets that exclude dairy (i.e., vegan, Paleo) can meet the calcium EAR by prioritizing high-bioavailability calcium sources such as Brassica family dark leafy greens, the use of fortified dairy alternatives, and certain nuts and legumes. Lower-carbohydrate dietary patterns can consume primarily plant-based fat sources and low carbohydrate vegetables to align more closely with food-based dietary patterns, reduce intakes of saturated fats (linked to higher LDL-C) and achieve higher fiber intakes. In individuals presenting on the spectrum of disordered eating behavior, care must be taken with regard to communication around popular diets to limit triggering language and the inadvertent promotion of existing disordered eating behaviors; practitioners should refer to Chapter 25, "Disordered Eating."

TABLE 6-1 · Glossary of common popular diets	
Anti-Inflammatory Diet	An anti-inflammatory diet is promoted as a remedy to "fight" inflammation in the body. Many nutrients are involved in the appropriate initiation and resolution of inflammation; proponents of anti-inflammatory diets typically emphasize some subset of these nutrients, with the common belief that "inflammation" is always bad. Although it produces unpleasant side effects, inflammation is actually a healthy response by our immune system.
Clean Eating	What it means will depend on who you ask. The terms *clean eating* and *clean diets* are not federally regulated in the United States, so interpretation by consumers and the marketing of "clean" products (typically lacking in specific ingredients) by the food industry can vary widely.
DASH Diet	The DASH (Dietary Approaches to Stop Hypertension) diet is a dietary approach that emphasizes food and nutrient intakes that lower blood pressure (e.g., high fruit, vegetable, dairy, and whole grain intakes; lower sodium intake). Accumulating evidence shows wide-ranging health benefits of this eating pattern beyond just blood pressure lowering.
Gluten-Free	A gluten-free diet eliminates all foods containing or contaminated with gluten. As the sole treatment for the 1%–2% of Americans who have celiac disease, this diet is not new. What is new—and driving these sales upward—is the use of a gluten-free diet for weight loss and nonspecific gastrointestinal symptoms.
Intermittent Fasting	Intermittent fasting is a diet regimen that cycles between brief periods of fasting, with either no food or significant calorie reduction, and periods of unrestricted eating. The most common methods are fasting on alternate days, for whole days with a specific frequency per week, or during a set time frame.
Ketogenic Diet	The ketogenic or "keto" diet is a low-carbohydrate, fat-rich eating plan that substantially increases serum ketone levels without the need for fasting. A carbohydrate- and protein-restricted version has been used for over a century to treat specific medical conditions. However, in recent years, a less restrictive version of the diet focused on restricting carbohydrates has gained considerable attention as a potential weight-loss strategy.
Mediterranean Diet	The Mediterranean diet is a primarily plant-based eating plan that includes daily intake of whole grains, olive oil, fruits, vegetables, beans and other legumes, nuts, herbs, and spices. Other foods like animal proteins are eaten in smaller quantities, with the preferred animal protein being fish and seafood. It does not specify portion sizes or specific amounts, as it is up to the individual to decide exactly how much food to eat at each meal.
MIND Diet	Dementia is the sixth-leading cause of death in the United States, driving many people to search for ways to prevent cognitive decline. The Mediterranean-DASH Diet Intervention for Neurodegenerative Delay, or MIND diet, targets the health of the aging brain.
Mindful Eating	This approach to eating focuses on the eating experience, body-related sensations, and thoughts and feelings about food, with heightened awareness and without judgment. Attention is paid to the foods being chosen, internal and external physical cues, and your responses to those cues.
Paleo Diet	The Paleolithic or "Paleo" diet seeks to address 21st-century ills by revisiting the way humans ate during the Paleolithic era more than 2 million years ago. Paleo proponents state that because our genetics and anatomy have changed very little since the Stone Age, we should eat foods available during that time to promote good health.

Adapted from Harvard's Nutrition Source and available online at: https://www.hsph.harvard.edu/nutritionsource/healthy-weight/diet-reviews/.

CONCLUSION

No single chapter can ever capture the diversity of popular diets presented to patients and clients. Popular diets are formulated, disseminated, interpreted, and further evolve in an increasingly dynamic information ecosystem that is informed by not only the updated science surrounding nutrition, medicine and disease, but also the social, cultural, political, economic, and religious factors that influence what and why consumers choose to eat. Within this chapter, we have aimed to arm practitioners with a structured way of thinking about popular diets, how to assess their potential safety and efficacy, and the importance of communicating with accuracy while respecting patient autonomy in determining their own food and nutrition choices.

CASE STUDY ANSWERS

1. **A, B, E;** Mr. Macro has a history of clinically severe malnutrition (lost > 5% weight loss in 1 month in the context of an acute illness or injury; 2012 AND/ASPEN guidelines) and a BMI towards the lower end of the normal range. Depending upon the rate of implementation, strictness of the ketogenic ratio, and variety of foods available, unintentional weight loss may occur with implementation of a ketogenic diet. Mr. Macro's diet is currently low in variety and this is unlikely to improve with a more restrictive ketogenic diet; this raises concerns about nutrient adequacy (e.g., protein, micronutrients, fiber) and may require nutrient supplementation. As Mr. Macro requires assisted feeding, his adherence to such a diet would depend upon the dietary planning and implementation of feeding provided by his family and full-time nurse, who would likely require education and counseling on how to implement a ketogenic diet. Mr. Macro does, however, have support in the form of his full-time nurse and daughter. Mr. Macro does not have strict food preferences.

2. **False;** While several mechanisms have been put forth as to why ketones such as beta-hydroxybutyrate might have beneficial effects in several neurological conditions including mild cognitive impairment, there is a need for strong clinical evidence to determine the required ketogenic ratio/serum ketone levels necessary to achieve such an effect (if a true clinical effect exists), the duration of the intervention required, the average clinical effect size of such an intervention, and potential side effects.

3. **B, C, D;** Practitioners should both limit their own biases (personal enthusiasm, anecdotal evidence) when providing counseling on a diet with limited evidence to facilitate patient-centered decision making and accurately informed consent. This can be done by acknowledging the existing data and its limitations and the current guidelines from respected medical organizations. Nutrients and foods contain numerous bioactive compounds and metabolic effects purported to improve an outcome, many of which have some small, positive evidence on intermediate biomarkers or potential mechanistic pathways. Noting that such evidence exists for many dietary patterns beyond the one that a patient saw advertised on social media may help better inform what dietary approach they wish to implement. In this instance, the interested family member of the patient may benefit from speaking with a knowledgeable registered dietitian to discuss the various ways ketogenic diets can be formulated, practical aspects of implementation, other elements of the ketogenic diet to consider that may have undesirable effects (e.g., high long-chain saturated fatty acid intake and elevated LDL-C), and blood/urinary ketone monitoring. Dismissing the idea of a ketogenic diet in this case is likely to limit patient-centered decision making and may degrade patient-provider trust.

REFERENCES

1. Marcus Cato on Agriculture. Accessed January 31, 2023. Available at: http://penelope.uchicago.edu/Thayer/E/Roman/Texts/Cato/De_Agricultura/K*.html.

2. Medicine: The Fat of the Land. TIME.com. Published January 13, 1961. Accessed January 31, 2023. https://content.time.com/time/magazine/article/0,9171,828721,00.html.

3. Stierman B, Ansai N, Mishra S, Hales CM. Special diets among adults: United States, 2015–2018. *NCHS Data Brief.* 2020;289:1-8.

4. Committee DGA, Dietary Guidelines Advisory Committee. Scientific Report of the 2020 Dietary Guidelines Advisory Committee: Advisory Report to the Secretary of Agriculture and Secretary of Health and Human Services. Published online 2020. doi:10.52570/dgac2020.

5. Lewis C. The "Poison Squad" and the advent of food and drug regulation. *FDA Consum.* 2002;36(6):12-15.

6. Willett WC, Sacks F, Trichopoulou A, et al. Mediterranean diet pyramid: a cultural model for healthy eating. *Am J Clin Nutr.* 1995;61(6 Suppl):1402S-1406S.

7. Tobias DK, Chen M, Manson JE, Ludwig DS, Willett W, Hu FB. Effect of low-fat diet interventions versus other diet interventions on long-term weight change in adults: a systematic review and meta-analysis. *Lancet Diabetes Endocrinol.* 2015;3(12):968-979.

8. Kazemi M, Hadi A, Pierson RA, Lujan ME, Zello GA, Chilibeck PD. Effects of dietary glycemic index and glycemic load on cardiometabolic and reproductive profiles in women with polycystic ovary syndrome: A systematic review and meta-analysis of randomized controlled trials. *Adv Nutr.* 2020;12(1):161-178.

chapter 7

Herbs and Dietary Supplements

Cora Collette Breuner MD, MPH, FAAP

Chapter Outline

CASE STUDY

A 17-year-old assigned female at birth is a competitive rower who wants to improve performance, brighten mood, and boost immune system. The patient has been having a hard time falling asleep and is feeling more depressed recently. The patient asked the primary care physician if it was OK if take creatine, melatonin, St John's wort, and echinacea. The patient wanted to use natural products as they thought they would be healthier and safer than any prescribed medication.

1. Are there evidence-based studies that support the use of creatine, melatonin, St John's wort, and echinacea for any of her symptoms (trouble falling asleep, depressed mood) and to obtain benefits desired (improve performance, "boost" immunity)?

2. How would you discuss the use of dietary herbs and supplements with the patient?

3. What are the regulations around herbs' and supplements' safety and health benefits?

INTRODUCTION

Complementary, holistic, and integrative medicine is used in the overall population, across the life course, both for health promotion and as a therapeutic intervention in those with chronic health conditions. In a study published in 2015, adults' use of natural products (dietary supplements other than vitamins and minerals) was reported to be 17.7%.[1] In one study of people approximately 60 years and older, 21% of respondents were taking at least one herbal product or dietary supplement, and there the potential for adverse drug reactions was apparent in 19%.[2] From an Italian study published in 2018, the interest in plant food supplements is approximately 22.7%.[3] From a study published in 2020, about 2.9 million American children and adolescents have used herbs and/or dietary supplements. Children with disabilities or who have substantial use of medical services, are more likely to use herbs and dietary supplements.[4]

Healthcare providers need to learn how to access information on herbs and dietary supplements from evidence based on up-to-date resources, in addition to becoming familiar with best practices regarding counseling patients and their families on herb and dietary supplement use.[5]

DEMOGRAPHICS OF USAGE OF HERBS AND DIETARY SUPPLEMENTS INCLUDING RACE, ETHNIC AND GENDER MINORITIES

Herbs and dietary supplement use is common across most socioeconomic, race, cultures, ethnic, and gender minority populations.[6] These practices may be justified through country of origin, cultures, and beliefs.[7–9]

From a systematic review of complementary medicine use including herbs and dietary supplements amongst ethnic minorities, 424 articles were identified from the database search and only 17 articles met the inclusion criteria regarding estimation of usage of herbs/supplements and the motivations behind their use. Herb and supplement use among ethnic minority populations was attributed to support for natural products and was concurrent with conventional medicine. The referral sources were usually family and friends and, importantly, patients under reported usage to their primary care providers about herb and supplement usage.[10]

In a study published in 2022, 1,653 gender minority individuals were recruited from The Population Research in Identity and Disparities for Equality. Appearance and performance-enhancing drugs and supplements (APEDS) use was common across groups (30.7% of gender-expansive people, 45.2% of transgender men, and 14.9% of transgender women) with protein and creatine supplements most commonly used. APEDS use is common in gender-expansive people and must be asked about when caring for this population.[11,12]

SAFETY

The Food and Drug Administration (FDA) has limited authority to protect patients from potential harm. Herbs and dietary supplements are unregulated, meaning that the manufacturer is not required to demonstrate manufacturing purity, safety, and/or efficacy. Importantly, herbs and dietary supplements are not allowed to be marketed as treatments, preventions, or cures for any disease. However, marketing from the manufacturers is often deceiving. For example, sales of dietary supplements marketed for immune health increased after the emergence of COVID-19 because many people hoped that these products might provide some protection or reduction of disease SARS-CoV-2 infection burden. Unfortunately, patients and families may not discuss herb and dietary supplement use with their primary healthcare provider, which can lead to safety issues due to contaminated product usage or interactions with prescribed treatments.[13]

Since the U.S. Congress passed the Dietary Supplement Health and Education Act (DSHEA) in 1994, use of herbal products has been increasing exponentially, from 4,000 products to over 90,000 products. Under the current regulatory system, herbs and dietary supplements are not tested for safety or effectiveness, as with over-the-counter and prescription drugs, and the Food and Drug Administration (FDA) has limited authority to protect Americans from potential harm.

Historic Perspective

The dangers of patent medicines in the late 19th century are well documented. One of the most powerful of these regulatory agencies was an early version of the Food and Drug Administration (FDA), created by the Pure Food and Drug Act of 1906. The legislation that created the FDA initially focused on (1) requiring that drugs meet standards of strength and purity; (2) creating definitions of "adulteration" and "misbranding"; and (3) prohibiting the shipment for sale of foods, drinks, and drugs that fit these definitions of adulterated or misbranded. In the 1950s and 1960s, the FDA, in collaboration with the American Medical Association, attempted to reign in misleading marketing of vitamins, including hosting two joint National Congresses on Medical Quackery. In response to this regulatory environment, a number of vitamin manufacturers joined the National Health Federation, which markets itself as being dedicated to promoting consumer choice. In 1976, this group promoted the passage of the Proxmire Amendment to the Food, Drug, and Cosmetics Act.[14]

This amendment prohibits the FDA from treating vitamins and other dietary supplements such as nonprescription medications and prevents any regulation unless they are inherently dangerous or are marketed with illegal claims regarding treatment or prevention of specific diseases. Although the Proxmire Amendment specifically deregulated vitamins, continued legislative efforts resulted in the 1994 Dietary Supplement Health and Education Act, which classified dietary supplements under the broad regulatory framework of food rather than drugs.

Efforts in congress to legislate safer regulations for the herb and supplement industry have been met with limited success, partly because of the industry's lobbying efforts.[15] The quality and safety of herbal plants, particularly those used for dietary supplement preparations, must be determined for consumer health protection. Importantly, toxicological data on the identification of genotoxic, carcinogenic, and tumorigenic ingredients in many raw herbs and their mechanisms of action is insufficient. Identification of carcinogenic components in herbal plants is timely and important.[16]

A retrospective observational study used adverse event reports (death, disability, life-threatening events, hospitalization, emergency room visit, and/or required intervention to prevent permanent disability) between January 2004 and April 2015 in the U.S. Food and Drug Administration Adverse Event Reporting System on food and dietary supplements database. The authors of the study quantified the relative risks for severe medical events of dietary supplements sold for various functions relative to vitamins among individuals aged between 0 and 25 years. Of 40,086 adverse events in people of all ages, the authors identified 977 single-supplement-related adverse event reports affecting individuals aged between 0 and 25 years over 11 years (50.6% female; age: mean = 16.5 years, standard deviation = 7.5 years). Supplements sold for muscle building, energy, and weight loss were associated with almost three times the risk for severe medical events compared with vitamins.[17]

EXAMPLES OF COMMON HERBS AND DIETARY SUPPLEMENTS

The next section highlights a few common herbs and dietary supplements, and herbs that many patients may discuss with their providers. Detailed information of a larger number of supplements and herbs can be found on the NIH—Office of Dietary Supplements website: https://ods.od.nih.gov/factsheets/list-all/#.[18]

Creatine

Creatine is an amine that plays a role in skeletal muscle energy metabolism. It is naturally produced in the body from amino acids in the kidney and liver. It is also found in the diet, most often in red meat and seafood. Ninety-five percent of creatine is stored in skeletal muscle, with the remainder stored mostly in the brain and cardiac muscle.

Uses Oral creatine monohydrate seems to modestly improve lower leg performance.[19] When combined with resistance training, creatine supplementation might help some athletes increase muscle mass and strength. However, those focused on endurance training will not experience the same improvements in performance, and the increase in body weight sometimes associated with creatine supplementation might even impair endurance sport performance.

Mechanism of Action Creatine enters the cytosol through creatine transporters to help maintain glycolytic adenosine triphosphate levels to help meet energy needs.

Clinical Studies In multiple reviews, there has been evidence to indicate that creatine supplementation during resistance training is more effective at increasing muscle strength and weightlifting performance than resistance training alone, although the response is highly variable.[20,21]

Adverse Effects Dehydration, diarrhea, gastrointestinal upset, muscle cramps, and water retention are usually observed.

Herb/Supplement Drug Interactions Taking creatinine supplements with nonsteroidal anti- inflammatory drugs (NSAIDs) may increase the risk of kidney disease.

St. John's Wort

Uses St. John's wort has historically been used for depression.

Mechanism of Action The two active ingredients are hypericin and hyperforin, which inhibit the reuptake of serotonin, norepinephrine, and dopamine as well as neurotransmitters.

Clinical Studies St. John's wort appears to be more effective than a placebo (an inactive substance) and as effective as standard antidepressant medications for mild and moderate depression. It's uncertain whether this is true for severe depression and for time periods longer than 12 weeks.[22]

Adverse Effects These include gastrointestinal (GI) symptoms, dizziness, and confusion. Phototoxicity may occur with ingestion of high doses.

Herb/Supplement—Drug Interactions There is a significant interaction with cyclosporine, oral anticoagulants, oral contraceptives, and certain antiretroviral agents including indinavir due to SJW ability to induce the cytochrome P450 3A4 enzyme system. The concomitant use of SJW with standard antidepressants is also contraindicated because of the risk of serotonergic syndrome.

Chamomile

Uses Chamomile has been used for GI discomfort, peptic ulcer disease, pediatric colic, mild anxiety, and insomnia.

Mechanism of Action Chamomile may act via binding to central benzodiazepine receptors and has anti-inflammatory and antioxidant effects.

Clinical Studies There is limited evidence about chamomile's effect on sleep quality and on insomnia. Based on a 2019 systematic review, chamomile might help improve the individual component of sleep quality over a 4-week period in people without insomnia, but the only study that specifically investigated the effect of chamomile in people experiencing insomnia did not find any benefit.[23]

Adverse Effects Several cases of significant allergic reactions to chamomile have been reported; no significant toxicity has been reported.

Herb/Supplement—Drug Interactions Reported interactions are known between chamomile and cyclosporine and warfarin and there are suspicions that chamomile might interact with other drugs as well. Patients should carefully review their list of medications with their primary care providers before using chamomile.

Elderberry (Sambucus)

Uses Elderberry has been popular for treating upper respiratory infections and fevers, and to help expectoration in bronchitis and asthma.

Mechanism of Action Elderberry inhibits H1N1 influenza activities by binding to H1N1 virions and blocking host cell recognition and entry. Elderberry showed mild inhibitory effect at the early stages of the influenza virus cycle, with considerably stronger effect in the post-infection phase. It blocks viral glycoproteins and increases the expression of interleukin 6, interleukin 8, and tumor necrosing factor.

Clinical Studies Elderberry may not reduce the risk of developing upper respiratory infections, but it may reduce the duration and severity of upper respiratory infections.[24]

Adverse Effects Adverse effects include nausea, vomiting, stomach cramps, dizziness, and weakness.

Herb/Supplement—Drug Interactions Elderberry has no known severe, serious, or moderate interactions with other drugs.

Echinacea (E. angustifolia, E. pallida, E. purpurea)

Uses *Echinacea* has been used for the treatment of upper respiratory infections, and as a topical analgesic for snake bites, stings, and burns. It has become popular as a natural immune booster.

Mechanism of Action *Echinacea* protects the integrity of the hyaluronic acid matrix and by stimulating the alternate complement pathway where it can promote nonspecific T-cell activation by binding to T cells and increasing interferon production. The polysaccharides arabinogalactan and echinacin are the active ingredients of *Echinacea* and therefore, may have immune-modulating effects on the body. Other ingredients include glycosides, alkaloids, alkylamides, polyacetylenes, and fatty acids that may inhibit viral replication, improve the motility of polymorphonuclear cells, and enhance phagocytosis.

Clinical Studies One Cochrane review of a total of 24 prevention and acute treatment studies on a large variety of echinacea monopreparations reported weak evidence that *Echinacea* can prevent or treat upper respiratory infections.[25] Individuals with progressive systemic diseases such as multiple sclerosis, tuberculosis, systemic lupus erythematosus, autoimmune diseases, and human immunodeficiency virus (HIV) infection should not use *Echinacea* because of its possible immunomodulation.

Adverse Effects These include skin rash, GI distress, and diarrhea.

Herb/Supplement—Drug Interactions *Echinacea* should not be used in individuals on immunosuppressant medications.

Melatonin

Uses Melatonin has been used for jet lag, insomnia, shift work disorder, circadian rhythm disorders in the individuals who are visually impaired, and to limit the symptoms of benzodiazepine and nicotine withdrawal.[26]

Mechanism of Action Melatonin appears to increase the binding of GABA to its GABA receptors.

Clinical Studies Melatonin improves sleep in subjects notably in those with attention deficit hyperactivity disorder, autism, and for individuals receiving cancer treatment.[27–29]

Adverse Effects These include inhibition of ovulation, impair glucose utilization, and a decrease in prothrombin activity. Concomitant use of melatonin with alcohol, benzodiazepines, or other sedative drugs might cause additive sedation.

Herb/Supplement—Drug Interactions Melatonin has no known severe, serious, or moderate interactions with other drugs.

Glucosamine

Uses People use glucosamine sulfate orally to treat osteoarthritis (OA) and other chronic joint conditions.[30]

Mechanism of Action Sulfate is required for articular cartilage glycosaminoglycan synthesis. Glucosamine sulfate might be responsible for its effect on osteoarthritis by increasing serum and synovial sulfate levels.

Clinical Studies Most studies showing symptomatic improvement secondary to glucosamine sulfate treatment were generally of lower quality and small sample size, making it difficult to draw conclusions. The remaining, larger studies hold a high probability of bias, as the majority appears to have been sponsored by corporations manufacturing these formulations. Moreover, the heterogeneity between studies examining the capacity of oral glucosamine sulfate as an OA therapy is prohibitive of pooling data and validating conclusions. The verdict regarding the use of the supplement as an adjunct osteoarthritis therapy remains unclear.[31]

Adverse Effects Bloating, constipation, cramps, diarrhea, heartburn, and nausea are some of the side effects noted and there have been rare reports of severe allergic reactions and hepatotoxicity.

Herb/Supplement—Drug Interactions It may increase the effects of warfarin, leading to an increase in bruising and serious bleeding. Glucosamine may interfere with certain cancer drugs, known as topoisomerase II inhibitors such as doxorubicin, etoposide, teniposide, mitoxantrone, and daunorubicin.

Probiotics

Uses Prokaryotic organisms are known as probiotics. In the gastrointestinal tract, these organisms help metabolize food and maintain intestinal health. Probiotics may be taken as supplements or found in foods. Probiotics are nonpathogenic, living microbes that are thought to provide a therapeutic benefit to the host. Probiotics are found in supplements, as well as in foods such as cheese, kefir, kimchi, kombucha, miso, sauerkraut, and yogurt.

Mechanism of Action Probiotics are thought to be able to block pathogenic bacteria from finding a spot on the host tissue to bind and grow. When taken orally, probiotics such as *Lactobacilli* pass through the gut and attach to the intestinal mucosa where they can persist for at least a week. Once the *Lactobacilli* latch on to and colonize the intestinal or urogenital tract, epithelial attachment by pathogenic bacteria is reduced. Potential mechanisms by which *Lactobacilli* may be having their beneficial effects are by increasing epithelial mucus production and competing with pathogens for mucosal binding sites.[32]

Clinical Studies Probiotics may produce bacteriocidal proteins (bacteriocins) as well as lactic acid, hydrogen peroxide, and acetic acid, which can interfere with bacterial colonization. Probiotics may have antidiabetic affect by producing short-chain fatty acids during the anaerobic fermentation of fiber. Short-chain fatty acids are thought to act like signaling molecules involved in the activation of glucagon-like peptide-1 and gut hormone peptide tyrosine-tyrosine, leading to insulin secretion and increased cellular uptake of glucose.[33]

Clinical studies have shown that probiotics may be effective for the treatment of abdominal pain, antibiotic-associated diarrhea, atopic dermatitis, bacterial vaginosis, clostridium difficile, colic, constipation, and *Helicobacter pylori*.[34]

Adverse Effects For most people with an intact immune system, probiotics do not carry the risk of infections. There have been rare occurrences where patients who took probiotics were subject to fungemia, bacteremia, and endocarditis, mostly in patients severely ill, immunocompromised, and/or with indwelling or central venous catheters. Research has revealed the most documented probiotics to cause fungemia to be *Saccharomyces cerevisiae* and *Saccharomyces boulardii*. Studies also show that bacteremia and sepsis resulted from various *Lactobacillus* strains, *S. boulardii*, *S. cerevisiae*, *Bacillus subtilis*, and *Bifidobacterium breve*. Endocarditis caused by probiotics may be caused by *Lactobacillus* and *Streptococcus*.[35]

Herb/Supplement—Drug Interactions Probiotics may interact with antibiotics and antifungals.

● CONCLUSION

Herbs and dietary supplements are frequently used in our patient populations. In addition to understanding the issues around regulation and safety, the following four take-home points will help the provider in creating a framework for discussing herbs and dietary supplements use with their patients and their families.

FOUR TAKE-HOME POINTS/TALKING WITH PATIENTS ABOUT HERBS AND DIETARY SUPPLEMENTS

1. **Be open-minded.** Most patients are reluctant to share information about their use of herbs and dietary supplements because they are concerned their healthcare providers will disapprove. By remaining open-minded, you can learn a lot about your patient's use of herbs and dietary supplements.

2. **Ask the question.** Ask every patient about their use of herbs and dietary supplements during routine history taking. One approach is simply to inquire, "Are you doing anything else for this condition?" It is an open-ended question that gives the patient the opportunity to tell you about their use of herbs and dietary supplements. Another approach is to simply ask, "Are you taking any over-the-counter remedies such as herbs or dietary supplements?"

3. **Do not dismiss any therapy as a placebo.** If a patient tells you about use of an herb or dietary supplement that you are unaware of, make a note of it in and schedule a follow-up visit after you have learned more—when you will be in a better position to provide accurate feedback. If you determine the use of an herb or dietary supplement might be harmful, you will have to ask the patient to stop using it. If it is not harmful and the patient feels better using it, you may want to consider incorporating the herb or dietary supplement into your documented care plan.

4. **Discuss herbs and dietary supplements with your patients at every visit.** People may change their use of herbs and supplements over time. Asking at every visit will alert your patient that you are interested and need to know what they are taking and it may also help alert you to potential complications before they occur.

CASE STUDY ANSWERS

1. **Yes;** There is some data to support the use of creatine (moderate level of evidence, modest effect on muscle mass/strength in combination with resistance training), melatonin (moderate level of evidence for insomnia in specific medical conditions, i.e., cancer patients, ADHD) and St. John's wort (moderate level of evidence for lowering depressive symptoms; however only studies short duration i.e., ≤12 weeks) but no consistent evidence for echinacea (weak evidence for efficacy on prevention or treatment of infectious diseases). Contraindications for creatine are preexisting renal disease, for melatonin people should avoid taking with concomitant use of prescribed sleep medication, and for St. John's wort it is contraindicated with a combined use of SSRIs.

2. As with all herbs and dietary supplements, the interaction with prescribed or over-the-counter medications should be discussed. The patient should be advised that the products used must be free from contaminants, consistently produced with quality control measures in place, with an option for child-proof caps and accurate labeling with an expiration date.

3. The Food and Drug Administration (FDA) has limited authority to protect patients from potential harm regarding supplements. Under the current regulatory system, i.e., the 1994 Dietary Supplement Health and Education Act (which classified dietary supplements under the broad regulatory framework of food rather than drugs), herbs and dietary supplements are not tested for safety or effectiveness.

REFERENCES

1. Clarke TC, Black LI, Stussman BJ, Barnes PM, Nahin RL. Trends in the use of complementary health approaches among adults: United States, 2002–2012. National health statistics reports; no 79. National Center for Health Statistics; 2015.

2. Marinac JS, Buchinger CL, Godfrey LA, Wooten JM, Sun C, Willsie SK. Herbal products and dietary supplements: a survey of use, attitudes, and knowledge among older adults. *J Am Osteopath Assoc.* 2007 Jan;107(1):13-20; quiz 21-3.

3. Restani P, Di Lorenzo C, Garcia-Alvarez A, et al. The PlantLIBRA consumer survey: findings on the use of plant food supplements in Italy. *PLoS One.* 2018;13(1):e0190915.

4. Stierman B, Mishra S, Gahche JJ, Potischman N, Hales CM. Dietary supplement use in children and adolescents aged ≤19 years—United States, 2017–2018. *MMWR Morb Mortal Wkly Rep.* 2020;69:1557-1562.

5. Cuff S, LaBotz M. Legal performance-enhancing substances in children and adolescents: why should we care? *Pediatrics.* 2020 sep;146(3):e2020012278.

6. Robinson N, Blair M, Lorenc A, Gully N, Fox P, Mitchell K. Complementary medicine use in multi-ethnic paediatric outpatients. *Complement Ther Clin Pract.* 2008;14(1):17-24.

7. Laiyemo MA, Nunlee-Bland G, Adams RG, Laiyemo AO, Lombardo FA. Characteristics and health perceptions of complementary and alternative medicine users in the United States. *Am J Med Sci.* 2015;349(2):140-144.

8. Chao MT, Wade CM. Socioeconomic factors and women's use of complementary and alternative medicine in four racial/ethnic groups. *Ethn Dis.* 2008;18(1):65-71.

9. Lee EL, Richards N, Harrison J, Barnes J. Prevalence of use of traditional, complementary and alternative medicine by the general population: a systematic review of national studies published from 2010 to 2019. *Drug Saf.* 2022 Jul;45(7):713-735.

10. Agu JC, Hee-Jeon Y, Steel A, Adams J. A systematic review of traditional, complementary and alternative medicine use amongst ethnic minority populations: a focus upon prevalence, drivers, integrative use, health outcomes, referrals and use of information sources. *J Immigr Minor Health.* 2019;21(5):1137-1156.

11. Nagata JM, McGuire FH, Lavender JM, et al. Appearance and performance-enhancing drugs and supplements, eating disorders, and muscle dysmorphia among gender minority people. *Int J Eat Disord.* 2022 May;55(5):678-687.

12. Nagata JM, McGuire FH, Lavender JM, et al. Appearance and performance-enhancing drugs and supplements (APEDS): lifetime use and associations with eating disorder and muscle dysmorphia symptoms among cisgender sexual minority people. *Eat Behav.* 2022;44:101595.

13. Shelley BM, Sussman AL, Williams RL, Segal AR, Crabtree BF. "They don't ask me so I don't tell them": patient-clinician communication about traditional, complementary, and alternative medicine. *Ann Family Med.* 2009;7(2):139-147.

14. Swann P. The history of efforts to regulate dietary supplements in the USA. *Drug Test Anal.* 2016;8:271-282.

15. Bravender T. Dietary supplements: caveat emptor redux. *J Adol Health.* 2019;65(4):433-434.

16. Fu PP, Chiang HM, Xia Q, et al. Quality assurance and safety of herbal dietary supplements. *J Environ Sci Health C Environ Carcinog Ecotoxicol Rev.* 2009 Apr;27(2):91-119.

17. Or F, Kim Y, Simms J, Austin SB. Taking stock of dietary supplements' harmful effects on children, adolescents, and young adults. *J Adolesc Health.* 2019;Oct;65(4):455-461.

18. https://ods.od.nih.gov/factsheets/list-all/#.

19. Lanhers C, Pereira B, Naughton G, Trousselard M, Lesage F, Dutheil F. Creatine supplementation and lower limb strength performance: a systematic review and meta-analyses. *Sports Medicine.* 2015;45(9):1285-1294.

20. Kreider RB, Stout JR. Creatine in health and disease. *Nutrients.* 2021;13(2):447.

21. Kreider RB, Kalman DS, Antonio J, et al. International society of sports nutrition position stand: safety and efficacy of creatine supplementation in exercise, sport, and medicine. *J Int Soc Sports Nutr.* 2017;14:18.

22. Linde K, Berner MM, Kriston L. St John's wort for major depression. *Cochrane Database Syst Rev.* 2008 Oct 8;2008(4):CD000448.

23. Hieu TH, Dibas M, Surya Dila KA, et al. Therapeutic efficacy and safety of chamomile for state anxiety, generalized anxiety disorder, insomnia, and sleep quality: a systematic review and meta-analysis of randomized trials and quasi-randomized trials. *Phytother Res.* 2019 Jun;33(6):1604-1615.

24. Wieland LS, Piechotta V, Feinberg T, et al. Elderberry for prevention and treatment of viral respiratory illnesses: a systematic review. *BMC Complement Med Ther.* 2021;21:112.

25. Karsch-Völk M, Barrett B, Kiefer D, et al. Echinacea for preventing and treating the common cold. *Cochrane Database Syst Rev.* 2014;2:CD000530.

26. www.nccih.nih.gov/health/melatonin-what-you-need-to-know.

27. Maras A, Schroder CM, Malow BA, et al. Long-term efficacy and safety of pediatric prolonged-release melatonin for insomnia in children with autism spectrum disorder. *J Child Adolesc Psychopharmacol.* 2018 Dec;28(10):699-710.

28. Esposito S, Laino D, D'Alonzo R, et al. Pediatric sleep disturbances and treatment with melatonin. *J Transl Med.* 2019 Mar 12;17(1):77.

29. Andersen LP, Gögenur I, Rosenberg J, Reiter RJ. The safety of melatonin in humans. *Clin Drug Investig.* 2016 Mar;36(3):169-175.

30. https://www.nccih.nih.gov/health/glucosamine-and-chondroitin-for-osteoarthritis.

31. Zhu X, Sang L, Wu D, Rong J, Jiang L. Effectiveness and safety of glucosamine and chondroitin for the treatment of osteoarthritis: a meta-analysis of randomized controlled trials. *J Orthop Surg Res.* 2018 Jul 06;13(1):170.

32. Shahrokhi M, Nagalli S. Probiotics [Updated 2022 Jul 4]. In: *StatPearls [Internet].* Treasure Island, FL: StatPearls Publishing; 2022 Jan. Available at: https://www.ncbi.nlm.nih.gov/books/NBK553134/.

33. Gomes AC, Bueno AA, de Souza RG, Mota JF. Gut microbiota, probiotics and diabetes. *Nutr J.* 2014 Jun 17;13:60.

34. Probiotics—Health Professional Fact Sheet (nih.gov).

35. Merenstein D, Pot B, Leyer G, et al. Emerging issues in probiotic safety: 2023 perspectives. *Gut Microbes.* 2023 Jan-Dec; 15(1):2185034.

Precision Nutrition

Jordi Merino, PhD / Andrew T. Chan, MD, MPH

Chapter Outline

CASE STUDY

A 26-year-old healthy female with a body mass index of 27.6 kg/m² (weight of 76 kg and height of 166 cm) gained 6 kg last year. She has no major medical conditions other than a history of appendicitis, for which she underwent an appendectomy when she was 15 years old. During her annual physical exam, she asked her primary care physician if she should follow a precision nutrition approach. Her mother was recently diagnosed with type 2 diabetes at age 53 and recalls that most of her relatives older than 60 have type 2 diabetes. Her parents emigrated from Jamaica, and she was born in the United States. She has a Ph.D. in economics, is unemployed, and lives with her fiancée. She heard about these new studies and scientific advances showing the importance of genetics and the gut microbiome in developing obesity and diabetes. She would like to determine if following a precision nutrition approach will help control her body weight and prevent type 2 diabetes in the future.

1. In which medical conditions is there robust evidence supporting precision nutrition?
2. How would you counsel this patient, given the current evidence on precision nutrition in her situation?
3. What are the pros and cons of following a precision nutrition approach?

● INTRODUCTION

What Is Precision Nutrition?

Precision nutrition is an emerging discipline that considers the health effects of diet in the context of human variation. That is, how nutrients, foods, and dietary patterns influence health outcomes based on differences in human biology, lifestyle and environmental variables, and social determinants, defined as the social, physical, and economic factors that impact health. To the extent that a nutrient, food, or diet is more likely to benefit individuals sharing similar characteristics, precision nutrition information may help in recommending specific nutrients, foods, or diets to the subgroup of the population most likely to benefit from exposure to them while limiting those that are potentially harmful.

Precision nutrition is not a new concept, but our ability to implement it effectively and rationally has only recently advanced in a meaningful way over the last decade. The concept of precision nutrition has evolved from an initial focus on individualized therapeutic strategies (personalized nutrition) to a more realistic notion that intends to convey the principle that, although dietary recommendations are rarely developed for single individuals, subgroups of individuals with unique features can be more rigorously defined and subsequently treated in more efficient ways. Indeed, nutrition science has historically focused on these concepts of categorizing and identifying subgroups of individuals. For example, a low-phenylalanine diet is the targeted dietary advice in phenylketonuria, a rare inherited metabolic disorder characterized by the inability to effectively metabolize the amino acid phenylalanine due to mutations affecting the phenylalanine hydroxylase gene. Likewise, the current nutritional treatment for individuals with galactosemia, a disease characterized by the partial incapacity to break down galactose due to genetic defects in the gene that encodes for the galactose-1-phosphate uridyl transferase enzyme, is to limit the intake of foods containing galactose. Aside from inborn errors of metabolism, nutritional stratification is primarily used as a blunt instrument in the general population, as reflected in the current dietary reference intake, in which, for example, recommended intake for vitamins and minerals varies according to age groups, sex, or physiological processes such as pregnancy. Subgroups and categories are increasingly refined due to the massive capture of data points across orthogonal axes of the molecular and environmental space.

Why Is Precision Nutrition Needed?

The sophisticated subgroup characterization consequence of increasing knowledge of disease susceptibility processes stresses the need for refinement and personalization of dietary advice. For example, a post-hoc analysis of the Look AHEAD (Action for Health in Diabetes) study, a multicenter randomized controlled trial designed to determine whether intentional weight loss reduces cardiovascular morbidity and mortality in overweight individuals with type 2 diabetes, showed that individuals with a specific diabetes subtype characterized by

poor baseline glycemic control were less likely to lose weight and benefit from a lifestyle intervention that included dietary modifications.[1] These results suggest that individuals with a diabetes subtype characterized by poor glycemic control could benefit from other therapeutic strategies. The Personalized REsponses to DIetary Composition Trail (PREDICT), a single-arm, multicenter study that enrolled 1,002 healthy individuals in a 14-day intervention consisting of test meal challenges of different nutritional content, found substantial differences between individuals in postprandial responses to identical foods. The population coefficient of variation, a parameter to quantify the dispersion of a measure, which is calculated based on the ratio of the standard deviation to the mean, in postprandial responses of blood glucose, triacylglycerol, and C-peptide was 68%, 103%, and 59%, respectively.[2]

These two examples illustrate how clinical decision making based on extrapolating average responses from clinical trials can often be misleading. While current treatment guidelines have been developed with the "average" patient in mind, there is now ample evidence supporting that the same intervention results in different effects and outcomes from one individual to another. As shown in Figure 8-1, for any given intervention, only a small proportion of people will likely respond in a manner that resembles the "average" patient. In principle, precision nutrition will eventually allow clinicians to determine the optimal nutritional intervention course for any given patient at any given time rather than providing nutritional recommendations based on the extrapolation of average responses.

The need for new or more efficient dietary and lifestyle approaches is magnified by the continuing rise of obesity and related complications, including diabetes and cardiovascular diseases, which are still the leading cause of death in the United States and worldwide. To combat this epidemic, dietary guidelines endorse dietary patterns rich in fruits and vegetables, whole grains, nuts, legumes, and seafood and recommend

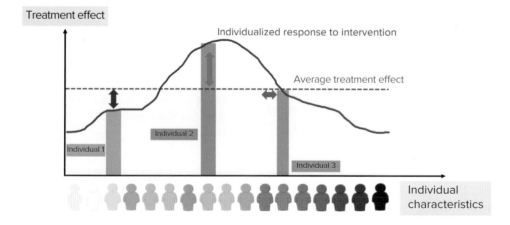

FIGURE 8-1 • Inter-individual differences lead to a variable response to current therapeutic strategies. This hypothetical figure illustrates how people with different characteristics respond to therapeutic interventions. The dotted red line represents the average intervention effect documented in clinical studies. Most people will either under- or over-respond to the intervention (defined as individuals #1 and #2 here). Only a small proportion of participants (represented as individual #3) respond in a manner that resembles the average response. Precision nutrition is needed to identify the characteristics that make people respond differently to dietary interventions and determine the optimal intervention course for any given patient at any given time.

reduced intakes of refined and ultra-processed foods to prevent and manage many diseases. However, the efficacy of diet interventions diminishes over time, and the initial cardiovascular benefit of adhering to a healthy diet is usually not sustained after 1 year. The large inter-individual variability in response to diet, combined with strong physiological adaptations that occur after weight loss and the perceived amount of effort, time, and resources needed to sustain a healthy diet in the current obesogenic environment, can explain the low long-term adherence to current dietary recommendations and the high rate of relapse among people who have initially lost weight (also see Chapter 17, "Overweight and Obesity"). However, precision nutrition could be applied to many other health conditions and preventative approaches.

● NEW TOOLS AND TECHNOLOGIES TO CAPTURE INTER-INDIVIDUAL VARIABILITY

Deep Molecular Profiling

The foundation for a new era of precision nutrition has been facilitated by recent technological advances in "'omics" and wearable monitoring that enable deep molecular, physiological, and lifestyle profiling. One early step toward the historical change in the global reach of biological inquiry started just a few decades ago with the Human Genome Project, whose major contribution was to provide the world with a complete resource of detailed information about the structure, organization, and function of human genes. Led by genomics, other high-throughput technologies have emerged recently, providing comprehensive information about the transcriptome, epigenome, proteome, microbiome, and metabolome.

Genome-wide association studies (GWASs) have identified hundreds of thousands of regions across the human genome associated with many complex diseases.[3] However, the underlying molecular mechanisms for most associations remain unclear. Many recent studies have investigated the molecular mechanisms through integrative analysis of GWAS and omics data. These integrative studies have helped prioritize putative causal variants, genes, molecular pathways, tissues, and cell types of action for GWAS associations. This information allows investigators to explore complementary biological axes in greater breadth and depth.

Wearable Devices

Metabolic diseases like diabetes are conditions in which real-time physiologic monitoring is essential for diagnosis and therapy. In diabetes, for example, logbooks have been historically used to monitor glucose levels, insulin doses, food intake, or exercise. Wearable, noninvasive biosensors for continuously monitoring glucose, metabolites, nutrients, or other analytes that change in response to environmental stimuli are key in realizing the promise of precision nutrition.

By measuring interstitial glucose every 5–15 minutes, continuous glucose monitors (CGMs) can provide a complete picture of individuals' dynamic glycemic profiles throughout the day. The in-depth glycemic insights and direct feedback provided by CGMs have proven efficacious in lowering elevated HbA1c and reducing the incidence of hypoglycemia in individuals with type 1 diabetes and type 2 diabetes. Further, metrics such as time in range (the percentage of time that a person spends with their blood glucose levels in a target range (70 to 140 mg/dl)), the 2-hour incremental area under the glucose curve (a metric broadly used to characterize glycemic responses to meals), peak glucose concentration, the number of peaks in each day, or the morphology of these peaks, can be used to investigate the impact of glycemic variability on health outcomes (Figure 8-2). For example, the time in range has been associated with the risk of developing microvascular complications among individuals with type 1 diabetes and represents a valuable metric for understanding glucose level fluctuations in response to external stimuli.

With the increased use and demand for CGMs for the management of diabetes, questions have been raised regarding their utility and value among healthy individuals. A 2018 study that included 57 healthy participants found that many individuals considered nondiabetic by standard measures showed high glucose variability.[4] The study found that severe glucose variability was present in one-quarter of normoglycemic individuals, with glucose levels reaching prediabetic ranges up to 15% of the duration of CGM recordings. A 2019 study including 153 healthy individuals with about 1 week of CGM monitoring found that participants spent 96% of the time within the normal glycemic range.[5] While the study reinforces the argument that there is, in fact, tight glucose control among healthy individuals, the study also showed that half of the included participants had at least one hyperglycemic event, defined as a glucose level above 180 mg/dL. These findings seem to support the notion that a better picture of glycemic variability and fluctuations could identify individuals at increased risk of developing diabetes and related metabolic abnormalities.

New tools and technologies are needed to monitor other biomarkers beyond glucose that change in response to diet. Human sweat has attracted attention as an important body fluid containing a wealth of chemicals that are reflective of nutritional and metabolic conditions, which can be used as a medium to indirectly reflect health status. A recent study using a wearable electrochemical biosensor of graphene electrodes enabled the real-time monitoring of amino acids, vitamins, metabolites, lipids, hormones, and drugs during physical exercise. While technology matures, wearables capable of monitoring temporal chemical variations upon food intake and supplements are excellent candidates to bridge the gap between digital and biochemical analyses for a successful precision nutrition approach.

Recent advances in wearable trackers and mobile phone applications enable the monitoring of dietary habits, physical activity, and sleep with great potential to influence behavioral changes. For example, in the PREDICT study, the use of a wearable device with a triaxial accelerometer to monitor activity and sleep showed that specific sleep features such as poor sleep efficiency and later bedtime were associated with more pronounced postprandial glycemic responses.[6] The study also

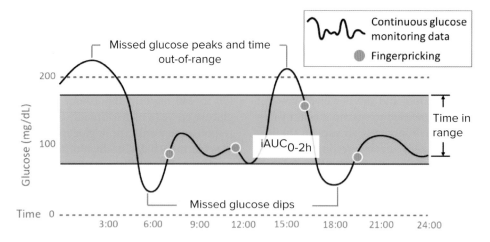

FIGURE 8-2 • Continuous glucose monitoring provides an in-depth characterization of glycemic response to external stimuli. By measuring interstitial glucose every 5–15 min, CGMs better characterize dynamic glycemic profiles than single time-in-point glucose measurements such as fingerpicking. A challenge for a single point-in-time glucose determination is that it provides a lack of information from one determination to the next. CGMs enable us to fill the gap of what's happening between determinations. In addition, to provide a dynamic view of glycemic variability throughout the day, CGM data can be used to explore additional metrics related to glycemic fluctuations, such as peak glucose concentration, the number of peaks in each day, or the morphology of these peaks, nadirs below baseline glucose, or time in range of optimal glucose levels. These features are beneficial for individuals with diabetes, primarily type 1 diabetes, as people can adjust medications based on this information. In addition, using CGMs in people without diabetes could provide a better picture of detrimental glucose response to specific exposures, which is linked to the risk of developing obesity, diabetes, and cardiovascular disease. (Adapted from Heo YJ, Kim S-H. Toward long-term implantable glucose biosensors for clinical use. *App Sci.* 2019;9(10):2158.)

showed that a person's deviation from their usual sleep pattern is associated with poorer glycemic responses. These findings underscore the importance of physical activity and sleep monitoring in developing predictive algorithms for precision nutrition.

Importance of the Postprandial State

The rationale to assess postprandial glucose and lipids has become increasingly evident due to initial epidemiological data showing that nonfasting determinations are an independent predictor of cardiovascular disease and, in some studies, more closely related to the risk of major cardiovascular events than glucose or triglycerides measured in the fasting state. For example, the Diabetes Epidemiology: Collaborative Analysis of Diagnostic Criteria in Europe (DECODE) study analyzed data from 10 prospective European cohort studies that included up to 22,000 participants. The authors concluded that 2-hour glucose values were a better predictor than fasting glucose of death from all causes and cardiovascular disease, with the most significant number of excess deaths being observed in patients showing impaired glucose tolerance after a 2-hour oral glucose test but normal fasting glucose levels.

Postprandial lipemia, characterized by a rise in triglyceride-rich lipoproteins after eating, is a dynamic, nonsteady-state condition with a rapid remodeling of lipoproteins in which humans spend most of their time. There are several lines of evidence suggesting that postprandial lipemia increases the risk of atherogenesis and cardiovascular complications. Mechanistic studies demonstrate that triglyceride-rich lipoprotein remnants may adversely affect the endothelium and penetrate the subendothelial space. Clinical data show the effect of remodeled postprandial lipoproteins on the progression of carotid atherosclerosis and coronary artery disease.

RECENT ADVANCES IN PRECISION NUTRITION

Evidence from Gene-Diet Interaction Studies

Previous studies have yielded convincing examples of how environmental pressures have enriched the human genome with specific variants that could affect an individual's response to therapeutic interventions. For example, a scan of Greenlandic Inuit genomes revealed signals at several loci for signatures of adaptation to a diet rich in polyunsaturated fatty acids, with the strongest signal located in a cluster of fatty acid desaturases (FADS). Due to a diet based on fatty fish, which is rich in long-chain polyunsaturated fatty acids (i.e., arachidonic acid and eicosapentaenoic acid), adaptation and selection have favored alleles that increase levels of short-chain polyunsaturated fatty acids (i.e., linoleic acid and α-linolenic acid) as these fatty acids were rarely incorporated by diet. Elsewhere, a common risk haplotype in the *SLC16A11* locus among people of Mexican or Latin American descent, but rare among Europeans and absent in Africa, is associated with ~a 20% increased T2D risk. Carriers of the risk haplotype have low plasma levels of monocarboxylate transporter 11 (the protein encoded by *SLC16A11*) in the plasma membrane of hepatocytes. Under energy overload, there is a metabolic shift toward triacylglycerol accumulation. Those with this gene variant might have been more efficiently able to store energy from the available food in times of food insecurity. This may have led to natural selection favoring those who carried this "thrifty" gene variant and could account for the notable frequency of the variant in contemporary Mexicans. While population-wide dietary advice to avoid energy-dense foods is beneficial in reducing the risk of obesity and diabetes, limiting energy intake could be particularly valuable among carriers of this risk haplotype.

Beyond specific genetic variants interacting with diet on the development of complex diseases, a critical question is whether genetic predisposition according to multiple common variants could be relevant to identifying groups of individuals more likely to benefit from targeted nutritional recommendations (Figure 8-3). Polygenic scores, also known as genetic risk scores, represent a quantitative measure of genetic risk to disease and thus could be used to identify individuals sharing similar characteristics. Polygenic scores are often generated by computing the sum of an individual's risk alleles, weighted by the risk allele effect sizes estimated in a genome-wide association study on the phenotype. Epidemiological studies have demonstrated that polygenic scores for virtually all diseases and conditions are independently associated with these outcomes and often can predict long-term risk above clinical factors. For example, individuals at the top 2–5% distribution of polygenic scores for type 2 diabetes, cancer, or cardiovascular disease have a ~threefold increased disease risk indicated by their respective polygenic risk scores.

Previous epidemiological studies support that certain dietary or lifestyle factors such as unhealthy dietary patterns, high consumption of sugar-sweetened drinks or fried foods, and levels of physical inactivity might modify how much someone with elevated polygenic scores for high BMI is at risk of developing obesity. These studies show, for example, that the genetic association with high adiposity appeared to be more pronounced with a greater intake of sugar-sweetened beverages.[7] The relative risk of obesity per 10 risk alleles in the polygenic score was five times higher among individuals consuming one or more sugar-sweetened beverages per day compared to those consuming less than one serving per month. These data suggest that individuals sharing an increased genetic predisposition to obesity are more susceptible to the deleterious effects of sugar-sweetened beverages than people at lower genetic risk, supporting the use of polygenic scores to identify subsets of individuals who would particularly benefit from reducing or avoiding sugar-sweetened beverages.

Contrary to obesity, evidence on the interaction of dietary and lifestyle exposures with polygenic scores for type 2 diabetes is less convincing. In a prospective study including male health professionals, the association between a polygenic score for type 2 diabetes and the risk of the disease was amplified by a Western dietary pattern, suggesting that individuals at increased genetic risk for type 2 diabetes could significantly benefit from avoiding a Western dietary pattern. However, no evidence of significant interactions was detected between genetic risk and the Mediterranean diet on the development of diabetes in the longitudinal study using data from the EPIC-InterAct consortia. Null findings were also reported in an individual-participant-data meta-analysis, including data from up to 102,000 individuals from 15 prospective studies followed during a median follow-up of 12 years. The study showed that genetic risk and dietary fat quality were each associated with the development of type 2 diabetes with no evidence of interactions. In the Diabetes Prevention Program, a lifestyle intervention effectively prevents type 2 diabetes, regardless of genetic susceptibility to diabetes or glycemic traits.[8] A recent observational study in UK Biobank showed that diet was associated with incident diabetes within and across genetic risk groups. These findings support the notion that genetic risk does not modify the beneficial effect of nutritional interventions. However, the lack of significant interactions reported in these studies could be attributed to the influence of a heterogenous mixture of genetic variants affecting divergent pathways into a single score.

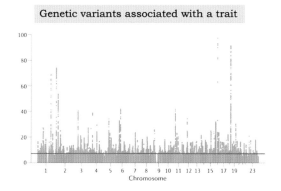

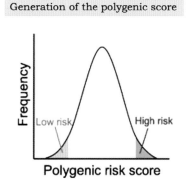

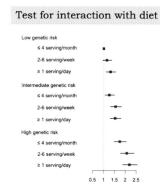

FIGURE 8-3 • Interplay between genetic and dietary factors in the development of metabolic diseases. Genome-wide association studies have identified genetic variants associated with metabolic traits and diseases. These genetic variants could be used to generate polygenic scores. Polygenic scores, which provide a quantitative measure of genetic risk, are often generated by computing the sum of an individual's risk alleles, weighted by the risk allele effect sizes estimated in a genome-wide association study on the phenotype (left panel). These polygenic scores (middle panel) could be used to investigate whether genetic susceptibility to a disease is either attenuated or amplified by specific dietary exposures. In this hypothetical example, consuming sugar-sweetened beverages amplified the genetic risk for obesity (right panel): individuals with similar genetic risk had higher disease risk when consuming ≥ 1 serving/day compared to ≤ 4 servings/month.

Studies in other complex diseases, such as cardiovascular disease, mental health disorders, or cancer, have reached similar conclusions. In a landmark study including 55,685 participants from three different epidemiological studies in Europe and the United States, genetic and lifestyle factors were independently associated with susceptibility to coronary artery disease. The study showed that a healthy lifestyle characterized by a healthy diet, no current smoking, no obesity, and regular physical activity was associated with a nearly 50% lower risk of coronary artery disease than an unhealthy lifestyle, regardless of genetic risk for coronary artery disease. Lourida et al. conducted a retrospective study to investigate whether a healthy lifestyle was associated with a lower risk of dementia and how genetic susceptibility to dementia modified these associations. The study included 196,383 participants of European ancestry aged at least 60 years without dementia at baseline. They found that participants with high genetic risk and unhealthy lifestyle had a twofold increased risk for dementia compared with participants with low genetic risk and a healthy lifestyle score. They also documented that a healthy lifestyle score was associated with a lower risk of dementia, and there was no significant interaction between genetic risk and a healthy lifestyle.

Research on the interplay between genetics and diet in cancer has also provided mostly null findings. A review of the literature investigating gene-diet interactions in five common cancers (breast, lung, prostate, colorectal, and stomach) concluded that there is null evidence for strong gene-diet interactions in most common cancer types, except for interaction between processed meat intake and the 10p14 locus (rs4143094, near *GATA3*) in colorectal cancer risk, which was classified as moderate certainty. In a recent study including 100,220 individuals from the China Kadoorie Biobank, both increased genetic risk and unhealthy lifestyle were independently associated with gastric cancer. The study showed that participants with a high genetic risk for gastric cancer, based on a polygenic score including 112 genetic variants, and a favorable lifestyle had ~50% lower risk of gastric cancer than those with high genetic risk and an unfavorable lifestyle after 10 years of follow-up. The study also failed to show evidence of significant interactions between genetic risk and lifestyle factors, suggesting that a healthy lifestyle is associated with a lower risk of gastric cancer regardless of genetic susceptibility. The same observations were reported in a study using polygenic scores for colon cancer, showing a risk gradient with increased genetic risk and unhealthy lifestyle components similar to the addition of each factor separately.[9]

In conclusion, while genetic and dietary factors may interact in ways that can be difficult to disentangle with current methods, these studies suggest that genetic variation alone is not enough to target dietary recommendations and that more holistic approaches through the integration of alternative biological, environmental, and social metrics are needed to target dietary advice.

Evidence from Diet and Gut Microbiome Studies

In parallel with the identification of genetic profiles for precision nutrition applications, there is a growing interest in discovering gut microbiota signatures that interact with or mediate the effect of diet on obesity and related complex diseases.

The human gut microbiome is a complex ecosystem consisting of tens of trillions of microorganisms, mainly bacteria, but also viruses, fungi, and protozoa.[10] A key feature of the gut microbiome is the dynamic nature of its composition, which allows it to facilitate adaptation to a range of environments. For example, a shift from animal to plant protein-based diets has increased the abundance of microorganisms that metabolize plant polysaccharides after only 5 days. Further, the pervasive influence of the microbiota on host physiology, together with resilience to temporal changes documented in dietary intervention studies, suggests some degree of host control in the gut microbiota.

Following the discovery in 2006 that a transferrable obesity-associated microbiota can induce weight gain in lean mice,[11] subsequent epidemiological studies have shown differences in the gut microbiota of humans with obesity and type 2 diabetes. A metagenome-wide association study showed that the abundance of Bacteroides thetaiotaomicron, a glutamate-fermenting commensal, was markedly decreased in individuals with obesity and was inversely correlated with serum glutamate concentration. A separate study showed that a shift in microbiome composition away from butyrate-production species is associated with an increased risk of diabetes even after adjusting for BMI and lifestyle characteristics. However, whether obesity-associated aberrant microbiota is involved in disease causation in humans or is a secondary phenomenon has been widely debated.

The Men's Lifestyle Validation Study, a sub-study of the long-running Health Professionals Follow-Up Study, represents one of the most comprehensive biorepositories to validate some of these previous observations and identify gut microbiota signatures that interact with or mediate the effect of diet on complex diseases. By leveraging longitudinal metagenomics and metatranscriptomics profiles from 307 healthy men, a recent study showed that the cardioprotective benefits of the Mediterranean diet are particularly relevant among individuals with decreased abundance of Prevotella copri in the gut.[12] The study documented that higher adherence to the Mediterranean diet was associated with a reduced risk of myocardial infarction only among those with decreased abundance of *P. copri*. In a separate study from the same cohort to investigate the links between diet, gut microbiome, and systematic inflammation, the authors showed that fiber intake was associated with significantly greater C-reactive protein (CRP) reduction in individuals carrying a low abundance of *P. copri* in the gut. In contrast, those with higher *P. copri* carriage maintained stable CRP levels regardless of fiber intake. In another study, there was evidence that a higher habitual intake of red meat was significantly associated with increased HbA1c levels only among participants with a microbial profile enriched with trimethylamine N-oxide (TMAO) producing bacteria. Elsewhere, a gut microbiome signature including 21 fiber-fermentation bacteria mediated 60% of the beneficial effect of a healthy diet on the risk of type 2 diabetes.

Emerging evidence also implicates the gut microbiota as an important effector in the relationship between diet and cancer. Recent data indicate that changes in the intestinal microbiome allow dietary and environmental risk factors to initiate and promote colorectal cancer, probably because changes in the microbiome affect metabolism and immune function. These studies suggest that increased consumption of whole grains is associated with a higher abundance of short-chain fatty acids (SCFA) producing bacteria, a lower abundance of proinflammatory bacteria, and higher levels of fecal SCFAs.[13] Given the shared microbes in the synthesis of SCFA and ferulic acid (the most abundant phenolic compound in whole grains), synergistic mechanisms might augment the production of beneficial metabolites and might account for the ability of whole grains to reduce colorectal cancer risk compared with other food sources of dietary fiber. Evidence linking colorectal cancer, gut microbiome, and other nutrients or foods is less convincing, as is evidence for microbiome associations with other cancers such as breast or prostate cancer. However, the recognition that dietary interventions can modify the gut microbiome and influence the efficacy and safety of novel immunotherapeutic drugs provides the framework to continue defining the optimal nutritional interventions that are specific to the rapidly emerging array of treatment regimens.

Observational studies have been complemented with fecal microbiota transplantation (FMT) studies demonstrating that transplantation of feces from twins discordant for obesity into germ-free mice transfers, in a diet-dependent manner, the phenotype of the human donor to the recipient animal. A previous study has found that FMT from lean donors to individuals with obesity and metabolic syndrome improves insulin sensitivity, a transient effect associated with changes in microbiota composition and fasting plasma metabolites. A recent randomized clinical trial to evaluate the efficacy and safety of autologous FMT in preventing weight regain over 14 months showed that diet-induced weight loss and glycemic control could be preserved for months after a diet via autologous FMT capsules.[14] In this randomized controlled trial, 90 obese participants were randomized into three different dietary interventions combined with an exercise regimen to induce weight loss over 6 months. Participants who lost weight in each of the three dietary groups provided a stool sample at the 6-month time point for the preparation of autologous FMT. Participants remained on their initial diets but included encapsulated autologous FMT or placebo every week for 8 months. Participants receiving the autologous FMT also maintained improvements in metabolic parameters, which was associated with a preservation of gut microbial changes that were seen 6 months after weight loss.

While these findings support the current body of evidence that gut microbiota has a role in weight gain and metabolism, many questions remain. There has been no evidence that FMT can induce weight loss in obese patients or prevent diabetes or cardiovascular disease among those at increased risk. Efforts should be undertaken to standardize further the FMT procedure (i.e., its dose-response, mode of delivery, pretreatment), donor-acceptor combination, or concomitant lifestyle or medication.

Evidence from Diet and Multiomics Studies

Beyond single omics approaches, clinical studies collecting personal, dense, and dynamic data inspire new venues for complex disease prevention and treatment through a better understanding of inter-individual variability (Table 8-1). Figure 8-4 shows a schematic representation of a precision nutrition study. Pioneering research led by Price and colleagues showed that targeted dietary and lifestyle recommendations based on data from the whole genome sequence, metabolomics, proteomics, microbiome, clinical tests, and daily activity tracking resulted in a modest improvement in glycemic control after a 9-month follow-up period.[15] The iPOP study (integrative Personalized Omics Profiling), a longitudinal prospective cohort including 109 participants at increased risk of type 2 diabetes, showed that deep longitudinal profiling could lead to actionable findings, such as improved characterization of the diabetes status by the identification of mechanisms of glucose dysregulation.[16]

The Personalized Nutrition Project showed that a machine learning algorithm synthesizing data from diverse sources, including blood biomarkers, diets, anthropometry, physical activity, and the gut microbiome, could predict individual glycemic responses to meals in 800 free-living individuals.[17] The algorithm, validated in an independent cohort of 100 participants, predicted individual postprandial glycemic responses better than models based on other approaches, such as carbohydrate counting or glycemic index scores. In a follow-up double-blinded randomized crossover trial, 26 individuals were randomly assigned to receive dietary recommendations from a clinical dietitian based on their expert interpretation of postprandial glucose response to meals during a profiling week or to receive dietary advice based on the machine learning algorithm. In both instances, participants were provided with a dietary recommendation for one week that was likely to be beneficial to postprandial glucose responses and one that was likely to be disadvantageous. The trial showed that some postprandial glucose response variables were lower during the week participants consumed the predicted beneficial diet based on the machine learning algorithm developed in the first phase.[17]

The recent PREDICT study showed a similarly wide variation in postprandial responses to identical foods. It demonstrated that people who display poor metabolic responses to a given food are likely to respond poorly to other similar foods.[2] Meal composition and genetic factors were the main predictors of postprandial glycemic responses. In contrast, serum lipid, glycemic markers, and gut microbiome explained the larger variation in postprandial lipid and c-peptide responses. Taken together, these results provide proof of concept that a precision nutrition approach is feasible and sets the stage for its application in different therapeutic areas.

While major scientific guidelines already emphasize flexible and culturally adapted healthy dietary patterns for the prevention and management of metabolic diseases, whether there are additional benefits of a precision nutrition approach based on differences in molecular, clinical, and social factors is currently unknown. A recent clinical study was designed to

TABLE 8-1 • Overview of main precision nutrition studies published to date

Author, year, journal	Participants	Study design/ intervention	Available data	Follow-up	Relevant findings
Zeevi D, 2015, *Cell*	Discovery cohort: 800 healthy and prediabetic participants Validation cohort: 100 healthy and prediabetic participants Clinical validation: 26 participants were randomized to a good/bad diet	Intervention study with standardized and election meals	Gut microbiota, blood tests, lifestyle and medication surveys, anthropometrics.	One-week follow-up for the discovery cohort. The clinical validation consisted of a 2-week intervention.	• High interpersonal variability in post-meal glucose • Implementation of a machine learning approach that accurately predicted glucose response in the validation cohort • Short-term personalized diet intervention successfully lowered post-meal glucose
Price N, 2017, *Nature Biotechnology*	108 individuals (ages 21–89+ years; 59% males, 41% females; 89% of European descent	Longitudinal study with behavioral coaching	Whole genome sequences; clinical tests, metabolomes, proteomes, and microbiomes at three time points	Nine-month follow-up	• Identification of putative biomarkers that can improve understanding of early transition to disease states. • Targeted dietary and lifestyle recommendations resulted in a modest improvement in glycemic control.
Schüssler-Fiorenza Rose SM, 2019, *Nature Medicine*	109 individuals with prediabetes	Longitudinal profiling	Multi-omics assessments, exercise testing, enhanced cardiovascular imaging, physiological testing, wearable sensor monitoring and lifestyle, demographic, and health surveys	Up to 8 years (median, 2.8 years)	• Discovered pathways associated with metabolic, cardiovascular, and oncology pathophysiology • Development of prediction models for insulin resistance using multi-omics • Participants improved diet and physical activity.
Berry SE, 2020, *Nature Medicine*	Discovery cohort: 1,000 healthy participants in the UK Validation cohort: 100 healthy participants in the United States	Clinical trials with standardized and ad libitum meals	Clinical and biochemical parameters, gut microbiome, genetics, metabolomics, meal composition, habitual diet, meal context, and anthropometrics	Two weeks of duration, including a full clinical day	• Population coefficient of variation in postprandial responses of blood triglyceride, glucose, and c-peptide following identical meals was 103%, 68%, and 59%, respectively. • Identification of person-specific factors underlying variable nutritional responses. • Development of a machine learning algorithm that accurately predicted glycemic responses in the validation cohort.
Ben-Yacov O, 2021, *Diabetes Care*	225 individuals with prediabetes	Randomized clinical trial. Personalized diet based on predicted glucose responses vs. Mediterranean diet	Main outcomes were changes in time in glucose >140 mg/dl, HbA1c, and OGTT	Six-month dietary intervention period with a 6-month post-intervention follow-up.	• The personalized diet was superior to the Mediterranean diet in terms of HbA1c reduction and daily time spent with glucose at 6 and 12 months.

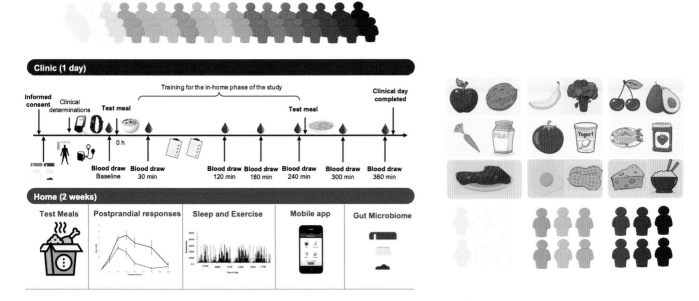

FIGURE 8-4 • Overview of a precision nutrition study.
Precision nutrition studies are often single-arm intervention studies involving the consumption of meals of different nutritional content. Participants usually spend the first day at the clinical center for deep phenotyping. These determinations typically include an array of questionnaires to obtain medical, lifestyle, and social information; anthropometric measurements; and collection of biospecimens for omics profiling. During the study, participants wear digital monitors (i.e., continuous glucose monitors or physical activity and sleep monitors). They are often instructed to record foods and drinks consumed via a phone application and collect additional biospecimens at regular intervals. Collected data would be fed into a predictive algorithm to identify nutrients, foods, and diets with optimal, neutral, or detrimental profiles (denoted as green, yellow, and red). For example (in right side of figure), based on the resulting algorithm, dark-purple individuals would benefit the most from cherries and avocados and should avoid cheese and rice.

address this specific question. The clinical trial included 225 adults with impaired fasting glucose randomized to either a personalized postprandial targeting diet based on a machine learning algorithm that predicted beneficial glucose responses or a Mediterranean diet in a 6-month dietary intervention period with a 6-month post-intervention follow-up.[18] The trial had three primary outcomes: the total time during the day when glucose measured by the CGM was above 7.8 mmol/l; HbA1c; and an oral glucose tolerance test (OGTT) undertaken at home. The between-randomized-group differences were statistically significant for glucose measured by the CGM and for HbA1c but not for the OGTT. The magnitude of the effect seen in the personalized diet group for A1c was 0.16% at six months, which was comparable with that reported in other behavioral intervention studies. Although these findings should be interpreted with caution, as there were marked differences in carbohydrate intake between study groups, this study highlights the potential of precision nutrition to improve glycemic control in prediabetes and reduce the unfavorable impact of postprandial glycemic responses on health outcomes.

FUTURE DIRECTIONS

Whether the promise of the precision nutrition approach is matched by evidence of the long-term beneficial impact remains uncertain. Still, interest and activity in this field are proliferating to identify factors underlying variable nutritional responses and develop algorithms to predict individual responses to nutrients, foods, and dietary patterns. However, important considerations are needed to address before precision nutrition can be implemented for complex disease prevention and care (Box 8-1). For example, precision nutrition should not overturn traditional broad-based nutrition guidelines but instead complement them and add to what we know about nutrition science to prevent and manage chronic diseases. In the same way, that promotion of physical activity and weight loss do not replace the need to adhere to a healthy diet, precision nutrition advice would not exclude the parallel goal of healthy dietary patterns nor replace other evidence-based strategies for decreasing the risk of complex diseases. However, the shift in emphasis to prioritize precision nutrition is essential to reflect the dynamic and divergent nature of responses to dietary interventions and the need to identify targeted strategies to reduce the burden of metabolic diseases.

Second, equitable access to practical precision nutrition advice should be ensured. Among the increasing prevalence of obesity, diabetes, and cardiovascular disease globally, three out of every four people live in low- and middle-income countries, and much of the disease burdens in high-income countries tend to be higher among ethnic minorities or people living in areas with higher deprivation.[19] Precision nutrition has the potential to reduce health disparities by embracing diversity in the design, implementation, and clinical validation of studies. Further, addressing upstream social determinants of health,

BOX 8-1

Top Ten Considerations for the Implementation of Precision Nutrition

- Precision nutrition should be an addition to the parallel goal of population-based nutritional dietary advice for preventing and managing chronic metabolic diseases such as obesity, diabetes, cancer, and cardiovascular disease.
- Scientific scrutiny should precede the introduction of emerging tools for precision nutrition.
- More research is needed to appreciate the clinical importance of glycemic fluctuations in individuals without diabetes and to define normal/abnormal nutritional responses.
- There is a need to go beyond changes in blood glucose levels and monitor other components that change in response to diet.
- Machine learning algorithms to predict nutritional responses may require more than 2 weeks of testing to capture the nuances of dynamic nutritional responses.

- Investment in research programs to depict molecular, behavioral, and social drivers of appetite regulation is needed to increase compliance with dietary advice.
- The success of precision nutrition will be parallel to the regulation of the modern food system and policies that support an environment enabling a healthy lifestyle
- Synergic approaches targeted to the population and individual level that address social determinants of health are needed to ensure equitable access to precision nutrition and reduce health disparities.
- New technologies and methods supporting precision nutrition require careful consideration of the ethical, regulatory, legal, and social implication.
- Collective responsibility is required for the effective implementation of precision nutrition.

particularly those related to the food environment, is critical for helping people sustain targeted dietary advice. Our food system is overflowing with energy-dense and highly palatable foods almost perfectly designed to maximize food reward properties and promote overconsumption. Policies that affect food pricing, sales, and advertising have successfully reduced the consumption of unhealthy foods, implying that the success of precision nutrition will be parallel to the implementation of strategies that modify the structural and environmental context in which eating behaviors occur.

Third, precise tools are needed for the eventual implementation of precision nutrition. Objective diet biomarkers are necessary to mitigate random and systematic errors from self-reported dietary assessment methods. High throughput metabolomics profiling has emerged as an agnostic approach to identifying biomarkers for nutritional exposures. Garcia-Perez and colleagues conducted a randomized crossover-controlled trial to identify metabolic signatures of diverse dietary patterns. They found 19 urinary metabolites to be present in higher concentrations after consumption of a healthy diet characterized by increased consumption of fruits, vegetables, whole grains, and dietary fiber and decreased intake of fats, sugars, and salt. Metabolomic signatures were replicated in two independent cohorts, suggesting that identified urinary metabolites could be good surrogates for different types of diets. However, the association between urine/blood biomarkers and foods reported in previous studies is generally modest and could partly be explained by the confounding effect of many variables. It is also possible that many foods and nutrients simply lack valid biomarkers. Further, the presence of identified biomarkers may not be specific to the dietary exposure of interest as it might reflect the consumption of other foods typically consumed together or substituted. Finally, the need to have multiple determinations to understand how these

diet biomarkers change over time and the progression from a healthy to a disease state has limited the implementation of diet biomarkers in clinical practice.

Fourth, the potential cost is a crucial consideration for precision nutrition in metabolic diseases. The extent to which deep phenotyping is superior to a simple clinical determination of traditional risk factors is uncertain. Recent studies have provided evidence that deep "omics" profiling could detect subtle changes in health markers at the earliest possible time, allowing early adoption of anticipatory prevention strategies targeted toward disrupted processes. In diabetes, for example, identifying actionable biomarkers of early alterations in insulin homeostasis is an unmet need, given that clinical tests such as the oral glucose tolerance test cannot characterize the nuances of glycemic and insulin fluctuations.[4] While the costs of deep phenotyping are greater than routine clinical testing, the pandemic of complex metabolic diseases is now a national priority. Cost-effectiveness studies have consistently shown that investing in obesity reduction and diabetes prevention is cost-effective,[20] opening the question of whether investing resources into acquiring deep phenotype data would be recouped by effective prevention, maybe by focusing resources on people at higher risk, or more likely to respond to these preventative interventions. However, no comprehensive attempts have been made to evaluate precision nutrition's cost-effectiveness.

Fifth, clinical trials specifically designed to capture the nuances of dynamic nutritional responses are needed for the eventual implementation of precision nutrition. Most precision nutrition evidence comes from post hoc analysis of clinical trials and observational studies, and independent replication in new intervention studies is usually lacking. Due to their short follow-up periods, these studies do not adequately capture the dynamic complexity of dietary and behavioral modification.

Sixth, it is unlikely that our increasing understanding of the pathophysiology of obesity, diabetes, cancer, or cardiovascular disease will translate into precision nutrition unless we can efficiently implement evidence from clinical studies in real-world interventions. This ongoing challenge of translating evidence of efficacy from preventive interventions into real-world interventions at scale has to do with how to deliver the intervention and identify individuals to whom it might be offered. The gold standard for providing dietary advice is following a standardized program consisting of group counseling and individualized advice. Advanced communication and education methods through mobile phone applications or medical portals are necessary to engage individuals in their care. The possibility to incorporate real-time data collection and provide real-time feedback has the potential to reinforce positive behaviors. In a new era of remote clinical testing and citizen science, in which various commercial companies are offering precision nutrition advice based on clinical, lifestyle, genetic, and gut microbiome variation, it is essential to address the current challenges by establishing a solid evidence base, protocols, and guidelines that could benefit individuals and populations.

THREE TAKE-HOME POINTS

1. The considerable etiological heterogeneity in metabolic diseases and the observed variability observed in response to dietary interventions stress the potential of precision nutrition. However, the science of precision nutrition is still in its infancy, and time and much more research are needed to tell if the initial prospects can be realized.

2. Precision nutrition sits uncomfortably in a false dichotomy between individual and social factors underlying disease risk. Shifting from population-based dietary advice to targeted recommendations would recognize the synergy between individual-level elements and social and environmental pressures shaping how people interact with and respond to foods.

3. New tools and technologies will continually improve our understanding of factors underlying inter-individual variation in response to therapeutic interventions and foster the implementation of precision nutrition as a frontline intervention for the prevention and management of metabolic diseases. However, many challenges remain to use these emerging tools effectively to prevent and manage chronic diseases and to disseminate the promise of precision nutrition equitably.

CASE STUDY ANSWERS

1. The best-known examples of the clinical application of precision nutrition have been about inborn errors of metabolism, which are monogenic diseases resulting from well-characterized, highly penetrant genetic variants, primarily in genetic coding regions that modify critical proteins in a metabolic pathway. Such monogenic disorders include phenylketonuria, galactosemia, and maple syrup urine disease. A diet low in phenylalanine, low in foods containing galactose, or a low-protein diet is the current nutritional treatment for individuals with these diseases.

   For common metabolic diseases such as obesity, type 2 diabetes, and certain types of cancer, evidence is less convincing about the role of highly personalized diets. While preliminary data support the benefit of a precision nutrition approach beyond a healthy dietary pattern, there is a need for large and long-term studies to investigate whether a precision nutrition approach can be sustained and is superior to other general healthy dietary recommendations for the prevention and management of common metabolic diseases.

2. There have been several recent studies investigating precision nutrition approaches targeted at one individual in the field of obesity and diabetes prevention. These studies demonstrate that people are likely to respond differently to the same food or meal based on their gut microbiome composition or genetic susceptibility. However, there is no robust and convincing evidence, especially related to long-term outcomes or among more vulnerable groups of the population, that a highly personalized diet would be of a higher benefit than meeting and following up with someone who has expertise in nutrition and can adapt general recommendations to specific preferences, cultural, or social contexts.

3. The potential benefits of following a precision nutrition approach lie in the premise that a better understanding of how people respond to diet will allow people to make more informed dietary choices. Further, it assumes that adopting a diet could be sustained in the long term and allow maintenance of healthier status for that individual. However, human behavior is very difficult to predict, and there needs to be evidence that a precision nutrition approach could be sustained in the long term. Preliminary evidence suggests that an individualized approach can help individuals adapt

(Continued)

CASE STUDY ANSWERS *(Continued)*

their diet to reduce glycemic fluctuations. Still, more research is needed to investigate whether a precision nutrition approach improves adherence to dietary advice and prevents diabetes and cardiovascular disease to a greater degree than general healthy diet recommendations.

The disadvantages of precision nutrition include the cost of obtaining detailed molecular, environmental, and social data; the participant's burden to collect biospecimens; or the anxiety resulting from knowing actionable or non-actionable health information such as genetic susceptibility to diseases. Further, the data captured to generate predictive algorithms are limited by other measurements that are more difficult to obtain, such as day-to-day variation in emotional aspects, motivation to eat healthily, or the social and environmental obstacles people might find to sustain targeted dietary advice.

REFERENCES

1. Bancks MP, Chen H, Balasubramanyam A, et al. Type 2 diabetes subgroups, risk for complications, and differential effects due to an intensive lifestyle intervention. *Diabetes Care.* 2021;44(5):1203-1210.

2. Berry SE, Valdes AM, Drew DA, et al. Human postprandial responses to food and potential for precision nutrition. *Nat Med.* 2020;26(6):964-973.

3. Claussnitzer M, Cho JH, Collins R, et al. A brief history of human disease genetics. *Nature.* 2020 Jan;577(7789):179-189.

4. Hall H, Perelman D, Breschi A, et al. Glucotypes reveal new patterns of glucose dysregulation. *PLoS Biol.* 2018;16(7):e2005143.

5. Shah VN, DuBose SN, Li Z, et al. Continuous glucose monitoring profiles in healthy nondiabetic participants: a multicenter prospective study. *J Clin Endocrinol Metab.* 2019;104(10):4356-4364.

6. Tsereteli N, Vallat R, Fernandez-Tajes J, et al. Impact of insufficient sleep on dysregulated blood glucose control under standardised meal conditions. *Diabetologia.* 2022;65(2):356-365.

7. Qi Q, Chu AY, Kang JH, et al. Sugar-sweetened beverages and genetic risk of obesity. *N Engl J Med.* 2012;367(15):1387-1396.

8. Florez JC, Jablonski KA, Bayley N, et al. TCF7L2 polymorphisms and progression to diabetes in the diabetes prevention program. *N Engl J Med.* 2006;355(3):241-250.

9. Carr PR, Weigl K, Jansen L, et al. Healthy lifestyle factors associated with lower risk of colorectal cancer irrespective of genetic risk. *Gastroenterology.* 2018;155(6):1805-1815.e5.

10. Turnbaugh PJ, Ley RE, Hamady M, Fraser-Liggett CM, Knight R, Gordon JI. The human microbiome project. *Nature.* 2007;449(7164):804-810.

11. Turnbaugh PJ, Ley RE, Mahowald MA, Magrini V, Mardis ER, Gordon JI. An obesity-associated gut microbiome with increased capacity for energy harvest. *Nature.* 2006 Dec 21;444(7122):1027-1031.

12. Abu-Ali GS, Mehta RS, Lloyd-Price J, et al. Metatranscriptome of human faecal microbial communities in a cohort of adult men. *Nat Microbiol.* 2018;3(3):356-366.

13. Martin-Gallausiaux C, Marinelli L, Blottière HM, Larraufie P, Lapaque N. SCFA: mechanisms and functional importance in the gut. *Proc Nutr Soc.* 2021;80(1):37-49.

14. Rinott E, Youngster I, Meir AY, et al. Effects of diet-modulated autologous fecal microbiota transplantation on weight regain. *Gastroenterology.* 2021;160(1):158173.e10.

15. Price ND, Magis AT, Earls JC, et al. A wellness study of 108 individuals using personal, dense, dynamic data clouds. *Nat Biotechnol.* 2017;35(8):747-756.

16. Schüssler-Fiorenza Rose SM, Contrepois K, Moneghetti KJ, et al. A longitudinal big data approach for precision health. *Nat Med.* 2019;25(5):792-804.

17. Zeevi D, Korem T, Zmora N, et al. Personalized nutrition by prediction of glycemic responses. *Cell.* 2015;163(5):1079-1094.

18. Ben-Yacov O, Godneva A, Rein M, et al. Personalized postprandial glucose response-targeting diet versus Mediterranean diet for glycemic control in prediabetes. *Diabetes Care.* 2021;44(9):1980-1991.

19. IDF [Internet]. [cited 2015 Sep 22]. Available at: https://www.idf.org/sites/default/files/EN_6E_Atlas_Full_0.pdf.

20. Diabetes Prevention Program Research Group. The 10-year cost-effectiveness of lifestyle intervention or metformin for diabetes prevention: an intent-to-treat analysis of the DPP/DPPOS. *Diabetes Care.* 2012;35(4):723-730.

Healthy and Sustainable Diets

Christopher D. Golden, PhD, MPH / Simone Passarelli, PhD, MS / Khristopher Nicholas, PhD / Jessica Fanzo, PhD

Chapter Outline

CASE STUDY

A 25-year-old medical student presents to your primary care clinic for a routine physical examination. They have been reading about food system sustainability and wish to change their diet to reduce their environmental impact. They are also training to run the Boston Marathon and have read that high-protein animal-sourced foods are needed after a strenuous strength training session, and that sugar is the preferred energy source to fuel endurance activity. As a medical student and amateur athlete, they are interested in nourishing their body with the right dietary sources to improve fitness and maintain a healthy lifestyle. As an environmentally conscious consumer, they are uncertain which dietary practices accomplish both goals and which trade-offs might occur when prioritizing one goal over the other.

1. If a patient wants to quantitatively appraise the environmental impacts of their diet, to which evidence-based approach might you direct them for additional information on specific foods?

2. If a patient wants to continue eating animal-sourced foods, what is the best advice you can provide to minimize their environmental impact?

A. Eat animal-sourced foods in moderation, and the type of meat doesn't really matter.
B. Focus on chicken, pork, and seafood, as their environmental impacts are roughly equal to a plant-based diet.
C. Avoid consuming red meats, and eat chicken and seafood in moderation.

3. The patient decides to limit consumption of red meat and simple sugars to training sessions and race days—which of the following environmental processes benefit from this decision?
A. Deforestation of primary forests and associated land tenure disputes.
B. Greenhouse gas emissions from livestock, farming, and transport.
C. Freshwater systems that are heavily taxed to provide crop irrigation and sustain livestock.
D. All of the above.

4. Why might the recommendations made to this patient be ill-tailored to another patient, despite its health and environmental benefits?

INTRODUCTION

Food systems, and the human diets produced by them, rely on functioning ecosystems. Without all of the critical inputs from ecosystems (e.g., freshwater, soil, biogeochemical cycles, pollinators, etc.), food systems would fail and human nutrition would be threatened. Yet, global food production is one of the largest forces driving ecosystem degradation and is responsible for one-third of anthropogenic greenhouse gas emissions.[1] There is a complex relationship whereby food production degrades ecosystems, and degraded ecosystems reduce the capacity for food production. This relationship has often been overlooked by an increasingly urbanized population that has become detached from its food systems. Given these trends, there have been calls for healthy and sustainable diets that can both nourish the global population and heal the planet.[2] By definition, a healthy diet must be nutritious (e.g., provide essential nutrients and prevent acute and chronic diseases) and safe; and a sustainable diet must be affordable, culturally acceptable, and cause low environmental impacts. But what should these diets look like? Let us first document current trends in planetary health to contextualize the issues that must be considered to construct these diets.

The current era in which we live is called the Anthropocene, an era characterized by human activity dominating the impacts on climate and the environment.[2] The Anthropocene began in 1950 at the start of the Great Acceleration, when trends in industrialization and economic growth began to sharply increase, pushing humanity to the limits of its planetary boundaries.[3] These planetary boundaries include climate change, biodiversity loss, biogeochemical cycles, ocean acidification, land use, freshwater use, ozone depletion, atmospheric aerosols, and chemical pollution. The trajectory of these planetary boundaries is shaped by human activity and driven by the product of three factors: human population size, the affluence of these populations, and the technologies that they use.

THE DEPENDENCE OF HUMAN FOOD PRODUCTION ON FUNCTIONING ECOSYSTEMS

Food availability, access, and stability within the global food supply chain are dependent on functioning ecosystems.[2] Roots reduce soil erosion, plants provide a natural filter for water and air, pollinators facilitate plant reproduction, and fungi decompose waste returning nitrogen to the soil. The extent to which ecosystems can sustain global food production depends largely on the demands a population makes on its dwindling natural resource reserves. This section outlines the importance of three ecosystem functions necessary for food production: freshwater systems, soil and biogeochemical cycles, and the role of pollinators.

Freshwater Systems

Agriculture represents the largest draw on global freshwater reserves.[4] Irrigated agriculture (using engineered water sources) represents only 20% of total cultivated land, yet contributes 40% of global food production.[5] Volatility in rainfall contributes significantly to crop failure. Anticipated increases in rainfall volatility due to climate change, rising costs, and higher levels of contamination from industrial runoff contribute to greater risks of water scarcity, furthering reliance on rainfed systems.[6]

Soil and Biogeochemical Cycles

Soil is a necessary substrate for most food production. Soil fertility and composition are determined by its porosity, water infiltration rate, organic matter, and nutrient provision.[7] As microorganisms in soil consume organic matter, they release excess nutrients (notably nitrogen and phosphorus) back into the soil through a process called *mineralization*.[7] Nitrogen and phosphorus are the most common rate-limiting nutrients in most agricultural systems and are the foundation of synthetic fertilizers.[8] Synthetic creation and widespread application of these nutrients in commercial chemical fertilizers are core inputs for many cropping systems.

Pollinators

Most crop species in the global food system rely on animal pollination; it is estimated that the absence of pollinators would lead to a decline in global agricultural production of up to 8%.[9] However, there is geographic variation in this theoretical decline. For example, farmers in West Africa produce over half of the world's stimulant crops (e.g., coffee, tea, cacao) and would experience a 90% harvest loss in the absence of pollinators.[10] Although most calories in human diets derive from cereals that rely on wind pollination, crops that depend on animal pollination account for the vast majority of dietary intake of vitamins A, C, lipids, calcium, and other key micronutrients and minerals.[11] Accordingly, a continued loss of pollinator stock may be associated with reduced dietary nutrient content in some settings. As with vulnerability to total food production, there is geographic variation in the vulnerability to micronutrient deficiencies. In some countries, estimates predict that pollinator loss may be associated with a 50% increase in populations at-risk of micronutrient deficiencies.[12]

FOOD PRODUCTION AS A DRIVER OF ENVIRONMENTAL CHANGE

As described above, food systems rely on natural resources and ecosystems to create the products that sustain us. The degree and type of environmental impacts that food production causes vary considerably depending on what is produced and how it is produced. Over 570 million farms around the world produce our food, ranging from small family-owned rice farms in Bangladesh to sprawling sheep farms in Australia.[13] The following section will describe the environmental impacts of food systems, including greenhouse gas emissions, deforestation, eutrophication (waterway pollution), biodiversity loss, and freshwater availability.

Greenhouse Gas Emissions

Global food production systems consist of all agriculture, livestock, aquaculture, and fishing that contribute to the food supply. Each of these systems uses energy to convert natural resources into the edible biomass that ends up on consumers' plates. Land use change—or the conversion of land into farmland—is responsible for about one-third of all food system emissions alone.[13] Once land is ready for farming, foods travel through the supply chain stages of production, processing, transport, packaging, retail, consumption, and disposal. The first step—food production—accounts for the greatest contribution to emissions at 40%,[1] due to the energy-intensive manufacturing of chemical fertilizers, pesticides, and antibiotics; the fossil fuels used to power farm machinery; the methane emissions from enteric fermentation by ruminants (17% of all food system emissions[13]); and from numerous other processes. The remaining stages of the food supply account for smaller shares of emissions, including processing (4%), transport (5%), packaging (5%), retail (4%), consumption (3%), and end of life, which consists of waste and disposal (9%).[13] Emissions vary substantially depending on the food; for example, producing 1 kg of beef creates over 30 times more carbon dioxide equivalents than the same amount of tofu, and over 230 times more than that same amount of nuts.[13]

Deforestation

Land-use change for agriculture accounts for the second highest share of greenhouse gas emissions in our food system.[13] When forests are cleared for crops or animal pasture, the immense sink of carbon stored in trees and other plant life is released into the atmosphere. Tilling farmland also breaks up and homogenizes soils that stored carbon in clumps, roots, and decaying matter. Today, about half of all the world's habitable land is used for agriculture.[14] Agriculture is the leading cause of deforestation, with cropland expansion accounting for about half of global deforestation, followed by clearing land for livestock grazing, which contributes 38%.[15] In 2021, over 25 million hectares of forest were lost—an area larger than the United Kingdom in 1 year. The amount of land required for food production depends on what is produced. The collective land used for pasture and livestock feed amounts to about two-thirds of all agricultural land, but animals contribute only 18% of the world's calories and 37 percent of protein.[14] Improvements in agricultural productivity could help to feed the planet's growing population without further increases in deforestation, especially by reducing our consumption of animal products in favor of plant-based products.[2]

Eutrophication

Eutrophication—or the pollution of inland and coastal waterways with excessive nutrients from runoff—is a phenomenon caused by anthropogenic activities like landscaping, wastewater discharge, and above all, agriculture. When nitrogen- and phosphorus-containing synthetic fertilizers, crops, animal feeds, or manures accumulate in soils in excessive amounts, erosion of these soils into waterways can have detrimental effects on aquatic ecosystems.[8] This over-enrichment of water can cause excessive growth of algae and marine plants, depleting oxygen in the system, stimulating the growth of harmful pathogens, causing fish kills, and threatening marine plant and animal life. One example of this can be seen in the hypoxic "dead zone" off the Gulf of Mexico caused by upstream agricultural production in the Mississippi River Basin. The consequences of eutrophication—including harming endangered or threatened species, devaluing property, limiting water for recreational uses, and damaging commercial fishing—has been estimated to cost billions of dollars per year in the United States alone. Optimizing the amounts of fertilizer applied, improving soil management to reduce runoff, and introducing mitigating measures like bivalves can help to minimize instances of eutrophication.

Biodiversity Loss

Agriculture is responsible for the majority of today's biodiversity loss.[2] Practices of land clearing, heavy tillage, and monocropping reduce the number of bird, plant, mammal, insect, and microbial species in landscapes. In marine ecosystems, destructive fishing practices like overfishing, bottom trawling, and bycatch, combined with climate change and other anthropogenic activities, threaten thousands of marine species.[16] Today, only nine crops account for 66% of all global production.[17] In the face of climate change, biodiverse ecosystems become even more important for regulating and mitigating climate impacts, while pollution and climate change will continue to be their own powerful drivers of biodiversity loss. Moreover, when we lose genetic diversity in plant life to extinction, we also lose opportunities to breed plants with more climate-resilient traits. By shifting diets away from high energy, nutrient-poor dietary patterns (so-called Western diets) towards more sustainable plant-based sources, by reducing food waste, preserving tracts of land for conservation, and practicing more nature-friendly practices like polyculture and integrated pest management, our food systems can help to preserve and promote biodiversity.[2]

Freshwater Availability

Our food system relies on a steady supply of water for irrigation, livestock consumption, production, and processing. Over 70% of all freshwater withdrawals globally are used for agricultural purposes.[2] Although the crops with the highest water footprint include stimulants (e.g. coffee and tea), rubber, and nuts—the majority of the world's water consumption is from cereal crops like wheat, rice, and maize, due to the massive quantities produced for animal and human consumption.[18]

Where and how foods are produced determines the degree of pressure that agriculture has on water resources. Water insecurity in agriculture is already a reality, with 28% of all cropland facing high or extremely high water stress, based on its withdrawals of renewable water resources being at unsustainable levels.[19] In the face of increasing human demands and increasingly unpredictable rainfall, freshwater scarcity will continue to pose a challenge. By 2050, an anticipated 50% increase in agricultural production will increase freshwater use by another 15%.[20] Consuming and producing foods with lower water footprints, improving soil management practices, and increasing the adoption of water-saving technologies can help to offset agriculture's high demand for water.

HOW WILL CLIMATE CHANGE AFFECT FOOD SYSTEMS?

We have now documented how food production relies on functioning ecosystems, with a proper balance of freshwater, atmospheric conditions, sunlight, temperature, and soil quality. Yet, the current methods of food production are driving all of the forms of environmental change mentioned in the prior section. This produces a negative feedback loop whereby growing populations and incomes will continue to increase global food demand and degrade the underlying biophysical conditions required to produce food on earth.

In addition to these environmental changes, climate change will also drastically alter the landscape of food production, shifting access to freshwater and changing the temperature and atmospheric conditions.[2] Climate change will lead to increased carbon dioxide in the atmosphere, generally increased temperatures, reduced precipitation in arid and semi-arid regions, and increased precipitation in polar regions. The Intergovernmental Panel on Climate Change found that our planet will reach or exceed 1.5°C of warming by 2050,[21] which showcases the rapid and intensifying trajectories underway. Every crop has a unique set of ideal growing conditions, but air temperatures above 30°C are typically associated with reduced yields in rain-fed crops.[22] Climate variability can explain at least 30% of annual variations in crop yield.[23] Globally increasing temperatures and increases in the number of days in a given growing season that exceed 30°C could lead to catastrophic losses and breadbasket failures.[24]

Increased carbon dioxide in the atmosphere may have a variety of impacts on agricultural production. On the one hand, there is a "fertilization effect," whereby higher rates of CO_2 actually increase rates of photosynthesis and water use efficiency,[25] leading to higher crop productivity. On the other hand, increasing CO_2 levels are reducing the nutrient composition of crops, with estimated declines of 5–15% in protein and micronutrient content of the edible portions of staple crops, particularly rice, wheat, barley, and potatoes.[26] Given these impacts, projected increases in atmospheric CO_2 are anticipated to decrease growth in the global availability of nutrients by 19.5% for protein, 13.6% for iron, and 14.6% for zinc by 2050.[27] The burden of this net negative effect will be borne by the poorest, highlighting issues of inequity that will arise from climate change.

Although staple crops provide the majority of dietary energy, increasing land and sea temperatures will threaten the supply of animal-sourced foods that provide critical supplies of protein and micronutrients. The impacts of climate change on terrestrial livestock production is not well characterized, though the effects are considered to be detrimental, affecting animal growth rates, dairy production, reproductive performance, morbidity and mortality.[28] Climate change affects all of these dimensions, particularly as they relate to heat stress and water scarcity.

Beyond terrestrial livestock, climate change is also reshaping the potential of aquatic food production in both marine and freshwater systems.[29] Of particular importance in marine systems, sea temperature rise will lead to the reduction of fish biomass, and will also lead to fisheries migration away from the equator and toward the poles.[30] This will drive subsistence populations in food-insecure regions to become more malnourished by reducing fish catch potential. Estimates suggest that this reduced access to seafood will leave 845 million people vulnerable to deficiencies in iron, zinc, and vitamin A and 1.4 billion people vulnerable to deficiencies of vitamin B12 and omega-3 long-chain polyunsaturated fatty acids.[29]

HOW TO EAT FOR PERSONAL AND PLANETARY HEALTH

Some research has shown that without drastic changes in our current dietary patterns, diets high in red meats, fats, and refined sugars could drive an 80% increase in greenhouse gas emissions.[31] Yet, the science behind quantifying the planetary impacts of foods can be complex, convoluted, and contradictory, as there are many touchpoints to consider. For instance, should local foods be prioritized? Or organic? Or fair trade? Or humanely produced to ensure better animal welfare? Each of these characteristics may be more or less environmentally friendly depending on a variety of issues related to where and how these foods are grown and what consumers value. Therefore, much of it relies on personal choices of what one chooses to prioritize. With that said, there are some clear rules of thumb on how to choose what to eat for optimal personal and planetary health. The most evidence-based approach to understanding the *environmental* impacts of diet uses a methodology called Life Cycle Assessment (Box 9-1).

General Rules of Thumb

The best available evidence we have on how to eat to maintain or improve human health, while staying within the boundaries of planetary sustainability, comes from the EAT-*Lancet* Commission Report on Health Diets from Sustainable Food Systems. This report was the first to comprehensively link human nutrition to the environment by setting scientific targets for what people should be eating, called the Planetary Health Diet (Figure 9-1).

1) **Double consumption of fruits, vegetables, nuts, and legumes.** Often termed the "Mediterranean diet," a major pattern in this diet includes increased consumption of fruits, vegetables, nuts, and legumes that are associated with a reduced incidence of cardiovascular disease, obesity, hypertension, diabetes, cognitive dysfunction, neurodegenerative disorders, and overall mortality.[38] Focusing on these food products can also lead to tremendous environmental and climate benefits, as these products generally require less land and freshwater, and cause fewer greenhouse gas emissions and eutrophication potential.[39] Food systems are responsible for roughly one-third of total human-caused GHG emissions.[1] In an analysis that compared dietary scenarios by 2050, transforming the global food system toward more plant-based diets could reduce global mortality by 6–10% and food system GHG emissions by 29–70%.[40]

Life Cycle Assessment

There are many metrics for assessing the sustainability of food production, from greenhouse gas emissions, to water footprints, to food miles. One commonly used method of quantifying the environmental impacts of products is known as life cycle assessment, or LCA. The official definition of LCA is the "compilation and evaluation of the inputs, outputs, and potential environmental impacts of a product or system throughout its life cycle."[32] The goal of LCA is to evaluate the environmental impacts of any product "from cradle to grave." Although LCA can be used for most consumable goods and processes—from your cup of coffee to your morning commute—for food production, an LCA would include farm inputs (e.g., fertilizers, pesticides), the agricultural stage (i.e., on-farm production), processing, distribution, consumption, and waste management.[33]

LCA typically occurs in four steps.[34] The first step is to define the objectives and scope of the analysis. For example, if you are assessing the environmental impacts of a cup of coffee, you would need to set boundaries like whether you will include the cup, the milk, the brewing method, etc. Your objective might be to either assess the overall environmental impacts of your morning cup of coffee, or it might be to compare different types of coffee to select the most sustainable option. At this stage, you also define which impacts you wish to assess quantitatively, like greenhouse gas emissions, eutrophication, and/or water use. Other types of LCA analyses have also included social (social LCA) and cost (life cycle cost) elements.[35]

The second step is known as inventory analysis.[34] In this stage, the assessor compiles the inputs and outputs of all processes involved in the production of the item and adds them together. The assessor would employ a database or software in order to inventory, for example, the greenhouse gas emissions associated with each stage in the production value chain. The inventory could include hundreds of contributing factors.[34]

In the third stage, known as life cycle impact assessment, the assessor selects the *impact categories* of interest (like climate change, human health consequences) and the indicators used to assess these categories (like CO_2 equivalents, disability-adjusted life years). The steps in the process are then *classified* into these impact categories (e.g., classifying CO_2 emission results under the climate change impact category), and then *characterized* by multiplying out how much each factory contributes to an indicator.[36] This would typically be done with software.

The last step of LCA is known as interpretation, in which the assessor interprets their results based on the objectives of the assessment. This step can be done as the last step, as well as continuously throughout the LCA.

LCA is not without its challenges and criticisms—it can be difficult to maintain comparability of items and processes across different economies of scale and geographies.[37] Boiling complex systems down to a single number will almost certainly fail to capture certain social, economic, financial, and environmental aspects. Nonetheless, LCA represents one useful way of guiding individual and policy choices toward more sustainable food systems.

2) **More than halve consumption of red meats.** Reducing our consumption of red meats is one of the single most important actions we can take to protect our planet and health. The consumption of red meats is associated with a higher incidence of coronary heart disease (CHD), type 2 diabetes, breast cancer, stroke, and overall mortality. Of all forms of food production, red meat production is the most environmentally damaging across various dimensions (GHG emissions, land use, terrestrial acidification, eutrophication, and scarcity-weighted freshwater withdrawals).[13]

3) **More than halve consumption of sugar.** Over the past half century, consumption of added sugars has more than tripled globally.[41] Increased consumption of added sugars is associated with a higher incidence of obesity, hypertension, diabetes, dental diseases, and cardiovascular disease mortality. Sugarcane production leads to increases in deforestation and land conversion, stress on water resources due to irrigation needs, air quality and GHG emissions from sugar cane burning, and increased runoff and eutrophication.[42]

4) **Reduce consumption of refined grains and ultra-processed foods (UPFs).** The consumption of UPFs (breakfast cereals, savory snacks, reconstituted meat products, pre-packaged frozen dishes, soft and/or sweetened drinks, distilled alcoholic beverages, and supplements) are highly associated with obesity and metabolic syndrome, and processed meats are associated with a higher incidence of diabetes and CHD. In parallel, UPFs are often manufactured from a handful of prolific crops (e.g., maize, wheat, soy, and oil crops) and industrial-farmed animals (which consume those crops as feed). These same crops, and the land they require, have been destructive to global biodiversity and biogeochemical cycles.[43]

5) **More consumption of sustainably harvested aquatic foods.** There is substantial evidence that consuming aquatic foods can benefit our health by both supplying critical long-chain omega-3 fatty acids, protein, and micronutrients, and reducing the risk of cardiovascular disease and all-cause mortality.[44] The environmental impacts of fish vary because

The Planetary Health Plate

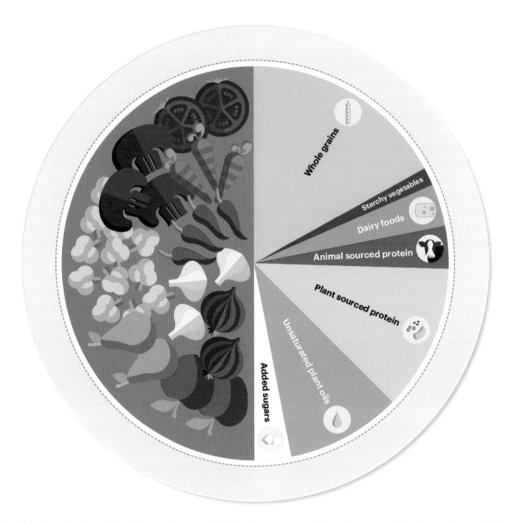

FIGURE 9-1 • The planetary health diet plate provides guidelines to a range of food consumption by category that will optimize human health and environmental sustainability. (Reproduced with permission from EAT Foundation.)

of their wide variety, sourcing and production systems.[45] Yet, aquatic foods can be sustainably produced, and there is the potential to increase the supply substantially, while remaining within planetary boundaries, especially by relying on sustainably farmed sources.[46]

6) **Moderate consumption of eggs, poultry, and dairy.** Eggs, poultry and dairy have lower environmental impacts than red meat, but higher impacts as compared to most plant-based foods and could be considered a more efficient substitute if vegetarianism is not an option.[47]

7) **Minimize food waste.** In the United States, nearly one-third of food produced is never eaten, and food waste contributes nearly one quarter of all landfilled solid waste.[48] More than 150 million people per year could meet their energy needs just by using American food waste.[48] Reducing the amount of food wasted by improving farming, transportation, market, and consumption practices will lead to major advances in reducing the food system's environmental impact.

8) **Recognize that not all of these food choices are actual *choices*.** There is a need for both top-down and bottom-up policy support to create healthy food environments that enable healthy eating for people and planet. Consumers can only operate within a range of possible choices, many of which are unhealthy.

These types of actions will benefit the planet and human health, especially considering nutritional deficiencies, cardiovascular diseases, diabetes, hypertension, cancers, and all-cause mortality.[39] Following the Planetary Health Diet could help to avert nearly 11 million premature deaths per year.[2] Although these dietary recommendations are broadly in alignment with many national food-based dietary guidelines, there are still many reforms that must be made at the national and city level, as current dietary guidelines are often incompatible with decarbonizing our planet.[49]

CASE STUDY ANSWERS

1. Life cycle assessments (LCA) aim to evaluate the environmental impacts of any product from production to consumption. For foods, this includes farming inputs all the way to commercial transportation.
2. C
3. D
4. The patient finds themselves in a well-resourced environment wherein they make food choices in a context of food abundance, have no limiting health conditions, and engage in physical activity for sport. For other individuals in the United States, factors such as age, sex, resource constraints, and health status may determine their specific dietary needs. Further still, other individuals globally may face limitations to food availability and/or accessibility. In short, clinical dietary recommendations should encompass environmental concerns while still maximizing the health of a specific individual.

REFERENCES

1. Crippa M, Solazzo E, Guizzardi D, Monforti-Ferrario F, Tubiello FN, Leip A. Food systems are responsible for a third of global anthropogenic GHG emissions. *Nat Food.* 2021;2(3):198-209.
2. Willett W, Rockström J, Loken B, et al. Food in the anthropocene: the EAT–Lancet Commission on healthy diets from sustainable food systems. *Lancet.* 2019;393(10170):447-492.
3. Rockström J, Steffen W, Noone K, et al. Planetary boundaries: exploring the safe operating space for humanity. *Ecol Soc.* 2009;14(2). doi:10.5751/ES-03180-140232.
4. Annual freshwater withdrawals, agriculture (% of total freshwater withdrawal). World Bank. Accessed July 25, 2022. Available at: https://data.worldbank.org/indicator/er.h2o.fwag.zs.
5. Rockström J, Karlberg L, Wani SP, et al. Managing water in rainfed agriculture—The need for a paradigm shift. *Agric Water Manag.* 2010;97(4):543-550.
6. Chen B, Han MY, Peng K, et al. Global land-water nexus: agricultural land and freshwater use embodied in worldwide supply chains. *Sci Total Environ.* 2018;613-614:931-943.
7. Bot A, Benites J. *The Importance of Soil Organic Matter: Key to Drought-Resistant Soil and Sustained Food Production.* Food and Agriculture Organization of the United Nations; 2005.
8. Guignard MS, Leitch AR, Acquisti C, et al. Impacts of nitrogen and phosphorus: from oenomes to natural ecosystems and agriculture. *Front Ecol Evol.* 2017;5:70. Accessed July 10, 2022. Available at: https://www.frontiersin.org/articles/10.3389/fevo.2017.00070.
9. Aizen MA, Garibaldi LA, Cunningham SA, Klein AM. How much does agriculture depend on pollinators? Lessons from long-term trends in crop production. *Ann Bot.* 2009;103(9):1579-1588.
10. Gallai N, Salles JM, Settele J, Vaissière BE. Economic valuation of the vulnerability of world agriculture confronted with pollinator decline. *Ecol Econ.* 2009;68(3):810-821.
11. Eilers EJ, Kremen C, Greenleaf SS, Garber AK, Klein AM. Contribution of pollinator-mediated crops to nutrients in the human food supply. *PLoS One.* 2011;6(6):e21363.
12. Ellis AM, Myers SS, Ricketts TH. Do pollinators contribute to nutritional health? *PLoS One.* 2015;10(1):e114805.
13. Poore J, Nemecek T. Reducing food's environmental impacts through producers and consumers. *Science.* 2018;360(6392):987-992.
14. Ritchie H, Roser M. Environmental impacts of food production. *Our World Data.* Published online January 15, 2020. Accessed July 25, 2022. Available at: https://ourworldindata.org/environmental-impacts-of-food.
15. Global Forest Resource Assessment 2020. FAO. www.fao.org. Accessed July 25, 2022. Available at: http://www.fao.org/forest-resources-assessment/2020.
16. O'Hara CC, Frazier M, Halpern BS. At-risk marine biodiversity faces extensive, expanding, and intensifying human impacts. *Science.* 2021;372(6537):84-87.
17. FAO C on GR for F and A. *The State of the World's Biodiversity for Food and Agriculture, 2019.* Accessed July 25, 2022. Available at: http://www.fao.org/state-of-biodiversity-for-food-agriculture/en/.
18. Mekonnen MM, Hoekstra AY. The green, blue and grey water footprint of crops and derived crop products. *Hydrol Earth Syst Sci.* 2011;15(5):1577-1600.
19. Aqueduct Water and Food Security Analyzer. Accessed July 25, 2022. Available at: https://www.wri.org/applications/aqueduct/food/#/.
20. Chart: Globally, 70% of Freshwater is Used for Agriculture. Accessed July 25, 2022. Available at: https://blogs.worldbank.org/opendata/chart-globally-70-freshwater-used-agriculture.
21. IPCC, ed. Summary for Policymakers. In: *Global Warming of 1.5°C: IPCC Special Report on Impacts of Global Warming of 1.5°C above Pre-Industrial Levels in Context of Strengthening Response to Climate Change, Sustainable Development, and Efforts to Eradicate Poverty.* Cambridge University Press; 2022:1-24. doi:10.1017/9781009157940.001.
22. Schlenker W, Roberts MJ. Nonlinear temperature effects indicate severe damages to U.S. crop yields under climate change. *Proc Natl Acad Sci U S A.* 2009;106(37):15594-15598.
23. Lobell DB, Field CB. Global scale climate–crop yield relationships and the impacts of recent warming. *Environ Res Lett.* 2007;2(1):014002. doi:10.1088/1748-9326/2/1/014002.
24. Gaupp F, Hall J, Hochrainer-Stigler S, Dadson S. Changing risks of simultaneous global breadbasket failure. *Nat Clim Change.* 2020;10(1):54-57.
25. Ainsworth EA, Long SP. 30 years of free-air carbon dioxide enrichment (FACE): what have we learned about future crop productivity and its potential for adaptation? *Glob Change Biol.* 2021;27(1):27-49.
26. Myers SS, Smith MR, Guth S, et al. Climate change and global food systems: potential impacts on food security and undernutrition. *Annu Rev Public Health.* 2017 Mar 20;38:259-277.
27. Beach RH, Sulser TB, Crimmins A, et al. Combining the effects of increased atmospheric carbon dioxide on protein, iron, and zinc availability and projected climate change on global diets: a modelling study. *Lancet Planet Health.* 2019;3(7):e307-e317.

28. Cheng M, McCarl B, Fei C. Climate change and livestock production: a literature review. *Atmosphere.* 2022;13(1):140.

29. Golden CD, Allison EH, Cheung WWL, et al. Nutrition: fall in fish catch threatens human health. *Nature.* 2016;534(7607):317-320.

30. Hastings RA, Rutterford LA, Freer JJ, Collins RA, Simpson SD, Genner MJ. Climate change drives poleward increases and equatorward declines in marine species. *Curr Biol.* 2020;30(8):1572-1577.e2.

31. Tilman D, Clark M. Global diets link environmental sustainability and human health. *Nature.* 2014;515(7528):518-522.

32. International Organization for Standardization (ISO). The New International Standards for Life Cycle Assessment: ISO 14040 and ISO 14044. ISO. Accessed July 25, 2022. Available at: https://www.iso.org/cms/render/live/en/sites/isoorg/contents/data/standard/03/84/38498.html.

33. Hauschild MZ, Rosenbaum RK, Olsen SI, eds. *Life Cycle Assessment.* Springer International Publishing; 2018. doi:10.1007/978-3-319-56475-3.

34. Hellweg S, Milà i Canals L. Emerging approaches, challenges and opportunities in life cycle assessment. *Science.* 2014;344(6188):1109-1113.

35. Guinée J. Life cycle sustainability assessment: what is it and what are its challenges? In: Clift R, Druckman A, eds. *Taking Stock of Industrial Ecology.* Springer International Publishing; 2016:45-68.

36. Hauschild MZ, Huijbregts MAJ, eds. Introducing liife cycle impact assessment. In: *Life Cycle Impact Assessment. LCA Compendium – The Complete World of Life Cycle Assessment.* Springer; 2015:1-16.

37. Sevigné-Itoiz E, Mwabonje O, Panoutsou C, Woods J. Life cycle assessment (LCA): informing the development of a sustainable circular bioeconomy? *Philos Trans A Math Phys Eng Sci.* 2021;379(2206):20200352.

38. Guasch-Ferré M, Willett WC. The mediterranean diet and health: a comprehensive overview. *J Intern Med.* 2021;290(3):549-566.

39. Jarmul S, Dangour AD, Green R, Liew Z, Haines A, Scheelbeek PF. Climate change mitigation through dietary change: a systematic review of empirical and modelling studies on the environmental footprints and health effects of `sustainable diets'. *Environ Res Lett.* 2020;15(12):123014.

40. Springmann M, Clark MA, Rayner M, Scarborough P, Webb P. The global and regional costs of healthy and sustainable dietary patterns: a modelling study. *Lancet Planet Health.* 2021;5(11):e797-e807.

41. Lustig RH, Schmidt LA, Brindis CD. The toxic truth about sugar. *Nature.* 2012;482(7383):27-29.

42. Verdade LM, Gheler-Costa C, Penteado M, Dotta G. The impacts of sugarcane expansion on wildlife in the state of Sao Paulo, Brazil. *J Sustain Bioenergy Syst.* 2012;2(4):138-144.

43. Leite FHM, Khandpur N, Andrade GC, et al. Ultra-processed foods should be central to global food systems dialogue and action on biodiversity. *BMJ Glob Health.* 2022;7(3):e008269.

44. Rimm EB, Appel LJ, Chiuve SE, et al. Seafood long-chain n-3 polyunsaturated fatty acids and cardiovascular disease: a science advisory from the American Heart Association. *Circulation.* 2018;138(1):e35-e47.

45. Gephart JA, Henriksson PJG, Parker RWR, et al. Environmental performance of blue foods. *Nature.* 2021;597(7876):360-365.

46. Gephart JA, Golden CD. Environmental and nutritional double bottom lines in aquaculture. *One Earth.* 2022;5(4):324-328.

47. Clark M, Tilman D. Comparative analysis of environmental impacts of agricultural production systems, agricultural input efficiency, and food choice. *Environ Res Lett.* 2017;12(6):064016.

48. Kirsten Jaglo, Shannon Kenny, Jenny Stephenson. *From farm to kitchen: The environmental impacts of U.S. food waste.* EPA.:113.

49. Ritchie H, Reay D, Higgins P. The impact of global dietary guidelines on climate change. *Glob Environ Change.* 2018;49:46-55.

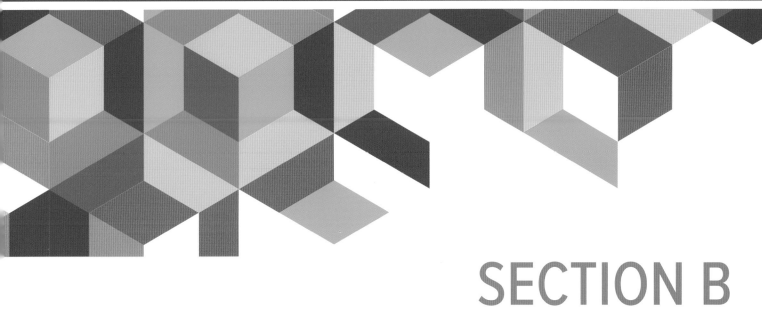

SECTION B

Nutrition and Metabolism in Disease

Specialized Nutrition Therapies

Katelyn Ariagno, MPH, RD, LDN, CNSC / Kris M. Mogensen, MS, RD-AP, LDN, CNSC

Chapter Outline

ADULT CASE STUDY

A 68-year-oldman presents to the Emergency Department after a fall. He was cleaning leaves out of the gutters of his home when he lost his footing, fell, and hit the concrete patio below. He was taking anticoagulation medication for a history of a myocardial infarction 2 years prior to this presentation. He was found to have a large subdural hematoma and was taken to the operating room for evacuation. Postoperatively, he required mechanical ventilation, and the ICU team is concerned that this may be a prolonged admission. A nutrition consult is ordered, and the team has requested guidance for the optimal route of feeding. You speak to the patient's nurse, who reports that the patient has low output from his orogastric tube, and the team plans to start using the tube for enteral medication delivery.

1. What is the optimal timing for starting nutrition support therapy?

2. How do you decide the best route of feeding for this patient?

3. The patient has a high intracranial pressure and was then noted to be vomiting his enteral nutrition around the orogastric tube. The nurse puts the orogastric tube to low wall suction and 1,500 mL of gastric contents are drained. An abdominal CT scan is ordered and reveals an ileus. You review the amount of enteral nutrition infused over the past week and the patient has received < 50% of his goal volume. You note that the patient has new temporal, pectoralis, quadriceps, and gastrocnemius muscle wasting and fat wasting at the triceps that was not present on admission. What are your next steps for nutrition therapy?

PEDIATRIC CASE STUDY

A 10-month-old infant is admitted to the hospital with newly diagnosed high-risk neuroblastoma. Family reports decreased interest and usual oral intake of human milk and age-appropriate purees/solids, and have attempted to maintain the infants' hydration with oral rehydration solution with symptoms of vomiting and diarrhea leading up to admission. Family also shares that the infant has fallen from the 25th to the 5th weight-for-age percentile over the past month. The primary team has initiated conditioning treatment for the underlying neuroblastoma, and the infant remains inpatient for close monitoring during treatment. The team is allowing the patient to resume their usual oral diet of human milk and age-appropriate purees/solids, however they anticipate ongoing symptoms of gastro-intestinal intolerance in response to the treatment. The patient currently has three peripheral IVs with a plan for a central line later this week.

1. What is your recommendation for initiation of nutrition support for this patient?
2. How do you decide whether this patient is appropriate for peripheral PN support?
3. What PN-associated complications should you be thinking about when considering PN for this patient?
4. What signs and symptoms are you looking for to determine whether initiation of EN support would be appropriate for this patient?

INTRODUCTION

Specialized nutrition therapies are used for patients who have limitations in consuming nutrition by mouth or who are unable to adequately digest and absorb nutrients. In these cases, enteral nutrition (EN) and/or parenteral nutrition (PN) are important therapies to provide nutrition to support appropriate growth and development, correct malnutrition, maintain nutrition status, and meet metabolic demands in times of stress that may alter nutrient needs.

NUTRITION ASSESSMENT

Assessing nutritional status by a trained dietitian is the first step in developing a nutrition care plan. Nutrition assessment is reviewed in detail in Chapter 3. In addition to the assessment tools discussed in Chapter 3, additional tools are available for adult malnutrition nutrition assessment, summarized in a recent review.[1] Key aspects of the nutrition assessment process will provide guidance for deciding appropriate timing, dose and, in some cases, the type of specialized nutrition therapy. For both adult and pediatric patients, the presence of malnutrition will increase the urgency of initiation of specialized nutrition support if oral intake is inadequate or impossible.

As with adults, a comprehensive pediatric nutrition assessment is a critical component of the care of the child. Specific to pediatrics, recent guidelines have been established to more uniformly define pediatric malnutrition in the hospital setting, supporting the importance of earlier detection of those patients deemed at greatest nutrition risk.[2] The nutrition assessment should aim to include a thorough dietary intake history, anthropometric and growth history, nutrition-focused physical exam, review of medications and biochemical values, as well as review of functional status. Upon completion of the nutrition assessment, the care team can develop an individualized nutrition plan aimed to meet the nutritional needs of the child, while also addressing concerns for potential nutritional deficiencies or excesses. The nutrition plan may include recommendations for EN or PN support, modifications to the child's diet, and/or supplementation of vitamins or minerals. Many hospitalized children are at risk for nutrition deterioration; therefore, regular nutrition reassessment is just as important as the initial nutrition assessment.[3]

Patients with malnutrition are at higher risk of complications including infections, surgical complications, prolonged hospital length of stay, higher hospital readmission rates, and mortality.[1,4] A careful approach to nutrition assessment in this patient population is important to assure timely and adequate provision of nutrition support therapy and may improve clinical outcomes.

Estimating energy needs is reviewed in Chapter 3; however, it remains crucial for providers involved in prescribing nutrition support to be vigilant in regards to both under- and over-feeding, to avoid potential deleterious side effects (Figure 10-1).

ROUTE AND TIMING OF NUTRITION SUPPORT

Enteral Nutrition

ASPEN defines enteral nutrition (EN) support as a system of providing nutrition directly into the gastrointestinal tract via a tube, catheter, or stoma that bypasses the oral cavity.[5] Enteral formulas used for EN support are typically commercially prepared and can be made of various protein sources, carbohydrates, and fats (Table 10-1). They are designed to be nutritionally complete to meet the calculated nutritional requirements for both adult and pediatric patients. The protein sources can be made of intact protein such as whey, casein, or soy protein. Hydrolyzed proteins to provide peptides or free amino acids may be used as a protein source, depending on the functional status of the gastrointestinal tract. Carbohydrate sources can be corn syrup solids, cornstarch, sucrose, or maltodextrin. Lactose is generally not used as a carbohydrate source to avoid intolerance in patients with lactose intolerance. Fat sources are typically a blend of canola oil, corn oil, medium chain

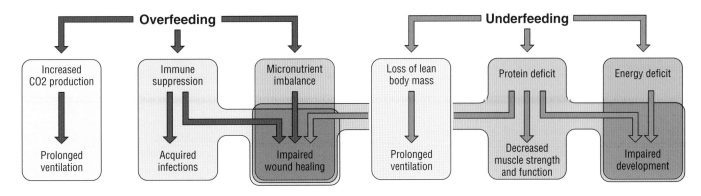

FIGURE 10-1 • Complications associated with underfeeding and overfeeding. (Ariagno K, Mehta NM. Care of the critically ill pediatric patient. In: Goday P, Waila, C, eds. *Pediatric Nutrition for Dietitians*. 1st ed. Boca Raton, FL: CRC Press; 2022:166.)

triglyceride (MCT) oil and/or fish oil (in selected products). Commercial ready-to-feed products can be packaged in large containers (e.g., 1L-1.5L total volume) or individual cartons ranging in volume from 237 to 355 mL each. Some specialized formula products are available in powdered form and must be reconstituted in sterile water prior to administration to the patient.[6-8]

It is becoming more common for patients and families to make their own homemade enteral formulas, often referred to as food-based or blenderized formulas. In some cases, the formula is the meal prepared for the entire family, blended with a liquid so it is thin enough to administer through an enteral feeding tube. Other patients make one large batch of formula to meet their needs for the entire day. These formulas may include animal proteins (e.g., beef, chicken, fish, egg, dairy), plant-based proteins (e.g., legumes or nuts), fruits, whole grains, vegetables, and oils, blended with water or broth to make a formula that this thin enough to administer through a feeding tube. Homemade enteral formulas can pose

a significant amount of work for a patient and/or caregiver and require safe food-handling practices to minimize microbial contamination. More recently, commercially made formulas made of "real" foods are available as an "off-the-shelf" alternative to gain the perceived benefits of a food-based formula without the labor required to prepare such a formula.[9]

Considerations for appropriate formula selection include the age of the patient, as well as their energy, protein, and fluid needs, underlying medical condition, and assessment of their GI function. The majority of adult and pediatric hospitalized patients requiring EN support can be initiated on a polymeric EN formula that contains intact protein, complex carbohydrates, fiber, and standard amounts of fat.[8] Compared to the composition of standard adult EN formulas, standard pediatric EN formulas have a higher percentage of calories from fat; 35-40% vs. 30%. Infant formulas, designed to mimic the nutrient composition of breastmilk, have the highest percent of calories from fat; 40–50%, to support the neurodevelopment of the growing infant.

TABLE 10-1 • Enteral nutrition formula types		
Formula type	Description	Indication
Polymeric	Intact protein, complex carbohydrate, fat	Functional GI tract with ability to digest and absorb nutrients
Disease specific	Modified in protein, carbohydrate, fat, and/or electrolytes to meet the needs of specific disease states	Products are available for patients with diseases including but not limited to: kidney disease, liver disease, diabetes, critical illness, genetic-metabolic disorders
Partially hydrolyzed protein source	Partially hydrolyzed protein and carbohydrate; fat provided as a blend of MCT and LCT oils	Malabsorption disorders
Amino acid-based protein source	Protein provided as free amino acids, partially hydrolyzed carbohydrate, very low fat with a large proportion as MCT	Severe malabsorption disorders
Modular	Single macronutrient product (protein, carbohydrate, or fat)	Used to increase delivery of a single macronutrient based on clinical need

GI, gastrointestinal; MCT, medium chain triglycerides; LCT, long-chain triglycerides.
Adapted from Roberts S, Kirsch R. Enteral nutrition formulations. In: Mueller CM, Lord LM, Marian M, McClave SA, Miller SJ, eds. *The ASPEN Adult Nutrition Support Core Curriculum*. 3rd ed. Silver Spring, MD: American Society for Parenteral and Enteral Nutrition; 2017:227-249.

Critically ill adult patients should not receive insoluble fiber because of the risk of intestinal obstruction. Soluble fiber supplements can be provided if required, for example, for patients with diarrhea.[10]

Indications for Specialized Formulas

Disease-specific enteral formulas may be appropriate for patients with certain conditions. Patients with malabsorptive conditions, liver disease, lymphatic disorders, or short bowel syndrome, may better tolerate formulas enriched with medium chain triglycerides. Specific formulas are available for patients with inborn errors of metabolic disease. Formulas restricted in fluid and electrolytes are available for patients with renal impairment and formulas with lower carbohydrate content are available for patients with diabetes. More recently, therapeutic additions to formula, such as both pre- and pro-biotics have been marketed to address GI symptoms such as constipation or diarrhea. There are also dietary components used in varied combinations aimed to attenuate the inflammatory response and support altered demands during periods of stress, such as omega-3 fatty acids, glutamine, arginine, and antioxidants. More research is needed to support the safety and efficacy of immunonutrition formulas.[4,8] Specialized EN formulas are typically more expensive and may not show a benefit to justify the cost. Guidelines from clinical nutrition societies may be helpful in determining the utility of specialty enteral formulas.

Indications for Enteral Nutrition Support

A major indication for EN is inability to safely consume nutrition by mouth.[11] Examples of patients in this category include those with severe dysphagia because of a neurological disorder (e.g., stroke) or those with head/neck cancer with severely impaired swallowing. Patients requiring mechanical ventilation with oral intubation also cannot take nutrition by mouth and require EN. Another indication is inability to take enough nutrition by mouth. This may be a patient with severe trauma or burn injury with very high energy and protein requirements. Patients with anorexia during times of disease or injury may also require supplemental EN to meet energy and protein requirements to support healing and recovery. A typical cutoff for when to start EN is in the adult or pediatric patient who cannot meet at least 60–75% of energy and protein requirements consistently with oral diet alone.[11] Pediatric patients share similar indications to the adult population, as to who would benefit from EN, while also having some unique indications (Table 10-2).

In critically ill adult and pediatric patients who are unable to take oral nutrition, EN should be started within the first 24–48 hours of ICU admission, regardless of their nutritional status.[11] Trophic feeding of just 10–20 mL/hr in adults or 10 mL/kg in pediatrics, can have beneficial effects including preservation of the intestinal epithelium barrier, stimulation of brush border enzyme activity, and preventing bacterial

TABLE 10-2 · Indications for enteral nutrition	
Adult	**Pediatric**

• **Inability to safely consume nutrition by mouth**
  ◦ Dysphagia
  ◦ Head/neck cancer
  ◦ Mechanical ventilation
• **Inability to take adequate nutrition by mouth**
• High nutrition demand (burn, trauma)
  ◦ Reduced appetite related to disease
  ◦ Malnutrition
  ◦ Malabsorption
  ◦ Need for specialized nutrients (e.g., genetic-metabolic disorder)
• **Altered gastrointestinal anatomy/function**
  ◦ Partial or total gastrectomy
  ◦ Esophagectomy
  ◦ Gastroparesis
  ◦ Pancreatitis
  ◦ Short bowel syndrome
	• **Functional**
	  ◦ Prematurity
	  ◦ Congenital malformations (Pierre Robin syndrome, tracheoesophageal fistula, cleft palate)
	  ◦ Dysphagia
	  ◦ Inability to consume adequate oral intake
	• **Psychological**
	  ◦ Disordered eating
	  ◦ Oral aversion
	• **Injury**
	  ◦ Trauma
	  ◦ Burns
	  ◦ Caustic ingestion
	  ◦ Sepsis
	• **Obstruction**
	  ◦ Invasive ventilation
	• **Impaired/Altered absorption/digestion**
	  ◦ Cystic fibrosis
	  ◦ Short bowel syndrome
	  ◦ Food allergies
	  ◦ Chronic liver disease
	  ◦ Solid organ transplantation
	• **Disease/disorder specific**
	  ◦ Metabolic disorders
	  ◦ Neurologic disorders
	  ◦ Congenital heart disease
	  ◦ Chronic kidney disease
	  ◦ Severe chronic lung disease

Adapted from Bechtold ML, Brown PM, Escuro A, et al. When is enteral nutrition indicated? *JPEN J Parenter Enteral Nutr.* 2022;46(7):1470-1496; Konek S, Becker P (eds). *Samour & King's Pediatric Nutrition in Clinical Care.* 5th ed. Burlington, MA: Jones & Bartlett Learning; 2020:202.

translocation.[10] For non-ICU patients, the nutrition assessment will help guide the decision regarding initiation of EN. Early EN can be deferred in patients who are assessed as well nourished or low risk, or who are anticipated to resume an oral diet within 5–7 days of hospital admission. The nutrition assessment will also help identify patients deemed to be at risk for the refeeding syndrome, in which EN initiation and advancement will need to be done cautiously to avoid unnecessary complications.[11] See Chapter 13 ("Severe Malnutrition and Refeeding Syndrome").

Enteral feeding algorithms are common in the hospitalized setting, and are designed to support a standardized advancement plan, in which the patient will reach their goal nutrition delivery in a timely fashion. They also prevent unnecessary interruptions and delays to EN delivery that can lead to greater nutrition deficits.

Enteral Nutrition Access Devices

Once a patient is identified as benefiting from initiation of EN support, an enteral access device must be selected to administer the EN formula to the patient. The decision process includes considerations of the patient's anatomy and the duration of time that the patient will require EN.[12] Once the enteral feeding device is determined and secured, the best mode of enteral nutrition delivery can be decided, either as a bolus/intermittent feeding or as a continuous infusion feeding (Table 10-3).

Short-term EN devices are typically placed through the nose and into either the stomach (nasogastric) or small bowel (nasoduodenal or nasojejunal). For adults and children, these tubes can stay in place for 4–12 weeks; longer courses can lead to sinusitis or damage to the nares. In critically ill patients requiring mechanical ventilation, orogastric tubes may be used to reduce the risk of sinusitis. Adequate sedation is necessary to avoid patient discomfort. The orogastric tube may be switched to a nasogastric or nasoenteric tube for comfort as sedation is lightened. These tubes are typically placed at the bedside, but for patients with complex anatomy, guidance from interventional radiology or placement in the operating room may be necessary.[12]

Long-term enteral access devices include those placed directly into the stomach (gastrostomy) or into the jejunum (jejunostomy). Long-term enteral access devices may be

TABLE 10-3 • Summary of enteral nutrition delivery methods					
Administration method	Description	Enteral access location	Indications	Advantages	Disadvantages
Continuous infusion	Formula infused via pump, continuously over 24 hours	Gastric or post-pyloric	- Typical feeding method when initiating EN - Delayed gastric emptying - Aspiration risk - Limited absorptive area	- Improved tolerance - Ease of administration for inpatient setting - Ease of monitoring feeding in inpatient setting	- Feeding pump required - Limits patient activity - May reduce appetite for patients also taking oral nutrition
Bolus infusion	A specific amount of formula is infused over a short period of time, multiple times during the day	Gastric only	- Need/desire for a simplified feeding schedule to accommodate school, work, appointments, etc - Supplemental feeding if intake at a meal is inadequate	- May be administered via syringe, limiting equipment required for feeding - More physiologic feeding schedule - Allows for increased patient mobility	- Potential for nausea, vomiting, or aspiration with large volume bolus - Risk of aspiration
Cyclic infusion	Formula infused via pump, over a restricted number of hours/day (e.g., 12–18 hours)	Gastric or post-pyloric	- Need/desire for time off the feeding pump, but unable to transition to bolus feeding - Allows development of an appetite during the day to promote oral intake/feeding	- Allows disconnection from the pump during the day to allow for activities of daily living, school, work, etc - For patients who are eating, nocturnal infusion allows for development of an appetite during the day	- Higher infusion rate may contribute to nausea, vomiting, and/or diarrhea - Interrupted sleep (for night-cycled feeding)

Adapted from Harshman SG, Fiechtner LG. Enteral nutrition. In: Goday P, Waila, C, eds. *Pediatric Nutrition for Dietitians*. 1st ed. Boca Raton, FL: CRC Press; 2022:102 and Doley J, Phillips W. Overview of enteral nutrition. In: Mueller CM, Lord LM, Marian M, McClave SA, Miller SJ, eds. *The ASPEN Adult Nutrition Support Core Curriculum*. 3rd ed. Silver Spring, MD: American Society for Parenteral and Enteral Nutrition. 2017;213-225.

considered early in a patient's course, depending on the clinical indication for EN. For example, a patient with a major resection for oral cancer may benefit from early placement of a gastrostomy tube. A patient who is undergoing an esophagectomy for esophageal cancer may benefit from placement of a feeding jejunostomy tube at the time of the esophagectomy. For patients with a short-term enteral access device in place, consideration of transition to a long-term device should be considered after 6–8 weeks with the short-term device in place. This may be the case for a patient requiring a nasogastric tube for EN because of swallowing difficulty after a stroke but without sufficient recovery of swallowing function to allow for removal of the short-term access device. These tubes can be placed in the operating room, GI endoscopy suite, or in interventional radiology.[12]

Enteral Nutrition Complications

Common complications associated with enteral nutrition involve the gastrointestinal tract. These complications include nausea and vomiting, diarrhea, and constipation. These complications need to be evaluated carefully to determine if the complication is associated with the patient's underlying disease, existing medical therapy, or the feeding itself. Aspiration of the enteral formula is another potential complication that may occur in patients with depressed neurological function or with a poor gag reflex. Keeping the head of the bed up at least 30 degrees will help reduce risk of aspiration; post-pyloric enteral access may also help reduce aspiration risk. Electrolyte derangements, dehydration, or volume overload are other potential complications that may occur in the patient receiving enteral nutrition. Appropriate monitoring of electrolyte levels and hydration status is essential to allow for early intervention and adjustment of the enteral formula, if indicated.[13]

Parenteral Nutrition

Parenteral nutrition (PN) is the intravenous infusion of nutrients. It is composed of crystalline amino acids, dextrose, lipid injectable emulsion, electrolytes, vitamins, trace elements, and sterile water. PN may be customized for individual patients, or premixed solutions are available for institutions that do not have the clinical expertise for managing customized solutions. PN is commonly termed as 3:1 or 2:1 solutions. In addition to all the other PN components, the 3:1 PN solutions contain all three macronutrients, whereas in the 2:1 solution, the lipid is provided separately from the rest of the PN components.[14] The 2:1 solution is more often utilized in the hospital setting, where the 3:1 solution is more common in patients who require PN support at home.

PN delivery is initiated as a 24-hour continuous infusion. Once a patient has demonstrated tolerance on a stable PN solution, the PN solution can be cycled over fewer hours as a way to offer time being disconnected to a continuous infusion.[15] This may also be a desirable practice when a patient is receiving intravenous medications that are incompatible with the PN solution. Extended PN cycling is better tolerated in older children and adults due to glucose metabolism and the ability to maintain euglycemia when cycled off the PN,

which contains dextrose.[16] Acceptable ranges for both glucose infusion rates (GIRs) and lipid infusion rates (LIRs) exist to help guide the clinician when determining the duration of the cycle.[17]

PN support is costly and is associated with complications, including mechanical and infectious central venous catheter complications, so careful patient selection is important. The type of intravenous access will dictate the type of PN solution ordered, either central PN or peripheral PN. Dextrose and amino acids are major contributors to the osmolarity of a PN solution, with electrolytes contributing to a lesser degree. Peripheral PN solutions may have an osmolarity up to 900 mOsm/L; solutions greater than 900 mOsm/L must be infused through a central venous catheter to avoid thrombophlebitis and other complications.[16,18] Peripheral PN solutions are more dilute compared to central PN solutions and require larger volumes and more lipid to meet energy requirements. Patients who need a fluid restriction (e.g., heart failure, renal disease, liver disease) may not benefit from peripheral PN solutions. As with EN, the nutrition assessment plays an important role in determining when a patient should be initiated on PN, as well as the specific dose of parenteral macronutrients, micronutrients, vitamins, and trace elements prescribed.[14,16]

Indications for Parenteral Nutrition

Indications for PN revolve around GI dysfunction and the patient's underlying nutritional status. Worthington et al.[16] provided key indications for both adults and pediatrics requiring PN support in the ASPEN consensus paper, "When is parenteral nutrition indicated?" Impaired absorption or loss of nutrients is a major indication for initiation of PN. These may include patients with various forms of intestinal failure, high-output intestinal fistula, or severe diarrhea. In some of these cases, EN may be attempted, but if there is evidence of intolerance or worsening of fistula output or diarrhea, PN should be considered. Mechanical bowel obstruction is another indication for PN; this is a clear indication where enteral nutrients are blocked from traveling normally down the GI tract. In some cases, a bowel obstruction may resolve spontaneously and in a short period of time; however, in cases of prolonged obstruction, PN is required to correct nutritional compromise. Bowel rest is another common reason for PN initiation; this may be for patients with ischemia bowel, severe pancreatitis, or chylothorax/chylous ascites (i.e., presence of chyle (lymphatic fluids and chylomicrons) in the chest or abdominal cavities). In some cases of severe inflammatory bowel disease requiring surgery, PN is used for preoperative nutritional optimization prior to surgery to reduce nutrition-related complications. Gastrointestinal motility disorders are another indication for PN; this may include postoperative ileus, scleroderma, or other underlying diseases that lead to reduced intestinal motility. Inability to achieve or maintain enteral access is another major indication for PN. Patients who are unable to have enteral access placed or used for feeding would fall into this category. Examples of this category include severe GI bleeding or severe epistaxis precluding placement of a nasoenteric tube. Patients who decline placement of enteral access but who still need specialized nutrition therapy would also fit in this category.[16]

Very low birth weight (VLBW: < 1,500 grams) and low birth weight (LBW: < 2,500 grams), and/or premature infants should be considered for PN initiation soon after birth to support glucose homeostasis and nitrogen balance. Starter PN solutions that contain amino acids, dextrose, and calcium are available in NICUs to support early protein delivery for this highly vulnerable patient population, while awaiting for initiation of full PN support. See Chapter 11 "Prematurity." Worthington et al.[16] recommend initiating PN in full-term infants within 1–3 days, and malnourished children/adolescents within 4–5 days if it is likely that they will have a delayed return of bowel function over an extended period of time. Well-nourished children and adolescents with an acute illness, in contrast, can delay PN initiation for 1 week.

ASPEN provides guidance on how a clinician should initiate and advance both adults and pediatric patients on PN support.[17] Implementation of quality improvement initiatives supporting best practice care bundles for insertion and maintenance of central venous catheters have reduced the incidence of central line-associated bloodstream infections (CLABSI) in the hospitalized setting.

Parenteral Nutrition Access

Like enteral access, consideration for parenteral access should be based on the patient's condition (acute or chronic), the primary indication for PN, as well as the anticipated duration for PN support. The type of intravenous access will dictate the type of PN solution ordered, either central PN or peripheral PN. As previously mentioned, peripheral PN support is often limited in the ability to meet a patients nutrition needs due to osmolarity restrictions not exceeding 900 mOsm/L. Central venous access allows for optimal delivery of hyperosmolar parenteral solutions, ideally at the junction of the distal superior vena cava and right atrium.[19]

Non-tunneled catheters, such as peripherally inserted central catheters (PICCs) are recommended for short-term PN use (Figure 10-2). They can be placed at the bedside or by interventional radiology and utilized for weeks to months. Tunneled catheters are designed for more long-term PN use, with a lower associated infection risk (Figure 10-3). They are more commonly placed in the operating room.[19]

Parenteral Nutrition Complications

Patients receiving parenteral nutrition must be monitored closely for complications while initiating therapy, then monitoring may be extended as stability is established.[20] The infusion of nutrients directly into the bloodstream contributes to the most common acute complications of PN: electrolyte imbalances and hyperglycemia. When PN is initiated, electrolytes should be monitored daily allowing for correction of abnormalities separately from the PN and for adjustments in the PN prescription. Blood glucose should be monitored daily and if a patient is hyperglycemic, more frequent blood glucose monitoring is warranted with regular insulin coverage. Regular insulin may be safely added to PN if necessary.[20]

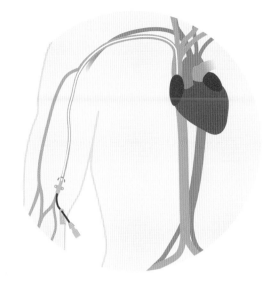

PERIPHERALLY INSERTED CENTRAL CATHETER (PICC LINE)

FIGURE 10-2 · Peripherally inserted central venous catheter. (Used with permission from Science Photo Library/Alamy Stock Photo.)

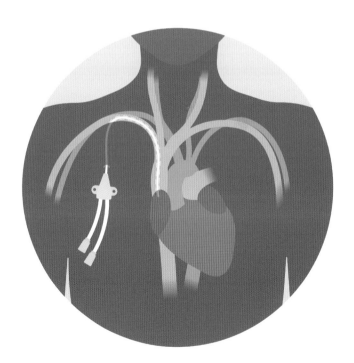

FIGURE 10-3 · Tunneled central venous catheter. (Used with permission from art4stock/Alamy Stock Photo.)

Patients requiring PN for long-term support are at risk for long-term complications including PN-associated liver disease and metabolic bone disease. Potential interventions to avoid PN-associated liver disease include avoidance of overfeeding, avoiding high doses of lipid emulsions that are comprised of

TABLE 10-4 • Recommended monitoring for parenteral nutrition		
Parameter	Initiation	Stable, long-term
Electrolytes: Na, K, Cl, CO2, Mg, Ca, phosphorus, BUN, Cr	Daily with PN advancement	Weekly
Serum glucose	Daily with PN advancement	Weekly
Capillary glucose	Every 6 hours initially in patients with hyperglycemia	If change in clinical management or status warrants closer monitoring
Serum triglycerides	Daily with IV lipid advancement	Weekly
CBC with differential	Day 1	Weekly
INR, PT, PTT	Day 1	Weekly
ALT, AST, ALP, total bilirubin, direct bilirubin	Day 1	Weekly to Monthly
Extended micronutrient panel	Not recommended	Periodically
Weight	Daily	2–3 × per week
Intake and output	Daily	Daily

Adapted from: Kumpf VJ, Gervasio J. Complications of parenteral nutrition. In: Mueller C, ed. *The ASPEN Adult Nutrition Support Core Curriculum.* 3rd ed. ASPEN; 2017:345-360.

Na, sodium; K, potassium; Cl, chloride; CO_2, carbon dioxide; Mg, magnesium; Ca, calcium; BUN, blood urea nitrogen; Cr, creatinine; PN, parenteral nutrition; IV, intravenous; CBC, complete blood count; INR, international normalized ratio; PT, prothrombin time; PTT, partial thromboplastin time; ALT, alanine transaminase; AST, aspartate aminotransferase; ALP, alkaline phosphatase

100% soybean oil, selecting lipid emulsions that contain fish oil, and cycling parenteral nutrition. Patients at risk for metabolic bone disease need adequate provision of calcium and vitamin D, reduction of aluminum in the PN admixture, and appropriate activities for bone health as the clinical condition allows. In-depth discussion of long-term complications of PN are covered elsewhere.[20]

A major, and potentially lethal, complication associated with PN is central-line associated bloodstream infection. Aseptic technique is essential when caring for central venous access devices and while connecting and disconnecting PN infusion. Even with the best efforts, infectious complications may occur. Clinicians must be aware of early signs and symptoms of infections, which include elevated white blood cell count, fever, chills, and malaise. Unexpected hyperglycemia may be an early sign of infection and should be evaluated promptly. Management of infectious complications is discussed in detail elsewhere.[19]

MONITORING AND EVALUATION

Both EN and PN require close monitoring by the entire healthcare team to ensure tolerance and continued appropriateness. Many studies have confirmed that safe and effective administration of advanced nutritional therapies is best performed in the setting of a multidisciplinary team.[21] The nutrition support plan should be tailored accordingly based on the changes in a patient's clinical status. The following components should be closely monitored for anyone receiving nutrition support:

- Serial anthropometric measurements
- Signs and symptoms of intolerance to EN or PN
- Biochemical data
- Physical examination for potential micronutrient deficiencies or edema

Table 10-4 outlines specific parameters to follow when initiating and maintaining a patient on PN support. Additionally, the team should monitor a patient's ability or readiness to transition from one mode of nutrition support to another. Patients initially requiring PN support may show evidence of return of adequate bowel function, in which they can be initiated/advanced on EN and wean off PN support. The same can occur for when a patient may be able to safely resume an oral diet. Generally, when a patient can meet > 50–75% of nutrition needs orally, PN or EN support can be weaned off. During these periods of transition, close monitoring of anthropometrics, as well as fluid and electrolyte status is important to be able to demonstrate the patient is meeting and tolerating their nutrition goals, while also staying adequately hydrated.

CONCLUSION

Both EN and PN provide life-sustaining modes of nutrition support to complex patients. EN is the preferred mode of nutrition support with a functioning GI tract. The timing, dose, and mode of delivery all need to be considered when nutrition support has been identified to benefit the patient. Nutrition therapies should be tailored to meet the individual needs of the patient and regularly reassessed to ensure the nutrition delivery remains appropriate.

THREE TAKE-HOME POINTS

1. The presence of malnutrition increases the urgency of starting specialized nutrition therapies in adult and pediatric patients who are unable to consume adequate food by mouth to meet metabolic demands of disease.
2. Enteral nutrition is the first choice for intervention in adult and pediatric patients who cannot eat by mouth or consume enough by mouth but otherwise have a functional gastrointestinal tract. Selection of enteral formula and delivery method should be individualized to the patient and their nutritional needs.
3. Parenteral nutrition is indicated in adult and pediatric patients with gastrointestinal dysfunction that impairs ability to absorb nutrients. Routine monitoring of patients on parenteral nutrition by a multidisciplinary nutrition support team can minimize associated complications.

ADULT CASE STUDY ANSWERS

1. The Society of Critical Care Medicine and the American Society for Parenteral and Enteral Nutrition recommend initiation of enteral nutrition within 24–48 hours of intensive care unit admission for patients who are unable to eat by mouth. Nutritional status is also an important factor in deciding how quickly to start nutrition support therapy. Presence of malnutrition increases the urgency of starting nutrition support therapy to minimize loss of lean body mass. In this case, the nutritional status is unknown, but a head injury requiring neurosurgery has a significant metabolic demand. Early nutrition support will be beneficial for this patient.

2. Assessment of the functional status of the GI tract is essential in determining the route of feeding. Patients with a functional GI tract and who can have enteral access placed can start enteral nutrition. In this case, the minimal output from the orogastric tube and using the tube for enteral medications are indicators that enteral nutrition can be started using the orogastric tube.

3. An ileus is a contraindication to enteral nutrition. In addition, the patient has been poorly fed over the past week and is showing signs of malnutrition: muscle and fat wasting. The next step in this case is to start parenteral nutrition until the ileus is resolved and enteral nutrition can be resumed.

PEDIATRIC CASE STUDY ANSWERS

1. Based on the patients decreased oral intake and weight loss leading up to this admission, the patient is assessed at increased nutrition risk, and initiation of nutrition support would be appropriate. With the anticipated GI side effects associated with the current treatment for neuroblastoma, parenteral nutrition support would be the preferred route of nutrition support at this time, to ensure consistent, adequate nutrition delivery (in addition to supporting oral intake as tolerated with use of anti-emetic agents).

2. Peripheral PN support would be appropriate in this patient, in the short term to allow for timely delivery of both macronutrients and micronutrients, also knowing it is a bridge to central PN once a central venous catheter is placed later in the week. Patient considerations with peripheral PN include making sure that the patient is not fluid restricted or requires increased electrolyte provision, given that the osmolarity cannot exceed 900 mOsm/L.

3. PN support (central and peripheral) is considered a high-risk medical therapy. Associated PN complications to consider for this patient include metabolic complications, such as electrolyte disturbances related to a side effect of medications or end-organ dysfunction. Infectious complications can also pose a risk, especially being immunocompromised, however central line care bundles have been implemented in many hospital care settings to reduce central line-associated bloodstream infections (CLABSI).

4. Depending on the duration of the treatment course and GI symptoms of vomiting and diarrhea, supplemental EN should be considered if oral intake remains suboptimal. Establishing enteral intake/tolerance is important to not only have to rely on PN support for longer than needed, but also to ensure a healthy GI tract. EN via a nasogastric or nasojejunal feeding tube would both be appropriate options to consider for this patient. Once the patient is demonstrating adequate intake > 60–75% of estimated energy/protein needs orally or via an enteral feeding tube, PN support would be appropriate to wean off.

REFERENCES

1. Malone A, Mogensen KM. Key approaches to diagnosing malnutrition in adults. *Nutr Clin Pract*. 2022;37(1):23-34.

2. Becker P, Carney LN, Corkins M, et al. Consensus statement of the Academy of Nutrition and Dietetics/American Society for Parenteral and Enteral Nutrition: indicators recommended for the identification and documentation or pediatric malnutrition (undernutrition). *Nutr Clin Pract*. 2015;30(1):147-161.

3. Mehta NM, Skillman HE, Irving SY, et al. Guidelines for the provision and assessment of nutrition support therapy in the pediatric critically ill patient: Society of Critical Care Medicine and American Society for Parenteral and Enteral Nutrition. *JPEN J Parenter Enteral Nutr*. 2017;41(5):706-742.

4. Bechard LJ, Duggan C, Touger-Decker R, et al. Nutritional status based on body mass index is associated with morbidity and mortality in mechanically ventilated critically ill children in the PICU. *Crit Care Med*. 2016;44(8):1530-1537.

5. Robinson D, Walker R. Adams SC, et al. American Society for Parenteral and Enteral Nutrition (ASPEN) definition of terms, style, and conventions used in ASPEN Board of Directors-approved documents. May 2018. Available at: https://www.nutritioncare.org/Guidelines_and_Clinical_Resources/Clinical_Practice_Library/Special_Reports/. Accessed 10/15/2022.

6. Boullata JI, Carrera AL, Harvey L, et al. ASPEN safe practices for enteral nutrition therapy. *JPEN J Parenter Enteral Nutr*. 2017;41(1):15-103.

7. Doley J, Phillips W. Overview of enteral nutrition. In: Mueller CM, Lord LM, Marian M, McClave SA, Miller SJ, eds. *The ASPEN Adult Nutrition Support Core Curriculum*, 3rd ed. American Society for Parenteral and Enteral Nutrition; 2017:213-225.

8. Roberts S, Kirsch R. Enteral nutrition formulations. In: Mueller CM, Lord LM, Marian M, McClave SA, Miller SJ, eds. *The ASPEN Adult Nutrition Support Core Curriculum*. 3rd ed. American Society for Parenteral and Enteral Nutrition; 2017:227-249.

9. Bennett K, Hjelmgren B, Piazza J. Blenderized tube feeding: health outcomes and review of homemade and commercially prepared products. *Nutr Clin Pract*. 2020;35(3):417-431.

10. McClave SA, Taylor BE, Martindale RG, et al. Guidelines for the provision and assessment of nutrition support therapy in the adult critically ill patient: Society of Critical Care Medicine (SCCM) and American Society for Parenteral and Enteral Nutrition (A.S.P.E.N.). *JPEN J Parenter Enteral Nutr*. 2016;40(2):159-211.

11. Bechtold ML, Brown PM, Escuro A, et al. When is enteral nutrition indicated? *JPEN J Parenter Enteral Nutr*. 2022;46(7):1470-1496.

12. Fang JC, Kinikini M. Enteral access devices. In: Mueller CM, Lord LM, Marian M, McClave SA, Miller SJ, eds. *The ASPEN Adult Nutrition Support Core Curriculum*. 3rd ed. American Society for Parenteral and Enteral Nutrition; 2017:251-264.

13. Malone AM, Seres DS, Lord LM. Complications of enteral nutrition. In: Mueller CM, Lord LM, Marian M, McClave SA, Miller SJ, eds. *The ASPEN Adult Nutrition Support Core Curriculum*. 3rd ed. American Society for Parenteral and Enteral Nutrition; 2017:265-284.

14. Patel R. Parenteral nutrition formulations. In: Mueller CM, Lord LM, Marian M, McClave SA, Miller SJ, eds. *The ASPEN Adult Nutrition Support Core Curriculum*. 3rd ed. American Society for Parenteral and Enteral Nutrition; 2017:297-320.

15. Ayers P, Adams S, Boullata J, et al. A.S.P.E.N. parenteral nutrition safety consensus recommendations. *JPEN J Parenter Enteral Nutr*. 2014;38(3):296-333.

16. Worthington P, Balint J, Bechtold M, et al. When is parenteral nutrition appropriate? *JPEN J Parenter Enteral Nutr*. 2017;41(3): 324-377.

17. American Society for Parenteral and Enteral Nutrition. Appropriate dosing for parenteral nutrition: ASPEN recommendations. Available at: https://www.nutritioncare.org/PNResources/. Accessed 4/30/2023.

18. Boullata JI, Gilbert K, Sacks G, et al. A.S.P.E.N. Clinical guidelines: parenteral nutrition ordering, order review, compounding, labeling, and dispensing. *JPEN J Parenter Enteral Nutr*. 2014;38(3): 334-377.

19. Neal AM, Drogan K. Parenteral access devices. In: Mueller CM, Lord LM, Marian M, McClave SA, Miller SJ, eds. *The ASPEN Adult Nutrition Support Core Curriculum*. 3rd ed. American Society for Parenteral and Enteral Nutrition; 2017: 321-344.

20. Kumpf VJ, Gervasio J. Complications of parenteral nutrition. In: Mueller CM, Lord LM, Marian M, McClave SA, Miller SJ, eds. *The ASPEN Adult Nutrition Support Core Curriculum*. 3rd ed. American Society for Parenteral and Enteral Nutrition; 2017:345-360.

21. Barrocas A, Schwartz DB, Bistrian BR, et al. Nutrition support teams: institution, evolution and innovation. *Nutr Clin Pract*. 2023;38(1):10-26.

chapter 11

Prematurity

Mandy Brown Belfort, MD MPH

Chapter Outline

CASE STUDY

A pregnant patient presents at 29 weeks of gestation with progressive preterm labor. She delivers a male infant weighing 1,200 grams (2 pounds, 10 ounces) with a body length of 38 cm and head circumference 26.5 cm. The infant is noted to have respiratory distress in the delivery room and is intubated. Upon arrival to the neonatal intensive care unit, a peripheral IV is placed and a continuous infusion of 10% dextrose is started. Initial blood glucose is 50. An umbilical venous catheter is placed and confirmed to be in a central location at the junction of the inferior vena cava and right atrium. Blood pressure is stable and in the normal range for gestational age. Once initial care is complete, the infant is placed in a humidified isolette. The mother intends to provide human milk for her infant and hand-expressed several drops of colostrum shortly after giving birth.

1. Using the online Fenton and Kim 2013 fetal growth reference, you determine that the infant's birth weight is at the 46th percentile for gestational age. How does one classify this infant's size at birth? (Choose one.)
   A. Small for gestational age
   B. Appropriate for gestational age
   C. Large for gestational age

2. What is the appropriate nutritional management in the first few hours after birth? (Choose all that apply.)
   A. Total fluids of 160 mL/kg/day
   B. Neonatal parenteral nutrition solution with dextrose and amino acids
   C. Mouth care with expressed colostrum
   D. Trophic feedings with maternal milk or pasteurized donor milk, 1.5 mL per gavage every 3 hours (10 mL/kg/day)
   E. NPO (no enteral feeding)

(Continued)

CASE STUDY   *(Continued)*

By day of life 14, the infant is feeding fortified human milk at 160 mL/kg/day, parenteral nutrition has been discontinued, and the central line has been removed. The baby's weight is now 1,056 grams, which represents the weight nadir thus far, with no weight gain observed in the past 3 days. Milk is being given via continuous infusion through a nasogastric tube due to previous spit-ups that have now resolved. Feedings comprise approximately half maternal milk and half donor milk. He is receiving vitamin D and iron supplements.

3. **How much weight has the infant lost as a percent of birth weight? (Choose one.)**
   A. 12%
   B. 14%
   C. 6%
   D. 7%

4. **Which of the following represents appropriate next steps in management? (Choose all that apply.)**
   A. Discontinue donor milk and start using preterm infant formula to supplement maternal milk.
   B. Check electrolytes and consider sodium supplementation.
   C. Ensure adequate lactation support is available for mother.
   D. Place a new central line to restart parenteral nutrition and continue until birth weight is regained.
   E. Add a modular liquid protein supplement.
   F. No change in current management is indicated.

5. **Which of the following represents the most appropriate discharge plan for this infant?**
   A. To ensure adequate fluid and caloric intake at home, the infant should receive all feedings by bottle as maternal milk fortified with formula powder or liquid concentrate.
   B. The infant should stop breastfeeding and transition to a postdischarge formula.
   C. The infant should directly breastfeed two to three times per day and receive the remainder of his feedings as expressed maternal milk fortified with formula powder or liquid concentrate, with close monitoring of weight gain.
   D. The infant should not be discharged until he weighs >2,500 grams.

EPIDEMIOLOGY OF PRETERM BIRTH, NUTRITIONAL STATUS, AND OUTCOMES

Each year in the United States, > 360,000 infants are born preterm (< 37 completed weeks of gestation). Preterm birth is the second-leading cause of neonatal mortality and confers an increased risk of short- and long-term morbidities among survivors. Although survival is now > 90%, infants born very preterm (< 32 weeks of gestation), and particularly those born extremely preterm (< 28 weeks), are vulnerable to serious medical complications due to their physiological immaturity and ongoing critical illness. These infants require intensive care therapies after birth and typically remain hospitalized in the neonatal intensive care unit (NICU) until approximately term equivalent age (40 weeks of postmenstrual age).[1] Even moderate- and late-preterm infants who do not require intensive care experience more complications after birth, such as feeding difficulties and jaundice, than full-term peers.[2] After discharge, preterm infants are at increased risk for rehospitalization and require continued management of chronic conditions, heightened developmental surveillance, and rehabilitative therapies to optimize long-term outcomes.

Preterm infants represent a nutritionally vulnerable population. Prenatally, nutrient deficits may accumulate in the setting of intrauterine growth restriction (IUGR), a pathological condition of pregnancy in which a fetus fails to meet its growth potential due to maternal, fetal, and/or placental factors including maternal hypertensive disorders, smoking, intrauterine infection, and fetal genetic disorders. IUGR and/or its underlying causes may contribute to preterm delivery. Postnatally, preterm infants typically experience impaired weight gain and stunted linear growth relative to the fetus, driven by the reduced accretion of fat-free mass and resulting in a higher body fat percent at NICU discharge.[3] These prenatal and postnatal growth impairments indicate deficits in nutrient accretion occurring during critical or sensitive periods in brain development. The past two decades have seen substantial improvements in growth outcomes at NICU discharge,[1] reflecting the effectiveness of clinical interventions. Despite these improvements, surveillance data indicate that the average body weight of a very preterm infant at hospital discharge is nearly a full standard deviation lower than that of a full-term newborn[1] and the average body length is more than a standard deviation lower.[4] Thus, preterm infants leave the NICU with accumulated nutrient deficits, making postdischarge nutritional management a critical element of care for this population.

NUTRIENT REQUIREMENTS FOR PRETERM INFANTS

Once preterm birth occurs and the placental circulation is abruptly removed, the infant depends on an exogenous supply of nutrients in the hospital setting. The overarching goal of nutritional care for hospitalized preterm infants is to provide the nutrients needed to achieve the rate of growth and composition of weight gain for a normal fetus while supporting healthy brain development.[5] Very preterm infants double or even triple their body weight during the NICU hospitalization, reflecting a rapid expansion of organs and tissues. Nutritional and non-nutritional factors related to critical illness may limit preterm infants from achieving their growth potential.

Ensuring that nutrient requirements are met is a key priority of overall clinical care. Recommended intakes to promote growth and prevent nutrient deficiencies cannot simply be extrapolated from healthy full-term newborns both because requirements may be substantially higher for preterm infants, and because preterm infants often face medical complications that alter nutrient requirements and/or limit the provision of nutritional support. Detailed recommendations for the nutritional management of preterm infants have been published.[5,6]

Fluid and Electrolyte Balance

In the fetus, total body water decreases sharply over gestation; for example, at 24 weeks, the fetus contains 90% water, whereas at 40 weeks the fetus contains 75% water. This change reflects, in part, the accumulation of fat stores over the third trimester. After full-term and preterm birth, extracellular water contracts; this contraction is more pronounced in preterm infants. Following an initial period of oliguria, a diuretic phase occurs. The preterm infant's weight typically falls by ~0.8 SD[7] or ~10–12% in the first 5 days due to fluid losses in urine and through an immature skin barrier. Skin losses can be reduced by the use of the humidified incubator. In the first several days after birth, the primary goals of fluid and electrolyte provision are to allow extracellular water to contract while preserving intravascular volume, and to allow a net negative sodium balance while maintaining normal serum sodium levels.[8] Initially, fluids and electrolytes are mainly parenteral while enteral nutrition is initiated at a low volume and slowly increased. Following a nadir in body weight, and as enteral nutrition becomes more established, weight gain resumes. Eventually, a stable growth pattern is reached that parallels the fetal curve, but with an offset reflecting the initial weight loss.

During all phases, the fluid volume required to provide optimal nutrients may exceed the minimum fluid volume needed for hydration. The common practice of limiting fluid intake in an attempt to improve the respiratory status of infants with bronchopulmonary dysplasia may limit growth while failing to improve pulmonary outcomes.[9] Sodium and chloride are required for stable growth. Hyponatremia and/or hypochloremia in the setting of growth faltering should prompt supplementation. Some evidence suggests that routine sodium chloride supplementation may be beneficial for human milk-fed preterm infants.[10]

Energy

Energy is needed to support metabolic processes and for growth. The energy balance equation is helpful in conceptualizing the components of gross energy intake, which is equal to energy expended + energy stored + energy excreted. Energy requirements are estimated from studies of energy metabolism, tissue accretion, and energy expenditure in human and animal models. Growth requires energy, in other words there is an "energy cost of growth" comprising the energy needed to create new tissue and the energy stored in the new tissue. Caring for infants in an incubator reduces energy expenditure. Enterally fed infants, as compared with parenterally fed infants, have greater energy expenditure due to the energy cost of absorbing nutrients and energy excretion through stool. At least 110 kcal/kg/day is recommended for enterally fed infants, and intakes of 130 kcal/kg/day or higher may be required for catch-up following a period of growth faltering *in utero* and/or postnatally. Recommended parenteral energy intakes for stable, growing infants are somewhat lower at 90 to 115 kcal/kg/day.[11]

Carbohydrate

Glucose is a major energy source and is particularly critical for the brain and heart. Glucose also contributes carbon for amino acid and fatty acid synthesis. In the fetus, all glucose is provided by the mother through passive diffusion across the placenta; endogenous glucose production (gluconeogenesis) does not occur. After preterm birth, glucose demands of the infant are met initially by continuous infusion of dextrose-containing fluids and increasingly through human milk and/or infant formula. Postnatally, gluconeogenesis occurs even with adequate intravenous glucose provision and is further stimulated by intravenous lipid provision.

Glucose utilization may be twice as high for extremely preterm and very preterm infants, as compared with full-term infants.[11] The rate of glucose utilization for the preterm infant is ~6–8 mg/kg/minute. At glucose higher infusion rates, glycogen and fat synthesis occur. The goals of meeting glucose requirements must be counterbalanced by the risk of hyperglycemia, particularly in extremely preterm infants. Hyperglycemia is driven both by exogenous glucose provision and endogenous gluconeogenesis. To prevent hyperglycemia, clinicians may initiate a lower glucose infusion rate and use serial serum glucoses to guide increases. The glucose infusion rate in *mg/kg/minute* is calculated as (infusion rate, *mL/hour* * dextrose concentration, *g/dL* * 1000 *mg/g*) / (weight, *kg* * 60 *minutes/hour*). Several online calculators are available to assist the clinician in calculating and adjusting the glucose infusion rate. Routine insulin treatment to prevent hyperglycemia carries risks and does not improve long-term outcomes.[12] Insulin is used to treat individual infants with refractory hyperglycemia, despite reducing the glucose infusion rate.

Glucose in enterally fed infants is produced by hydrolysis of lactose in human milk or glucose polymers contained in formula. Other important carbohydrates are galactose, inositol, and human milk oligosaccharides. Galactose is released in the intestine, easily absorbed into the portal circulation, and stored as glycogen. Human milk oligosaccharides but support the growth of commensal bacteria such as *Bifidobacterium* and *Lactobacillus* and may protect against NEC.[13]

Protein

Protein intake is the main driver of lean body mass growth. Protein also has many functions within the infant, including cell structure, cell signaling (enzymes and hormones, transporters, receptors), and immune function. For growth to occur, protein synthesis must outweigh degradation. Excess amino acids that are not incorporated into new tissue are oxidized into carbon dioxide and ammonia, releasing 4 kcal/g of energy, as well as ammonia, which is detoxified by the liver into urea and excreted in the kidney. Of the 20 amino acids, some are essential, some are non-essential, and some are conditionally essential for the preterm infant, meaning that endogenous synthesis is present but not adequate to meet requirements. Thus, in addition to the requirement for total protein intake, the quality of dietary protein is important. Certain amino acids have been investigated specifically for beneficial effects in this population. Taurine is a conditionally essential amino acid that is important for neural tissue growth and to conjugate with bile salts to facilitate fatty acid absorption.[14] Cysteine is another commonly supplemented amino acid in parenteral nutrition. Neither enteral nor parenteral glutamine supplementation appear to improve long-term outcomes,[15] whereas arginine may reduce risk of NEC[16] by altering intestinal epithelial blood supply.

Actual protein requirements for the preterm infant differ from the fetus. The fetus receives approximately 3.5 to 4 g/kg/day of protein as a continuous infusion across the placenta, of which one-third is oxidized as energy and the remainder is accreted into tissues. Overall, accounting for normal fetal accretion, protein oxidation, and immature intestinal function, very preterm infants require 4–4.5 g/kg/day of protein to achieve intrauterine growth of 20 g/kg/day, provided that energy and other nutrients are not limiting.[17] Because protein synthesis requires adequate energy intake, amino acids will be oxidized if adequate energy is not available. Preterm infant formula provides 3.9 to 4.7 g/kg/day of protein. Human milk does not meet protein requirements for preterm infants when fed at typical volumes and must be fortified. The protein content of preterm human milk is higher than that of full-term milk, but declines over time.

Fat

For preterm infants, fat serves as a major energy source and supplies essential fatty acids and bioactive components such as the structural lipids within cell membranes. At birth, the very preterm infant has very little stored body fat. A normal fetus accretes approximately 400 grams of lipid between 24 weeks of gestation and term birth, and stored lipid represents 75% of total stored energy. Achieving this high level of fat deposition while also meeting requirements for essential fatty acids requires a robust dietary lipid supply. Fat intake of human milk-fed infants varies, whereas formula provides a consistent supply. A reasonable range for fat intake is 4.1 to 7.4 g/100 kcal which translates to approximately 37% to 67% of energy as fat.[18]

Human milk fat comprises saturated, monounsaturated, and polyunsaturated fatty acids (PUFAs). The balance of fatty acids in human milk depends in part on the maternal diet. Medium chain triglycerides, which are widely used in preterm infant formulas, are easily absorbed and enter the portal circulation. Palmitic acid is the most abundant saturated fatty acid in human milk. Essential fatty acids are linoleic acid (LA) and alpha-linolenic acid (ALA), which compete for desaturase and elongase enzymes in PUFA conversion pathways. Downstream of LA and ALA are arachidonic (ARA) acid and docosahexaenoic acid (DHA), which in the normal fetus are transferred across the placenta in large amounts during the third trimester. ARA and DHA are conditionally essential in the preterm infant. DHA supplementation may improve neurodevelopment[19] although respiratory outcomes may be worsened.[20]

Vitamins and Minerals

Preterm infant bone health depends on an adequate supply of calcium, phosphorus, magnesium, and vitamin D. These nutrients also play diverse roles in the functioning of other organ systems. Most mineral deposition into bones occurs during the third trimester. Fetal accrual of calcium is 100–136 mg/kg/day, phosphorus 60–81 mg/kg/day, and magnesium 3–5 mg/kg/day. In the first few days after birth, preterm infants may experience hypophosphatemia if parenteral phosphorus delivery is not adequate to support intracellular metabolism and tissue accretion alongside parenteral amino acid delivery. Longer term, preterm infants are at risk for developing metabolic bone disease, and this risk is highest among infants born at the lowest gestational ages. Fortified human milk and preterm formula provide recommended intakes of calcium and phosphorus, whereas unfortified human milk and full-term infant formula do not meet requirements for preterm infants. Routine vitamin D supplementation likely improves early growth outcomes and reduces vitamin D deficiency in preterm infants.

Micronutrients such as iron, zinc, and iodine play diverse roles in physiological functioning including direct or indirect roles in brain development.[21] Iron is the most well-studied micronutrient in the very preterm infant. Iron status is impacted by iron stores at birth, delayed umbilical cord clamping, phlebotomy losses, and red blood cell transfusions. Iron supplementation may reduce long-term behavioral problems in this population.[22] Zinc supplementation at a pharmacologic level may reduce morbidity and mortality[23] but is not yet practiced routinely. Iodine supplementation may benefit those with low serum thyroxine.[24]

Requirements for vitamins may be different for the preterm vs. full-term infant. For some vitamins, supplementation trials and/or observational studies support preterm infant-specific recommendations. Other recommendations are based on guidance for full-term infants, many of which derive from concentrations of vitamins in mature milk which may underestimate true requirements given the rapid growth and critical illness of the preterm infant. Current preterm infant formulas and human milk fortifiers are not associated with any known deficiency, implying that they meet minimum requirements. A vitamin K injection is given at birth to prevent hemorrhagic disease of the newborn, with a lower dose recommended for very preterm infants.[25] Vitamin A plays important roles in fetal lung development and intramuscular supplementation reduces the risk of bronchopulmonary dysplasia.[26]

NUTRITIONAL ASSESSMENT OF THE PRETERM INFANT

Anthropometry

Serial anthropometric assessment is the primary approach to nutritional assessment in the hospitalized preterm infant. At birth and with repeated assessments over time, infants are compared in weight, length, and head circumference with a reference population representing the fetus of equivalent postmenstrual age. An example is the Fenton and Kim 2013 growth charts (available online at the University of Calgary-sponsored Fenton Preterm Growth Chart site and at the PediTools website) comprising sex-specific charts constructed through meta-analysis of size-at-birth data from nearly 4 million births in six countries including the United States.[27] These curves were smoothed with the World Health Organization Growth Standard after 36 weeks and cover a postmenstrual age range from 22–50 weeks, enabling their use in the NICU and for continued growth monitoring after discharge.

To classify nutritional status at birth, growth charts are used to compare the newborn's size to a fetal reference. Newborns are classified as small for gestational age (SGA, weight < 10th percentile for gestational age), appropriate for gestational age (AGA, weight at least 10th percentile and < 90th percentile), or large for gestational age (LGA, weight 90th percentile or higher). SGA status may reflect IUGR (discussed above) however IUGR does not always result in an SGA newborn. Conversely, an SGA newborn may be constitutionally small, rather than pathologically small due to IUGR. SGA status indicates an increased risk of neonatal complications such as hypoglycemia and hypothermia, and SGA preterm infants are at heightened risk for complications such as necrotizing enterocolitis (NEC) and bronchopulmonary dysplasia. Symmetrically small size e.g., weight, length, and head circumference all below the 10th percentile may indicate a genetic disorder or early congenital infection; asymmetric small size, e.g., SGA for weight but AGA for head circumference (known as "head sparing") is often seen in the context of third-trimester placental insufficiency. LGA status most commonly results from maternal diabetes and places the newborn at risk for birth injuries and hypoglycemia.

Newborn size differs by race and ethnicity, which largely reflects social inequity rather than genetic determinants; thus, we do not recommend using race-specific newborn size references.[28]

Following an initial assessment of size at birth, monitoring of preterm infant growth over time facilitates the identification of growth faltering. Consensus definitions of indicators for neonatal malnutrition[29] include definitions for mild, moderate, and severe malnutrition based on time to regain birth weight, weight gain and linear growth velocities, and changes in weight and length z-scores. After the initial weight loss, preterm infants should regain and begin to surpass birth weight by 10–14 days of age. For infants who remain below birth weight, the percent difference from birth weight is calculated as [(birth weight) – (current weight) / (birth weight)]. Weight gain velocity is a convenient and commonly used indicator in clinical practice, with a target of 15–20 g/kg/day recommended through 36 weeks of postmenstrual age.[30]

Biochemical Indicators

Biochemical indicators provide more specific information to complement routine growth assessment. Blood urea nitrogen provides information about protein status and toxicity and can be used to adjust protein fortification. Calcium, phosphorus, alkaline phosphatase, and vitamin D levels can guide interventions to support bone health. Hematocrit, reticulocyte count, and ferritin provide information about iron status. Whether biochemical indicators should be monitored routinely, or only if symptoms arise, is currently unknown.

NUTRITIONAL THERAPY

Water Requirements

Water requirements are higher for preterm as compared with full-term infants and vary based on gestational age, with more immature infants requiring higher volumes due to insensible losses. Table 11-1 shows typical initial total daily fluid volumes by gestational age for infants cared for in humidified incubators to limit insensible fluid losses; volumes are higher for infants on radiant warmers. Total fluid volumes are typically increased by 10–20 mL/kg daily to a goal of 160 mL/kg/day. Extremely immature infants may transiently require fluid intakes of 200 mL/kg/day or more to compensate for large insensible losses.

Parenteral Nutrition

Very preterm infants are born with limited nutrient stores, and the gastrointestinal tract is immature and not immediately able to receive, digest, and absorb adequate nutrients to support physiological functions and rapid growth. Providing parenteral nutrition immediately after birth can minimize the interruption of nutrient delivery that previously occurred across the placenta. The goal is to transition the infant from parenteral to enteral nutrition over a period of several days to 2 weeks of age, depending on the degree of immaturity and tolerance of enteral feeding. Prolonged parenteral nutrition can be lifesaving for infants with significant gastrointestinal pathology such as NEC that precludes enteral feeding.

Parenteral nutrition should be provided via a central venous catheter, most often an umbilical venous catheter (UVC) or a peripherally inserted central catheter. Routine parenteral nutrition is recommended for infants born < 1,500 grams or < 32 weeks of gestation.[31] Neonatal parenteral nutrition solutions

TABLE 11-1 • Recommended initial total fluid intake by gestational age

Gestational age, weeks	Initial fluid intake, mL/kg/day
< 28	90–120
28–34	80–100
> 34	60–80

Data from Steven Ringer, MD, PhD. Fluid and electrolyte therapy in newborns. *UpToDate*. 2023.

contain more essential amino acids than solutions intended for older children and adults, although the amino acid composition may not be optimized for the extremely preterm or critically ill newborn. Target amino acid intakes are 3.5–4 g/kg/day. Because protein synthesis is energy-demanding, adequate energy provision must accompany protein. Hypophosphatemia can occur in growth-restricted infants due to a refeeding-like syndrome that can be mitigated by adequate phosphorus administration provided in an equimolar dose with calcium.[32] Parenteral lipid emulsions provide essential fatty acids and a concentrated energy source. Target lipid intakes are 3 g/kg/day. Short-term complications of parenteral nutrition include hyperglycemia, elevation of blood urea nitrogen, and hypertriglyceridemia. Longer term, cholestasis can occur and is mainly related to the lipid.[33] Complications can also occur from the central venous catheter, including infection and thrombosis.

Enteral Nutrition

Human Milk Maternal milk is the recommended enteral diet for virtually all newborns, including those born preterm.[34] Pasteurized donor human milk is widely available in U.S. NICUs. Maternal milk is preferred over donor milk because donor milk is typically lower in protein and other nutrients. However, when maternal milk is in short supply or unavailable, donor milk is preferred over infant formula. One reason that human milk (maternal and/or donor) is preferred over infant formula is that, in addition to nutrients, human milk contains myriad non-nutritive bioactive components with important functions in the newborn such as the promotion of gastrointestinal development and protection of from infection and inflammation. Some human milk bioactives have specific benefits for preterm infants. For example, the human milk oligosaccharide disallyllacto-N-Tetraose (DSLNT) reduces the incidence and severity of NEC in both animal models and human studies, in part by altering the composition of the gastrointestinal microbiome.[13] Maternal milk feeding, as compared with formula, is associated with improved neurodevelopmental outcomes in preterm infants, with strongest associations in the most immature infants.[35] Currently, human milk bioactives are not routinely supplemented and clinical trials evaluating the effectiveness of human milk bioactive supplementation for preterm infants have generally yielded null results. Therefore, promoting and supporting lactation after preterm birth, and providing donor milk to infants when maternal milk is not available, are the only effective current strategies by which preterm infants can benefit from human milk bioactives.

Milk Fortification Unfortified human milk and standard full-term infant formula do not meet nutrient requirements of the growing preterm infant when fed at standard volumes (~140–160 mL/kg/day). Some key nutrient requirements are not met even when unfortified milk is fed at higher volumes (~180–200 mL/kg/day). Multicomponent human milk fortification is standard practice. When human milk is not available, specialized preterm infant formula, rather than full-term infant formula, should be used. Several sterile liquid preterm formulas and human milk fortifiers are commercially available in the United States and are recommended over powdered products due to the risk of *Cronobacter sakazakii* contamination. Both fortified human milk and preterm infant formula promote weight gain, linear growth, and head growth more effectively unfortified milk. Data are lacking on the extent to which these fortified diets improve neurodevelopmental outcomes.[36] Very preterm infants fed predominantly fortified maternal milk have similar growth patterns and outcomes to infants fed preterm formula.[4]

Initiation and Advancement of Enteral Nutrition Due to critical illness and immaturity of the preterm infant gastrointestinal tract, enteral nutrition is initiated at low volume (trophic feeding or gut priming) and advanced over several days. Results from a large, multi-center randomized trial (Speed of Increasing Milk Feeds, SIFT)[37] suggest that faster, as compared with slower advancement, is not harmful and reduces parenteral nutrition use. Gastric residuals should not be checked routinely, instead infants should be monitored for specific signs of feeding intolerance and/or more serious pathology such as NEC.

Although there is no universally agreed-upon practice for establishing enteral nutrition in preterm infants, following standardized practice guidelines improves nutrition-related outcomes and reduces the incidence of NEC.[38] Table 11-2 indicates volumes for initiation and advancement from SIFT and in our center. Our practice is birthweight based to account for both immaturity and fetal growth restriction. We initiate maternal milk or donor milk as soon as possible after birth unless there are absolute contraindications such as hypotension and fortify human milk with a commercially available liquid fortifier once the infant is tolerating 60 mL/kg/day of unfortified milk. We continue to increase the volume to a goal of 150–160 mL/kg/day.

Route of Feeding The route of enteral feeding depends on the infant's developmental and clinical status. Developmentally, the ability to coordinate suck, swallow, and breathe emerges ~ 32–34 weeks and does not become safe and efficient until at least 34–35 weeks. Before then, preterm infants require exclusive gavage tube feeding. Bolus rather than continuous feedings are preferred to prevent nutrient loss in the tubing, including > 40% loss of fat.[39] Infants who require respiratory support,

TABLE 11-2 • Initiation and advancement of enteral nutrition for newborn infants

Birth weight (g)	Initial volume, mL/kg/day	Volume increase, mL/kg/day per 12 hours	
		Our center	SIFT trial[a]
1,000 or less	10	10	15
1,001–1,500	20	15	15
1,501–1,800	30	15-20	N/A
1,801–2,500+	30-40	20	N/A

[a]SIFT is Speed of Increasing Milk Feeds.[37]
Source: Dorling J, Abbott J, Berrington J, et al. Controlled trial of two incremental milk-feeding rates in preterm infants. *N Engl J Med.* 2019;381(15):1434-1443.

such as high flow nasal cannula or continuous positive airway pressure are at increased risk for aspiration when fed orally[40] and may benefit from continued gavage tube feeding with concurrent developmental feeding support.

● POSTDISCHARGE CONSIDERATIONS

National data indicate that preterm infants leave the NICU lighter, shorter, and with smaller heads than full-term peers.[1] After discharge, they experience accelerated weight gain and linear growth, which allows catch up with full-term peers within the first 2 years.[41] Nutrient intakes after NICU discharge must address deficits and support normal post-term growth. In addition to high nutrient requirements, another challenge is ongoing oral feeding difficulties. Further, excess weight gain may contribute to the development of childhood obesity and related complications.[42] Thus, preterm infants require close nutritional monitoring postdischarge.

Between 40–75% of infants are still receiving human milk at NICU discharge, with notable inequities by race and ethnicity.[43] Donor milk is not typically used outside the hospital setting, nor are commercial human milk fortifiers. Optimal postdischarge fortification of maternal milk needs to balance nutritional requirements of the infant with practical challenges of continued milk expression, and the use of bottles to provide fortified milk which limits infant feeding at the breast. Commonly used strategies include fortifying expressed milk with transitional formula powder or liquid concentrate and supplementing an unfortified maternal milk diet with 2–3 bottles per day of postdischarge formula. If maternal milk is not available, postdischarge formulas are commonly used although evidence of their effectiveness is limited.[44]

Growth patterns guide nutritional management after NICU discharge. Growth monitoring may be accomplished through collaboration of visiting nurses, primary care providers, academic follow-up programs, and specialized growth and nutrition programs. We recommend the World Health Organization (WHO) Child Growth Standard, which aligns with the Fenton and Kim 2013 reference. Plotting measurements for both chronologic and adjusted (corrected) age provides insight about postdischarge catch-up growth. An adjusted age calculator can be found at the NICHD Neonatal Research Network website under Tools.

THREE TAKE-HOME POINTS

1. Overarching goal of nutritional care in preterm infants is to provide the nutrients needed to achieve the rate of growth and composition of weight gain for a normal fetus while supporting healthy brain development.

2. Calorie, protein, and micronutrient needs are higher in preterm infants compared to full-term infants.

3. Maternal milk is the recommended enteral diet for virtually all newborns. Maternal milk needs to be fortified to meet the energy and micronutrient needs of preterm infants.

CASE STUDY ANSWERS

1. **B;** Using the Fenton and Kim 2013 growth reference, this male infant's weight of 1,200 grams at 29 weeks of gestation represents the 46th percentile, which falls between the 10th and 90th percentiles and is therefore considered appropriate for gestational age. Note that percentiles for body length and head circumference at birth should also be determined.

2. **B, C, D;** Very preterm birth is a nutritional emergency. Initial fluid requirements vary by gestational age. A typical 28-week infant receiving care in a humidified isolette would require approximately 80 mL/kg/day of total fluids in the first day after birth. Infants weighing below 1,500–1,800 grams should receive parenteral nutrition with dextrose and amino acids as soon as possible after birth. Mouth care with expressed colostrum provides the infant with protective maternal antibodies. Early initiation of enteral nutrition with maternal milk or

donor milk is indicated unless there is an absolute contraindication such as hypotension or other clinical instability. Because the infant in this case does not have any absolute contraindications, low volume enteral feedings (known as "trophic feedings") should be initiated. NPO is not appropriate because there are no absolute contraindications to enteral feeding.

3. **A;** The percent weight loss from birth weight is calculated as [(birth weight) – (current weight) / (birth weight)]*100.

4. **B, C, E;** This infant has lost > 10% of birth weight and has not yet started re-gaining weight by 2 weeks of age, suggesting inadequate nutrient intake. Human milk is variable in its sodium content and donor milk may have less sodium and protein as compared with maternal milk or preterm formula. Therefore, in addition to ensuring adequate lactation support to maximize the availability

(Continued)

CASE STUDY ANSWERS *(Continued)*

of maternal milk and reduce the use of donor milk, sodium chloride supplementation if hyponatremia is identified and empiric additional protein fortification of milk may both improve weight gain; both interventions can be initiated simultaneously. Preterm formula should only be considered if weight gain is poor despite maximum fortification, which has not yet been achieved in this case. The risk of placing a new central line is not justified in this case in which additional fortification is likely to be effective in improving weight gain.

5. **C;** Continued fortification postdischarge is indicated for this infant given nutrient deficits indicated by a weight percentile of 14. He has established weight gain on a combination of direct breastfeeding and fortified expressed milk feedings via bottle, and the mother desires to continue direct breastfeeding. Therefore, it is reasonable to continue this plan after discharge with close monitoring by the pediatrician. Discontinuing direct breastfeeding, and switching to formula, both do not align with the mother's goal for feeding. There is no absolute NICU discharge requirement for body weight.

REFERENCES

1. Edwards EM, Greenberg LT, Ehret DEY, Lorch SA, Horbar JD. Discharge age and weight for very preterm infants: 2005-2018. *Pediatrics.* 2021;147(2):e2020016006.

2. Escobar GJ, Clark RH, Greene JD. Short-term outcomes of infants born at 35 and 36 weeks gestation: we need to ask more questions. *Semin Perinatol.* 2006;30(1):28-33.

3. Johnson MJ, Wootton SA, Leaf AA, Jackson AA. Preterm birth and body composition at term equivalent age: a systematic review and meta-analysis. *Pediatrics.* 2012;130(3):e640-e649.

4. Soldateli B, Parker M, Melvin P, Gupta M, Belfort M. Human milk feeding and physical growth in very low-birth-weight infants: a multicenter study. *J Perinatol.* 2020;40(8):1246-1252.

5. American Academy of Pediatrics Committee on Nutrition. Nutritional needs of preterm infants. In: Kleinman RE, Greer FR, eds. *Pediatric Nutrition.* 8th ed. American Academy of Pediatrics; 2019.

6. Koletzko B, Cheah FC, Domellöf M, Poindexter BB, Vain N, van Goudoever JB. *Nutritional Care of Preterm Infants: Scientific Basis and Practical Guidelines.* Karger Medical and Scientific Publishers; 2021.

7. Landau-Crangle E, Rochow N, Fenton TR, et al. Individualized postnatal growth trajectories for preterm infants. *JPEN J Parenter Enteral Nutr.* 2018;42(6):1084-1092.

8. Fusch C. Water, sodium, potassium, and chloride. *World Rev Nutr Diet.* 2021;122:103-121.

9. Travers CP, Wang T, Salas AA, et al. Higher- or usual-volume feedings in infants born very preterm: a randomized clinical trial. *J Pediatr.* 2020;224:66-71.e1.

10. Segar DE, Segar EK, Harshman LA, Dagle JM, Carlson SJ, Segar JL. Physiological approach to sodium supplementation in preterm infants. *Am J Perinatol.* 2018;35(10):994-1000.

11. Huff KA, Denne SC, Hay WW Jr. Energy requirements and carbohydrates in preterm infants. *World Rev Nutr Diet.* 2021;122:60-74.

12. Alsweiler JM, Harding JE, Bloomfield FH. Tight glycemic control with insulin in hyperglycemic preterm babies: a randomized controlled trial. *Pediatrics.* 2012;129(4):639-647.

13. Masi AC, Embleton ND, Lamb CA, et al. Human milk oligosaccharide DSLNT and gut microbiome in preterm infants predicts necrotising enterocolitis. *Gut.* 2021;70(12):2273-2282.

14. Verner A, Craig S, McGuire W. Effect of taurine supplementation on growth and development in preterm or low birth weight infants. *Cochrane Database Syst Rev.* 2007;(4):CD006072.

15. Moe-Byrne T, Brown JVE, McGuire W. Glutamine supplementation to prevent morbidity and mortality in preterm infants. *Cochrane Database Syst Rev.* 2016;4:CD001457.

16. Shah PS, Shah VS, Kelly LE. Arginine supplementation for prevention of necrotising enterocolitis in preterm infants. *Cochrane Database Syst Rev.* 2017;4:CD004339.

17. van den Akker CHP, Saenz de Pipaon M, van Goudoever JB. Proteins and amino acids. *World Rev Nutr Diet.* 2021;122:75-88.

18. Koletzko B, Lapillonne A. Lipid requirements of preterm infants. *World Rev Nutr Diet.* 2021;122:89-102.

19. Makrides M, Gibson RA, McPhee AJ, et al. Neurodevelopmental outcomes of preterm infants fed high-dose docosahexaenoic acid: a randomized controlled trial. *JAMA.* 2009;301(2):175-182.

20. Collins CT, Makrides M, McPhee AJ, et al. Docosahexaenoic acid and bronchopulmonary dysplasia in preterm infants. *N Engl J Med.* 2017;376(13):1245-1255.

21. Volpe JJ. Iron and zinc: nutrients with potential for neurorestoration in premature infants with cerebral white matter injury. *J Neonatal Perinatal Med.* 2019;12(4):365-368.

22. Berglund SK, Chmielewska A, Starnberg J, et al. Effects of iron supplementation of low-birth-weight infants on cognition and behavior at 7 years: a randomized controlled trial. *Pediatr Res.* 2018;83(1-1):111-118.

23. Staub E, Evers K, Askie LM. Enteral zinc supplementation for prevention of morbidity and mortality in preterm neonates. *Cochrane Database Syst Rev.* 2021;3:CD012797.

24. Williams FLR, Ogston S, Hume R, et al. Supplemental iodide for preterm infants and developmental outcomes at 2 years: an RCT. *Pediatrics.* 2017;139(5):e20163703.

25. Agostoni C, Buonocore G, Carnielli VP, et al. Enteral nutrient supply for preterm infants: commentary from the European Society of Paediatric Gastroenterology, Hepatology and Nutrition Committee on Nutrition. *J Pediatr Gastroenterol Nutr.* 2010;50(1):85-91.

26. Darlow BA, Graham PJ, Rojas-Reyes MX. Vitamin A supplementation to prevent mortality and short- and long-term morbidity in very low birth weight infants. *Cochrane Database Syst Rev.* 2016;2016(8):CD000501.

27. Fenton TR, Kim JH. A systematic review and meta-analysis to revise the Fenton growth chart for preterm infants. *BMC Pediatr.* 2013;13:59.

28. Belfort MB, Wheeler SM, Burris HH. Health inequities start early in life, even before birth: why race-specific fetal and neonatal growth references disadvantage Black infants. *Semin Perinatol.* 2022 Dec;46(8):151662.

29. Goldberg DL, Becker PJ, Brigham K, et al. Identifying malnutrition in preterm and neonatal populations: recommended indicators. *J Acad Nutr Diet.* 2018;118(9):1571-1582.

30. Fenton TR, Anderson D, Groh-Wargo S, Hoyos A, Ehrenkranz RA, Senterre T. An attempt to standardize the calculation of growth velocity of preterm infants-evaluation of practical bedside methods. *J Pediatr.* 2018;196:77-83.

31. Van Goudoever JB, Carnielli V, Darmaun D, Sainz de Pipaon ME; ESPEN/ESPR/CSPEN Working Group on Pediatric Parenteral Nutrition. ESPGHAN/ESPEN/ESPR/CSPEN guidelines on pediatric parenteral nutrition: amino acids. *Clin Nutr.* 2018 Dec;37 (6 Pt B):2315-2323.

32. Galletti MF, Brener Dik PH, Fernandez Jonusas SA, et al. Early high amino-acid intake is associated with hypophosphatemia in preterm infants. *J Perinatol.* 2022;42(8):1063-1069.

33. Frazer LC, Gura KM, Bines JE, Puder M, Martin CR. Prevention and management of parenteral nutrition-associated cholestasis and intestinal failure-associated liver disease in the critically ill infant. *World Rev Nutr Diet.* 2021;122:379-399.

34. Parker MG, Stellwagen LM, Noble L, et al. Promoting human milk and breastfeeding for the very low birth weight infant. *Pediatrics.* 2021;148(5):e2021054272.

35. Belfort MB, Knight E, Chandarana S, et al. Associations of maternal milk feeding with neurodevelopmental outcomes at 7 years of age in former preterm infants. *JAMA Netw Open.* 2022;5(7): e2221608.

36. Brown JV, Lin L, Embleton ND, Harding JE, McGuire W. Multi-nutrient fortification of human milk for preterm infants. *Cochrane Database Syst Rev.* 2020;6:CD000343.

37. Dorling J, Abbott J, Berrington J, et al. Controlled trial of two incremental milk-feeding rates in preterm infants. *N Engl J Med.* 2019;381(15):1434-1443.

38. Kaplan HC, Poindexter BB. Standardized feeding protocols: evidence and implementation. *World Rev Nutr Diet.* 2021;122: 289-300.

39. Paulsson M, Jacobsson L, Ahlsson F. Factors influencing breast milk fat loss during administration in the neonatal intensive care unit. *Nutrients.* 2021;13(6):1939.

40. Ferrara L, Bidiwala A, Sher I, et al. Effect of nasal continuous positive airway pressure on the pharyngeal swallow in neonates. *J Perinatol.* 2017;37(4):398-403.

41. Belfort MB, Rifas-Shiman SL, Sullivan T, et al. Infant growth before and after term: effects on neurodevelopment in preterm infants. *Pediatrics.* 2011;128(4):e899-e906.

42. Simon L, Hadchouel A, Arnaud C, et al. Growth trajectory during the first 1000 days and later overweight in very preterm infants. *Arch Dis Child Fetal Neonatal Ed.* Published online August 25, 2022. doi:10.1136/archdischild-2022-324321.

43. Parker MG, Greenberg LT, Edwards EM, Ehret D, Belfort MB, Horbar JD. National trends in the provision of human milk at hospital discharge among very low-birth-weight infants. *JAMA Pediatr.* 2019;173(10):961-968.

44. Young L, Embleton ND, McGuire W. Nutrient-enriched formula versus standard formula for preterm infants following hospital discharge. *Cochrane Database Syst Rev.* 2016;12:CD004696.

Critical Illness

Nilesh M. Mehta, MD, FASPEN

CASE STUDY

A previously healthy 4-year-old boy was admitted to the pediatric intensive care unit (PICU) with recently diagnosed bacterial pneumonia. His symptoms have progressed to acute respiratory distress syndrome and respiratory failure, requiring mechanical ventilatory support. On Day 2 in the PICU, the patient is sedated, and chemically muscle relaxed, on high ventilator settings. His temperature is 102°F. He has a central venous catheter in place, a nasogastric sump (he is NPO), and his endotracheal tube is secure. His weight of 13 kg is a z-score of −2.0 and his height of 97 cm is a z-score of −1.2.

1. Describe some of the variables (patient, disease, and therapeutic factors) that will increase or decrease the energy expenditure in this patient.

2. What are the available methods for determining energy requirement in this patient? What are the limitations and advantages of these methods?

3. Protein metabolism in this child is best represented by: (Choose most appropriate option.)

A. Increased protein synthesis; decreased protein breakdown; positive protein balance
B. Decreased protein synthesis; Increased protein breakdown; negative protein balance
C. Increased protein synthesis; Increased protein breakdown; negative protein balance

4. After determining nutrition goals, what is the optimal nutrient delivery strategy? Describe some considerations for choosing enteral versus parenteral route in this patient.

A. Early enteral nutrition (EN); advance stepwise as tolerated; use of supplemental parenteral nutrition (PN) only if goal feeding not possible by EN after 4–5 days.
B. Early PN to achieve nutrition delivery goals; initiate EN late and advance as tolerated; discontinue PN after EN delivery is established.
C. Early EN; advance stepwise as tolerated; no role for supplemental PN

BASIC EPIDEMIOLOGY—NUTRITIONAL STATUS, INTAKE AND OUTCOMES

Over 250,000 children are admitted to pediatric intensive care units (PICUs) in the United States annually. Nutritional status on admission, nutrient delivery, and subsequent nutritional deterioration are important factors that are associated with outcomes in critically ill children.[1,2] In low-resource areas, lack of adequate nourishment due to socioeconomic factors is a major cause of malnutrition and is associated with morbidity and mortality. In high-income countries, the predominant reasons for imbalance between nutrient requirement and delivery are illness-related, including excessive nutrient losses, increased energy expenditure, decreased nutrient intake, and altered nutrient absorption or utilization. Malnutrition is prevalent in hospitalized children; it has been reported in 5%–50% of admissions.[3] Preexisting malnutrition has been associated with altered physiologic responses and it influences outcome during critical illness. Malnourished, hospitalized patients have a higher rate of infectious complications, increased mortality, longer stay in the hospital, increased resource utilization, and increased hospital costs.

Furthermore, critical illness may increase metabolic demand on the patient and when this is combined with suboptimal nutrient intake, patients are at risk for worsening nutritional status with increased morbidity. A vast majority of children in the pediatric intensive care unit (PICU) with respiratory failure experience muscle atrophy.[4] Immobilized children with respiratory failure are particularly vulnerable, incurring 1.5%–7.0% muscle loss daily.[4–6] Thus, careful nutritional status assessment on admission and serially during the ICU course helps early identification of vulnerable patients in whom nutritional therapies might help improve outcomes.

In 1,622 mechanically ventilated critically ill children, enrolled over two prospective international studies, our group explored the influence of admission nutritional status, as assessed by BMI z-score, on important clinical outcomes.[7] Suboptimal nutritional status (underweight, overweight, or obesity) was documented in nearly half (46%) the cohort at admission to the PICU. Being underweight was associated with significantly higher odds of 60-day mortality and hospital-acquired infections, fewer ventilator-free days, and lower likelihood of discharge. Obesity was significantly associated with higher odds of hospital acquired infections and longer hospital stay among survivors. Underweight status has been shown to predict outcomes in a variety of critically ill pediatric populations in multiple studies. Therapies aimed at alleviating the underlying conditions along with attention to optimal nutrient intake for individual patients may be important in reversing or in some cases preventing nutritional deterioration.

Nutrient Intake and Outcomes

A variety of barriers impede the delivery of optimal nutrition ICU, resulting in failure or delay in reaching nutrition goals.[8] Suboptimal nutritional intake results in cumulative deficits in energy and protein, with loss of lean body mass and bone density.[9] In a large multicenter study of nutrient delivery in 500 mechanically ventilated children from 31 PICUs, we reported suboptimal delivery of energy and protein.[1] The adequacy of enteral energy intake was significantly associated with 60-day mortality in that cohort, and an increase in energy intake from 33% to 66% of the prescribed goal was associated with lower mortality (OR: 0.27; 95% CI: 0.11, 0.67; P = 0.002). In our second multicenter study, including 1,245 mechanically ventilated children from 59 PICUs, delivery of at least 60% of the prescribed protein goal was directly correlated with lower mortality, independent of energy intake and severity of illness.[2] These studies suggest that delivery of at least 60% of the prescribed energy and protein goal may be a valid target during the acute phase of a pediatric critical illness. These studies highlight the importance of careful assessment of energy and protein needs, and individualized prescription with prudent targets of nutrient delivery for potential improvement in clinical outcomes in this vulnerable cohort.

RELEVANT PATHOPHYSIOLOGY

The Metabolic Stress Response

The stress response to critical illness or surgery has provided evolutionary advantages to humans. As hunter-gatherers, prehistoric humans depended on this response to overcome periods of illness or injury when extrinsic nutrients were not available. In this preagricultural age, humans relied on a stereotypic stress response that was driven by a cascade of neurohormonal and cytokine pathways. With stress, serum levels of insulin, glucagon, cortisol, catecholamines, and proinflammatory cytokines increase and result in breakdown of endogenous stores of protein, carbohydrate, and fat. Protein breakdown is the *sine qua non* of this stress response, and results in availability of free amino acids that can be channeled through the liver (Figure 12-1).[10] The carbon skeletons of amino acids are used for gluconeogenesis to produce glucose, the preferred energy substrate for the brain, erythrocytes, and renal medulla. The amino acids are also reprioritized to assist with tissue repair, or to produce acute-phase reactant proteins and inflammatory proteins that help address the infectious pathology.

However, if the protein breakdown is prolonged, it far outstrips the capacity of the body to synthesize protein and can result in a large net negative balance with loss of critical lean body mass. Protein catabolism continues to be a predominant feature of the metabolic stress response in the modern day. Energy requirement may also be increased but this increase is unpredictable. The expected increase in energy expenditure is often offset by sedation, assisted ventilation and muscle relaxation in the PICU, and therefore often lower than baseline (hypometabolism) in some cases. This presents a unique problem where patients can be unintentionally underfed (from underestimation of their energy requirement) or overfed in some cases (due to overestimation of their energy requirement).[11] The use of an indirect calorimeter (metabolic cart) allows accurate assessment of energy expenditure and may be used in order to assess individual requirements and energy prescription in critically ill patients.[12]

METABOLIC RESPONSE TO STRESS

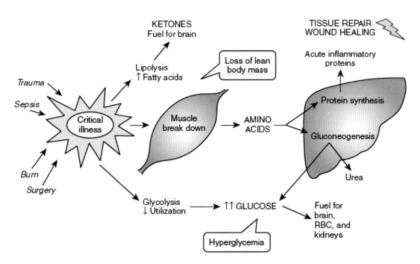

FIGURE 12-1 • Pathways of metabolic stress response.[10]
(From Mehta NM, Jaksic T. The critically ill child. In: Duggan CP, Walker W, eds. *Nutrition in Pediatrics.* 4th ed. B. C. Decker Inc; 2008: 663-673. Courtesy of Dr. Nilesh Mehta and Dr. Christopher Duggan.)

Starvation Versus Metabolic Stress Response

The stress response is distinct from the metabolic effects of starvation (Table 12-1). Unlike the protein catabolism (early) and hypermetabolism (increased basal metabolic rate) seen in many critically ill patients, starvation results in a reduction in BMR in an effort to preserve energy. Protein and other tissues do eventually breakdown to provide substrate late in the setting of sustained starvation. One of the principal differences between the two processes is that protein breakdown from prolonged starvation can be stopped with the provision of calories/nutrients. However, the protein breakdown seen in critical illness does not respond to nutrient provision.

Gastrointestinal Function During Critical Illness

The impact of critical illness and its therapies on gastrointestinal function is multifactorial. Both gastrointestinal motility and absorptive functions may be impeded in this group.

TABLE 12-1 • Basic differences between starvation and metabolic stress response		
	Metabolic stress	**Starvation**
Basal metabolic rate	Increased ++	Unchanged or decreased
Protein breakdown	+++	+ or unchanged
Lean body mass loss	Early	Late
Response to caloric intake	Protein catabolism continues	Protein catabolism halted
Insulin, cortisol, catecholamines	Increased ++	Decreased
Ketones	Increased ++	Unchanged
Gluconeogenesis	Increased ++	Decreased

Inflammation, trauma and surgery are known to decrease GI motility. Gastric emptying is further impeded by side effects of sedative and analgesic medications that are routinely administered in critically ill patients. A variety of medications used in the ICU have anticholinergic properties that disrupt the balanced autonomic control of gastrointestinal motility. As a result, delayed gastric emptying, ileus, constipation, diarrhea, emesis, and aspiration of stomach contents may be encountered in this population. Furthermore, absorptive capacity of the GI tract may be affected, resulting in unpredictable absorption of nutrients and medications administered enterally. Finally, impaired permeability of the intestinal epithelium can result in translocation of bacteria into the blood stream. The GI dysfunction in critical illness is associated with higher morbidity and has implications for safe and optimal enteral nutrient delivery.

● NUTRITIONAL THERAPY IN CRITICAL ILLNESS

The role of nutrition during critical illness is to offset the metabolic burden from the stress response by providing optimum amounts of energy and protein using the safest delivery strategy. Assessment of baseline nutritional status allows identification of vulnerable patients, such as those with severe preexisting malnutrition, who might benefit from early nutritional optimization. This includes metabolic assessment to determine the individual energy requirements, preferably using indirect calorimetry, and age-based protein requirements. When indirect calorimetry is not available or feasible, estimation equations (Schofield or FAO/WHO/UNU equations) may be used *without* the addition of stress factors to estimate energy expenditure.[13] Multiple cohort studies have demonstrated that most published predictive equations are inaccurate in the setting of critical illness. These equations were developed in healthy populations and therefore may result in unintended underfeeding or overfeeding in critically ill patients. The Harris-Benedict equations and the Recommended Daily Allowances (RDA), which are suggested by the Dietary Reference Intakes, should not be used to determine energy requirements in critically ill children. Tables 12-2A and 12-2B highlight some of the recommendations from recent guidelines for adult and pediatric critical care nutrition guidelines.[13,14] The recommendations were developed through an iterative process, after extensive review and systematic grading of the available evidence. These two references are recommended for more details on the evidence and the process of guidelines development. Of note, a majority of the recommendations are based on low to moderate grade of evidence, and we need further research that will help guide best practices.

Following assessment, the next step is accurate prescription of macronutrients and micronutrients individualized to each patient. There are two main considerations for the delivery of prescribed nutrition targets in critically ill patients; the *route* of nutrient delivery and the *timing* of achieving the delivery targets.

Route of Nutrient Delivery: Enteral Nutrition

Enteral nutrition (EN) is preferred and often the first choice in critically ill patients. Despite the prevalence of GI dysfunction during critical illness, a majority of patients can be fed via the enteral route in the ICU. There are several observational studies in large cohorts that have shown associations between EN and improved outcomes in critically ill patients.[15] Based on large cohort studies, early initiation of EN (within 24–48 hours of ICU admission) and achievement of up to two-thirds of the nutrient goal in the first week of critical illness has been associated with improved clinical outcomes.[13] Delivery of EN into the stomach (gastric feeding) via feeding tubes is preferred. However, in some patients, gastric feeding is either contraindicated (e.g., high risk or history of aspiration) or has not been tolerated. In these cases, several centers have described successful feeding into the small intestine (post-pyloric EN). Enteral nutrition may be delivered intermittently as boluses, or as a continuous infusion. In a recent

	Clinical question	Recommendation	Evidence grade	Strength of recommendation
	TABLE 12-2A • Recent recommendations for nutrition delivery in critically ill adult patients[14]			
1.	Does provision of higher vs. lower energy intake impact clinical outcomes?	No significant difference in clinical outcomes was found between patients with higher vs. lower levels of energy intake. We suggest feeding between 12 and 25 kcal/kg (i.e., the range of mean energy intakes examined) in the first 7–10 days of ICU stay.	Moderate	Weak
2.	Does provision of higher vs. lower protein intake impact clinical outcomes?	There was no difference in clinical outcomes in the relatively limited data. Because of a paucity of trials with high-quality evidence, we cannot make a new recommendation at this time beyond the 2016 guideline suggestion for 1.2–2.0 g/kg/day.	Low	Weak
3.	In adult critically ill patients who are candidates for EN, does similar energy intake by PN vs. EN as the primary feeding modality in the first week of critical illness impact clinical outcomes?	There was no significant difference in clinical outcomes. Because similar energy intake provided as PN is not superior to EN and no differences in harm were identified, we recommend that either PN or EN is acceptable.	High	Strong
4.	In adult critically ill patients receiving EN, does provision of SPN, as compared with no SPN during the first week of critical illness, impact clinical outcomes?	There was no significant difference in clinical outcomes. Based on findings of no clinically important benefit in providing SPN early in the ICU admission, we recommend not initiating SPN prior to day 7 of ICU admission.	High	Strong
5.	In adult critically ill patients receiving PN, does provision of mixed-oil ILEs (ie, medium-chain triglycerides, olive oil, FO, mixtures of oils), as compared with 100% soybean-oil ILE, impact clinical outcomes?	Because of limited statistically or clinically significant differences in key outcomes, we suggest that either mixed-oil ILE or 100% soybean-oil ILE be provided.	Low	Weak
6.	In adult critically ill patients receiving PN, does provision of FO-containing ILE, as compared with non–FO-containing ILE, impact clinical outcomes?	We suggest that either FO- or non–FO-containing ILE be provided to critically ill patients who are appropriate candidates for initiation of PN	Low	Weak

Adapted from Compher C, Bingham AL, McCall M, et al. Guidelines for the provision of nutrition support therapy in the adult critically ill patient: The American Society for Parenteral and Enteral Nutrition. *JPEN J Parenter Enteral Nutr.* 2021.

TABLE 12-2B • Recent recommendations for nutrition delivery in critically ill pediatric patients			
	Clinical question	Recommendation	Evidence grade	Strength of recommendation
1.	What is the recommended energy requirement for critically ill children?	On the basis of observational cohort studies, we suggest that measured energy expenditure by IC be used to determine energy requirements and guide prescription of the daily energy goal. If IC measurement of resting energy expenditure is not feasible, we suggest that the Schofield or Food Agriculture Organization / World Health Organization/United Nations University equations may be used without the addition of stress factors to estimate energy expenditure.	Low	Weak
2.	What is the target energy intake in critically ill children?	On the basis of observational cohort studies, we suggest achieving delivery of at least two-thirds of the prescribed daily energy requirement by the end of the first week in the PICU. Cumulative energy deficits during the first week of critical illness may be associated with poor clinical and nutrition outcomes.	Low	Weak
3.	What is the minimum recommended protein requirement for critically ill children?	On the basis of evidence from RCTs and as supported by observational cohort studies, we recommend a minimum protein intake of 1.5 g/kg/d. Protein intake higher than this threshold has been shown to prevent cumulative negative protein balance in RCTs.	Moderate	Strong
4.	What is the optimum method for advancing EN in the PICU population?	On the basis of observational studies, we suggest the use of a stepwise algorithmic approach to advance EN in children admitted to the PICU. The stepwise algorithm must include bedside support to guide the detection and management of EN intolerance and the optimal rate of increase in EN delivery.	Low	Weak
5.	What is the best site for EN delivery: gastric or small bowel?	Existing data are insufficient to make universal recommendations regarding the optimal site to deliver EN to critically ill children. On the basis of observational studies, we suggest that the gastric route be the preferred site for EN in patients in the PICU. The post-pyloric or small intestinal site for EN may be used in patients unable to tolerate gastric feeding or those at high risk for aspiration. Existing data are insufficient to make recommendations regarding the use of continuous vs. intermittent gastric feeding.	Low	Weak
6.	What is the indication for and optimal timing of PN in critically ill children?	On the basis of a single RCT, we do not recommend the initiation of PN within 24 hours of PICU admission.	Moderate	Strong
7.	What is the role of PN as a supplement to inadequate EN?	The threshold for and timing of PN initiation should be individualized. Based on a single RCT, supplemental PN should be delayed until 1 wk after PICU admission for patients with normal baseline nutrition state and low risk of nutrition deterioration. On the basis of expert consensus, we suggest PN supplementation for children who are unable to receive any EN during the first week in the PICU. For patients who are severely malnourished or at risk of nutrition deterioration, PN may be supplemented in the first week if they are unable to advance past low volumes of EN.	Low	Weak

Adapted from Mehta NM, Skillman HE, Irving SY, et al. Guidelines for the provision and assessment of nutrition support therapy in the pediatric critically ill patient: Society of Critical Care Medicine and American Society for Parenteral and Enteral Nutrition. *Pediatr Crit Care Med: A journal of the Society of Critical Care Medicine and the World Federation of Pediatric Intensive and Critical Care Societies.* 2017 Jul;18(7):675-715.

randomized control trial (RCT) that compared the two methods of EN delivery, there were no clinically significant differences in nutrient delivery or complications.[16]

A variety of barriers impede EN delivery in the PICU setting.[8] During the care of a critically ill patient, other interventions often compete with nutrient delivery. Elective procedures, unplanned interventions, or diagnostic tests often require a fasted state requiring interruption of EN. In addition, EN intolerance or contraindications to enteral feeding related to the disease processes may require feeds to be held or discontinued in the PICU. In addition to these unavoidable factors, patients are often deprived of EN due to avoidable factors, such as, suboptimal prescription, delayed initiation of EN early, or frequent and prolonged interruptions to enteral feeding. Despite the early and successful initiation of EN in most patients, a high rate of subsequent EN interruptions have been reported widely in the intensive care setting, resulting in suboptimal nutrient delivery and failure to achieve caloric goal or reliance on PN. Most centers have adopted guidelines to initiate early EN in eligible patients, stepwise algorithms to advance EN by addressing feed intolerance.[17] The use of such stepwise guides has allowed optimal. Parenteral nutrition (PN) may have a role in children with true EN intolerance or in patients with unavoidable EN interruptions. In these cases, PN may substitute or supplement EN to achieve nutrient intake goals.

Route of Nutrient Delivery: Parenteral Nutrition

In patients tolerating EN, stepwise advancement of nutrient delivery via the enteral route allows achievement of prudent targets and decreases the need for PN. PN may have a role in those with true EN intolerance or with unavoidable EN interruptions. In these cases, PN may substitute or supplement EN to achieve nutrient intake goals. When EN is inadequate or contraindicated during the first week of ICU admission, supplemental PN is often used. The timing of introducing supplemental PN to prevent cumulative nutrient deficits was recently examined in pediatric and adult trials. In a large, randomized trial in children admitted to three PICUs, early PN initiation (< 24 hours after admission) was compared to late PN initiation (after 7 days) as a supplement to insufficient EN, aiming for delivery of at least 80% of the prescribed energy target [Early versus Late Parenteral Nutrition in the Pediatric Intensive Care Unit (PEPaNIC) trial].[18] The late PN strategy was associated with lower rates of infection, as well as shorter intensive care unit and hospital stays, compared with the early PN approach.

At our center, PN is used in 1 of every 5 patients admitted to the ICU, mostly in the setting of no (or minimal) simultaneous EN. Supplemental PN is initiated with simultaneous EN in < 5% of patients, when EN nutrient delivery is minimal. In our recent international cohort study (PINS 3), conducted 3 years after publication of the PEPaNIC trial, PN continues to be used in an individualized fashion as a supplement to EN between 24 hours and 7 days of PICU admission. It is initiated mostly in the setting of minimal to no EN and is generally discontinued when EN has advanced to approximately half the prescribed target. Indeed, prudent use of PN with strict attention to asepsis, normoglycemia and other safety precautions has not been associated with higher rate of complications. Based on the above single RCT, supplemental PN should be delayed until 1 week after PICU admission in patients with normal baseline nutritional state and low risk of nutritional deterioration. Based on expert consensus, PN supplementation has been recommended in children who are unable to receive any EN during the first week in the PICU.[13] In patients who are severely malnourished or at risk of nutritional deterioration, PN may be supplemented in the first week if they are unable to advance past low volumes of EN. In adults, the available data suggest a more conservative approach. Supplemental PN to achieve target nutrient delivery may be delayed up to 1 week in the absence of underlying malnutrition.

Timing of Nutrient Delivery

There is a complex interplay between the right dose, safe route, and timing of delivery of nutrients in critically ill patients. The time required to achieve nutrient delivery targets may influence cumulative nutrient imbalance and consequentially impact clinical outcomes. In our most recent multicenter prospective observational study in 1,844 mechanically ventilated children from 77 PICUs, delayed achievement of macronutrient targets beyond 7 days in the PICU was associated with significantly greater mortality, after adjusting for key covariates.[19] In this study, we used a prudent macronutrient target of 60% of the prescribed goal. Achieving this target before 7 days (but not before 3 days) after admission to the PICU was associated with lower mortality, with no associated worsening of ventilator-free days (VFDs) or acquired infections. This association was seen in patients who achieved their targets via EN alone or via EN with supplemental PN. Since, achieving targets within 3 days was not superior to achieving nutrient delivery targets by Days 4–7, aggressive efforts to escalating nutrient delivery soon after admission may not be necessary. However, our observations also suggest that routinely delaying achievement of nutrient targets after until after 7 days following PICU admission cannot be recommended.

SUMMARY

Based on the concepts and evidence discussed in this chapter, Figure 12-2 represents a prudent approach to providing nutrition therapy for the 4-year-old patient described in our vignette. The patient is vulnerable to poor outcomes due to preexisting undernutrition as evidenced by his anthropometry on admission. Z-scores are used to assess weight and height/length for age and help identify patients with suboptimal nutrition. In addition, this patient has significant disease severity with inflammation (pneumonia, fever) that might be associated with increased energy expenditure. However, sedation, muscle relaxation and assisted ventilation may offset this and result in lower than expected energy expenditure. Since energy expenditure estimations are frequently inaccurate, accurate measurement of his resting energy expenditure must be attempted using an indirect calorimetry. The increased protein breakdown seen in metabolic stress response would indicate a higher protein requirement. In addition to energy and protein targets, dietitians account for total fluid requirement and micronutrient needs when developing an individualized nutrition prescription for this child.

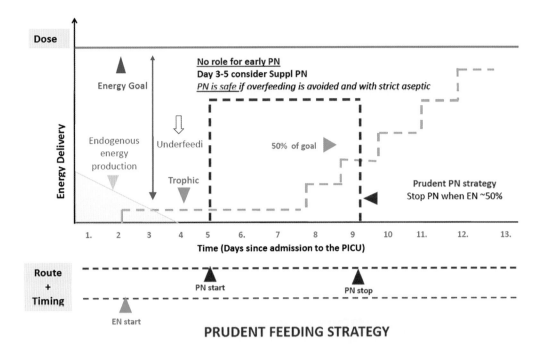

FIGURE 12-2 • Prudent feeding strategy in the PICU.[20]
*In critically ill adults without underlying malnutrition, nutrition intake may be delayed up to one week. Supplemental PN may be started after this period if EN delivery is not feasible or tolerated.
Source: https://healthmanagement.org/c/icu/issuearticle/emerging-concepts-in-nutritional-therapy-for-the-critically-ill-child.

Once the patient is stabilized, enteral nutrition must be initiated early, via a nasogastric feeding tube that is placed at the bedside and the tip confirmed by radiograph. Enteral feeding is initiated, may be small volume (trophic) initially, and then advanced in a stepwise fashion. Careful monitoring for signs of intolerance is essential component of the stepwise EN advancement algorithm. If EN is not tolerated and advancement is not possible for an extended period, there is risk of underfeeding. Prudent use of PN, considered after 4 days, might be indicated in that case in order to achieve nutrient delivery targets. After careful and individualized custom PN prescription, it is provided via the existing central venous catheter, under strict aseptic precautions and careful monitoring. PN may be discontinued once EN is tolerated and able to be advanced. During this period, serial weight and body composition measurements will help monitor for nutritional status changes in this patient.

In adults in the ICU, data from recent trials suggest harm from aggressive feeding. Despite a number of trials examining different strategies for energy and protein prescription, use of early EN or supplemental PN, and different intralipid emulsion, no definitive evidence-based recommendations can be made.[14] Hence, clinicians are advised to use their judgment to prescribe individualized strategies. Energy overfeeding is concerning and must be avoided. The optimal protein dose during acute critical illness in adults is not known and requires further investigation. The nutrition prescription for energy, protein, and intralipids must take into account the individual patient's tolerance to these macronutrients. In an average critically ill adult, without malnutrition, delaying nutrition intake up to 7 days may be reasonable. If EN is not feasible, supplemental PN may be used during the first week in patients with malnutrition and low lean body mass.

THREE TAKE-HOME POINTS

1. The metabolic stress response to critical illness is characterized by variable and unpredictable energy requirement. Failure to accurately estimate or measure energy expenditure during critical illness may result in unintended underfeeding or overfeeding, with consequential poor outcomes.
2. Protein breakdown is accelerated during critical illness, is greater than protein synthesis, and may result in loss of lean body mass in critically ill patients. Thus,

routine measures of anthropometric status (weight, height, BMI; and in infants, head circumference) on admission and serially is vital.
3. The delivery of optimal nutrition in this group requires individualized assessment of macronutrient and micronutrient needs, prescription of prudent goals, and the selection of a safe route and timing of nutrient delivery to achieve the prescribed goals.

CASE STUDY ANSWERS

1. Disease severity, premorbid conditions, nutritional status, fever (may increase energy expenditure). Sedation, muscle relaxation, assisted ventilatory support, temperature and humidity control, pain relief (may decrease energy expenditure).

2. Indirect calorimetry (using a metabolic cart or indirect calorimeter)

3. C

4. Early enteral nutrition (EN); advance stepwise as tolerated; use of supplemental parenteral nutrition (PN) only if goal feeding not possible by EN after 4–5 days.

REFERENCES

1. Mehta NM, Bechard LJ, Cahill N, et al. Nutritional practices and their relationship to clinical outcomes in critically ill children—an international multicenter cohort study*. *Crit Care Med*. 2012;40(7):2204-2211.

2. Mehta NM, Bechard LJ, Zurakowski D, Duggan CP, Heyland DK. Adequate enteral protein intake is inversely associated with 60-d mortality in critically ill children: a multicenter, prospective, cohort study. *Am J Clin Nutr*. 2015;102(1):199-206.

3. Joosten KF, Hulst JM. Prevalence of malnutrition in pediatric hospital patients. *Curr Opin Pediatr*. 2008;20(5):590-596.

4. Johnson RW, Ng KWP, Dietz AR, et al. Muscle atrophy in mechanically-ventilated critically ill children. *PLoS One*. 2018;13(12): e0207720.

5. Breen L, Stokes KA, Churchward-Venne TA, et al. Two weeks of reduced activity decreases leg lean mass and induces "anabolic resistance" of myofibrillar protein synthesis in healthy elderly. *J Clin Endocrinol Metab*. 2013;98(6):2604-2612.

6. Bury C, DeChicco R, Nowak D, et al. Use of bedside ultrasound to assess muscle changes in the critically ill surgical patient. *JPEN J Parenter Enteral Nutr*. 2021 Feb;45(2):394-402.

7. Bechard LJ, Duggan C, Touger-Decker R, et al. Nutritional status based on body mass index is associated with morbidity and mortality in mechanically ventilated critically ill children in the PICU. *Crit Care Med*. 2016;44(8):1530-1537.

8. Mehta NM, McAleer D, Hamilton S, et al. Challenges to optimal enteral nutrition in a multidisciplinary pediatric intensive care unit. *JPEN J Parenter Enteral Nutr*. 2010;34(1):38-45.

9. Hulst JM, van Goudoever JB, Zimmermann LJ, et al. The effect of cumulative energy and protein deficiency on anthropometric parameters in a pediatric ICU population. *Clin Nutr*. 2004;23(6): 1381-1389.

10. Mehta NM, Jaksic T. The critically ill child. In: Duggan CP, Walker W, eds. *Nutrition in Pediatrics*. 4th ed. Hamilton, ON: B. C. Decker Inc; 2008:663-673.

11. Mehta NM, Bechard LJ, Leavitt K, Duggan C. Cumulative energy imbalance in the pediatric intensive care unit: role of targeted indirect calorimetry. *JPEN J Parenter Enteral Nutr*. 2009;33(3): 336-344.

12. Mehta NM, Smallwood CD, Graham RJ. Current applications of metabolic monitoring in the pediatric intensive care unit. *Nutr Clin Pract: official publication of the American Society for Parenteral and Enteral Nutrition*. 2014;29(3):338-347.

13. Mehta NM, Skillman HE, Irving SY, et al. Guidelines for the provision and assessment of nutrition support therapy in the pediatric critically ill patient: Society of Critical Care Medicine and American Society for Parenteral and Enteral Nutrition. *Pediatr Crit Care Med: a journal of the Society of Critical Care Medicine and the World Federation of Pediatric Intensive and Critical Care Societies*. 2017;18(7):675-715.

14. Compher C, Bingham AL, McCall M, et al. Guidelines for the provision of nutrition support therapy in the adult critically ill patient: The American Society for Parenteral and Enteral Nutrition. *JPEN J Parenter Enteral Nutr*. 2022 Jan;46(1):12-41.

15. Mikhailov TA, Kuhn EM, Manzi J, et al. Early enteral nutrition is associated with lower mortality in critically ill children. *JPEN J Parenter Enteral Nutr*. 2014;38(4):459-466.

16. Brown AM, Irving SY, Pringle C, et al. Bolus gastric feeds improve nutritional delivery to mechanically ventilated pediatric medical patients: results of the COntinuous vs. BOlus (COBO2) Multi-Center Trial. *JPEN J Parenter Enteral Nutr*. 2022 Jul;46(5):1011-1021.

17. Hamilton S, McAleer DM, Ariagno K, et al. A stepwise enteral nutrition algorithm for critically ill children helps achieve nutrient delivery goals*. *Pediatr Crit Care Med: a journal of the Society of Critical Care Medicine and the World Federation of Pediatric Intensive and Critical Care Societies*. 2014;15(7):583-589.

18. Fivez T, Kerklaan D, Mesotten D, et al. Early versus late parenteral nutrition in critically ill children. *N Engl J Med*. 2016;374(12): 1111-1122.

19. Bechard LJ, Staffa SJ, Zurakowski D, Mehta NM. Time to achieve delivery of nutrition targets is associated with clinical outcomes in critically ill children. *Am J Clin Nutr*. 2021;114(5):1859-1867.

20. Mehta NM. Emerging concepts in nutritional therapy for the critically ill child. *ICU Management & Practice*. 2019;19(3). Available at: https://healthmanagement.org/c/icu/issuearticle/emerging-concepts-in-nutritional-therapy-for-the-critically-ill-child.

chapter 13

Severe Malnutrition and Refeeding Syndrome

Robert Bandsma, MD, PHD / Mary Flanagan, MB BCh BAO, BPharm

Chapter Outline

I. Case Studies
II. Definitions
   a. Nutritional Status Assessment
   b. Diagnostic Criteria for Malnutrition
   c. Wasting/Acute Malnutrition
   d. Malnutrition in High Resource Settings
   e. Micronutrient Deficiency
   f. Sarcopenia
   g. Epidemiology
   h. Pathophysiology
III. Nutrition as Primary Prevention for Severe Malnutrition
IV. Nutrition as Therapy for Malnutrition and Refeeding Syndrome
V. Case Studies Answers

CASE STUDY 1

A 12-month-old boy is brought to his local health clinic in Malawi due to anorexia and swelling in his lower limbs. He is mostly breastfed (on demand, but his mother reports no difference in intake from what her older children took at the same age) and eats some porridge once daily. Due to floods in the area this year, there have been multiple crop failures with low supplies of food for the whole community. His mother describes that he was born a usual size but his weight and size started to falter a few months ago. His lower limb swelling started a couple of weeks ago but is progressively worsening in the last few days and now involves his hands, too. After appropriate evaluation, including a urine dipstick that was negative for proteinuria, providers at his local health clinic diagnose him with severe malnutrition.

1. What are the two classical phenotypes of severe acute malnutrition? List one or two clinical signs of each phenotype.

2. List a pathophysiological change in five organ systems associated with severe acute malnutrition.

3. How is severe acute malnutrition in children diagnosed according to the World Health Organization Guidelines?
   A. Body Mass Index (BMI)
   B. A combination of weight-for-height z-score, mid-upper-arm-circumference, and/or presence of nutritional edema
   C. Use of functional assessment tools
   D. Sustained dietary inadequacy

CASE STUDY 2

A 15-year-old girl with a 5-year history of Crohn's disease, poor adherence to management plans, and poor attendance for follow-up presents to the Emergency Department. She is carried in by her father and is hemodynamically unstable with hypotension, tachycardia, tachypnea, and hypothermia. A focused history reveals a month-long history of decreasing oral intake, no solid intake in the previous 2 to 3 days, a 2-week history of bloody diarrhea, and no ambulation for the past week due to increasing dyspnea. On examination, she weighs 35 kg, is cachectic, and dehydrated. Her vitals respond to a slow fluid bolus. She is admitted with a diagnosis of Crohn's disease flareup and severe malnutrition.

1. Two days after commencing nutritional therapy in conjunction with her Crohn's disease, electrolyte imbalances are identified on her laboratory blood work diagnostic of refeeding syndrome. Which of the following electrolyte changes are most in keeping with a diagnosis of refeeding syndrome?
   A. Hypophosphatemia
   B. Hypokalemia
   C. Hypomagnesemia
   D. All of the above
   E. None of the above

2. Which serum vitamin level is reduced in refeeding syndrome due to its involvement in glucose metabolism, thus requiring supplementation?
   A. Vitamin A
   B. Vitamin B1 (thiamine)
   C. Vitamin C
   D. Vitamin D
   E. Vitamin E

3. How would you approach initial nutritional therapy for this patient?
   A. Use enteral feeding route
   B. "Start low & go slow"; e.g., start intake at 50% of calorie needs and increase calories slowly, as tolerated
   C. Consider thiamine supplementation
   D. Monitor closely for electrolyte imbalance and replenish electrolytes if needed
   E. All of the above

● DEFINITIONS

Nutritional Status Assessment

As reviewed in Chapter 3 ("Nutritional Assessment"), anthropometric measurements are noninvasive measurements of the body, which provide valuable assessments of a patient's nutritional status. The main anthropometric measurements include weight, height, body mass index (BMI), head circumference, waist/hip/limb circumferences, limb lengths, and skinfold thickness. Routine and repeated collection and interpretation of anthropometric data are critically important steps to diagnose and assess patients with severe acute malnutrition. Although undernutrition focuses mainly on weight, height, and mid-upper-arm-circumference (MUAC), a comprehensive assessment of all anthropometric measurements across at least two timepoints is more beneficial for diagnostic purposes. Functional assessments, though performed far less commonly, also provide meaningful information on the nutritional state of a child or adult. *Frailty*, the term given to progressive functional decline across multiple physiological systems, was previously reserved for those aged ≥ 65 years, is now felt to be applicable to all patient age groups and has recently been applied to pediatric patients.[1] A range of frailty diagnostic/functional assessment tools exist; however, the 2001 Fried Frailty Criteria are the most commonly used five measures to define frailty, including weakness (grip strength), slowness (6-minute walk test), shrinkage (unintentional weight loss), exhaustion, and diminished physical activity.[1]

Diagnostic Criteria for Malnutrition

Malnutrition is defined as any condition in which deficiency, excess or imbalance of energy, protein or other nutrients adversely affects body function and/or clinical outcome. (Overnutrition is of growing global concern, but for the purposes of this chapter will not be discussed; see Chapter 17, "Overweight and Obesity.") Undernutrition can indiscriminately affect any age group, with infants, children, pregnant women and those over the age of 65 years being most at risk. In children under 5 years of age, undernutrition is an umbrella term, which includes wasting, stunting, underweight, and micronutrient deficiencies. Children who are thin for their height are referred to as wasted or acutely malnourished, which often occurs due to an acute food shortage or illness. Low height for age is known as stunting and is characteristic of chronic or recurrent undernutrition. Children with low weight-for-age are known as underweight. A child who is underweight may be stunted, wasted, or both. Undernutrition in adults, in general, refers to being underweight or having micronutrient (trace element, vitamin or mineral) deficiencies. Disease-related malnutrition, referring to the complex interplay of inadequate intake and disease-related systemic inflammatory responses, plays a major role in both adult and child malnutrition. Unsurprisingly any child who is undernourished is not only at risk of macronutrient (protein, lipid and carbohydrate) deficiency but also of micronutrient deficiencies or indeed both. This chapter will discuss undernutrition with particular focus on wasting/acute malnutrition.

Wasting/Acute Malnutrition

Wasting or acute malnutrition is measured using a weight-for-height z-score (WHZ-score), mid-upper arm circumference (MUAC) (Figure 13-1[2]) or by the presence of bilateral pitting edema. Based on cut off parameters for each of these measurements it can be further divided into moderate- and severe acute malnutrition (MAM or SAM) (Table 13-1). Due to the multifactorial etiology and pathophysiology of acute malnutrition, the term *SAM* replaced the older terminology of protein-energy malnutrition including marasmus and kwashiorkor.[3] However, there is growing debate about the term *SAM* as severe malnutrition rarely is an acute problem but rather commonly develops over weeks to months. Some are arguing, and we agree, to use simply "severe malnutrition" or alternatively "severe wasting" and "nutritional edema" or "edematous malnutrition."[4] The typical characteristics of these phenotypes are illustrated in Figure 13-2.[5] Severe wasting gives a skeletal or "wizened" appearance with loss of muscle and subcutaneous fat. Edematous malnutrition describes the phenotype of bilateral edema of the lower limbs/edema of the face, often associated with cutaneous signs including shiny or cracked skin, burn-like appearance along with discolored and brittle hair. In infants less than 6 months of age severe malnutrition is felt to be, at least in part, related to strikingly low worldwide rates of breastfeeding and is defined using a WHZ-score alone.[6] In order to guide treatment type and location the WHO further classifies severe malnutrition as either complicated or uncomplicated severe malnutrition, depending on the presence/absence of appetite, severe edema or medical complications (including high fever, severe anemia, pneumonia, or seizures). Children with complicated severe malnutrition are at an even higher risk of morbidity and mortality and thus require initial stabilization in an inpatient setting.

TABLE 13-1 • Types of acute malnutrition in children aged 6–59 months		
Type of acute malnutrition	Measure	Cut off values
Moderate (MAM)	WHZ-score	Between -2 to -3 SD
	and/or	
	MUAC	115-125 mm
Severe (SAM) – also known as Severe Wasting or Nutritional Edema	WHZ-score	< -3 SD
	and/or	
	MUAC	<115 mm
	and/or	
	Bilateral pitting edema	

WHZ score, weight-for-height z-score; MUAC, mid-upper-arm-circumference.

Malnutrition in High Resource Settings

Though the same anthropometric parameters used to diagnose acute malnutrition in low resource settings are also used in countries with higher resources, often additional anthropometric parameters, anthropometric calculators and functional assessments are also used in nutritional status assessment of children and adults in high-resourced settings. Due to more extensive laboratory testing capabilities, micronutrient deficiencies are often tested for in patients at risk of malnutrition in high resource settings.

The term *failure to thrive* (FTT) in children is often used instead of acute malnutrition in industrialized countries. However, this term is vague, without a general consensus on its definition and it does not support or encourage a quantitative approach to nutrition for physicians. Some define FTT as a weight for age < 5th centile on multiple occasions or a weight deceleration that crosses two major percentile lines on a growth

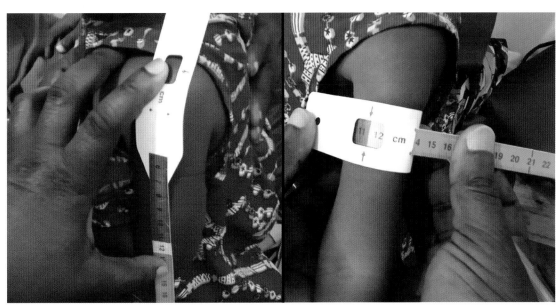

Mid Upper Arm Circumference (MUAC) Measurement: measure arm circumference at midpoint of shoulder tip to bent elbow

FIGURE 13-1 • Mid-upper arm circumference measurement[2]

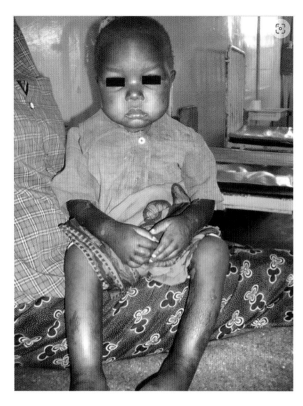 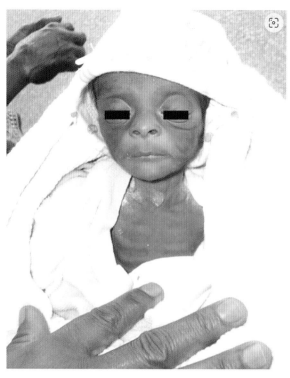

FIGURE 13-2 • Phenotypes of severe malnutrition: Nutritional edema (also known as kwashiorkor and edematous malnutrition) and severe wasting (also known as marasmus). (Reproduced with permission Langston SM, Bales BD. Protein-energy malnutrition—Kwashiorkor and Marasmus. In: Knoop KJ, Stack LB, Storrow AB, Thurman RJ, eds. *The Atlas of Emergency Medicine*. 5th ed. New York, NY: McGraw-Hill; 2021. Photo contributor: Meg Jack, MD.)

chart. We recommend that a combination of anthropometric criteria rather than a single parameter be used to assess those at risk of malnutrition, and that more definitive terminology such as acute malnutrition/wasting, stunting, underweight and micronutrient deficiency be used.

Similarly, in adults, no single clinical parameter or laboratory test is diagnostic of malnutrition. Nor indeed is there a standardized diagnostic approach to malnutrition diagnoses in adults. Instead, various diagnostic approaches include a range of characteristics to identify both adults at risk of malnutrition and those who are already malnourished including assessment of all or some of the following indicators: unplanned weight loss, inadequate energy intake, low BMI, muscle mass loss, fat mass loss, functional status, edema, presence of disease severity, neuropsychological problems, and GI symptoms.[7] The details of these characteristics can also be used to decipher the degree and chronicity of malnutrition.[7] Hospital inpatients' nutritional status can deteriorate while in hospital for a variety of reasons, including scheduled fasting for testing, disease related loss of appetite, digestive system dysfunction, and suboptimal nutrition management.[8] Malnutrition in older patients is associated with an increased risk of morbidity and mortality, longer hospital stays, functional decline and an increased risk of readmission to hospital.[7,8]

Micronutrient Deficiency

Clinical symptoms and signs of micronutrient deficiencies are not always enough to allow for diagnosis, and instead biochemical laboratory testing is required to ascertain deficiency states (see Chapter 2, "Micronutrient Metabolism"). Certain populations are more likely to suffer from specific micronutrient deficiencies. Children and young people with autism, due to food refusal, limited dietary repertoire and high frequency single food intake, have been shown to be more likely to suffer from deficiencies in vitamins A, C, D, and iron.[9] Children and adults who follow a vegan diet are at risk of vitamin B12 deficiency and to a lesser extent calcium, zinc, and/or selenium deficiency if they are not supplemented in their diet.[10] Micronutrient status is not routinely assessed in children with severe malnutrition in low resource settings. However, studies in this population show a high prevalence of abnormalities in a variety of electrolytes, minerals, and vitamins.[11–13]

Sarcopenia

Sarcopenia, defined as loss of muscle strength and impaired physical function, is considered a biologic correlate of frailty and is associated with significant morbidity and mortality. The diagnosis of sarcopenia requires measurement of a combination of muscle mass, muscle strength and physical performance. Muscle strength is typically tested by measuring grip strength, understanding that other causes for decreased strength apart from sarcopenia should be considered including hand arthritis and neurological disorders. Muscle mass is generally estimated using dual energy X-ray absorptiometry (DXA) but other imaging modalities such as bioelectrical impedance analysis,

CT, MRI, and ultrasound have also been used. Physical performance assessment involves function of the whole body and depends on skeletal muscle along with intact and integrated musculoskeletal and neurological systems. Measures of physical performance vary from single tests such as a 400-meter timed walk test or more complex tests such as a short physical performance battery test.[14]

Epidemiology

Malnutrition remains an important global health problem. The most recent data (2021) from the joint UNICEF/WHO/The World Bank Group estimate that about 45 million (6.7%) children are wasted, compared to around 52 million a decade earlier, indicating a modest improvement in the absolute prevalence during this time. Currently 13.6 million (2%) children are reportedly severely wasted.[15] It is important to realize that the prevalence of edematous malnutrition is not included in these reports, but can comprise more than half of children presenting with severe malnutrition in some regions.

Importantly, malnutrition is common in hospitalized children in both low- as well as high-resource settings.[16] For example, a study in Turkey reported a prevalence of 32% of malnutrition among hospitalized children.[17] A UK study reported a prevalence of 27%,[18] whereas a European report showed a range of malnutrition between 6% and 12%.[19] However, definitions of malnutrition differed between these reports and severe wasting likely represents a small proportion of hospitalized children with malnutrition in high resource settings. It is important to realize that hospitalization commonly worsens nutritional status in already nutritionally vulnerable populations, such as children and adults with chronic illnesses.

Though the prevalence of adults being underweight (BMI < 18.5 kg/m^2) over the past four decades has also declined; 462 million adults are underweight, with an age-standardized global prevalence of 8.8% in men and 9.7% in women.[20] The prevalence of malnutrition among the > 65 years of age population varies depending on the diagnostic approach taken but in general is considered to be very common, with studies showing approximately one-third of adult patients admitted to hospital are malnourished or are at risk of malnutrition.[7]

Pathophysiology

Malnutrition affects almost every organ system in the body;[21] there are also specific impairments found in edematous forms of malnutrition. An overview of the main systems affected in severe malnutrition is shown in Table 13-2 and highlights which impairments are generally more pronounced in edematous malnutrition compared to severe wasting.

Malnutrition is associated with several endocrinological and metabolic changes in both children and adults. In disease-related malnutrition, endocrine changes including lower testosterone and thyroid hormone levels, higher cortisol levels, peripheral growth hormone resistance, and cellular insulin resistance contribute to catabolism. Reduced insulin responses affect glucose homeostasis specifically, making children and adults susceptible to hyperglycemia. Glucose synthesis is also impaired, likely exacerbated in edematous malnutrition, making these children

TABLE 13-2 • Systemic effects of severe malnutrition

Organ system	Pathophysiological changes	Functional consequences
Intestine	Villous blunting Inflammation Dysbiosis Dysmotility Impaired barrier function	Malabsorption Feeding intolerance Bacterial translocation
Liver	Impaired metabolism Mitochondrial dysfunction	Steatosis[a] Reduced synthesis of glucose and proteins[a] Reduced bile secretion
Renal	Reduced glomerular filtration rate Tubular dysfunction	Unclear
Pancreas	Atrophy	Impaired lipid digestion Glucose dysregulation
Brain	Altered serotonin metabolism	Lethargy Irritability[a] Impact on child development
Cardiac	Cardiac muscle atrophy	Likely mostly preserved at least in non-severely sick children

[a]Specifically pronounced in nutritional edema/edematous malnutrition.

in particular vulnerable to hypoglycemic events. Apart from disturbed glucose homeostasis, protein and lipid metabolism is also affected, and is reportedly more pronounced in children with edematous malnutrition with an overall reduction in oxidation of these macronutrients and reduced synthesis of proteins, such as albumin.[21]

Nutrient digestion and absorption are affected in malnourished children and adults. Digestion is, in part, controlled by bile acids and pancreatic enzymes and there is direct evidence linking malnutrition to reduced biliary secretion and exocrine pancreatic insufficiency. Intestinal function is also affected in children with severe malnutrition, characterized by blunting of small intestinal villi, impaired intestinal barrier function, and intestinal inflammation. The combination of impairments in nutrient digestion and intestinal dysfunction is thought to limit absorptive capacity, but direct evidence is limited. Similarly in adults decreased intestinal motility and absorption due to disease is thought to contribute further to malnutrition. Diarrhea is common, especially in children, and is primarily osmotic and can thus be driven by feeding beyond absorptive capacity.

On the specific pathophysiology of edematous malnutrition, multiple hypotheses have been generated over the last decades but none of these hypotheses have been proven. Historically, edema was thought to be caused by low concentrations of albumin, but although low albumin might be required, it is likely not sufficient to lead to edema. This is supported by observations that edema generally resolves before serum albumin has shown significant improvement. In addition, children with low albumin without overt edema have been reported.[22] Oxidative stress has been associated with edematous malnutrition but whether it is causally related to the development of edema or many of the pathophysiological changes remains to be proven. Mitochondrial dysfunction has also been linked to edematous malnutrition and suggested to be related to impaired hepatic synthetic function, i.e., of albumin or glucose, and could be related to the observed oxidative stress. Finally, exogenous toxins, in particular aflatoxins, produced by molds, particularly *Aspergillus* species, have also been hypothesized to be responsible for the development of edematous malnutrition.[23]

NUTRITION AS PRIMARY PREVENTION FOR SEVERE MALNUTRITION

In general, a proactive approach to ensure adequate nutrition is critical to prevent any form of malnutrition at any age. It should start as early as conception in the pregnant mother, continue through into infancy and indeed throughout a person's life span.

A number of interventions have been reported to positively affect the nutritional status in infants and children, which include promotion and support of breastfeeding, improving hygiene, and nutrition supplementation programs for pregnant mothers and infants. In humanitarian settings, blanket or targeted supplementary feeding programs are generally implemented to prevent moderate and severe malnutrition in children. However, it is important to realize that prevention in very impoverished settings or in humanitarian crises has proven to be challenging and is thought to be most effective when programs are introduced in a holistic manner. In the global context, this translates into interventions that target malnutrition directly, such as breastfeeding support and supplementary feeding interventions, but also indirectly, such as improving financial status, social safety nets, enhanced agricultural methods, improving access to water, sanitation and hygiene (WASH), and enhancing healthcare access and quality.

Interventions that are also relevant for people of any age include identification of at-risk populations through malnutrition screening tools such as the Pediatric Nutritional Screening Score (PNSS) or the Screening Tool for Risk on Nutritional Status or Growth in children[24] or similar tools in adults such as the Subjective Global Assessment Tool, the Malnutrition Universal Screening Tool and the Global Leadership Initiative on Malnutrition criteria.[7] Early involvement of dietitians in the care of these at-risk children can support a subsequent detailed nutritional assessment and provision of adequate and tailored nutrition throughout the hospitalization.

NUTRITION AS THERAPY FOR MALNUTRITION AND REFEEDING SYNDROME

The mainstay of treatment for malnutrition is nutritional rehabilitation. The quantity and form of nutritional rehabilitation prescribed depends largely on patient age, weight, and the medical and nutritional resources available but broadly follows the same approach (see Figure 13-3[25]). Nutrition is started at a low rate and increased gradually in a manner of "start low, go slow" to ensure medical stabilization and prevent refeeding syndrome (see below). This may also assist in not overstretching the absorptive capacity of the malnourished intestine and reducing the chances of causing osmotic diarrhea. In those at high risk of refeeding syndrome, such as patients with anorexia nervosa, initial feeding should start at as low a rate as 10–20 kcal/kg, especially if there is a history of significant rapid weight loss, a BMI < 13 kg/m^2, fluid refusal, or hemodynamic instability. Simple age, weight, and disease-based formulas exist to guide goal/target intake amounts (e.g., 25–30 kcal/kg body weight in malnourished adults or 60 kcal/kg body weight in patients with anorexia nervosa). Nutritional intake should be reassessed every 24–48 hours and escalation of enteral to parenteral feeding should only be considered if a significant proportion of energy and protein targets cannot be reached after 5–7 days, which is a major change from how nutrition was approached in critically ill patients in the past.[8,26] This newer approach results in shorter length of intensive care unit stay, shorter hospital stays, and reduced rates of new airway and bloodstream infection.[27,28]

In the 1990s, in order to combat the strikingly high mortality rate associated with severe malnutrition, therapeutic milks and feeds were pioneered and implemented globally for the nutritional treatment of severe malnutrition in children 6–59

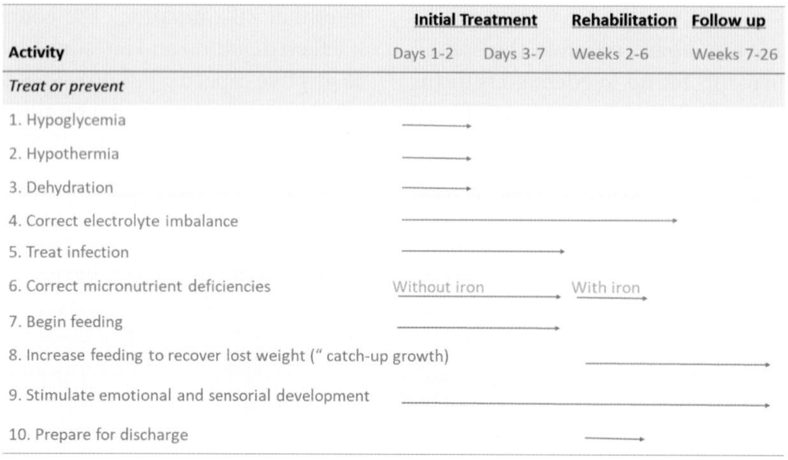

Activity	Initial Treatment		Rehabilitation	Follow up
	Days 1-2	Days 3-7	Weeks 2-6	Weeks 7-26
Treat or prevent				
1. Hypoglycemia	———→			
2. Hypothermia	———→			
3. Dehydration	———→			
4. Correct electrolyte imbalance	——————————————→			
5. Treat infection	———————→			
6. Correct micronutrient deficiencies	Without iron ————→	With iron ————→		
7. Begin feeding	———————→			
8. Increase feeding to recover lost weight (" catch-up growth)			——————————→	
9. Stimulate emotional and sensorial development		————————————————————→		
10. Prepare for discharge			————————→	

FIGURE 13-3 • General approach to severe malnutrition[25]

months of age. Currently, only those with "complicated severe malnutrition," i.e., being unwell, are treated in inpatient settings in a phased manner.[3] The aim of the first phase is medical stabilization, not weight gain. Nutritional therapy in this stabilization phase is a milk-based formulation (F75–75 kcal/100 ml), which is noticeably lower in calories with more calories coming from fat rather than protein and carbohydrates when compared to the maintenance nutritional therapy. Children in this phase of treatment are provided with 80–100 kcal/kg/day spread out over 8–12 meals/day for approximately 3 days. Oral feeds are the mainstay of therapy for the vast majority of children with severe malnutrition, with nasogastric feeds reserved for those with poor intake, severe lethargy, etc. Once a child's appetite returns, they are medically stable and their edema is subsiding, they are transitioned gradually to the maintenance phase of therapy. This transition period utilizes either a higher calorific milk-based therapy (F100–100 kcal/100 mL) or a solid based nutrition (RUTF–Ready-to-use-therapeutic-food), which is also the food used at home once patients are discharged. RUTF are specially formulated pastes, bars or biscuits that provide high energy (approximately 200 kcal/kg/day) with the objective of weight gain and catch-up growth. RUTF is designed to require no preparation and due to its low moisture content does not have specific storage requirements allowing ease of use in the outpatient setting. It can be made locally or bought preformulated and consists mainly of peanuts enriched with sugar, powdered milk, vegetable oil, vitamins, and mineral salts. Children are encouraged to eat additional food on top of their prescribed RUTF.[3] Of note infants less than 6 months of age who have severe malnutrition are treated differently, with an emphasis on breastfeeding and lactation support.[6]

Provision of continued nutritional support beyond the hospitalization period when patients transfer back to their home environment is also of large importance. This includes regular monitoring of nutritional parameters including growth and early interventions when and where needed.

Concurrent Empiric Therapy

Antibiotics Epidemiological data has shown a high prevalence of infection in children with severe malnutrition.[29] All patients with severe malnutrition, whether admitted to an inpatient or outpatient therapeutic feeding center are prescribed a 5-day course of broad-spectrum antibiotics. The rationale for empiric antibiotic administration, in the absence of infectious symptoms or signs, comes from studies in both complicated and uncomplicated severe malnutrition patients, in which antibiotics improved both the mortality rate and the rate of nutritional recovery.[30–32] Though these studies are of low quality, expert opinion concurs with the sound and rational basis of empiric antibiotics for all children with severe malnutrition.[33] Similarly malnourished adults also experience increased rates of infection but empiric therapy is not recommended and instead targeted antibiotics are recommended if there are symptoms or signs of infection.

Micronutrient Supplementation

F-75, F-100, and RUTF all contain added micronutrients to prevent or resolve deficiencies, reduce risk of refeeding syndrome, and promote homeostasis.[3,21] The supplementary dose of micronutrients to therapeutic feeds is based largely on expert opinion rather than evidenced based. Despite the overall paucity of quality information on micronutrient deficiency, there are studies showing persistent thiamine, iron, and vitamin D deficiency despite supplemented nutritional therapy,[34–36] suggesting that even higher doses or lengthier durations of micronutrient supplementation may be required. Further studies are needed in this area.

Outside of low resource settings an assessment of micronutrient status in terms of both intake and clinical and biochemical evidence of status is recommended to target therapy instead of empiric micronutrient supplementation. Exceptions apply to those at risk of refeeding syndrome where prophylactic electrolyte, thiamine, and multivitamin supplementation is recommended[8,37] or in adults whose enteral nutrition provides < 1,500 kcal/day where micronutrient supplements are recommended.[8]

Fluids

Children with severe malnutrition frequently present with a history of diarrhea and dehydration. Large-scale studies have shown the prevalence of diarrhea in children with severe malnutrition to be ~45%.[11,29] Due to changes in skin elasticity, wasting, and edema, it can often be difficult to diagnoses acute dehydration in severely malnourished children. Due to concerns regarding total body sodium retention in children with complicated severe malnutrition with inferred implications of cardiac dysfunction, a specific electrolyte solution with low sodium, high potassium content (ReSoMal, 45 mmol/L Na+) is used in inpatient settings instead of the typical oral rehydration salts (ORS, 70 mmol/L Na+) normally recommended for diarrhea and dehydration.[3] ORS rather than ReSoMal is used in children with severe malnutrition treated in the community. ORS is also recommended in children hospitalized concurrently with severe malnutrition and cholera due to cholera's ability to induce high fecal sodium losses. Along the same rationale of concerns regarding fluid overload and sodium excess, the use of intravenous fluids in children with severe malnutrition is strongly advised against by the WHO unless there are signs of hypovolemic shock or severe dehydration.[25]

Refeeding Syndrome

Refeeding syndrome is defined by The American Society for Parenteral and Enteral Nutrition (ASPEN) as a measurable reduction in levels of one or any combination of phosphorus, potassium, and/or magnesium, or the manifestation of thiamin deficiency, developing shortly (hours to days) after initiation of calorie provision to an individual who has been exposed to a substantial period of undernourishment.[38] Though initially described in the 1940s following the unexpected death and disability of prisoners of war and concentration camp survivors, the pathophysiology of refeeding syndrome is not yet entirely understood. It is thought that prolonged undernutrition and starvation deplete total body levels of energy, vitamins, and electrolytes. In this setting, an intake of glucose causes a switch from catabolism to anabolism, a rise in

TABLE 13-3 • Systemic effects of refeeding syndrome[39]	
Hypophosphatemia Anorexia Anemia Proximal muscle weakness Skeletal effects (bone pain, rickets, and osteomalacia) Increased infection risk Paresthesia, ataxia, and confusion	*Hypokalemia* Mild: constipation, fatigue, muscle weakness, and malaise Moderate to severe: polyuria, encephalopathy, glucose intolerance; muscular paralysis, poor respiration, and cardiac arrhythmias. Severe: altered muscle contraction and cardiac function
Hypomagnesemia Mild: loss of appetite, nausea, vomiting, fatigue, and weakness. Moderate: paresthesia, muscle contractions and cramps, seizures, personality changes, abnormal heart rhythms, and coronary spasms Severe: hypocalcemia or hypokalemia	*Thiamine Deficiency* Beriberi (peripheral neuropathy, wasting, rarely congestive heart failure). Wernicke-Korsakoff syndrome: 1st acute, and life-threatening stage = Wernicke's encephalopathy (peripheral neuropathy), 2nd chronic stage = Korsakoff's psychosis (severe short-term memory loss, disorientation, and confabulation)

insulin levels resulting in increased utilization of phosphate for glucose metabolism, and a drive of electrolytes intracellularly, which can lead to a drop in serum electrolyte levels with subsequent effects on multiple body systems[39] (Table 13-3). Refeeding syndrome can also result in thiamine deficiency due to increased demand for glucose dependent metabolic pathways. In addition to malnutrition, various other chronic disease states increase the risk of refeeding syndrome including, but not limited to, anorexia nervosa, acquired immunodeficiency syndrome, esophageal dysmotility, malabsorptive states, and cancer.[38] The incidence of refeeding syndrome is largely unknown, partly due to differing cut off values for definition but also due to the difficulty in identifying all patients at risk of refeeding syndrome.

Guidance varies depending on the institution regarding how to mitigate the risk of refeeding syndrome but in general the advice is to start feeds at a low rate (max ~50% goal rate, but may be as low as 10–20 kcal/kg body weight if there is a high risk of refeeding syndrome) with particular attention paid to glucose intake along with consideration for empiric thiamine and electrolyte administration. The risk of refeeding syndrome is greatest in the first 72 hours of feed initiation, during which time guidelines recommend twice daily electrolyte checks and generous electrolyte replenishment if low levels are identified.[37,38]

Outcomes

Malnutrition Outcomes in Low-Resource Settings Ideally once a child reaches the rehabilitation phase of severe malnutrition treatment the ideal weight gain for catch up growth is > 10 g/kg/day. The criteria for discharge from a nutritional treatment program and severe malnutrition recovery is defined by the WHO as weight-for-height/length z-score (WHZ) ≥ −2 or mid-upper-arm circumference ≥ 125 mm and no edema for at least 2 weeks.[3] At discharge from nutritional rehabilitation programs parents/guardians are educated to continue frequent feeds with energy and nutrient dense foods and provide play therapy, in addition to recommendations to bring their child back for regular follow-up checks, immunizations, and vitamin A boosters.

Despite the introduction of standardized nutritional therapy and supportive care in nutritional rehabilitation units, mortality in severe malnutrition remains high. During hospitalization mortality rates vary from 10% to 23%.[11,40,41] A systematic review of 28 studies showed that HIV infection, diarrhea, pneumonia, shock, lack of appetite, and lower WHZ-scores are independent predictors of inpatient mortality in children with severe malnutrition.[42] Postdischarge mortality continues to be an issue with a further 11–25% of deaths in children with severe malnutrition occurring after normal program discharge.[40,41] In this cohort HIV seropositivity, age < 12 months, severity of malnutrition at admission and disability (mostly neuro-disability such as cerebral palsy) were associated with an increased risk of death.[40]

Though long-term survivors show good catch-up growth in terms of weight-for-height, the same does not apply to linear growth with minimal height-for-age catch up at 1 year and lower, though improved, height-for-age scores 7 years post treatment end when compared to control children/siblings.[40,43] Physical function, measured by grip strength and steps-per-hour, is also reduced in child severe malnutrition survivors. Although one study has shown no significant difference in cardiorespiratory function or metabolic function between child survivors of severe malnutrition and control children 7 years postdischarge from inpatient nutritional treatment,[43] the accepted hypothesis is that early life malnutrition increases the risk of long-term metabolic consequences and noncommunicable diseases such as type 2 diabetes mellitus, nonalcoholic fatty liver disease, etc. A study of adult survivors of childhood severe malnutrition with a median age of 28.4 +/− 8.8 years showed different metabolic profiles via metabolomic analysis when compared to community controls.[44]

Despite the high prevalence of severe malnutrition globally and its high mortality rate, many questions about severe malnutrition remain unanswered. Further research is needed to help identify earlier those at a higher risk of mortality, so that targeted interventions can be identified and implemented. Additionally, the role that singular or compound micronutrient deficiencies and their treatment may have in this population requires closer attention.

Malnutrition Outcomes in High-Resource Settings

Unsurprisingly malnutrition is associated with adverse outcomes even in high-resource settings with higher rates of morbidity and mortality, functional decline, and prolonged hospital stays independent of the underlying medical illness. Data on the impact of nutritional therapy for malnourished patients or those at risk of malnutrition varies but some larger studies have shown improvements in inpatient and 90-day mortality along with lower hospital readmission rates.[8]

CASE STUDY 1 ANSWERS

1. Severe acute malnutrition phenotypes	Clinical sings of phenotypes
Severe wasting (also known as marasmus)	Skeletal/"wizened" appearance Muscle & fat loss
Nutritional edema (also known as edematous malnutrition or kwashiorkor)	Bilateral limb edema Facial edema Shiny/cracked skin Burn-like skin Discoloured and/or brittle hair

2. Organ system	Pathophysiological changes
Intestinal	Villous blunting Inflammation Dysbiosis Dysmotility Impaired barrier function
Hepatic	Impaired metabolism Mitochondrial dysfunction
Renal	Reduced glomerular function rate Tubular dysfunction
Pancreatic	Atrophy
Brain	Impaired serotonin metabolism
Cardiac	Cardiac muscle atrophy

3. B

CASE STUDY 2 ANSWERS

1. D

2. B

3. E

REFERENCES

1. Fried LP, Tangen CM, Walston J, et al. Frailty in older adults: evidence for a phenotype. *J Gerontol A Biol Sci Med Sci*. 2001;56(3):146-157.

2. Powell C, Butterly JR. Chapter 7. Nutrition. In: Markle WH, Fisher MA, Smego RA, eds. *Understanding Global Health*. 2nd ed. The McGraw-Hill Companies; 2014. Available at: http://accessmedicine.mhmedical.com/content.aspx?aid=57933638.

3. World Health Organization. *Guideline: Updates on the Management of Severe Acute Malnutrition in Infants and Children*; 2013. doi:9789241506328.

4. Kerac M, McGrath M, Connell N, et al. "Severe malnutrition": thinking deeplyS, communicating simply. *BMJ Glob Health*. 2020;5(11):1-4.

5. Langston SM, Bales BD. Protein-Energy malnutrition—Kwashiorkor and Marasmus. In: Knoop KJ, Stack LB, Storrow AB, Thurman RJ, eds. *The Atlas of Emergency Medicine*. 5th ed. McGraw-Hill; 2021. Available at: http://accessmedicine.mhmedical.com/content.aspx?aid=1181051461.

6. Kerac M, Tehran I, Lelijveld N, Onyekpe I, Berkley J, Manary M. *Inpatient treatment of severe acute malnutrition in infants aged <6 months*. Executive summary commissioned for WHO. Published online 2012.

7. Malone A, Mogensen KM. Key approaches to diagnosing malnutrition in adults. *Nutr Clin Prac*. 2022;37(1):23-34.

8. Schuetz P, Seres D, Lobo DN, Gomes F, Kaegi-Braun N, Stanga Z. Management of disease-related malnutrition for patients being treated in hospital. *Lancet*. 2021;398(10314):1927-1938.

9. Kinlin LM, Birken CS. Micronutrient deficiencies in autism spectrum disorder: a macro problem? *Paediatr Child Health (Canada)*. 2021;26(7):436-437.

10. Bakaloudi DR, Halloran A, Rippin HL, et al. Intake and adequacy of the vegan diet. A systematic review of the evidence. *Clin Nutr*. 2021;40(5):3503-3521.

11. Bandsma RHJ, Voskuijl W, Chimwezi E, et al. A reduced-carbohydrate and lactose-free formulation for stabilization among hospitalized children with severe acute malnutrition: a double-blind, randomized controlled trial. *PLoS Med*. 2019;16(2):1-19.

12. Iannotti LL, Trehan I, Manary MJ. Review of the safety and efficacy of vitamin A supplementation in the treatment of children with severe acute malnutrition. *Nutr J*. 2013;12(1):125.

13. Ali SQ, Dhaneria M. Study of serum vitamin D levels in severe acute malnutrition and moderate acute malnutrition from 6 months to 59 months of age: a hospital based study. *Indian J Appl Res*. 2021;11(4):60-62.

14. Cruz-Jentoft AJ, Sayer AA. Sarcopenia. *Lancet.* 2019;393(10191): 2636-2646.

15. UNICEF/WHO/WORLD BANK. *Levels and trends in child malnutrition UNICEF/WHO/World Bank Group Joint Child Malnutrition Estimates Key findings of the 2021 edition.* World Health Organization. Published online 2021:1-32.

16. Joosten K, Hulst J. Nutritional screening tools for hospitalized children: methodological considerations. *Clin Nutr.* 2014; 33(1):1-5.

17. Oztürk Y, Benal B, Arslan N, Ellidokuz H. Effects of hospital stay on nutritional anthropometric data in Turkish children. *J Trop Pediatr.* 2003;49(3):189-190.

18. Pichler J, Hill S, Shaw V, Lucas A. Prevalence of undernutrition during hospitalisation in a children's hospital: what happens during admission? *Eur J Clin Nutr.* 2014;68:730-735.

19. Huysentruyt K, De Schepper J, Bontems P, et al. Proposal for an algorithm for screening for undernutrition in hospitalized children. *J Pediatr Gastroenterol Nutr.* 2016;63(5):e86-e91.

20. Di Cesare M, Bentham J, Stevens GA, et al. Trends in adult body-mass index in 200 countries from 1975 to 2014: a pooled analysis of 1698 population-based measurement studies with 19.2 million participants. *The Lancet.* 2016;387(10026):1377-1396.

21. Bhutta ZA, Berkley JA, Bandsma RHJ, Kerac M, Trehan I, Briend A. Severe childhood malnutrition. *Nat Rev Dis Primers.* 2017;3:17067.

22. Gonzales GB, Njunge JM, Gichuki BM, et al. The role of albumin and the extracellular matrix on the pathophysiology of oedema formation in severe malnutrition. *EBioMedicine.* 2022;79:103991.

23. Soriano JM, Rubini A, Morales-Suarez-Varela M, Merino-Torres JF, Silvestre D. Aflatoxins in organs and biological samples from children affected by kwashiorkor, marasmus and marasmic-kwashiorkor: a scoping review. *Toxicon.* 2020;185:174-183.

24. Hulst JM, Huysentruyt, Koena B, Joosten KF. Pediatric screening tools for malnutrition: an update. *Curr Opin Clin Nutr Metab Care.* 2020;23(3):203-209.

25. Ashworth A, Khanum S, Jackson A, Schofield CE. *Guidelines for the Inpatient Treatment of Severely Malnourished Children;* 2003. Available at: https://www.ncbi.nlm.nih.gov/books/NBK190324/%0A.

26. Singer P, Blaser AR, Berger MM, et al. ESPEN guideline on clinical nutrition in the intensive care unit. *Clin Nutr.* 2019;38(1):48-79.

27. Eulmesekian P. Early versus late parenteral nutrition in critically ill children. *Arch Argent Pediatr.* 2016;114(4):e274-e275.

28. Jones Q, Walden A. Early versus late parenteral nutrition in critically ill adults. *J Intensive Care Soc.* 2011;12(4):338-339.

29. Maitland K, Berkley JA, Shebbe M, Peshu N, English M, Newton CRJC. Children with severe malnutrition: can those at highest risk of death be identified with the WHO protocol? *PLoS Med.* 2006;3(12):2431-2439.

30. Trehan I, Goldbach HS, LaGrone LN, et al. Antibiotics as part of the management of severe acute malnutrition. *N Engl J Med.* 2013;368(5):425-435.

31. Trehan I, Amthor RE, Maleta K, Manary MJ. An evaluation of the routine use of amoxicillin as part of the home-based treatment of severe acute malnutrition. *Trop Med Int Health.* 2010;15(9):1022-1028.

32. Lazzerini M, Tickell D. Antibiotics in severely malnourished children: systematic review of efficacy, safety and pharmacokinetics. *Bull World Health Organ.* 2011;89(8):593-606.

33. Jones KDJ, Berkley JA. Severe acute malnutrition and infection. *Paediatr Int Child Health.* 2014;34(sup1):S1-S29.

34. Hiffler L, Adamolekun B, Fischer PR, Fattal-Vavleski A. Thiamine content of F-75 therapeutic milk for complicated severe acute malnutrition: time for a change? *Ann N Y Acad Sci.* 2017;1404(1):20-26.

35. Saleem J, Zakar R, Zakar MZ, et al. High-dose vitamin D 3 in the treatment of severe acute malnutrition: a multicenter double-blind randomized controlled trial. *Am J Clin Nutr.* 2018; 107(5):725-733.

36. Kangas ST, Salpéteur C, Nikièma V, et al. Vitamin A and iron status of children before and after treatment of uncomplicated severe acute malnutrition. *Clin Nutr.* 2020;39(11):3512-3519.

37. Royal College of Psychiatrists. Medical emergencies in eating disorders (MEED) Guideance on recognition and management. Published online 2022.

38. da Silva JSV, Seres DS, Sabino K, et al. ASPEN consensus recommendations for refeeding syndrome. *Nutr Clin Prac.* 2020; 35(2):178-195.

39. National Institutes of Health. *Dietary Supplement Fact Sheets.* Available at: https://ods.od.nih.gov/factsheets/.

40. Kerac M, Bunn J, Chagaluka G, et al. Follow-up of post-discharge growth and mortality after treatment for severe acute malnutrition (FuSAM Study): a prospective cohort study. *PLoS One.* 2014;9(6):e96030.

41. Diallo AH, Sayeem Bin Shahid ASM, Khan AF, et al. Childhood mortality during and after acute illness in Africa and south Asia: a prospective cohort study. *Lancet Glob Health.* 2022;10(5): e673-e684.

42. Karunaratne R, Sturgeon JP, Patel R, Prendergast AJ. Predictors of inpatient mortality among children hospitalized for severe acute malnutrition: a systematic review and meta-analysis. *Am J Clin Nutr.* 2020;112(4):1069-1079.

43. Lelijveld N, Seal A, Wells JC, et al. Chronic disease outcomes after severe acute malnutrition in Malawian children (ChroSAM): a cohort study. *Lancet Glob Health.* 2016;4(9):e654-e662.

44. Thompson DS, Bourdon C, Massara P, et al. Childhood severe acute malnutrition is associated with metabolic changes in adulthood. *JCI Insight.* 2020;5(24):1-17.

Infectious Diseases

Christopher R. Sudfeld, ScD

Chapter Outline

I. Introduction

II. Mechanisms for the Cyclic Relationship of Undernutrition and Infectious Disease
   a. Barrier Impairment
   b. Impaired Immunity
   c. Infection Increases the Risk of Nutrient Deficiency

III. Mechanisms for the Relationship of Overnutrition with Infectious Diseases
   a. Barrier Impairment

   b. Impaired Immunity
   c. Altered Physiology
   d. Comorbid infections

IV. Examples of the Relationship of Nutrition with Infectious Diseases
   a. Protein Energy Malnutrition
   b. Micronutrients
   c. Obesity

V. Conclusion

CASE STUDY 1

Ten-month-old child who weighs 5 kg (<3rd% for age and sex) presents to your clinic with a 10-day history of diarrhea. The child was born at home and has not received any immunizations or growth monitoring. She is only receiving human milk as a source of nutrition. She has edema on both of her feet and hands.

1. Important nutritional concerns about her infectious illness include:

A. Being substantially underweight.
B. Zinc deficiency
C. Protein insufficiency
D. Malabsorption of nutrients in the setting of diarrhea
E. A, C, and D
F. A, B and D
G. A, B, C, and D

CASE STUDY 2

You are evaluating a 65-year-old man in the Emergency Department who has a 2-day history of cough, rhinorrhea, and a 1-day history of dyspnea. His body mass index is 41 kg/m². A nasopharyngeal swab comes back positive for SARS-COVID-19.

1. His obesity places him at risk of all of the following complications of this respiratory infection, except:
A. Death
B. ICU admission
C. Respiratory failure
D. All of the above

● INTRODUCTION

In 1968, Scrimshaw, Gordon, and Taylor published a World Health Organization (WHO) monograph that described the potential pathways and interactions between undernutrition and infection.[1] The monograph included evidence from animal and human studies that showed that malnutrition, including protein-energy malnutrition and micronutrient deficiencies, was associated with increased incidence and severity of infectious diseases, and that in turn, infectious illnesses have negative effects on nutritional status.[1] Over the past 50 years, our knowledge of the relationship between nutrition and infectious disease has greatly expanded, including the links between overnutrition and infections, but the pathways that link malnutrition and infection presented in the WHO monograph remain foundational.

Figure 14-1 presents an updated framework presenting our current understanding of the cyclic relationship between undernutrition and infection. Undernutrition (macronutrient or micronutrient deficiencies) can increase the risk of new infections or the severity of infectious disease and in turn, infections can increase the risk for many nutritional deficiencies. The major pathways linking undernutrition and infection are barrier impairment and impaired immunity, while infections can increase the risk of undernutrition through decreased appetite,

increased energy demands, nutrient loss, and malabsorption. The cyclic relationship between undernutrition and infectious disease is most well studied in children and the elderly, but these cyclic relationships can occur in individuals of all ages.

There is also growing appreciation of the relationship between overnutrition, including obesity and associated comorbidities, with infection. Figure 14-2 presents a general framework that links overnutrition to infection. In contrast to the cyclic relationship for undernutrition, the relationship between overnutrition and infection appears to be more one-directional. There are multiple mechanisms through which overnutrition can increase the incidence and severity of infectious disease including barrier impairment, impaired immunity, altered physiology, and comorbidities (i.e., type 2 diabetes). Generally, most infections are associated with weight loss, which does not lead to a cyclical relationship between overnutrition and infection. However, there may be some exceptions to the framework, including Adenovirus-36 infection, that may be associated with weight gain.[2]

In this chapter, we present the mechanisms and provide clinical examples of the relationships between both undernutrition and overnutrition with infectious diseases. However, it is important to note that these are generalized frameworks and the examples do not necessarily apply to all nutrients and infectious diseases.

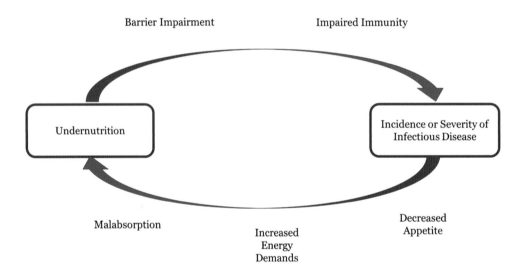

FIGURE 14-1 · Framework for the cyclical relationship of undernutrition with infectious disease

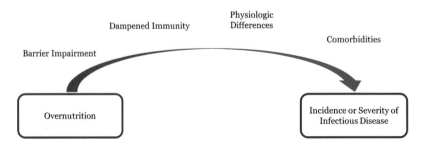

FIGURE 14-2 · Framework for the relationship of overnutrition with infectious disease

MECHANISMS FOR THE CYCLIC RELATIONSHIP OF UNDERNUTRITION AND INFECTIOUS DISEASE

The cyclic relationship between undernutrition with infection is well established.[3] In the early 20th century, research generally focused on the epidemiology and biology of children with protein energy malnutrition (PEM).[4] PEM is defined as an imbalance between the supply of protein or energy that does not meet demands for optimal growth. Severe forms include marasmus, which is characterized by severe wasting and kwashiorkor, which is notable for the presence of edema.[4] See Chapter 13, "Severe Malnutrition and Refeeding Syndrome." More recent research has elucidated the role of other macronutrient and micronutrient deficiencies in infectious diseases. While the consequences of PEM and micronutrient deficiencies are often different, both generally increase the risk of infection through barrier impairment and impaired immunity. Infections can then increase the risk of nutrient intake through effects on the intake and absorption of energy, protein, macronutrient, and micronutrients.

Barrier Impairment

Physical and chemical barriers, which are considered the first-line defense of the innate immune system, can prevent infectious pathogens from entering the body or establishing infection.[5] Undernutrition can impair multiple barrier systems, including the skin, mucosal membranes of the gastrointestinal tract, and epithelial cells of the respiratory tract.[6] Children with PEM have been noted to have atrophy of skin layers and some children can present with dermatosis, which causes the skin to resemble "peeling paint," which increases the risk of infection. PEM can also lead to changes in the intestinal mucosa that lead to increased gut permeability.[6] Biopsy studies of the small intestine among children with PEM have found thinning of the intestinal mucosa, deceased villous height, and lymphocyte infiltration, findings that have been termed *environmental enteric dysfunction*. PEM may also lead to altered microbial colonization of the gut which can increase the risk of infection.[6] In addition, nutrient deficiencies can also independently impair barrier function. For example, vitamin A is important for the normal differentiation of epithelial cells, particularly in the skin, and is also involved in intestinal immune responses that support the integrity of the gut and respiratory tract.[7]

Impaired Immunity

Animal and human studies conducted since the early 20th century have documented a wide range of negative effects of PEM on the immune system and more recent research also characterized the negative effects of micronutrient deficiencies on immunity.[3] PEM has been shown to have negative effects on both innate and adaptive immunity.[6] In terms of innate immunity, PEM is associated with increased inflammatory biomarkers, decreased neutrophil chemotaxis and phagocytosis, reduced leukocyte phagocytosis, decreased natural killer (NK) cell numbers, impaired responsiveness to interferon (IFN)-γ, and altered complement system function.[6] PEM also

has multiple effects on adaptive immunity, including atrophy of the thymus, decreased B-cells, and altered cytokine production.[4] Thymic atrophy in PEM primarily leads to changes in the lymphoid compartment of the thymus and leads to the loss of immature CD4+CD8+ cells and decreased CD4 to CD8 ratio. Importantly, it appears that thymic atrophy due to PEM is reversible with treatment.[3]

Macronutrients and micronutrient deficiencies, beyond insufficient energy intake, can also impair immunity. Macronutrients and micronutrients can have differential effects on innate and adaptive immunity. In terms of innate immunity, vitamin A is involved in the regulation of NK cell proliferation, while vitamin B6, vitamin B12 vitamin C, vitamin E, folate, and zinc can alter NK cell cytotoxic activity.[7] Vitamin D has been shown to have important biological effects on innate antimicrobial immune responses by way of effects on the proliferation and function of monocytes and macrophages.[8] Nutrients can also modify oxidative and inflammatory stress.[7] Vitamin A reduces the production of the proinflammatory cytokines IL-2 and TNF-α, while zinc reduces the proliferation of proinflammatory Th17 and Th9 cells, reduces IL-2 and TNF-α production, and has antioxidant effects on reactive oxygen (ROS) and nutrition species (NOS).[7] Dietary lipids also have notable anti-inflammatory effects, including n-3 polyunsaturated fatty acids (PUFAs), which inhibit eicosanoids, proinflammatory cytokines (i.e., TNF-α and IL-6), promote anti-inflammatory cytokines (IL-10), and have antioxidant properties.[8] Overall, macronutrients and micronutrients can have wide-ranging and differential effects on immunity.

Infection Increases the Risk of Nutrient Deficiency

Infections can increase the risk of undernutrition through multiple pathways. Loss of appetite (anorexia) and reduced food intake are well documented as common among individuals with infectious illnesses. It has been hypothesized that anorexia during infection is beneficial to host adaptations to restrict nutrient availability for pathogens. It is estimated that energy intake decreases between 8% and 22% in children with diarrheal disease, malaria, or acute respiratory infections.[9] During infection, proinflammatory cytokines cause a catabolic shift in metabolism, including increases in IL-1 and TNF-α, which lead to increased leptin concentrations and appetite suppression.[10] Inflammatory markers, including CRP, are also associated with increased leptin concentrations.[10] In addition, energy requirements are increased during infection due to increased metabolic needs to respond to infection. It is estimated that fever increases energy expenditure for children by 7–11% per degree Celsius increase in body temperature.[11] It is theorized that fatigue due to infection is an adaptation to conserve energy due to these increases in energy expenditure. Infections can also directly cause nutrient malabsorption. Diarrheal pathogens can also damage epithelial cells in the gut and directly impair absorption during infection. Environmental enteric dysfunction (EED), an acquired subclinical condition characterized by villous atrophy and crypt hyperplasia, is also common among individuals living with unimproved water and sanitation and can cause nutrient malabsorption.

MECHANISMS FOR THE RELATIONSHIP OF OVERNUTRITION WITH INFECTIOUS DISEASES

Research on the mechanisms that link overnutrition, primarily obesity, with the risk and severity of infections, is rapidly increasing. The major pathways that link overnutrition with the risk and severity of the infection that has been characterized include barrier impairment, impaired immunity, altered physiology, and comorbidities.

Barrier Impairment

Obesity is associated with disrupted microcirculation in the skin and decreased wound healing which can increase the risk of infection.[12] Obese children have been noted greater transepidermal water loss which may be associated with an increased risk for cutaneous infections. Deep skin folds associated with obesity can also create an environment for the overgrowth of pathogenic bacteria and fungi.[12] Obesity and its complications, including diabetes mellitus, are also associated with impaired intestinal barrier function which may increase the risk of infection.[12]

Impaired Immunity

Obesity is also characterized by chronic, low-grade inflammation and is also generally associated with dampened immune responses.[13] There is growing evidence of dysregulation of both innate and adaptive immunity in obesity including impaired chemotaxis, altered differentiation of macrophages, and altered cytokine production.[13] Obesity is associated with increased neutrophils, mast cells, proinflammatory macrophages, and decreased number of eosinophils in adipose tissue.[13] Reduced levels of adiponectin and prolonged exposure to leptin in obesity are also associated with suppressed NK cell cytotoxicity.[14] Obese individuals also have greater production of proinflammatory cytokines in adipose tissue.[14] It has been hypothesized that among obese indivudals, chronic exposure to proinflammatory cytokines may desensitize the immune system to inflammatory responses.

Altered Physiology

Obesity and excess weight change organ physiology that can increase the risk and severity of infection.[15] Obesity is associated with reductions in functional residual capacity and expiratory reserve volume of the lungs, and lung and chest wall compliance that may impact the severity of outcomes of respiratory infections.[16] Skin folds due to excess weight can also increase the risk of infection.[16] Further, altered lymphatic systems among obese individuals can cause delayed wound healing.[15]

Comorbid Infections

Obesity is a risk factor for multiple comorbidities that may increase the risk of infection through independent mechanisms. Type 2 diabetes is associated with an increased risk of lower respiratory tract infections, including pulmonary tuberculosis and pneumonia, urinary tract infections, skin infections, and soft tissue infections.[17] Hyperglycemia due to insulin resistance or deficiency may impair immunity through multiple mechanisms, including NK cell, neutrophil, and macrophage dysfunction, impaired pathogen recognition, altered cytokine production, and other pathways.[17] Further, metabolic abnormalities, retention of uremic solutes, impaired immunity, urologic disease, immunosuppressive therapy, and other comorbidities associated with obesity, including kidney disease, may also increase the risk of infection.[18]

EXAMPLES OF THE RELATIONSHIP OF NUTRITION WITH INFECTIOUS DISEASES

Protein Energy Malnutrition

Decades of research have characterized clinical presentation and infection outcomes associated with PEM and these studies were foundational in the 1960 Scrimshaw, Gordon, and Taylor WHO monograph.[1] The majority of these studies were conducted in pediatric populations due to the burden of PEM experienced by this age group due to increased caloric requirements and susceptibility to infections.[19] PEM is associated with major barrier and immunologic deficits that significantly increase the risk for a range of infections. For example, *Pneumocystis carinii* pneumonia, a well-characterized HIV-related opportunistic, was documented among malnourished children after World War II.[20] Children with severe acute malnutrition are more likely to present to care with infection danger signs and have diarrheal infections associated with bacterial pathogens as compared to non-malnourished children.

Micronutrients

Evidence on the relationship between micronutrient deficiency or supplementation with infection has largely been conducted among children and pregnant women, especially in low- and middle-income countries; however, other populations, including the elderly also have a growing evidence base on the relationship between micronutrients and infection.[21] In this section, we provide summaries of the relationship of vitamin A, zinc, and iron with selected infectious diseases.

Vitamin A plays a crucial role in epithelial cell integrity and is also important in many aspects of innate and adaptive immunity.[22] In addition, to epithelial barrier impairment, vitamin A deficiency causes impairment of multiple innate immune cell function, including neutrophils, macrophages, and natural killer cells.[23] Vitamin A is also important for the differentiation of T-cells and B-cells and deficiency causes a shift from Th2 to Th1 responses. Vitamin A had long been recognized to be important in eye health due to its link with night blindness, but research on vitamin A in broader health and infectious disease rapidly increased after an observational study published in 1983 determined that Indonesian children with xerophthalmia (night blindness or Bitot's spots) had about four times increased risk of death as compared to non-xerophthalmic children.[24] Over 40 randomized controlled trials of vitamin A supplementation for children followed and the most recent systematic review found that vitamin A supplementation reduces the risk of all-cause mortality by 12%.[25] As a result, the World Health Organization currently recommends that all children aged 6–59 months receive routine vitamin A supplementation if they live in a community where vitamin A deficiency is a public health problem.[26] The World Health Organization also currently recommends vitamin A treatment for all children with acute measles. Vitamin A deficiency is rare in the United States (0.3% in the general population) and other high-income country settings and therefore routine vitamin A supplementation is not recommended.[27] However, vitamin A treatment is recommended by the American Academy of Pediatrics (AAP) for the treatment of children with severe measles (e.g., hospitalized children).[28]

Zinc is an essential trace element that catalyzes over 100 enzymes, enables protein folding, and plays an important role in the regulation of DNA and RNA synthesis.[29] Zinc is also required for the development and proper functioning of the innate and adaptive immune system with zinc deficiency being associated with thymic atrophy, reduced B-cells and antibody production, reduced polymorphonuclear cell chemotaxis, reduced phagocytosis, and increased inflammation.[29] Randomized clinical trials have shown that zinc supplementation for children with acute diarrhea shortens the duration of diarrhea, reduces stool output, and decreases the risk of persistent diarrhea.[30] The World Health Organization currently recommends that children with diarrhea receive 20 mg of zinc per day for 10–14 days in addition to standard oral rehydration solution treatment.[31] Zinc supplements have also been shown to prevent and treat respiratory tract infections. Zinc supplements reduce the duration of the common cold by approximately 2 days among adults.[32] Preventive zinc supplementation for children 2–59 months of age has also been shown to reduce the incidence of pneumonia.[33]

Iron is a critical nutrient for humans given its central involvement in many cellular processes including energy generation, oxygen transport, and DNA replication.[34] Iron is a similarly essential nutrient for the cellular processes of pathogenic bacteria and fungi.[35] Humans tightly control iron metabolism to reduce availability to pathogens and during infection greater iron sequestration occurs.[34] In turn, pathogens have developed different strategies to obtain host iron including siderophores and iron acquisition from heme, hemoglobin, transferrin, and other proteins.[35] Therefore, iron has a complex relationship with infectious diseases and much research has focused on the potential negative health effects of iron supplementation. The relationship between iron and malaria disease has long been a concern. A randomized trial of routine prophylactic iron supplementation for children 1–35 months conducted in malaria endemic Pemba Island in Zanzibar found that children who received iron were 12% more likely to die or be hospitalized, a 16% increased risk for severe adverse events due to clinical malaria, and a 22% increased risk of cerebral malaria.[36] These findings have led to challenges in anemia control for children globally, given anemia itself is a risk factor for child mortality and poor developmental outcomes. The World Health Organization updated its guidelines in 2016, and now

recommends that daily prophylactic iron supplementation be provided to infants and children 6–59 months of age in settings where anemia is a severe public health problem (> 40% prevalence) and in malaria-endemic settings it is essential to provide iron supplements in combination with interventions to prevent, diagnose, and treat malaria.[37] There is also evidence of the negative effects of iron supplements on non-malarial infections. A recent meta-analysis of 154 randomized trials conducted among individuals of all ages in all settings found that intravenous iron, primarily for the treatment of anemia, was associated with a 16% increase in the risk of infections.[38]

Obesity

The relationship between obesity and respiratory infections has received greater attention because of the severe acute respiratory syndrome coronavirus-2 (SARS CoV-2) and H1N1 influenza pandemics. However, obesity has also been linked to increased risk and severity of other infections including skin infections, urinary tract infections, and surgical site infections.[16]

In terms of respiratory tract infections, obesity has also been linked to increased risk and greater disease severity from influenza A infection.[16] During the 2009 H1N1 pandemic, obesity was identified as a key risk factor for hospitalization, requirement for ventilator support, and death.[39] Among patients hospitalized with pandemic H1N1, a body mass index ≥ 40 kg/m^2 was associated with twice the odds of being admitted to an intensive care unit or death.[40] Studies have also identified obesity as a risk factor for seasonal influenza in the general population.[39] There is also evidence that obesity may affect influenza vaccine response. A study conducted among adults vaccinated with the trivalent inactivated influenza vaccine in North Carolina found that obese adults were twice as likely to develop confirmed influenza or influenza-like illness as compared to healthy-weight adults.[41] Obesity was identified as a risk factor for severe disease early in the SARS CoV-2 pandemic with researchers in Wuhan, China reporting that each 1 kg/m^2 increase in BMI was associated with a 12% greater risk of severe SARS CoV-2 disease and that obesity was associated with three times the risk of severe disease.[42] The exact mechanisms linking obesity to more severe SARS-CoV-2 disease are not fully understood, but it is hypothesized to be related to inflammation and immune dysregulation.

Obesity is associated with an increased risk of multiple types of skin infections.[16] A cohort study of over 170,000 adults in South Korea found that a BMI >30 kg/m^2 was associated with a 19% greater risk of cellulitis and almost five times the risk of cellulitis-related hospital admission as compared to normal-weight adults.[43] Obesity is also a risk factor for UTIs among individuals admitted to intensive care units and postoperatively.[16] In the general population, higher BMI in women is also associated with a greater risk of recurrent UTIs, as well as UTIs among pregnant and postpartum people.[44] The mechanisms that predispose obese individuals to UTIs are not fully understood, but it is suspected that differences in immune responses, physiologic differences, and other pathways including glycosuria among obese diabetic individuals may be contributors.[16] Surgical site infections (SSIs) are also more common among obese individuals, and it is thought this relationship is attributable to suboptimal wound healing which may be a result of reduced flood flow and dampened immune responses.[16] A cohort study of ~75,000 U.S. adult patients who underwent elective colorectal surgery found that obesity class I (BMI 30.0–34.9 kg/m²) and obesity class III were associated with 1.5 and 2.1 times the risk of SSI as compared to normal weight individuals, respectively.[45]

CONCLUSION

Decades of research have shown clear cyclical links between undernutrition and the risk of infection, particularly in children. In low- and middle-income countries there remains a large burden of undernutrition and it is estimated that nearly half of remaining deaths among children under 5 years of age are attributable to undernutrition. Hospitalized patients are also at high risk of malnutrition and infectious morbidities. In addition, there is a growing appreciation for the role of obesity in the risk and severity of infections, particularly respiratory infections, but it is also important to note that multiple types of infections including skin, urinary tract, and SSIs are more common among individuals with high BMI. Given continuing increases in the prevalence of overweight and obesity in the United States and high-income settings as well as increases in low- and middle-income settings, the role of obesity in infection is a growing health priority.

THREE TAKE-HOME POINTS

1. Undernutrition (deficiency in energy or nutrients) and infectious diseases have a cyclical relationship whereby undernutrition increases the risk of infectious diseases and infections, in turn, have negative effects on nutritional status
2. Protein-energy malnutrition can profoundly increase the risk of infections but micronutrient deficiencies can also alter barrier function and impair immune responses to increase the risk and severity of infection.
3. Obesity is classically associated with low-grade inflammation; however, it also leads to altered barriers, dampened immune responses, and physiologic changes and comorbidities that can increase the risk and severity of respiratory, skin, urinary tract, SSIs, and other infections.

CASE STUDY 1 ANSWERS

1. G; All of the nutrient deficiencies (energy, protein, zinc, and many nutrients that are not well absorbed during diarrhea place this child at higher risk of nutritional and medical complications.

CASE STUDY 2 ANSWERS

1. D; Obesity increases the COVID-related risks of death, respiratory failure, and ICU admission.

REFERENCES

1. Scrimshaw NS, Taylor CE, Gordon JE. Interactions of nutrition and infection. *Monogr Ser World Health Organ.* 1968;3-329.
2. da Silva Fernandes J, Schuelter-Trevisol F, Cancelier ACL, et al. Adenovirus 36 prevalence and association with human obesity: a systematic review. *Int J Obes (Lond).* 2021;45(6):1342-1356.
3. Chandra RK, Kumari S. Nutrition and immunity: an overview. *J Nutr.* 1994;124(8 Suppl):1433s-1435s.
4. Chandra RK. Protein-energy malnutrition and immunological responses. *J Nutr.* 1992;122(3 Suppl):597-600.
5. Janeway CA Jr, Travers P, Walport M, Shlomchik MJ. Principles of innate and adaptive immunity. In: *Immunobiology: The Immune System in Health and Disease.* 5th ed. Garland Science; 2001.
6. Rytter MJ, Kolte L, Briend A, Friis H, Christensen VB. The immune system in children with malnutrition—a systematic review. *PLoS One.* 2014;9(8):e105017.
7. Gombart AF, Pierre A, Maggini S. A review of micronutrients and the immune system–working in harmony to reduce the risk of infection. *Nutrients.* 2020;12(1):236.
8. Wu D, Lewis ED, Pae M, Meydani SN. Nutritional modulation of immune function: analysis of evidence, mechanisms, and clinical relevance. *Front Immunol.* 2018;9:3160.
9. Bresnahan KA, Tanumihardjo SA. Undernutrition, the acute phase response to infection, and its effects on micronutrient status indicators. *Adv Nutr.* 2014;5(6):702-711.
10. Sarraf P, Frederich RC, Turner EM, et al. Multiple cytokines and acute inflammation raise mouse leptin levels: potential role in inflammatory anorexia. *J Exp Med.* 1997;185(1):171-175.
11. Stettler N, Schutz Y, Whitehead R, Jéquier E. Effect of malaria and fever on energy metabolism in Gambian children. *Pediatr Res.* 1992;31(2):102-106.
12. Yosipovitch G, DeVore A, Dawn A. Obesity and the skin: skin physiology and skin manifestations of obesity. *J Am Acad Dermatol.* 2007;56(6):901-916; quiz 17-20.
13. Muscogiuri G, Pugliese G, Laudisio D, et al. The impact of obesity on immune response to infection: plausible mechanisms and outcomes. *Obes Rev.* 2021;22(6):e13216.
14. Tilg H, Moschen AR. Adipocytokines: mediators linking adipose tissue, inflammation and immunity. *Nat Rev Immunol.* 2006;6(10):772-783.
15. Koenig SM. Pulmonary complications of obesity. *Am J Med Sci.* 2001;321(4):249-279.

16. Pugliese G, Liccardi A, Graziadio C, Barrea L, Muscogiuri G, Colao A. Obesity and infectious diseases: pathophysiology and epidemiology of a double pandemic condition. *Int J Obes (Lond)*. 2022;46(3):449-465.

17. Berbudi A, Rahmadika N, Tjahjadi AI, Ruslami R. Type 2 diabetes and its impact on the immune system. *Curr Diabetes Rev*. 2020;16(5):442-449.

18. Dalrymple LS, Go AS. Epidemiology of acute infections among patients with chronic kidney disease. *Clin J Am Soc Nephrol*. 2008;3(5):1487-1493.

19. Batool R, Butt MS, Sultan MT, Saeed F, Naz R. Protein-energy malnutrition: a risk factor for various ailments. *Crit Rev Food Sci Nutr*. 2015;55(2):242-253.

20. Cegielski JP, McMurray DN. The relationship between malnutrition and tuberculosis: evidence from studies in humans and experimental animals. *Int J Tuberc Lung Dis*. 2004;8(3):286-298.

21. Eggersdorfer M, Berger MM, Calder PC, et al. Perspective: role of micronutrients and omega-3 long-chain polyunsaturated fatty acids for immune outcomes of relevance to infections in older adults—a narrative review and call for action. *Adv Nutr*. 2022;13(5):1415-1430.

22. Stephensen CB. Vitamin A, infection, and immune function. *Annu Rev Nutr*. 2001;21:167-192.

23. Huang Z, Liu Y, Qi G, Brand D, Zheng SG. Role of vitamin A in the immune system. *J Clin Med*. 2018;7(9):258.

24. Sommer A. Vitamin a deficiency and clinical disease: an historical overview. *J Nutr*. 2008;138(10):1835-1839.

25. Imdad A, Mayo-Wilson E, Haykal MR, et al. Vitamin A supplementation for preventing morbidity and mortality in children from six months to five years of age. *Cochrane Database Syst Rev*. 2022;3(3):CD008524.

26. Organization WH. *Guideline: Vitamin A Supplementation in Infants and Children 6-59 Months of Age*. World Health Organization; 2011.

27. Pfeiffer CM, Sternberg MR, Schleicher RL, Haynes BM, Rybak ME, Pirkle JL. The CDC's second national report on biochemical indicators of diet and nutrition in the U.S. population is a valuable tool for researchers and policy makers. *J Nutr*. 2013;143(6):938s-947s.

28. Kimberlin DW. Red Book: 2018-2021 report of the committee on infectious diseases: Am Acad Pediatrics; 2018.

29. Saper RB, Rash R. Zinc: an essential micronutrient. *Am Fam Physician*. 2009;79(9):768-772.

30. Lukacik M, Thomas RL, Aranda JV. A meta-analysis of the effects of oral zinc in the treatment of acute and persistent diarrhea. *Pediatrics*. 2008;121(2):326-336.

31. World Health Organization. *Clinical Management of Acute Diarrhoea*. World Health Organization; 2004.

32. Wang MX, Win SS, Pang J. Zinc supplementation reduces common cold duration among healthy adults: a systematic review of randomized controlled trials with micronutrients supplementation. *Am J Trop Med Hyg*. 2020;103(1):86-99.

33. Lassi ZS, Moin A, Bhutta ZA. Zinc supplementation for the prevention of pneumonia in children aged 2 months to 59 months. *Cochrane Database Syst Rev*. 2016;12(12):CD005978.

34. Cassat JE, Skaar EP. Iron in infection and immunity. *Cell Host Microbe*. 2013;13(5):509-519.

35. Caza M, Kronstad JW. Shared and distinct mechanisms of iron acquisition by bacterial and fungal pathogens of humans. *Front Cell Infect Microbiol*. 2013;3:80.

36. Sazawal S, Black RE, Ramsan M, et al. Effects of routine prophylactic supplementation with iron and folic acid on admission to hospital and mortality in preschool children in a high malaria transmission setting: community-based, randomised, placebo-controlled trial. *Lancet*. 2006;367(9505):133-143.

37. World Health Organization. *Guideline Daily Iron Supplementation in Infants and Children*. World Health Organization; 2016.

38. Shah AA, Donovan K, Seeley C, et al. Risk of infection associated with administration of intravenous iron: a systematic review and meta-analysis. *JAMA Netw Open*. 2021;4(11):e2133935.

39. Mertz D, Kim TH, Johnstone J, et al. Populations at risk for severe or complicated influenza illness: systematic review and meta-analysis. *BMJ*. 2013;347:f5061.

40. Fezeu L, Julia C, Henegar A, et al. Obesity is associated with higher risk of intensive care unit admission and death in influenza A (H1N1) patients: a systematic review and meta-analysis. *Obes Rev*. 2011;12(8):653-659.

41. Neidich SD, Green WD, Rebeles J, et al. Increased risk of influenza among vaccinated adults who are obese. *Int J Obes (Lond)*. 2017;41(9):1324-1330.

42. Gao F, Zheng KI, Wang XB, et al. Obesity is a risk factor for greater COVID-19 severity. *Diabetes Care*. 2020;43(7):e72-e74.

43. Cheong HS, Chang Y, Joo EJ, Cho A, Ryu S. Metabolic obesity phenotypes and risk of cellulitis: a cohort study. *J Clin Med*. 2019;8(7):953.

44. Bamgbade OA, Rutter TW, Nafiu OO, Dorje P. Postoperative complications in obese and nonobese patients. *World J Surg*. 2007;31(3):556-560; discussion 61.

45. Wahl TS, Patel FC, Goss LE, Chu DI, Grams J, Morris MS. The obese colorectal surgery patient: surgical site infection and outcomes. *Dis Colon Rectum*. 2018;61(8):938-945.

chapter 15

Oral Conditions

Sondos Alghamdi, BDS, MMSc, FRCDC / Catherine Hayes, DMD, SM, DMSc / Nadine Tassabehji, PhD, RDN, LDN

Chapter Outline

CASE STUDY 1: DENTAL CARIES AND XEROSTOMIA

A 37-year-old female with asthma and allergic rhinitis presented to the clinic for her routine check-up for asthma control. The patient manages her asthma with a combination of albuterol and inhaled corticosteroids (ICS). Her physician checked her lab results and oral cavity for side effects and oral manifestations and found that she is experiencing xerostomia. She was referred to her dentist, who detected multiple active dental carious lesions. She brushes twice a day and does not floss; however, when asked about her lifestyle and dietary habits, she reported that she eats on the go, snacks frequently (pastries and baked products), and drinks more than two cups of coffee with cream and artificial sweeteners as she reports that helps to sustain her busy work schedule.

1. List the risk factors that lead to this patient developing multiple active carious dental lesions.

2. What dietary recommendations would you give to this patient to control
   A. Xerostomia?
   B. Dental caries?

CASE STUDY 2: PERIODONTAL DISEASE AND UNCONTROLLED DIABETES

A 54-year-old male with type II diabetes visited the dental clinic, complaining of pain in his oral cavity. The oral exam and radiographs showed he had a periodontal abscess with generalized periodontal inflammation and gingival bleeding. He brushes a few times a week and flosses occasionally. The dentist plans drainage to relieve the pain, followed by periodontal treatment; however, the dentist referred him to his physician for his uncontrolled diabetes to adjust his oral hypoglycemic agents (OHAs), so the patient can maximize the periodontal treatment. The patient's HbA1c level is 9.2%, and his BMI is 35. The patient is taking Metformin and Glibenclamide. He reported that he has not been adhering to the diabetic diet he was advised to follow, and he mainly follows a liquid diet (due to tooth loss) with frequent consumption of carbohydrates and sugar-sweetened beverages.

1. List dietary and other risk factors that are associated with this patient's uncontrolled diabetes and periodontal condition.

2. List some dietary interventions or adjustments the patient can follow to optimize the outcome of the periodontal treatment.

INTRODUCTION

Oral diseases and conditions affect more than 3.5 billion individuals globally; they are a significant public health concern and are closely connected to overall health, ultimately contributing to a higher burden of disease.[1] The importance of nutrition for oral health cannot be overstated. Consuming a healthy diet and calcium-rich foods, adequate protein, high in fruits and vegetables, while limiting sugary snacks and drinks can prevent the development of dental caries. In addition to this, drinking enough water keeps your mouth clean by flushing away food particles.[2] This chapter covers some of the common oral conditions and the role of nutrition in oral health that are important for all healthcare providers.

OVERALL HEALTH AND ORAL HEALTH

Oral health is an integral component and key indicator of overall health. The association between oral and overall health has been investigated in the scientific literature.[2] Many conditions manifest their signs and symptoms in the oral cavity first, allowing for early detection and diagnosis of some medical conditions.[2] Evidence has shown that poor oral health can lead to various systemic diseases. For example, periodontal pathogens have been found to be in higher concentrations in the bloodstream after that patient has undergone periodontal procedures, especially for patients with increased dental plaque accumulation on teeth surfaces. This can lead to developing bacteremia, which can increase the risk of systemic complications. The presence of *Porphyromonas gingivalis* in the bloodstream is found to be linked to multiple conditions, including stroke, cardiovascular event, and rheumatoid arthritis.[3]

Many diseases and chronic conditions have oral manifestations. It has been noted that Sialadenosis (swelling of the salivary glands) occurs in up to 25% of patients with bulimia.[4] Irreversible dental erosion in the palatal surfaces of the upper anterior teeth and the lingual surfaces of the lower posterior teeth can be a sign of gastroesophageal reflux disease (GERD) or recurrent vomiting.[5] Other pathologic changes that manifest in the oral cavity include periodontal inflammation or bleeding, mucosal swelling or pallor, glossitis, and cheilitis. These can be the initial signs that lead to the diagnosis of many systemic conditions, including endocrine, autoimmune, inflammatory, and neoplastic diseases.[6]

Chronic use of certain medications and polypharmacy can impact the oral cavity. Tongue, oral mucosal ulcerations and candidiasis are commonly seen in asthmatic patients who are using inhalation therapy due to the immune suppression of the treatment.[7] Anticholinergics have been found to cause hyposalivation; several studies showed that they could lead to xerostomia in patients who were treated for overactive bladder.[8,9] Other medications that cause xerostomia includes anti-depressants, diuretics, blood pressure medication such as enalapril, and nifedipine, and over-the-counter decongestants like pseudoephedrine.[8,9] The discomfort that accompanies the dry mouth can result in the discontinuation of the medication by the patients, which was reported to be one of the reasons in 40% of the cases that led patients to discontinue the use of their prescribed medication.[9] Xerostomia can also lead to decreased food intake and eventually malnutrition. Gingival hyperplasia is another side effect of certain medications, including seizure medications and calcium channel antagonists.[10]

The healthcare provider's understanding of this connection ensures the best care delivery and management of the condition to reach the optimum health outcome for patients. These connections extend to nutritional intake and dietary patterns. For example, an individual who experiences dry mouth often avoids consuming certain types of food (meat and vegetables), due to a lack of saliva, which is essential for chewing, swallowing, and ingestion.[8,9] These same patients may resort to consuming high carbohydrate-rich foods that can increase the risk of dental caries. Decreased salivary flow alone, is an independent risk factor for a faster rate of caries development and tooth cavitation. The presence of saliva in sufficient quantities increases the ability of the tooth surfaces to neutralize the effect of enamel demineralization by aiding in the remineralization process of the affected tooth structures.[11] Another area where nutrition comes into play is evidence, that shows consuming a balanced diet rich in essential key nutrients, such as calcium and vitamin C and D, can help strengthen the developing teeth and surrounding tissues as well as the healing process in the oral cavity.[1]

RELEVANT PHYSIOLOGY AND PATHOPHYSIOLOGY

This section of the chapter will focus on the most common oral conditions; dental caries and periodontal disease.

Dental Caries, Oral Microbiome, Saliva, and Dietary Patterns

Dental caries has been presented in the literature as a multifactorial and potentially reversible process that involves the bacterial biofilm in the oral cavity and on tooth surfaces (dental plaque). These factors include: first, oral microbiome, bacterial microorganisms, and their virlence. Second, the nature of the tooth structure and morphology (some teeth have thinner enamel and are more prone to cavitation, such as deep bits and fissures as part of the natural tooth anatomy, or weaker enamel composition in cases of enamel hypoplasia). Third, contributing factors involve diet (consumption of carbohydrates, sugars, frequency of consumption), fluoride exposure, and salivary factors that are heavily influenced by dietary patterns (pH, flow rate, composition, and buffering capacity).[12] The bioavailability of the consumed fermentable carbohydrates in saliva and oral tissues plays a large role in this process. The contact time the oral cavity and dental structures are exposed to the cariogenic conditions is an integral component of the caries development process.[13,14] The dietary component can potentially facilitate the demineralization process of enamel and dentin. Sugars consumption is an important dietary factor in dental caries development, specifically the type of sugar (fermentable) and frequency of consumption.[14,15]

The "Ecological Plaque Hypothesis",[16] which has been widely accepted by dental scholars and clinicians, can illustrate the role of diet in caries development. When sugars are consumed and thus are present in the oral cavity for prolonged periods of time, the microorganisms present in the dental plaque that are primarily responsible for the development of dental caries predominate. The acidogenic (acid-producing) and aciduric (acid-tolerating) bacteria, more specifically, the mutans streptococci (*Streptococcus mutans*) and lactobacilli, metabolize the sugars and produce acids as a byproduct which creates an acidic oral environment and lead to a drop in the salivary pH. A change in the pH of the saliva below the critical level of 5.5 results in enamel demineralization and leads to tooth cavitation over time.[15,17] Demineralization involves loss of key minerals such as fluoride, phosphate, and calcium from the tooth structure. These bacteria are able to tolerate acidic environments, whereas the bacteria associated with healthy enamel are more sensitive to low pH.[15–18] The higher frequency of sugar consumption, mainly sucrose/glucose, acts to nurture these acidogenic bacteria (i.e., *S. mutans*), which maintains the status of low salivary pH and the acidic oral environment resulting in multiple active dental carious lesions over time[15,17,18] (Figure 15-1).

Periodontal Diseases, Inflammation, and the Role of Diet

Periodontitis is an inflammatory disease affecting the supporting tissues surrounding the teeth. It can be prevented with proper oral hygiene, routine preventive dental care, diet, and the management of chronic conditions. The equilibrium between microbial activity and the host immune system is essential in maintaining periodontal health. It is generally managed and treated by periodontal scaling and root planing. However, some patients do not respond well to this treatment. The onset and progression of the disease depend on a multitude of risk factors, such as the presence of periodontal pathogens (*Porphyromonas gingivalis, Tannerella forsythia,* and *Aggregatibacter actinomycetemcomitans*), smoking, diabetes, obesity, genetics, stress, and inflammatory diseases.[19]

The mechanism by which diet, more specifically unhealthy dietary patterns, contributes to inflammation has been investigated by many scholars, as it ties closely with the development of some chronic conditions. Evidence shows that nutritional status has been associated with various inflammatory diseases and conditions, including cardiovascular diseases, rheumatoid arthritis, and type II diabetes, all of which have been associated with periodontal disease.[20] It has been reported that treatment and management of the periodontal disease can lead to improvement in glycemic control and decrease hemoglobin A1c levels. On the other hand, increased inflammation from periodontal disease can affect systemic inflammation and adversely affect patients with chronic inflammatory conditions such as heart disease.[6,21]

Systemic inflammation markers, C-reactive protein (CRP), interleukin (IL-6), and tumor necrosis factor-alpha (TNF-α), are found to be correlated with intake of pro-inflammatory diet.[21–23] These markers are elevated in gingival crevicular fluid (GCF) and subgingival plaque in individuals with periodontal disease and infection.[21–23] A key driver of chronic inflammation is oxidative stress, which results from the imbalance between reactive oxygen species (ROS), "oxidants, and antioxidants" in tissues at any part of the body, in this case, the periodontal tissues.[24] This disruption in the balance creates an excess of oxidant load with reduced antioxidant activity, leading to pathological changes and local tissue damage, and can further result in tooth loss due to loss of integrity of the tooth-supporting structures. The oxidative stress mechanism is associated with the production of advanced glycation end products (AGEs), which result from irreversible nonenzymatic glycation and oxidation of lipids and proteins by adding sugar to their polypeptide chain, altering their structure.[25] This further leads to an increase in inflammatory markers associated with periodontal disease. Diet plays a major role in managing oxidative stress and the inflammatory process. Diets that are rich in fruits and vegetables have high antioxidant capacity and can create an anti-inflammatory effect and possess the potential to slow the progression or reverse cellular damage and injury.

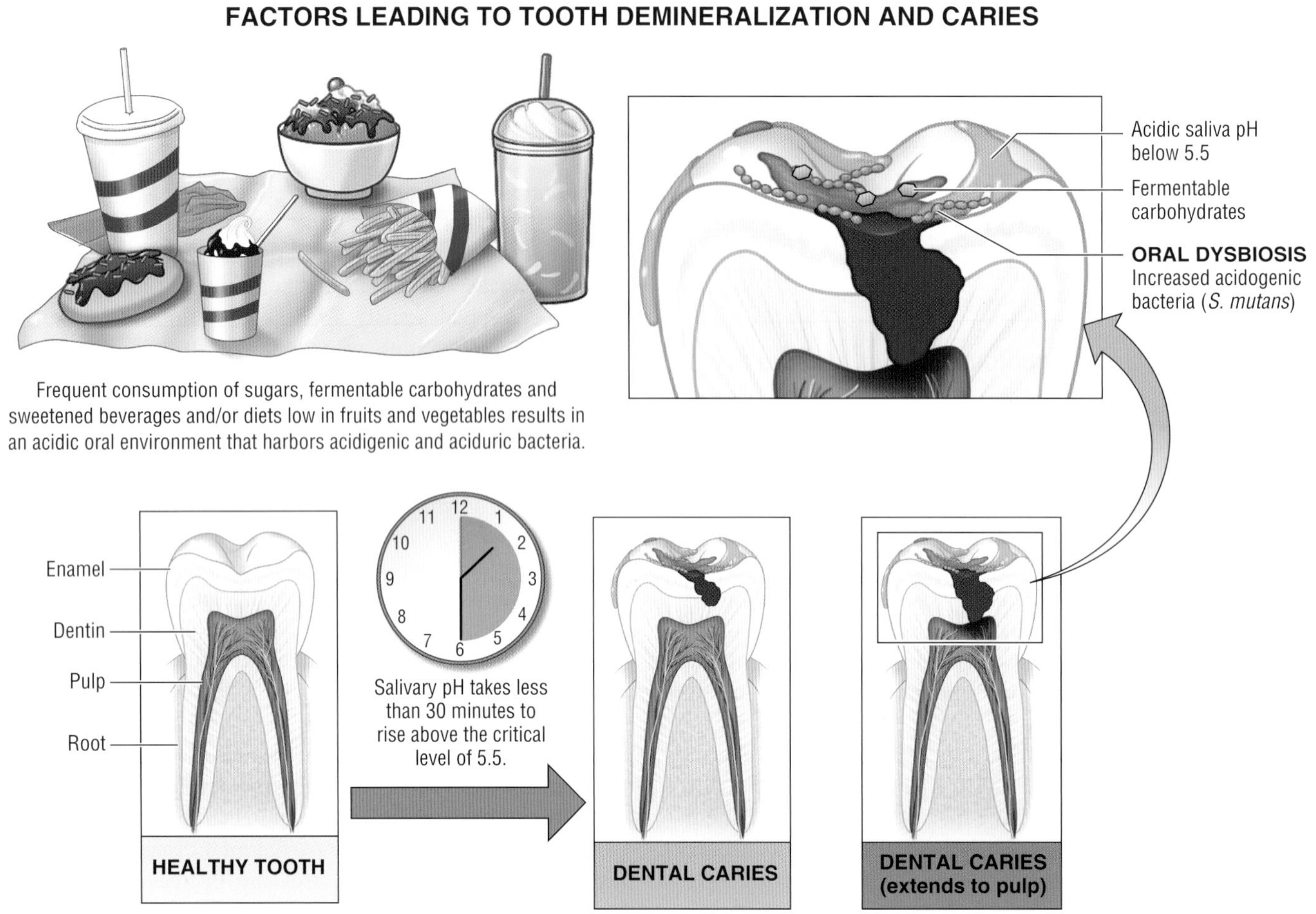

FACTORS LEADING TO TOOTH DEMINERALIZATION AND CARIES

Frequent consumption of sugars, fermentable carbohydrates and sweetened beverages and/or diets low in fruits and vegetables results in an acidic oral environment that harbors acidigenic and aciduric bacteria.

Acidic saliva pH below 5.5

Fermentable carbohydrates

ORAL DYSBIOSIS
Increased acidogenic bacteria (*S. mutans*)

Enamel

Dentin

Pulp

Root

HEALTHY TOOTH

Salivary pH takes less than 30 minutes to rise above the critical level of 5.5.

DENTAL CARIES

DENTAL CARIES
(extends to pulp)

FIGURE 15-1 • The role of diet in the development of dental caries.

Whereas processed food and animal products that are high in fat and processed simple sugars content can increase the production of advanced glycation end products (AGEs), contributing to the oxidative stress and inflammation of the tissues[21–25] (Figure 15-2).

● BIDIRECTIONAL RELATIONSHIP BETWEEN ORAL HEALTH AND NUTRITION

Good nutrition is essential for maintaining good oral and overall health. Consuming a balanced diet that is low in sugar and high in complex carbohydrates, protein, fiber, fruits, and vegetables that are high in vitamins and minerals can help to reduce the risk of developing dental caries and periodontal disease. Foods that are high in calcium, such as dairy products, edamame, and almonds can help to strengthen teeth and bones and remineralize tooth enamel. Vitamin C is important for oral health, as it helps in reducing gingival inflammation and promoting healing, whereas its deficiency can lead to gingival bleeding. Nutritional deficiencies manifest in the oral cavity, as they can lead to developing oral tissue inflammation, bleeding, and interference with wound healing. Oral manifestations of nutritional deficiencies are summarized in Table 15-1.[26,27]

TABLE 15-1 • Oral manifestations of common nutritional deficiencies[26,27]	
Vitamin/mineral	**Oral manifestations of deficiency**
Vitamin B3, B6, and B12	Angular cheilitis Glossitis Magenta color tongue
Folic Acid—Folate (Vitamin B9)	Superficial ulceration in the tongue and oral mucosa
Vitamin C	Gingival bleeding
Vitamin D and Calcium	Reduced bone density, reduced immune response
Iron	Pallor of lips and oral mucosa (Plummer Vinson Syndrome)
Zinc	Altered taste, smell, poor wound healing, impaired immune response

Moreover, because of the integral relationship between nutrition and oral health, it is important for all health providers, including physicians and dentists, to be aware of the potential effects of food insecurity; some of these effects can be first observed in the oral cavity. Studies have found that individuals

FACTORS LEADING TO PERIODONTAL DISEASE

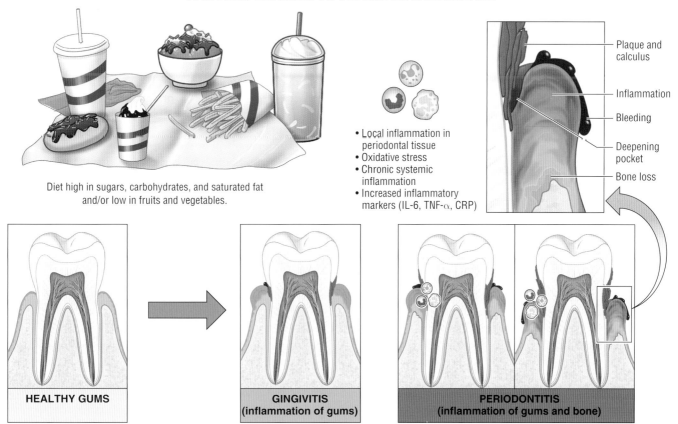

Diet high in sugars, carbohydrates, and saturated fat and/or low in fruits and vegetables.

- Local inflammation in periodontal tissue
- Oxidative stress
- Chronic systemic inflammation
- Increased inflammatory markers (IL-6, TNF-α, CRP)

Plaque and calculus

Inflammation

Bleeding

Deepening pocket

Bone loss

HEALTHY GUMS

GINGIVITIS (inflammation of gums)

PERIODONTITIS (inflammation of gums and bone)

FIGURE 15-2 · Role of diet in periodontal disease.

with household food insecurity have worse oral health status, specifically children and pregnant women, which could be mediated by dietary and other socioeconomic factors.[28] It is essential for all healthcare providers to identify these factors and make the proper recommendations and required referrals in their practice.

Dental Caries

Individuals with rampant caries or deep active carious lesions close to the dental pulp find it more difficult to eat certain types of food leading to fluctuations in their weight and affecting their dietary habits and nutrition status.[29,30] Scientific evidence has highlighted that one of the diagnostic criteria for cases with dental pulp inflammation is pain elicited by consuming sweets or cold or hard food.[29,30] The pain or discomfort constricts their dietary choices. It makes them more inclined to avoid eating until their dental condition is managed and relieved, whether it would require simple restoration or more complex management such as direct or indirect pulp capping, root canal treatment, or extraction of the symptomatic tooth. Discomfort comes from inflammation of the pulp which interferes with chewing ability leading to a less nutritious diet.[29–31] Evidence shows that the cariogenic potential of the diet plays a significant role in the development of dental caries more than its impact on the bacterial count (*S. mutans*) in the oral cavity, indicating the higher value of the diet in that process.[31,32]

In addition, it has been reported that the effect of sucrose rinse and dental biofilm accumulation changes the bioavailability of fluoride and calcium in the saliva; both of these components are essential to maintaining the health of the enamel and dentin and play a role in the remineralization process of tooth structure.[12,13]

Low-caloric sugar substitutes such as Xylitol play a large role in caries prevention via several anti-cariogenic effects: inhibition of the synthesis of the insoluble glucan from sucrose by *Streptococcus mutans;* decrease in *S. mutans* numbers in saliva and dental plaque; increase in the buffering capacity of Ph and dental plaque; interference and interruption of demineralization; and promoting enamel remineralization.[31,32]

Some dietary components, such as Eugenol, have the ability to alleviate dental pain, as it regulates ion channel signaling involved in pain sensation. It is naturally found in several plants and has high concentrations in clove oil as it is the main constituent of the extracted oil. Eugenol serves several uses in dentistry as an analgesic and antiseptic agent[33]; however, it is essential to note that its use must be regulated due to its toxic potential when administered or consumed in high doses.[33]

Periodontal Diseases

Gingival bleeding and periodontal inflammation are strongly correlated with dietary patterns and the nutrients that are consumed, especially for individuals who struggle with obesity and those with chronic conditions such as diabetes and cardiovascular disease.[24,34] Evidence shows that a healthy diet that includes the majority or all the essential dietary components and anti-inflammatory diets have a role in promoting and maintaining healthy periodontal tissue.[34,35] On the other hand, unhealthy, high consumption of processed foods and pro-inflammatory diets that are high in carbohydrates, unsaturated fat, total fat, trans-fat, protein, and cholesterol, have a higher score of the dietary inflammatory index (E-DII), are found to increase the risk of developing periodontal disease and chronic systemic inflammation.[20,35] In addition, it has been reported that periodontal disease is associated with less intake of fruits and vegetables and increased intake of processed foods.[20,34,35]

Individuals with periodontitis have been found to have lower levels of specific vitamins and minerals, including vitamin C and calcium, further re-enforcing the relationship between periodontitis and dietary habits.[20,34,35] Studies have investigated the effects of vitamin D on periodontal tissues and found that it can have preventive properties because of its direct relation with bone metabolism and anti-inflammation properties.[26,27,36,37] Taking into consideration these effects by the healthcare practitioners in the management of periodontal conditions can prevent further complications and improve clinical outcomes for the patient.

Tooth Loss

Tooth loss beyond the functional minimum of natural dentition that affects mastication, or complete edentulism can have further implications on digestion, diet, and nutritional status. This loss can be most detrimental for the elderly population, as they are already at risk of malnutrition, and tooth loss puts them at even greater risk. Evidence suggests that a nonfunctioning dentition of fewer than 20 teeth is associated with lower survival rates and a higher rate of hospitalizations and morbidity.[38] Individuals suffering from tooth loss or complete edentulism find it difficult to chew certain food such as whole fruits and vegetables or nuts. As a result, they would be limited to choose softer food alternatives such as soups, juices, liquid, blended, or mashed vegetables; soft-cooked rice and pasta; or soft bread, where the carbohydrate content is higher.[38] These soft dietary alternatives can negatively impact individuals' oral health and overall health as they contain a lower variety of macro- and micro-nutrients and reduce the intake of essential nutritional components like protein.

Moreover, individuals with less than 20 teeth and those without a functional dentition have been found at significantly higher risk of developing cardiovascular disease and diabetes,[26,38] both of which are highly associated with diet and metabolic syndrome.[39] Systemic inflammation associated with a pro-inflammatory diet can have an effect on the periodontal tissue and surrounding oral structures and has been found to be associated with tooth loss. On the other hand, adherence to an anti-inflammatory diet has been found to be associated with fewer missing teeth.[20,24,36,40]

● NUTRITIONAL AND ORAL HEALTHCARE RECOMMENDATIONS

Nutritional Recommendations

The effects of nutrition on oral and overall health have gained considerable attention, with the increased emphasis on nutritional research as it relates to oral health. Healthcare providers' ability to identify these associations between different dietary factors and health conditions, in addition to following the standard of care, will ensure the optimum clinical outcomes for the patient. Some recommendations for the medical professionals include:

- Identify unhealthy dietary patterns such as frequent snacking for sugars and carbohydrates and sweetened beverages high in sucrose and their effects on the oral cavity.
- Provide dietary counseling to limit snacking or suggest healthy food alternatives such as whole fruits and vegetables, whole wheat, and drinking water to flush the food particles that get stuck in the teeth if tooth brushing is not feasible.
- Identify signs of gingival and periodontal inflammation, such as gingival bleeding, redness, and swelling, and provide oral health recommendations to manage inflammation, such as avoiding processed food and a diet high in carbohydrates and sugars.
- For patients with functional tooth loss, provide sources for patients to be able to receive their required dietary intake of all essential components.
- Identify drug-induced side effects in the oral cavity with the prescribed medications, such as xerostomia, gingival enlargement, and altered taste in the mouth. Provide nutritional recommendations to the patient, such as to advise sufficient water consumption, chewing sugar-free gum to promote the production of saliva to alleviate the effects of dry mouth, or prescribing sialogogues.
- Topical fluoride application and using sugar-substitute chewing gums such as xylitol can be helpful in preventing dental caries.
- Screen for signs of nutritional deficiencies and unhealthy dietary patterns that could manifest in the oral cavity during a physical examination or reported by the patient such as angular cheilitis, glossitis, gingival bleeding, periodontal inflammation, altered taste, and multiple active dental carious lesions.
- Recognize the function nutrients have on oral tissues along with their dietary sources (Table 15-2).[26,36]
- Evaluate fluoride sources available to the patient (such as whether they live in a water-fluoridated area) and prescribe topical and dietary fluoride supplements for high caries-risk children, following the American Dental Association recommendations[37] (Table 15-3).
- Make the required referral to either a registered dietitian or oral health professional based on the oral health conditions present.

TABLE 15-2 • Food sources and impact of vitamins and minerals on oral health[26,36]

Vitamin/mineral	Food sources	Oral effect
Vitamin B3, B6, and B12	Leafy greens, Meat, fish, wheat flour, eggs, oats, and cheese	Accelerates healing of periodontal tissues
Vitamin C	Guava, citrus fruits, bell peppers, and strawberries	Enhances bone healing and promotes collagen synthesis and antioxidant
Vitamin D	Cod liver oil, and salmon, mushrooms, sunlight	Calcium homeostasis
Folic Acid	Dark green vegetables, beans, liver, and whole grains	Aids in growth and development of tissues
Calcium	Dairy products, soy milk, almonds, chia seeds, and edamame	Development of dentition
Iron	Organ meats, poultry, lentils, and dark chocolate	Promotes tissue repair
Zinc	Shellfish, legumes, pork and poultry, hemp, and pumpkin seeds and quinoa	Builds protein and aids in the healing process of tissues, and supports immune function

TABLE 15-3 • Fluoride supplement (Tablets and Drops) dosage schedule 2010 (Approved by the American Dental Association Council on Scientific Affairs)[37]

Age	Fluoride Ion level in drinking water (ppm)[a]		
	< 0.3	0.3–0.6	> 0.6
Birth–6 months	None	None	None
6 months–3 years	0.25 mg/day[b]	None	None
3–6 years	0.50 mg/day	0.25 mg/day	None
6–16 years	1.0 mg/day	0.50 mg/day	None

[a]1.0 part per million (ppm) = 1 milligram per liter (mg/L).
[b]2.2 mg sodium fluoride contains 1 mg fluoride ion.

Oral Healthcare Recommendations

For patients with or at risk of developing dental caries, gingival or periodontal disease, advise teeth brushing at least twice per day with fluoride toothpaste, clean in between the teeth with dental floss, and make referrals when necessary. It is essential to ensure that the patient's oral health is in good condition, as it is tightly connected with overall health. Any complications that might arise in the oral cavity might hinder the treatment process or lead to discontinuation of some of the prescribed medications, such as patients reporting discontinuing anti-choolinergics due to discomfort from dry mouth, which ultimately could result in less than the optimum prognosis of the outcome of the managed case.

- Recommend a soft toothbrush, tooth floss, or interdental brush to clean all surfaces of the teeth.
- Advise regular biannual visits to the oral health professional. Patients with periodontal disease are advised to visit oral health professionals more than healthy individuals to maintain their oral health and prevent the progression of these diseases and lower their impact on overall health.
- Professional fluoride varnish application on teeth is recommended to ensure that patients are receiving the required basic dental preventive services.
- Recommend that patients visit their dentist frequently and follow up with dental cleanings. For those patients, who require referrals to a specialized dentist such a periodontist, their general dentist should be able to make these referrals.

THREE TAKE-HOME POINTS

1. Oral conditions affect more than 3.5 billion individuals worldwide. However, the two most common two oral conditions (dental caries and periodontal disease) can be prevented by following simple oral hygiene practices (toothbrushing and flossing) and lifestyle approaches, such as following a healthy diet.
2. Oral and overall health are tightly connected; the health condition of one affects the other. Local oral microbes and oral tissue inflammation can progress further to impact systemic inflammation.
3. Physicians have a significant role identifying oral conditions and recommending dental visits. This can be of great value for patients who do not have an established dental home, or patients who do not visit the dentist regularly.

● ANSWERS TO QUESTIONS FOR THE CASES

CASE STUDY 1 ANSWERS

1.
- The oral flora, and presence of oral microorganisms
- Tooth nature and morphology (such as deep pit and fissures)
- Salivary factors (pH, flow rate, composition, and buffering capacity); in this case, reduced salivary flow caused by her medication
- Dietary factors (fermentable carbohydrates and sugars, frequency of consumption, and food composition)
- Bioavailability of these substrates in the body
- Time, such as frequent snacking prolongs the exposure to cariogenic food increase the probability of caries development

2.

A. Xerostomia
- Drinking water frequently, especially with and after meals

- Sugar-free or sugar substitute chewing gums such as Xylitol, and sugarless candy to stimulate saliva production
- Sialogogues and artificial saliva

B. Dental caries
- Limit snacking or substitute with healthy alternatives
- Fluoride in water, toothpaste and rinses, and fluoride varnish
- Oral hygiene practices
- Calcium in dairy products or other sources such as chia seeds, soy milk, almonds, and other minerals such as phosphates
- Noncariogenic diet. High in protein, low in fermentable carbohydrates, healthy fat food (plant-based and omega-3 is anti-inflammatory and anti-bacterial), cheese (which has Casein protective for teeth), avocado, nuts, and seeds.

CASE STUDY 2 ANSWERS

1.
- Not adhering to the recommended diabetic diet
- High and frequent consumption of carbohydrates and sugar-sweetened beverages
- Increased inflammation from uncontrolled diabetes and periodontal disease
- Poor oral hygiene practices (occasional brushing and flossing).

2.
- Diet high in protein and omega-3 fatty acids and dietary fibers
- Limit sugar consumption and processed foods
- Use sugar substitutes such as alcohol sugar
- Oral hygiene practices
- A patient who is at high risk of developing such as in this case, is advised to visit the oral health professional more frequently
- Better diabetes management

REFERENCES

1. Peres MA, Macpherson LMD, Weyant RJ, et al. Oral diseases: a global public health challenge. *Lancet.* 2019;394(10194):249-260.

2. Varoni EM, Rimondini L. Oral microbiome, oral health and systemic health: a multidirectional link. *Biomedicines.* 2022;10(1):186.

3. Horliana AC, Chambrone L, Foz AM, et al. Dissemination of periodontal pathogens in the bloodstream after periodontal procedures: a systematic review. *PLoS One.* 2014;9(5):e98271.

4. Riad M, Barton JR, Wilson JA, Freeman CPL, Maran AGD. Parotid salivary secretory pattern in bulimia nervosa. *Acta Otolaryngol.* 1991;111(2):392-395.

5. Valena V, Young W. Dental erosion patterns from intrinsic acid regurgitation and vomiting. *Aus Dent J.* 2002;47(2):106-115.

6. Porter SR, Mercadante V, Fedele S. Oral manifestations of systemic disease. *Brit Dent J.* 2017;223(9):683-691.

7. Khaled S, Ayinampudi B, Gannepalli A, Pacha V, Kumar J, Naveed M. Association between oral manifestations and inhaler use in asthmatic and chronic obstructive pulmonary disease patients. *J Dr NTR University of Health Sciences.* 2016;5(1):17. https://doi.org/10.4103/2277-8632.178950.

8. Thomson WM, Smith MB, Ferguson CA, Moses G. The challenge of medication-induced dry mouth in residential aged care. *Pharmacy.* 2021;9(4):162.

9. Wolff A, Joshi RK, Ekström J, et al. A guide to medications inducing salivary gland dysfunction, xerostomia, and subjective sialorrhea: a systematic review sponsored by the world workshop on oral medicine VI. *Drugs R D.* 2016;17(1):1-28.

10. Hughes FJ. Increasing awareness of drug induced gingival enlargement. *BMJ.* 2021;373:n1571.

11. Guggenheimer J, Moore PA. Xerostomia. *J Am Dent Assoc.* 2003;134(1):61-69.

12. Sheiham A, James WPT. Diet and dental caries. *J Dent Res.* 2015;94(10):1341-1347.

13. Idkaidek NM. Comparative assessment of saliva and plasma for drug bioavailability and bioequivalence studies in humans. *Saudi Pharm J.* 2017;25(5):671-675.

14. Naumova EA, Kuehnl P, Hertenstein P, et al. Fluoride bioavailability in saliva and plaque. *BMC Oral Health.* 2012;12(3). https://doi.org/10.1186/1472-6831-12-3.

15. Moynihan PJ, Kelly SAM. Effect on caries of restricting sugars intake. *J Dent Res.* 2013;93(1):8-18.

16. Rosier BT, De Jager M, Zaura E, Krom BP. Historical and contemporary hypotheses on the development of oral diseases: are we there yet? *Front Cell Infect icrobiol.* 2014;4:92.

17. Alghamdi SB, Togoo RA, Bahamdan GK, et al. Changes in salivary pH following consumption of different varieties of date fruits. *J Taibah Univ Med Sci.* 2019;14(3):246-251.

18. Colombo APV, Tanner ACR. The role of bacterial biofilms in dental caries and periodontal and peri-implant diseases: a historical perspective. *J Dent Res.* 2019;98(4):373-385.

19. Van der Velden U, Kuzmanova D, Chapple ILC. Micronutritional approaches to periodontal therapy. *J Clin Periodontol.* 2011;38: 142-158.

20. Li A, Chen Y, Schuller AA, Sluis LWM, Tjakkes GE. Dietary inflammatory potential is associated with poor periodontal health: a population-based study. *J Clin Periodontol.* 2021;48(7):907-918.

21. Carrizales-Sepúlveda EF, Ordaz-Farías A, Vera-Pineda R, Flores-Ramírez R. Periodontal disease, systemic inflammation and the risk of cardiovascular disease. *Heart Lung Circ.* 2018;27(11):1327-1334.

22. Dommisch H, Kuzmanova D, Jönsson D, Grant M, Chapple I. Effect of micronutrient malnutrition on periodontal disease and periodontal therapy. *Periodontology 2000.* 2018;78(1):129-153.

23. Bretz WA, Weyant RJ, Corby PM, et al. Systemic inflammatory markers, periodontal diseases, and periodontal infections in an elderly population. *J Am Geriatr Soc.* 2005;53(9):1532-1537.

24. Milward M. The role of diet in periodontal disease. *Dent Health.* 2013;52(3):18.

25. Sczepanik FSC, Grossi ML, Casati M, et al. Periodontitis is an inflammatory disease of oxidative stress: we should treat it that way. *Periodontology 2000.* 2020;84(1):45-68.

26. Cagetti MG, Wolf TG, Tennert C, Camoni N, Lingström P, Campus G. The role of vitamins in oral health. A systematic review and meta-analysis. *Int J Environ Res Public Health.* 2020; 17(3):938.

27. Marshall TA, Mobley CC. Impact of dietary quality and nutrition on general health status. In: *Nutrition and Oral Medicine.* Springer, Imprint: Humana Press; 2014;3-17.

28. Weigel MM, Armijos RX. Food insecurity is associated with self-reported oral health in school-age ecuadorian children and is mediated by dietary and non-dietary factors. *Public Health Nutr.* 2022;26(1368-9800):1-10.

29. Zhang M, Xiong Y, Wang X, et al. Factors affecting the outcome of full pulpotomy in permanent posterior teeth diagnosed with reversible or irreversible pulpitis. *Sci Rep.* 2022;12(1). https://doi.org/10.1038/s41598-022-24815-0.

30. Quandt SA, Chen H, Bell RA, et al. Food avoidance and food modification practices of older rural adults: association with oral health status and implications for service provision. *Gerontologist.* 2010;50(1):100-111.

31. van Palenstein Helderman WH, Matee MIN, van der Hoeven JS, Mikx FHM. Cariogenicity depends more on diet than the prevailing mutans streptococcal species. *J Dent Res.* 1996;75(1):535-545.

32. Matsukubo T, Takazoe I. Sucrose substitutes and their role in caries prevention. *Int Dent J.* 2006;56(3):119-130.

33. Akshaya R, Somasundaram J, Anjali AK. Eugenol as potential medicine—Review. *Annals of the Romanian Society for Cell Biology.* 2021;25(3):6250-6260.

34. Jauhiainen LM, Ylöstalo PV, Knuuttila M, Männistö S, Kanerva N, Suominen AL. Poor diet predicts periodontal disease development in 11-year follow-up study. *Community Dent Oral Epidemiol.* 2019;48(2):143-151.

35. Kinane DF, Stathopoulou PG, Papapanou PN. Periodontal diseases. *Nature Reviews Disease Primers.* 2017;3(1). https://doi.org/10.1038/nrdp.2017.38.

36. Najeeb S, Zafar M, Khurshid Z, Zohaib S, Almas K. The role of nutrition in periodontal health: an update. *Nutrients.* 2016;8(9):530.

37. Rozier RG, Adair S, Graham F, et al. Evidence-based clinical recommendations on the prescription of dietary fluoride supplements for caries prevention. *J Am Dent Assoc.* 2010;141(12):1480-1489.

38. Zhu Y, Hollis JH. Tooth loss and its association with dietary intake and diet quality in american adults. *J Dent.* 2014;42(11):1428-1435.

39. Lutsey PL, Steffen LM, Stevens J. Dietary intake and the development of the metabolic syndrome. *Circulation.* 2008;117(6):754-761.

40. Kotsakis GA, Chrepa V, Shivappa N, et al. Diet-borne systemic inflammation is associated with prevalent tooth loss. *Clin Nutr.* 2018;37(4):1306-1312.

chapter 16

Diseases of the Gastrointestinal Tract

Denis Chang, MD

Chapter Outline

I. Case Study
II. Introduction
III. Diseases of Malabsorption
    a. Celiac Disease
    b. Inflammatory Bowel Disease

IV. Non-IgE Mediated GI Disease
    a. Eosinophilic Esophagitis
    b. Food Protein Induced Allergic Proctocolitis
V. Disorders of the Gut Brain Interaction

CASE STUDY

A 15-year-old female presents with a history of abdominal pain, non-bloody diarrhea, and weight loss over the last month. She denies any specific association with meals or activities. Her labs are notable for iron deficiency anemia, normal serum inflammatory markers, and an elevated tissue transglutaminase IgA antibody level. An endoscopy is performed, and the small intestinal biopsies are notable for intraepithelial lymphocytosis, crypt hyperplasia, and villous atrophy, consistent with a diagnosis of celiac disease.

1. Which of the following statements are TRUE:
   A. Nutritional deficiencies can cause both a macro- and microcytic anemia
   B. Cow's milk is the most common food trigger for eosinophilic esophagitis
   C. Intestinal malabsorption can affect multiple systems in the body
   D. All of the statements are true

2. In addition to a gastroenterologist, what other members of the healthcare team should be involved in your patient's care and why?

3. Her symptoms resolve after starting a strict gluten free diet. She comes back for follow-up after a year, and she reports experiencing abdominal pain and constipation for the last three months. She denies any known gluten ingestion. Following your evaluation, you suspect irritable bowel syndrome (IBS). Which diet-based therapy would you recommend for IBS treatment?

● INTRODUCTION

The gastrointestinal tract is the primary system by which the body absorbs and metabolizes nutrients from the diet. Subsequently, diseases of the gastrointestinal system can lead to malabsorption and associated comorbidities. This chapter will review various gastrointestinal diseases and discuss both the nutritional consequences of each disease in addition to the role diet plays in their pathogenesis and/or treatment.

● DISEASES OF MALABSORPTION

Celiac Disease

Celiac disease (CeD) is a chronic, immune-mediated enteropathy triggered by gluten in genetically predisposed individuals.[1] Pooled global prevalence of biopsy confirmed CeD is estimated to be 0.7% although this varies based on geographic location, with a prevalence as high as 3% in some European countries. Genetic susceptibility is determined by the presence of either human leukocyte antigen (HLA)-DQ2 and/or DQ8, which is present in approximately 40% of the North American and European population. However, genetic risk alone is insufficient to develop the disease as the prevalence is far less common.

Dietary exposure to gluten, a storage protein found in wheat, barley, and rye, is central to the pathogenesis of CeD. When ingested, gluten is digested into gluten peptides (e.g., gliadin and glutenins), which undergo deamidation by tissue transglutaminase resulting in a T-cell mediated immune response in affected individuals.[1] Clinical presentation can manifest as either gastrointestinal or extra-intestinal symptoms. In early childhood, "classic" symptoms of malabsorption, such as abdominal pain, diarrhea, abdominal distension, and growth failure, are common. However, in older children and adults, "non-classic" symptoms (e.g., headaches, iron deficiency anemia, arthralgias), are more common, with some individuals experiencing no symptoms at all.[1] Initial screening is performed by assessing for autoantibodies such as tissue transglutaminase IgA in the blood, followed by confirmatory testing via upper GI endoscopy. The presence of histopathologic findings in the small intestine (including intraepithelial lymphocytosis and villous atrophy) in combination with autoantibodies in an individual on a gluten-containing diet confirms the diagnosis.

Since gluten is the main inflammatory trigger in CeD, a strict lifelong gluten-free diet (GFD) is currently the only effective treatment.[1] Successful adoption and adherence to a GFD results in symptom resolution, normalization of serology, and intestinal healing in most individuals. In addition to a GFD, assessing for micronutrient deficiencies at the time of diagnosis is crucial since deficiencies in iron, vitamin D, zinc, and selenium may be present. Notably, most deficiencies improve following adoption of a GFD.[2] Table 16-1 lists common micronutrient deficiencies and their clinical manifestations that are present in malabsorptive disorders.

TABLE 16-1 • Clinical findings in intestinal malabsorption		
Organ system	**Clinical feature**	**Cause**
Gastrointestinal tract	Diarrhea	Nutrient malabsorption; small intestinal secretion of fluid and electrolytes; action of unabsorbed bile acids and hydroxy-fatty acids on colonic mucosa
	Weight loss	Nutrient malabsorption; decreased dietary intake
	Flatus	Bacterial fermentation of unabsorbed dietary carbohydrates
	Abdominal pain	Distention of bowel, muscle spasm, serosal and peritoneal involvement by disease process
	Glossitis, stomatitis, cheilosis	Iron, riboflavin, niacin deficiency
Hematopoietic system	Anemia, microcytic	Iron, pyridoxine deficiency
	Anemia, macrocytic	Folate, vitamin B_{12} deficiency
	Bleeding	Vitamin K deficiency
Musculoskeletal system	Osteopenic bone disease	Calcium, vitamin D malabsorption
	Osteoarthropathy	Not known
	Tetany	Calcium, magnesium, and vitamin D deficiency
Endocrine system	Amenorrhea, impotence, infertility	Generalized malabsorption and malnutrition
	Secondary hyperparathyroidism	Protracted calcium and vitamin D deficiency
Skin	Purpura	Vitamin K deficiency
	Follicular hyperkeratosis and dermatitis	Vitamin A, zinc, essential fatty acids, niacin deficiency
	Edema	Protein-losing enteropathy, malabsorption of dietary protein
	Hyperpigmentation	Secondary hypopituitarism and adrenal insufficiency
	Vesicular eruption	Dermatitis herpetiformis
Nervous system	Xerophthalmia, night blindness	Vitamin A deficiency
	Peripheral neuropathy	Vitamin B_{12}, thiamine deficiency

Reproduced with permission from Friedman S, Blumberg RS, Saltzman JR. *Greenberger's CURRENT Diagnosis & Treatment Gastroenterology, Hepatology, & Endoscopy, Intestinal Malabsorption & Nutrition.* 4th ed. New York, NY: McGraw Hill; 2022.

Since CeD is a chronic disease and given the primary treatment being diet-based, involvement of a registered dietitian with expertise in the GFD in addition to a gastroenterologist is essential in its management.[3] Dietitians can provide counseling on identifying sources of gluten, especially as ongoing (unintentional) gluten consumption is a common reason for persistent symptoms, while also monitoring for potential deficiencies/excesses while on the diet.[4] Although a GFD is essential for individuals with CeD, the diet is not inherently "healthy." Compared to an unrestricted diet, the GFD can be deficient in several micronutrients and trace elements such as iron, B vitamins, and zinc.[4] Furthermore, gluten enriched grains are a common source of fiber, and their elimination may lead to constipation. Finally, many gluten-free products are processed or have additional additives to improve palatability and to replace the viscoelastic property of gluten. Consequently, many gluten-free foods have a higher glycemic index, fat content, and calories.[5]

Inflammatory Bowel Disease

Inflammatory bowel disease (IBD) is a chronic inflammatory condition of the gastrointestinal tract and consists of two subtypes: ulcerative colitis (UC) and Crohn's disease (CD). While most cases present with gastrointestinal symptoms, some may experience extraintestinal symptoms first, such as arthritis and erythema nodosum.[6,7] The global incidence over the years in both children and adults has been increasing. The pathogenesis involves the complex interplay between genetics, the gut microbiome, immune system, and the environment, including diet.[6,7]

Several mechanisms by which diet may factor into the pathogenesis of IBD have been proposed.[8] For example, the Western diet (high in the dietary intake of red meats, processed foods, saturated fats, and refined sugars) compared to the Mediterranean diet (high intake of fruits and vegetables, whole grains, and seafood) appears to have more of a detrimental effect on the gut microbiome and epithelial barrier function.[8] Additionally, both ultra-processed foods, which are high in additives, and sugar-sweetened beverage intake have been linked to intestinal inflammation, increasing IBD risk.[9]

Subsequently, several types of diets have been studied for their potential therapeutic role. Exclusive enteral nutrition (EEN), which entails replacing a regular food-based diet with exclusively formula for at least 6–12 weeks, has been extensively investigated in the treatment of mild to moderately severe CD, especially in children.[10] Potential mechanisms of action include alterations in the gut microbiota and luminal metabolites, reduction in antigenic load, and potential anti-inflammatory effects.[11] In comparison to systemic corticosteroids, EEN is as effective in inducing remission, particularly when small intestinal disease is present, and thus considered a first line treatment in pediatric CD.[10] Additionally, advantages of EEN over other medical therapies include avoidance of medication-related side effects such as immunosuppression, and nutritional supplementation, especially in the presence of malnutrition. One of the limitations of EEN, however, is the challenge of being on a formula-only diet for several weeks, which in some cases, require the placement of a feeding tube, such as a nasogastric tube.[11] Furthermore, while EEN is effective during the induction phase of treatment, it is not a feasible long-term treatment resulting in most individuals ultimately being started on a form of medication to maintain remission.

While other diets, such as the Crohn's Disease Exclusion Diet (CDED), Specific Carbohydrate Diet, and the Mediterranean diet, have also been studied in the treatment of IBD, their efficacy is not as promising.[11] One study found that when two diets were combined—partial enteral nutrition (PEN) and the CDED—this resulted in not only a higher rate of sustained steroid-free remission, but also increased tolerability compared to EEN suggesting a potential role in combining other diets to improve efficacy.[12]

In both CeD and IBD, chronic intestinal inflammation affects both the absorptive capacity of the gastrointestinal system along with the increased utilization of energy, resulting in risk for malnutrition. Furthermore, associated and/or exacerbation of symptoms with eating results in limited dietary intake, further increasing this risk. Many individuals at the time of diagnosis present with some degree of malnutrition, in addition to several micronutrient deficiencies, underscoring the importance of a proper nutritional assessment both at diagnosis and during follow-up.[11]

● NON-IGE MEDIATED GI DISEASE

Eosinophilic Esophagitis

Eosinophilic esophagitis (EoE) is a chronic immune mediated inflammatory disease of the esophagus triggered by allergens. The prevalence in Europe and North America is approximately 34.4/100,000 people, although the global incidence is increasing.[13] Symptoms of esophageal dysfunction such as dysphagia, heartburn, chest pain, and food impaction, are common in older children and adults; however, in young children, EoE can present with a variety of nonspecific symptoms including feeding difficulty, vomiting, and failure to thrive.[13] The diagnosis is made endoscopically (e.g., presence of esophageal furrows, exudates, or strictures) and/or histologically (e.g., 15 or more eosinophils per high power field in the esophageal mucosa). As esophageal eosinophilia can be seen in other conditions, such as gastroesophageal reflux disease, these must be excluded prior to confirming the diagnosis.[14]

Unlike classic food allergies, which results from a rapid-onset, IgE-mediated type 1 hypersensitivity, EoE results from a non-IgE mediated, type 2 hypersensitivity, with symptoms developing over weeks to months. However, there is some overlap between the two, as individuals with atopic conditions, such as asthma, eczema, and IgE-mediated food allergies are at increased risk of developing EoE.[15] Food allergens serve as triggers for esophageal inflammation in EoE, which supports the reason why elimination diets can lead to mucosal healing.[15] Pharmacologic therapies, such as proton pump inhibitors or topical steroids, are treatment options when an elimination diet is not desired and/or ineffective. In some cases, a combination of the two is required for adequate therapy.

Several different diets for the treatment of EoE have been studied with variable efficacy. An elemental (amino acid–based) formula diet, which consists entirely of innately hypoallergenic components, yields the highest response rates (85–95%) though its restrictive nature and poor palatability limits its adoption.[16] Targeted elimination diets based on allergy testing, such as a skin prick test or serologic testing for allergen specific IgE levels, are often more feasible though the sensitivity and positive predictive value for these tests in EoE are low.[16] Empiric elimination diets, which involves the removal of one or more of the most common food allergens (animal milk, wheat, egg, soy, nuts, and seafood), have subsequently become the more widely used approach.[17] Although the immediate effectiveness of elimination diets is well known, their durability in maintaining mucosal healing over time is less certain.

While elimination diets avoid the potential for medication induced side effects, some potential drawbacks exist. Depending on the number of different food allergens that are removed, restrictive diets can be challenging and negatively impact quality of life, and in the absence of appropriate dietary counseling and monitoring, can lead to various nutritional deficiencies. In cases where several different food allergens are removed and mucosal healing is achieved, the long-term goal of dietary therapy in EoE is to identify and remove only those causative allergens while reintroducing the foods that are tolerated. This is achieved by gradually reintroducing foods, usually one at a time, followed by monitoring for symptomatic alongside endoscopic and/or histologic recurrence via repeat endoscopies. This limits the appeal of the diet-based approach as it not only leads to the potential for symptom recurrence as foods are gradually reintroduced, but also requires repeat procedural sedation.[13] While non-sedating testing modalities, such as trans-nasal endoscopy, are currently being investigated, these are not yet widely available. Finally, diet-based therapies may pose a higher financial burden and undue stress on individuals as they are often not covered by insurance, resulting in a greater cost than other available medical therapies.[16]

Food Protein Induced Allergic Proctocolitis

Food protein induced allergic proctocolitis (FPIAP) is another non-IgE mediated food allergy that primarily affects infants. The prevalence is not well known and varies widely, with some studies reporting as low as 1–2% of infants, while other report rates that are much higher.[18] Cow's milk protein is the most common trigger, which is the reason for FPIAP commonly being referred to as a "cow milk protein allergy," though other proteins, such as soy, eggs, and wheat, can also induce inflammation.[18] FPIAP typically presents during the first few months of life in both breastfed and formula fed infants, and most commonly presents with blood (gross or occult) or mucus in the stool, though other less specific symptoms including irritability and worsening reflux can be seen.[19] In some cases, a more acute and severe presentation—Food Protein-Induced Enterocolitis Syndrome (FPIES)—can occur, which is characterized by recurrent vomiting, lethargy, pallor, dehydration, and even hypotension.[20] Similar to FPIAP, the treatment for

FPIES is the avoidance of the culprit food along with supportive measures during the period following an exposure.

The diagnosis of FPIAP is made based on symptom improvement following the removal of the food protein(s) from the infant's diet in suspected cases. This is accomplished by maternal dietary restriction in breast-fed infants or transitioning from a cow-milk based formula to an extensively hydrolyzed formula in formula-fed infants.[21] If symptoms persist while on a hydrolyzed formula, an amino acid-based formula is often used. While other formulations of "milk," such as rice, almond, or coconut, are available, these do not meet an infant's nutritional needs and so should not be used in treating FPIAP.[19]

Most infants will be able to tolerate cow's milk by 12 months of age, although some may require ongoing restriction into early childhood.[18] In those cases, individualized nutritional counseling with a dietitian is essential to ensure adequate nutritional intake to support normal growth as dietary requirements change over time.[19] Strategies for food reintroduction widely vary as more studies are needed to determine the optimal and safest approach. In most cases, this is accomplished slowly with close observation for any return of symptoms, starting as early as 6 months but often closer to 9, if not 12 months.[19] In more severe cases, such as with FPIES, an oral food challenge is often performed in a hospital or office setting rather than at home.

In addition to the infant, both mothers and caretakers of infants with non-IgE mediated allergies are often affected by the change in diet. Breastfeeding mothers avoiding allergens need to meticulously monitor their intake and read ingredient labels to ensure avoidance of all sources of dairy or other dietary proteins for their infant. This leads to both nutritional and lifestyle changes that may potentially be detrimental to their well-being. Dairy elimination places breastfeeding mothers at risk of inadequate calcium or vitamin D intake, requiring additional supplementation or intake through other sources.[18] Studies in other non-IgE mediated food allergies, such as EoE, have demonstrated the negative effects dietary restrictions can have not only on those following the diet, but also the entire household.[18] Consequently, it is important to consider these factors when choosing between dietary therapies and other treatment options, if available, in children with FPIAP or other non-IgE mediated food allergies.

● DISORDERS OF THE GUT BRAIN INTERACTION

While gastrointestinal symptoms can often be caused by underlying inflammation, this is not always the case, especially when symptom persist for months to years. Formerly known as "functional gastrointestinal disorders," disorders of the gut brain interaction (DGBI) encompass a variety of non-inflammatory gastrointestinal disorders that are common in both children and adults.[22] While the specific pathophysiology is still being explored, the etiology is believed to be multifactorial involving early life experiences, psychosocial factors, and physiologic changes, termed the biopsychosocial conceptual model.[22] This results in visceral hypersensitivity, along with alterations in motility, mucosal and immune function, gut microbiota, and central nervous system processing, leading to symptoms. DGBIs are very common, with global epidemiologic studies reporting a prevalence as high as 40%, with a greater preponderance in females. The diagnosis is made based on the presence of specific symptoms, known as the Rome criteria, with the most recent iteration (Rome IV) last revised in 2016.[22] As multiple factors contribute to its pathogenesis, treatment is built on a multimodal, multidisciplinary framework, which can include dietary elimination of potential food triggers.[22]

The functions of diet as both a trigger and treatment for DGBIs have been studied.[23] Several mechanisms by which food may contribute to symptoms include maldigestion, allergic and immunologic, food-microbiota interactions, and gut-brain signaling.[24] The most studied dietary intervention is the low FODMAP (fermentable oligosaccharides, disaccharides, monosaccharides, and polyols) diet (LFD), particularly in the treatment of irritable bowel syndrome (IBS). FODMAPs can provoke symptoms through their effect on osmotic overload, resulting in an increase in intraluminal fluid and gas, bacterial fermentation leading to increased gas production, and gut dysbiosis[24] (Figure 16-1). Additionally, localized food-induced immune activation that is distinct from IgE- or non-IgE mediated food allergies is also thought to play a role. Due to the significantly restrictive nature of the LFD, implementation includes several phases: 1) restriction, 2) reintroduction of FODMAPs, and 3) personalization based on the results from reintroduction. The goal of the LFD is to identify and eliminate only the specific foods that are contributing to symptoms.[25] Like any other diet, involvement of a dietitian during this process is crucial.

Beyond the LFD, other diet-based approaches, such as the gluten-free diet, Mediterranean diet, and the low carbohydrate diet, have not yielded the same efficacy in treating IBS or other DGBIs.[26] Subsequently, exclusion diets should only be reserved for those who demonstrate food-related symptoms or have

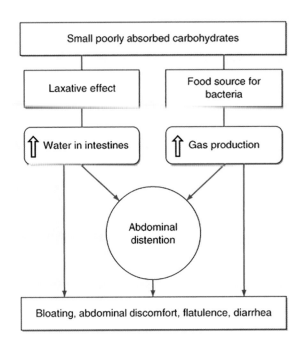

FIGURE 16-1 • Pathogenesis of FODMAP-related symptoms. (Reproduced with permission Localzo J, Fauci A, Kasper D, Hauser S, Longo D, Jameson JL. *Harrison's Principles of Internal Medicine.* 21st ed. New York, NY:McGraw Hill; 2022.)

clear benefit after the presumed trigger is removed. In many individuals, a healthy lifestyle along with a balanced diet may be adequate in treating symptoms.[26] Certain populations, such as those at risk for malnutrition or with a history of an eating disorder, may be poor candidates for dietary intervention. In those cases, diet-based therapies should be avoided, and other treatment strategies should be considered. Finally, there are many psychosocial factors to weigh when considering dietary therapies, many of which are not trivial and may even lead to more harm than benefit.

FOUR TAKE-HOME POINTS

1. Diet has a role in both the pathophysiology as well as the treatment of various gastrointestinal diseases.
2. Mechanisms by which food and diet contribute to gastrointestinal symptoms widely vary and are still under investigation.
3. Appropriate and regular assessments of nutritional status is essential and should be performed by an experienced dietitian.
4. The psychosocial impact of diet-based therapies should always be considered prior to implementation.

CASE STUDY ANSWERS

1. **Correct Answer: D;** Nutritional deficiencies can cause both a macro- (vitamin B12 or folate) or microcytic (Iron) anemia. While cow's milk is the most common food trigger for eosinophilic esophagitis, other common foods include wheat, egg, soy, peanuts, and shellfish. Intestinal malabsorption can lead to multi-systemic symptoms, based on the deficiency. Nutritional deficiencies and the clinical manifestations associated with intestinal malabsorption are detailed in Table 16-1.

(Continued)

CASE STUDY ANSWERS   *(Continued)*

2. In addition to a gastroenterologist, involvement of a registered dietitian with expertise in the gluten free diet (GFD) is vital in the management of celiac disease as the treatment is a strict lifelong GFD. Dietitians provide education on sources of gluten as well as safe gluten free options for individuals with celiac disease. Regular nutritional assessments are integral as the GFD has lower micronutrient content compared to a gluten-containing, unrestricted diet such as B vitamins, calcium, iron, and zinc, including fiber. Furthermore, dietitians can help identify potential unintentional gluten sources especially in individuals who are having persistent symptoms and/or elevated celiac auto-antibody levels despite adherence to a GFD.

3. The low FODMAP diet can be an effective dietary therapy to treat IBS in some individuals. Proposed mechanisms for FODMAP induced symptoms include osmotic overload resulting in an increase in intraluminal fluid and gas, bacterial fermentation leading to increased gas production, and gut dysbiosis. Adoption of a low FODMAP diet consists of three phases: 1) restriction of FODMAPs, followed by 2) gradual reintroduction of FODMAPs, and then 3) personalization based on the results of the reintroduction phase. Other dietary therapies have been investigated however are not as effective.

REFERENCES

1. Lindfors K, Ciacci C, Kurppa K, et al. Coeliac disease. *Nat Rev Dis Primers*. 2019;5(1):3.

2. See JA, Kaukinen K, Makharia GK, Gibson PR, Murray JA. Practical insights into gluten-free diets. *Nat Rev Gastroenterol Hepatol*. 2015;12(10):580-591.

3. Rubio-Tapia A, Hill ID, Semrad C, Kelly CP, Lebwohl B. American college of gastroenterology guidelines update: diagnosis and management of celiac disease. *Am J Gastroenterol*. 2023;118(1):59-76.

4. Dennis M, Lee AR, McCarthy T. Nutritional considerations of the gluten-free diet. *Gastroenterol Clin North Am*. 2019;48(1):53-72.

5. Sue A, Dehlsen K, Ooi CY. Paediatric patients with coeliac disease on a gluten-free diet: nutritional adequacy and macro- and micronutrient imbalances. *Curr Gastroenterol Rep*. 2018;20(1):2.

6. Kobayashi T, Siegmund B, Le Berre C, et al. Ulcerative colitis. *Nat Rev Dis Primers*. 2020;6(1):74.

7. Roda G, Ng SC, Kotze PG, et al. Crohn's disease. *Nat Rev Dis Primers*. 2020;6(1):22.

8. Khalili H, Chan SSM, Lochhead P, Ananthakrishnan AN, Hart AR, Chan AT. The role of diet in the aetiopathogenesis of inflammatory bowel disease. *Nat Rev Gastroenterol Hepatol*. 2018;15(9):525-535.

9. Lo CH, Khandpur N, Rossato SL, et al. Ultra-processed foods and risk of Crohn's disease and ulcerative colitis: a prospective cohort study. *Clin Gastroenterol Hepatol*. 2022;20(6):e1323-e1337.

10. van Rheenen PF, Aloi M, Assa A, et al. The medical management of paediatric Crohn's disease: an ECCO-ESPGHAN guideline update. *J Crohns Colitis*. 2020:jjaa161. doi: 10.1093/ecco-jcc/jjaa161. Epub ahead of print. PMID: 33026087.

11. Fitzpatrick JA, Melton SL, Yao CK, Gibson PR, Halmos EP. Dietary management of adults with IBD - the emerging role of dietary therapy. *Nat Rev Gastroenterol Hepatol*. 2022.

12. Levine A, Wine E, Assa A, et al. Crohn's disease exclusion diet plus partial enteral nutrition induces sustained remission in a randomized controlled trial. *Gastroenterology*. 2019;157(2):440-450.e8.

13. Muir A, Falk GW. Eosinophilic esophagitis: a review. *JAMA*. 2021;326(13):1310-1318.

14. Dellon ES, Liacouras CA, Molina-Infante J, et al. Updated international consensus diagnostic criteria for eosinophilic esophagitis: proceedings of the AGREE conference. *Gastroenterology*. 2018;155(4):1022-1033.e10.

15. O'Shea KM, Aceves SS, Dellon ES, et al. Pathophysiology of eosinophilic esophagitis. *Gastroenterology*. 2018;154(2):333-345.

16. Cotton CC, Durban R, Dellon ES. Illuminating elimination diets: controversies regarding dietary treatment of eosinophilic esophagitis. *Dig Dis Sci*. 2019;64(6):1401-1408.

17. Chang JW, Kliewer K, Haller E, et al. Development of a practical guide to implement and monitor diet therapy for eosinophilic esophagitis. *Clin Gastroenterol Hepatol*. 2023 Jul;21(7):1690-1698.

18. Meyer R, Chebar Lozinsky A, Fleischer DM, et al. Diagnosis and management of non-IgE gastrointestinal allergies in breastfed infants-An EAACI Position Paper. *Allergy*. 2020;75(1):14-32.

19. Koletzko S, Niggemann B, Arato A, et al. Diagnostic approach and management of cow's-milk protein allergy in infants and children: ESPGHAN GI committee practical guidelines. *J Pediatr Gastroenterol Nutr*. 2012;55(2):221-229.

20. Nowak-Węgrzyn A, Chehade M, Groetch ME, et al. International consensus guidelines for the diagnosis and management of food protein-induced enterocolitis syndrome: executive summary-Workgroup Report of the Adverse Reactions to Foods Committee, American Academy of Allergy, Asthma & Immunology. *J Allergy Clin Immunol*. 2017;139(4):1111-1126.e4.

21. Burris AD, Burris J, Järvinen KM. Cow's milk protein allergy in term and preterm infants: clinical manifestations, immunologic pathophysiology, and management strategies. *Neoreviews*. 2020;21(12):e795-e808.

22. Drossman DA. Functional gastrointestinal disorders: history, pathophysiology, clinical features and Rome IV. *Gastroenterology*. 2016. doi:10.1053/j.gastro.2016.02.032.

23. Tack J, Tornblom H, Tan V, Carbone F. Evidence-based and emerging dietary approaches to upper disorders of gut-brain interaction. *Am J Gastroenterol*. 2022;117(6):965-972.

24. Van den Houte K, Bercik P, Simren M, Tack J, Vanner S. Mechanisms underlying food-triggered symptoms in disorders of gut-brain interactions. *Am J Gastroenterol*. 2022;117(6):937-946.

25. Chey WD, Hashash JG, Manning L, Chang L. AGA clinical practice update on the role of diet in irritable bowel syndrome: expert review. *Gastroenterology*. 2022;162(6):1737-1745.e5.

26. Singh P, Tuck C, Gibson PR, Chey WD. The role of food in the treatment of bowel disorders: focus on irritable bowel syndrome and functional constipation. *Am J Gastroenterol*. 2022; 117(6):947-957.

17

Overweight and Obesity

Sara Saliba, MD, RD, LDN / W. Scott Butsch, MD, Msc, FTOS

Chapter Outline

CASE STUDY

A 35-year-old woman presents to your office interested in losing weight. She reports fatigue and recent weight gain, but is otherwise healthy. Prior medical history includes depression, with her symptoms improved and currently stable under pharmacotherapy. She briefly tried following a ketogenic diet after researching it online, but found it difficult to maintain and stopped after two weeks. She feels frustrated and knows she needs "to do better," blames herself for "not having enough willpower" to see the diet through. She reports no family history of obesity, and states her weight for the past 10 years has remained stable around 165 pounds. She has gained 15 pounds over the past few months and doesn't know what caused her to gain weight.

When asked about her diet, she reports it's not healthy. She is a nurse at a hospital and tends to snack on whatever is in the nurse's lounge throughout the day (usually bagels, donuts, cookies, etc.). She skips breakfast and reports larger portioned, but well-balanced dinners (i.e., roasted chicken, brown rice, and roasted vegetables). She denies any significant stressors, but typically has nighttime sweets as she "winds down." She is active at work but does not engage in physical activity outside of work. She takes public transport to work, and the bus stop is only 5 minutes of walk from her house. Her sleep is adequate, but she

sometimes picks up weekend night shifts. She was started on citalopram for depression a few months ago and receives subcutaneous medroxyprogesterone for contraception.

Vitals: BP 140/90, HR 85, O2 sat 97%. She is 5′4″ and weighs 195 pounds. Her body mass index (BMI) is 33.5 kg/m². Waist circumference is 35 inches. The rest of the physical exam does not reveal any anomalies.

1. What are some limitations of body mass index (BMI)?

2. What are possible contributors to her weight gain?

3. What medical conditions would you screen her for given her history?

4. What type of intervention would recommend and why?

5. She wants to know what the most effective diet for weight loss is and if she should return to the ketogenic diet. What do you advise?

6. How would you advise her on the timing of results and what your plan is if she does not lose weight?

7. At 3 months, the patient returns to your office and is excited that she has lost 10 pounds. She continues with her plan and returns at the 6-month mark, frustrated because her weight has plateaued despite continued intervention. What do you tell her?

DEFINITIONS OF OBESITY

Obesity is a chronic, relapsing, progressive disease, defined as a state of excess accumulation of body fat that impairs health. In 2013, the American Medical Association (AMA) House of Delegates recognized obesity as a disease state, marking a key milestone in progress towards its recognition as a disease and advancing obesity treatment and prevention. Body mass index (BMI), which correlates with total body fat, is used to classify overweight (also known as pre-obesity) and obesity. BMI is calculated by dividing an individual's weight (kilograms) by height (meters squared), and provides the most useful population-level measurement of obesity. However, it has limitations in predicting excess body fat and associated health risks on an individual basis. Historically, literature has proposed that BMI is preferable over other relative weight indices for this reason as well as generalizability given the simplicity of the calculation.[1]

KEY POINTS

- Overweight (Pre-Obesity): BMI of 25 to 29.9 kg/m²
  - Obesity: BMI ≥30 kg/m²
    - Class I: BMI 30–34.9 kg/m²
    - Class II: BMI 35–39.9 kg/m²
    - Class III (Severe Obesity): BMI ≥ 40 kg/m²
- BMI is a screening tool, used with other health risk assessments to best determine a clinical diagnosis of obesity. It does not measure individual health alone
- Limitations of BMI:
  - Not a direct measure of body fat
  - Unable to capture fat distribution
  - Does not distinguish between fat and lean muscle mass
  - Associations with health risks vary by ethnic group (e.g., China: Obesity BMI > 28 kg/m²)
  - Cut-offs vary in children and adolescents (BMI ≥ 95 percentile)
  - BMI >30 with high specificity but low sensitivity (40–50%) to identifying excess adiposity
- EOSS (Edmonton Obesity Staging System): 5-stage classification system used clinically in practice management; better predictor of mortality than BMI (Stage 0, no obesity-related risk factors, to Stage 4, severe disabilities from obesity-related chronic disease).[2]
- Waist circumference is the most practical measure of abdominal fat (> 40 inches in men, > 35 in women) and correlates with visceral adiposity
- Waist-to-height ratio (WHR) has been proposed as substitute to BMI but has measurement challenges
- BIA (bioelectric impedance analysis) measures body water and provides measurement of body fat mass vs. fat-free mass, however has large interindividual variation.

EPIDEMIOLOGY

The statistics speak for themselves with more than 1 billion people globally with obesity in 2016.[3] The numbers continue to increase with more than half of American adults projected to have obesity and nearly a quarter to have severe obesity by 2030. Recent data shows that the prevalence of obesity among children and adolescents ages 2 to 19 has increased from 17.7% in 2011–2012 to 21.5% in 2017–2020. There remains a widening disparity in prevalence, with the largest increase in Mexican American men, all equal increases in all race/ethnic groups of women. Trends show widening disparities between urban and rural areas in severe obesity in men.

Obesity represents a major health challenge because of its numerous complications including cardiometabolic disease (e.g., myocardial infarction, hypertension, type 2 diabetes mellitus, non-alcoholic fatty liver disease, dyslipidemia, stroke), gastroesophageal reflux disease, obstructive sleep apnea (and obesity hypoventilation syndrome), musculoskeletal conditions (e.g., chronic lower back pain, arthralgias, rheumatoid arthritis), mental health conditions (e.g., depression, anxiety), and several types of cancers (e.g., esophageal, pancreatic, hepatic, colorectal, breast, endometrial, and renal).[3,4] Obesity is associated with several factors (i.e., unemployment, reduced productivity), which lead to an economic burden in addition to healthcare cost.[4] The increased costs and poor health outcomes are in part a result of inadequate care of people with obesity and a more systemic weight bias intrinsic to our current health care.[3]

ETIOLOGIES

Historically, obesity was believed to be simply the result of poor lifestyle behaviors. However, science has elucidated the complexity of this disease and the diverse contributions, from a genetic and biological basis intertwined with psychological and environmental factors.[4] An obesogenic environment can bring about biological changes conducive to obesity by promotion of convenience, sedentary behaviors, poor sleep hygiene, and the consumption of readily available, highly processed foods.[4] However, there is a strong genetic component underlying the large individual variability of body weight in its response to this environment. The relative contributions of each of these factors have been studied, however, will not be extensively covered in this chapter.

PATHOPHYSIOLOGY

Weight Regulation

The control of food intake and energy expenditure, or energy regulation, is achieved by a highly coordinated, complex system that connects central executive, reward and autonomic circuits to the peripheral hormones (derived from adipose tissue and the gut) that signal changes in energy stores and nutrition status.[5] Autonomic regulation of energy balance primarily involves the hypothalamus nuclei which are the primary integrators of nutritional information and are sensitive to circulating hormones and metabolites. These neuron populations include orexigenic peptides; neuropeptide Y (NPY) and agouti-related protein (AGRP); and anorexigenic peptides, proopiomelanocortin (POMC), and cocaine-amphetamine-regulated transcript (CART), which are located in the arcuate nucleus. Peripheral hormone players include glucagon-like 1 (GLP-1), peptide YY (PYY), glucose dependent insulinotropic polypeptide (GIP), glucagon, insulin, neurotensin, pancreatic polypeptide (PP), ghrelin, and leptin.[6]

Adiposity Set Point and Metabolic Adaptation

Adiposity is tightly regulated, much like multiple other systems in the body including blood volume, glucose, urine output, etc. Despite ingesting nearly 1 million calories a year, energy intake and output are matched within 0.17% over a decade. Early animal studies demonstrated regulation of body weight, more recently known as the "weight set-point," regardless of the variability in energy intake and expenditure is orchestrated in the hypothalamus.[7] This tightly regulated system can be better understood in studies on metabolic adaptation.[8] When weight loss occurs, compensatory mechanisms promoting an increase in energy intake (increased hunger, cravings, increased preference for calorically dense foods, etc.), and a decrease in mitochondrial efficiency and energy expenditure are in place to defend the body fat stores. A real-life example of metabolic adaption is perhaps best exemplified in the television show, *The Biggest Loser*, which followed the journey of individuals with obesity competing to lose weight via drastic caloric deficits and increases in physical activity. Studies of contestants demonstrated a profound slowing of metabolism in individuals following significant weight loss that was not restored with weight regain.[9] It has been theorized that this phenomenon occurs for the purpose of minimizing changes to total energy expenditure in order to maintain energy balance and remain close to an individual's set weight. As a result, contestants who lost significant amounts of weight had to adhere to an extremely low-calorie intake in order to maintain their weight loss. In the same way, weight cycling due can be detrimental to one's metabolism. While behaviors such as drastic dieting lead to short-term weight loss, it can also lead to relatively more weight gain or more difficulty maintaining weight loss in the long term.

Genetics

It is important to appreciate the significant role of genetics in body weight regulation and the process of metabolic adaptation against weight loss. Genetic variations associated with obesity are located in the central nervous system, muscle, liver, and microbiota of the gut and include the processes of adipocyte differentiation, food sensing and digestion, and lipid metabolism.[4]

Obesity is often separated into two categories: a rare monogenic obesity that presents with early onset, severe obesity, and polygenic obesity, known as common obesity. Monogenic causes of obesity (e.g., mutations of *LEP, LEPR, PSCK1, POMC*), which involve the leptin-melanocortin pathway, are extremely rare. The most common is mutation on the melanocortin-4 receptor (*MC4R*) gene, which is regulated by leptin. It accounts for approximately 5% of severe obesity in childhood.[4,10]

Circadian Rhythm

Centrally regulated by the suprachiasmatic nuclei in the anterior hypothalamus, the circadian rhythm, comprised of a network of molecular clocks throughout the body, is primarily synchronized to the 24-hour day, and influenced by light, temperature, and feeding. It anticipates and adapts to daily environmental changes, therefore inherently is important in obesity and metabolic diseases.[11] Both animal and human studies have shown altered circadian rhythms (e.g., sleep deprivation, night-shift work) are correlated with weight gain and altered glucose metabolism and thought to contribute to the development of certain chronic diseases. One study found individuals under simulated shiftwork conditions have reduced daily energy expenditure with associated decrease in levels of satiety hormones. Thus, an understanding of the alignment of feeding/fasting cycles to the clock-regulated metabolic changes and the bidirectional relationship between the microbiota and the circadian rhythm is critical in the consideration of nutrition interventions for the treatment of obesity.[7]

● DEFINING AND STAGING OBESITY

Currently, BMI is still considered as the only clinical measurement by which to assess obesity. Unfortunately, there are limitations to using BMI for this purpose. Primarily, BMI does not distinguish whether weight is associated with muscle versus fat. Moreover, it does not identify body fat distribution, which is a major determinant of metabolic risk.[4] Additionally, BMI cutoffs vary by country. Thus, a one-size-fits-all approach is not sufficient for the assessment and management of obesity. A more individualized approach is warranted to improve the health of individuals with the most severe health conditions to ensure they receive optimal obesity treatment.

Health Consequences of Obesity

The phenotype "metabolically healthy obesity" (MHO) describes individuals who meet the standard BMI cutoff point for obesity but lack the elements that comprise metabolic syndrome, for which the diagnostic criteria by organization are listed in Table 17-1.[12] For a given BMI, these individuals have lower levels of visceral fat and a relatively low degree of systemic inflammation.[8]

Healthcare providers should view MHO as a transient state that can over time develop into an unhealthy phenotype. Similarly, obesity in children tends to track into adulthood. Given that the severity of obesity will likely worsen with weight gain over time, the likelihood of developing cardiometabolic disease as an adult is high.[13] This can occur regardless of good metabolic health when the individual is a child or adolescent with obesity and must be acknowledged by the healthcare provider.

TABLE 17-1 • Clinical diagnosis criteria for metabolic syndrome by organization

Clinical indicator	WHO (1998)	EGIR (1999)	NCEP-ATP III (2001)	AACE (2003)	IDF (2005)
Insulin Resistance	IGT, T2DM, IFG + 2 from below	Plasma insulin > 75th percentile + 2 from below	None + 3/5 from below	IGT, IFG + 1 from below	None
Waist Circumference or BMI	W:H > 0.90 in men; W:H > 0.85 in women; and/or BMI > 30 kg/m²	WC ≥ 94 cm in men or ≥80 cm in women	WC ≥ 40 inches in men or ≥ 35 inches in women	BMI ≥ 25 kg/m²	Increased WC (population specific) + 2 from below
Blood Pressure	≥ 140/90 mm Hg	≥ 140/90 mm Hg or on medication for hypertension	≥ 130/85 mm Hg	≥ 130/85 mm Hg	SBP ≥ 130 mm Hg or DBP ≥ 85 mm Hg or on medication for hypertension
Glucose	IGT, IFG, or T2DM	IGT or IFG (excluding DM)	> 100 mg/dL (includes DM)	IGT or IFG (excluding DM)	≥ 100 mg/dL (includes DM)
Lipids	TG ≥ 150 mg/dL and/or HDL < 35 mg/dL in men or < 39 mg/dL in women	TG ≥ 150 mg/dL and/or HDL < 39 mg/dL in men or women	TG ≥ 150 mg/dL and HDL < 40 mg/dL in men or < 50 mg/dL in women	TG ≥ 150 mg/dL and HDL < 40 mg/dL in men or < 50 mg/dL in women	TG ≥ 150 mg/dL or on medication and HDL < 40 mg/dL in men or < 50 mg/dL in women or on medication
Other	Microalbuminuria			Other features of insulin resistance	

AACE, American Association of Clinical Endocrinologists; DM, diabetes mellitus; EGIR, European Group for Study of Insulin Resistance; HDL, high-density lipoprotein cholesterol; IDF, International Diabetes Foundation; IFG, impaired fasting glucose; IGT, impaired glucose tolerance; mg/dL, milligrams per deciliter; mmHg, millimeters of mercury; NCEP-APT III, National Cholesterol Education Program, Adult Treatment Panel III; T2DM, type 2 diabetes mellitus; TG, triglycerides; WC, waist circumference; W:H, waist-hip ratio; WHO, World Health Organization.
Modified from table in Grundy SM, Cleeman JI, Daniels SR, et al. Diagnosis and management of the metabolic syndrome: an American Heart Association/National Heart, Lung, and Blood Institute scientific statement. *Circulation.* 2005;112(17):2735-2752.

● APPROACH: OBESITY THERAPIES

"Eat less and move more" has historically been the common approach to treating obesity. However, our understanding of the complex pathophysiology of obesity has grown and our approach to the individual with obesity has changed. It is essential to recognize that the treatment of chronic disease of obesity requires an individualized and often multimodal approach. Treatments thus need to be long term, and may require combinations of nutrition, physical activity, pharmacologic, endoscopic, or surgical interventions.[3,4,13] Figure 17-1 was adapted from the Obesity Care Path at the Cleveland Clinic and is just one example of an obesity treatment standard of care.[3,4] Currently, there is no standard of care for obesity and guidelines from several professional organizations have not reached a consensus. When considering a nutrition strategy to treat obesity, these guidelines vary and remain vague. Factors to consider when selecting a diet, duration of treatment, and criteria to measure effectiveness have not been clearly stated. It is clear, however, a true individualized approach is warranted.

Barriers to Treatment

While there exist effective treatments for obesity, they are unfortunately underutilized.[3] The Awareness, Care, and Treatment in Obesity (ACTION) management study, demonstrated that most healthcare providers viewed obesity as a disease, however, reported several barriers to care including lack of time and having more important issues to discuss.[14] However nearly one-quarter report not initiating a discussion about weight because of the belief that patients are not motivated, not interested, or not emotionally/physically ready to lose weight. Thus, it comes as little surprise that the average of 6 years has been reported to be the time between a patient's initial struggle with weight and initiation of a conversation with their physician.[4] It has been shown that patients view even a brief intervention consisting of advice on behavioral change from their primary care provider to be helpful and motivating.[4]

The aforementioned barriers coupled with the lack of medical knowledge surrounding availability and efficacy of obesity treatment prove that there is significant room for improvement through education of healthcare providers. It has been shown that both medical schools and residency training programs are remarkably lacking in obesity education.[3] The resulting lack of knowledge leads to misconceptions that interfere with initiating obesity treatment as healthcare providers. Efforts to reduce these educational, social, and financial barriers are crucial to obesity treatment moving forward.

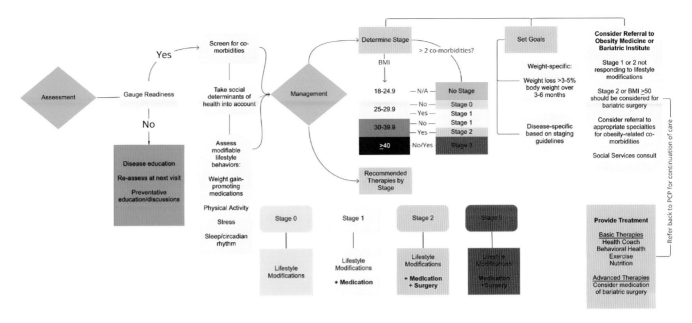

FIGURE 17-1 · Approach to obesity assessment and management

Implications of Weight Bias

The impact of obesity on one's health extends beyond the physical realm. Studies have shown that many healthcare providers, specifically physicians, hold strong negative attitudes and stereotypes about people with obesity.[15] Weight bias primarily stems from the primary belief that obesity is a character flaw, a behavioral condition that exists in weak individuals compared to their normal weight counterparts. This bias can have real health consequences including less preventative cancer screening, less clinical encounter time, and increased stress levels.[15]

Weight bias is defined as discriminatory behaviors and negative attitudes directed towards individuals with obesity. Implicit bias refers to attitudes or stereotypes that affect our understanding, actions and decisions in an unconscious manner. On the other hand, explicit bias refers to attitudes and beliefs we have about a person or group in a conscious manner. Examples of the latter weight bias include receiving insulting comments/criticisms from others, facing job discrimination, and exposure to derogatory media representations of obesity.

Unfortunately, these negative experiences with medical providers have a profound mental health implication on patients with obesity. Historically, the medical community has taken a "tough love" approach, blaming the patient to motivate positive behavior changes. However, weight bias may lead to disordered eating (e.g., extreme dieting, frequent binge eating, meal skipping, fasting, etc.), unhealthy physical activity habits (from compulsive exercise to exercise avoidance), poor health quality (e.g., low treatment adherence, avoiding medical care, etc.), and further precipitating a vicious cycle leading to worsening psychological stress and further weight gain.

The most concerning consequence of weight bias presenting the greatest challenge to providers is weight bias internalization. This self-directed stigma is reflected in the findings of the ACTION study (discussed later in this chapter) where

surveyed patients with obesity reported that the most significant barrier to bringing up obesity treatment was feeling that it was their responsibility to lose weight. Other barriers frequently reported by patients included lacking financial means to begin a weight loss program.[14]

The existing literature suggests an adverse impact of weight stigma on both psychological and physiological outcomes in adults with overweight and obesity. Findings from a systematic review focusing on these relationships showed that frequent experiences of weight stigma were associated with more depressive symptoms, higher anxiety levels, panic disorder, lower self-esteem, and higher levels of body dissatisfaction.[15] It is thus critical to acknowledge and educate the public about the impact of weight stigma and obesity on mental health.[3,4]

Nutrition Therapy

Despite decades of studies, no single diet (i.e., Mediterranean, low fat, low carbohydrate, etc.) has emerged as "the best" or most effective nutrition treatment for obesity. Recommendations have historically focused on caloric daily deficits with the belief that treatment of obesity is simply mathematical, with caloric reduction leading to consistent weight loss over time. However, as our knowledge of complexity of weight regulation has expanded, macronutrient composition and diet quality, not solely caloric intake, have played more significant roles in nutrition strategies for obesity. A small, randomized, controlled trial investigated 20 inpatient adults who had consumed an isocaloric diet of either ultra-processed or unprocessed foods. Despite being matched to the unprocessed diet for calories, fat, sugar, sodium, fiber, and macronutrients, the ultra-processed diet led to increased ad libitum energy intake (>500 kcal/d), increased fat mass (0.7 kg), and weight gain (1.8 kg) in the 14-day study.[16] Dozens of lifestyle intervention trials to treat obesity have been conducted; however, a few landmark

TABLE 17-2 • Landmark trials for nutrition interventions in weight management

Trial name	Study groups	Primary outcome	Duration	Weight loss effect
DPP	N = 3234, pre-diabetes with obesity 3 study groups: metformin vs. lifestyle intervention vs. placebo	Weight Loss, physical activity	10 years	At 2.8 years: Placebo: −0.1 kg Metformin: −2.1 kg Lifestyle: −5.6 kg
Look AHEAD	N = 5145, type 2 diabetes with obesity 2 study groups: lifestyle intervention vs. diabetes support and education group	Weight Loss, physical activity	9.6 years	At 1 year, % initial body weight lost: Lifestyle: −8.6% DSE: −0.7%
POUNDS Lost	N = 811, with overweight or obesity 4 study groups: - fat 40%/protein 15%, 45% carbs - fat 40%/protein 25%, 35% carbs - fat 20%/protein 15%, 65% carbs - fat 20% protein 25%, 55% carbs	Weight change	2 years	At 2 years: Fat 40%/protein 15%: −3.1 kg Fat 40%/protein 25%: −3.5 kg Fat 20%/protein 15%: −2.9 kg Fat 20% protein 25%: −3.8 kg
Comparison of the Atkins, Ornish, Weight Watchers, and Zone Diets for Weight Loss and Heart Disease Risk Reduction	N = 160 with overweight or obesity and known hypertension, dyslipidemia, or fasting hyperglycemia 4 study groups: Atkins diet, Ornish Diet, Weight Watchers, and Zone Diet	Weight change, change in cardiovascular risk factors, self-reported dietary adherence rates	1 year	At 1 year: Atkins Diet: 2.1 kg Ornish Diet: 3.3 kg Weight Watchers: 3.0 kg Zone Diet: 3.2 kg
DietFits	N = 609 with overweight or obesity 2 study groups: healthy low fat diet (HLF) vs. healthy low carbohydrate diet (HLC)	Weight change	1 year	At 1 year: HLF: 5.3 kg HLC: 6.0 kg

Carbs, carbohydrates; DPP, diabetes prevention program; DSE, diabetes support and education; Look AHEAD, action for health and diabetes; POUNDS lost, preventing obesity using novel dietary strategies.

randomized controlled trials are listed in Table 17-2.[3,17,18] Of note, while long-term weight loss in these trials refers to 1–2 years, weight management is a lifelong effort for patients with obesity. The American Association of Clinical Endocrinologists (AACE) recommendations also highlighted that most successful weight loss interventions included multidisciplinary components, with structured behavioral support to adopt and maintain the dietary modifications and most often a physical activity component.

The evidence supporting the efficacy of multi-components behavioral lifestyle intervention is supported by data from two landmark, large randomized clinical trials—the Diabetes Prevention Program (DPP) and the Look AHEAD trial (included in Table 17-2).[3] In both trials, lifestyle interventions that included caloric reduction, physical activity, and behavioral support led to relatively significant weight loss, compared to "control" usually with minimal education. There are also major studies that have looked at weight changes in response to dietary interventions with varying macronutrient compositions, including the POUNDS Lost and Dietfits studies.[17,19] While these studies did not reveal significant differences in weight loss between study groups, all study groups exhibited weight loss by the end of both studies, further supporting the efficacy of nutrition intervention in the management of overweight and obesity. It is crucial to determine what is sustainable for the patient, which often varies among individuals with obesity. As providers, we need to appreciate the heterogeneity in treatment response.

Recent Popular Nutrition Interventions

Nutrition interventions for obesity come with mixed messages, where "popular" diets, or "fad diets" (seen in Chapter 6, "Popular Diets") often cloud what is evidence-based in the literature. Both intermittent fasting and the ketogenic diets have more recently received attention in their use in the treatment of obesity.

Intermittent Fasting

Intermittent fasting (IF) is a dietary strategy characterized by alternating periods of eating with fasting periods up to 24 hours for 1–5 days a week. Animal studies have demonstrated IF results in favorable redistribution of adipose tissue, a metabolic switch, in which the body alternates between circulation-derived glucose during eating periods to ketones derived from adipose cells during periods of fasting.[20,21] The theory posits on that periods of fasting stimulate adaptive cellular responses including increased resistance to oxidative and metabolic stress, improved regulation of glucose, and suppression of inflammation. In most animal studies, the metabolic health benefits of IF have been observed with minimal weight changes. Long-term trials with large study populations are warranted.[21]

The three most common types of IF are time-restricted feeding (TRF), intermittent energy restriction, and alternate day fasting (ADF). TRF consists of a daily eating window (e.g., 8 or 10 hours) and fasting for the remainder of the day. ADF includes fasting for 24 hours 1 or 2 days per week and intermittent energy restriction includes various fasting schedules (e.g., a modified alternate day fasting, where "fasting" days include a very low caloric intake). While existing literature suggests various metabolic and aging benefits of IF, its association with weight loss outcomes is less clear. Conclusions are also difficult to make given that multiple types of intermittent fasting schedules exist. A recent study analyzed existing meta-analyses and IF trial on health outcomes in obesity and found a modified ADF and the 5:2 diet were the only IF types associated with significant weight loss of more than 5% in adults with overweight or obesity. In contrast, ADF and TRE were not.[20]

The mechanisms of the weight loss effect in IF studies appear to be caloric restriction. In contrast, TRF appears to embrace the contributory role of circadian rhythm on metabolism and weight loss. Small randomized controlled trials have demonstrated that meal-timing interventions facilitate weight loss (and fat loss) via reductions in appetite, not an increase in energy expenditure.[22]

Possible clinical applications of IF may be to consider TRF in people with circadian dysfunction or IF to help with caloric restriction in patients who are less likely/unable to use other methods of tracking food intake. This further highlights the need for individualized tailored interventions.

Ketogenic Diet

The ketogenic diet involves reducing daily total carbohydrate intake to less than 50 g per day and can be as low as 20 g per day. Typical ketogenic diets are relatively high in fat (average 70–80% of total daily calories), low in carbohydrate (5–10%) and protein (10–20%). The protein levels are intentionally lower as overconsumption of protein can prevent ketosis.[23] The available literature on the ketogenic diet demonstrates beneficial short-term (average duration 6 months) weight loss along with metabolic changes including improvements in insulin resistance, blood pressure, and elevated cholesterol and triglycerides.[23]

The mechanism by which the ketogenic diet promotes weight loss is not well understood; however, various theories have been proposed including decreased cravings and appetite (from the high fat content and ketone body formation), decreased production of the appetite-stimulating hormones insulin and ghrelin, and increased caloric expenditure (from the metabolic conversion of protein and fat to glucose).[23] While the ketogenic diet boasts weight loss alongside reductions in BMI and waist circumference, research investigating this relationship remains unclear. Limitations of existing studies include small study groups, lack control groups, or short duration.[23]

Clinical application of ketogenic diets varies, but adherence to a high fat intake and its associated adverse effects (headache, nausea, vomiting, constipation, and orthostatic hypotension) is challenging.[23]

APPROACH: NUTRITION ASSESSMENT AND MANAGEMENT IN PRIMARY CARE

There are multiple barriers to initiating a discussion about weight management in the primary care setting. The process should begin with a routine assessment of the patient with anthropometric measurements including height, weight, BMI, waist circumference. It is important to jointly agree on the patient's weight status prior to bringing up the topic of weight-related intervention. This can be done by reviewing anthropometric measurements with the patient while using respectful language in relation to weight.[4] Table 17-3 provides examples of terminology preferred by patients when referring to their weight.[24] After introducing the topic, the provider should ask the patient's permission to discuss next steps in taking action—there are various ways to do this which are listed in Table 17-4.[24] The patient should subsequently be asked to identify their support systems, motivating factors, and perceived barriers to change. It is in this way that the clinician can encourage the patient to acknowledge his/her intent to change. Examples of such questions include, "How would improving your health make your life better?".

Once the decision has been made to move forward with taking action, the healthcare provider should elicit a weight history from the patient.[3,4,24] This should include onset of weight issues, precipitating factors, perceived impact on quality of life, past weight loss attempts, and weight patterns. Potential factors underlying weight issues include a family history of weight issues, childhood overweight/obesity, major life events, medications that induce weight gain, medical conditions such as Cushing's syndrome, and lifestyle (dietary and activity) factors.[3,4]

Medications associated with weight gain include glucocorticoids, sulfonylureas, thiazolidinediones, selective serotonin reuptake inhibitors/selective norepinephrine reuptake inhibitors, tricyclic antidepressants, atypical antidepressants, mood stabilizers, antipsychotics, anticonvulsants, hormonal contraceptives, and beta blockers. If two or more of the above medications are present and can be safely switched, this should be done. After identifying potential contributors, weight-related complications—both physical and mental—should be considered and screened for.[3,4,13,24]

TABLE 17-3 • Terminology preferred by patients when referring to weight	
Preferred	**Not preferred/stigmatizing**
The patient has obesity or overweight	The patient is obese or overweight
The patient with obesity	The obese patient
Weight problem, unhealthy weight or body mass index, excess weight	Fat, extra-large, chubby, curvy, plus size, large, heavy
Severe obesity	Morbidly obese/Morbid obesity, extremely obese, super obese

TABLE 17-4 • Opening questions for weight-related discussions	
General	• Tell me about what brought you in today. • Are there any other health concerns you would like to discuss? • Would it be alright if we discuss your weight?
Tie to Other Health Problems	• Do you feel that your weight may be contributing the problem you're having? • Carrying excess weight can cause some of your health concerns. Would it be alright if we discuss how weight management can help?
Based on Clinical Markers	• Would it be alright if we discussed how weight management could help improve these results in the future? • I noticed you have a high body mass index, which means you are carrying excess weight for a person your height. This can impact your health. Would it be alright if we talk about your weight?[25]
Motivational Interviewing	• How would improving your health make your life better? • Do you feel that your weight is impacting your daily life and if so, how? • Have you ever discussed your weight with a health care professional in the past? Why or why not?[25]

SMART Goals and Successful Weight-Loss Habits (See also Chapter 26, "Introduction to Behavior Change")

Patient engagement is perhaps best achieved by the setting of SMART (specific, meaningful, action-based, realistic, and timely) goals. SMART goals are effective in reducing weight, improving eating behavior, and increasing physical activity. For example, setting a goal of "losing weight" or "being more active" is too broad a statement. Rather, a goal made applying the SMART framework would be "I will go for a jog Tuesdays and Thursdays in the park for 20 minutes for the next month." Application of the SMART Goals should be developed by the patient with clinician guidance rather than prescribed by the clinician.

Reviews on evidence-based weight loss interventions identified process predictors (behaviors associated with more favorable weight loss outcomes) and baseline assessments from studies ultimately associated with greater weight loss.[13] Such information can be used by the clinician to help further guide individualized therapy and discussion. Process predictors associated with weight loss included program adherence, high number of patient-provider contacts, self-weighing, self-monitoring food intake, self-monitoring physical activity, experiencing initial weight loss, and increasing physical activity. Eating patterns included regular breakfast intake, availability of healthy foods at home, increased vegetable intake, restricting sugary foods, high healthy food diversity index scores, regulation of circadian rhythms (sleeping for at least 8 hours nightly, limiting feeding time to less than 10 hours and eating earlier in the day), and low carbohydrate/high fiber diets for individuals with diabetes.[13]

Pharmacological Therapies

Table 17-5 shows the medications currently FDA-approved for the treatment of obesity.[3] Criteria for initiating obesity medications include BMI $\geq$ 30 or $\geq$ 27 kg/m^2 with an obesity-related co-morbidity, such as T2DM, hypertension, dyslipidemia, and sleep apnea). Decisions regarding medications for obesity should take into account patient preference, insurance coverage, safety issues, and particular characteristics driving food behaviors (i.e., food cravings, emotional eating, binge eating, etc.).[3,4] Of note, individual responses to medications greatly vary. Trials have suggested average efficacy of pharmacotherapy in assuming that obesity is a single disease entity. However, there exist various obesity phenotypes. Thus, treatment with an anti-obesity medication may result in no weight loss, weight loss of 5%–10% total body weight (TBW) or even exceeding 10%–20% of TBW. Healthcare providers should consider intensifying treating or switching to a different medication if the patient experiences < 5% weight loss after 3 months of initiation.[24]

Endoscopic Bariatric Therapies and Devices

Endoscopic interventions and devices that target the stomach and small bowel have emerged as an adjunctive therapy to treat mild to moderate obesity (BMI 30–40 kg/m^2) in individuals who have not responded to lifestyle therapies. The effectiveness of the FDA-approved space-occupying intragastric balloons (gas- or fluid-filled) and the endoscopic sleeve gastroplasty (ESG) is primarily dependent on caloric restriction. The temporary duration of the balloons (6–12 months) limits the long-term effectiveness while the ESG appears to be more durable. Oral hydrogels in the form of capsules taken prior to a meal also intend to reduced caloric intake, however appear to be less effective than the aforementioned minimally invasive procedures. The subcutaneously placed vagal nerve-blocking device intermittently blocks gastric vagal signals to the brain that regulate appetite and caloric intake. Other duodenal interventions (e.g., duodenal mucosal resurfacing or duodenal-jejunal bypass liner) are not FDA-approved but give some promise to devices that work through another mechanism of action.

Surgical Therapies

Metabolic and bariatric surgery (MBS) is the most effective, durable treatment for severe obesity. Although the mechanisms of MBS are not completely understood, studies have demonstrated both weight-dependent and weight-independent effects on metabolic complications of obesity, in particular type 2 diabetes.[26] The four main procedures and average weight outcomes are described in Table 17-6; however, response to a surgical intervention varies greatly.[3,13] The vertical sleeve

TABLE 17-5 • FDA-Approved medications for the treatment of obesity

Drug *Mechanism of action*	Additional conditions to consider	Average TBWL*	Side effects	Contraindications
Liraglutide *GLP1 receptor agonist*	Type 2 Diabetes CVD Renal Diseae	8%	- Nausea - Vomiting - Diarrhea - Constipation - HA - Injection site reaction	- Personal or family history of MEN 2 of medullary thyroid cancer - Pancreatitis - Untreated or acute gallbladder disease
Naltrexone/Bupropion SR *Opioid receptor antagonist/NE, DA reuptake inhibitor*	Depression Smoking Cessation	6.4%	- Insomnia - Dizziness - Nausea - Vomiting - Diarrhea - Constipation - Dry mouth - Increased BP/HR - Mood changes - HA	- Uncontrolled hypertension - Seizure disorder - Chronic opioid use - Bulimia nervosa - Anorexia nervosa - MAOI use - Alcohol/drug withdrawal - Uncontrolled mood disorders
Orlistat *Gastric and pancreatic lipase inhibitor*	Hyperlipidemia	> 10%	- Flatulence - Steatorrhea - Cholelithiasis - Vitamin deficiency	- Cholestasis - Malabsorptive conditions
Phentermine *Sympathomimetic, releases NE, DA, 5-HT*[127]	N/A	7.4%	- Insomnia - Increased BP/HR - Anxiety - Agitation - Dry mouth - Constipation - HA	- Cardiovascular disease - Stroke history - MAOI use - Untreated close angle glaucoma - Uncontrolled hyperthyroidism or hypertension
Phentermine/Topiramate CR *Sympathomimetic, releases NE, DA, 5-HT/ GABA receptor modulator*	HA	10.9%	- See phentermine above - Topiramate: - Mental fog - Dysgeusia - Word finding difficulty - Nephrolithiasis - Paresthesia - Drowsiness - Dry mouth - Constipation	- See Phentermine above - Topiramate: - Uncontrolled depression - Nephrolithiasis
Semaglutide 2.4 mg *GLP-1 receptor agonist*	Type 2 Diabetes CVD Renal Disease	14.9%	- Nausea - Vomiting - Diarrhea - Constipation - Headache - Injection site reaction	- Personal or family history of MEN 2 of medullary thyroid cancer - Pancreatitis - Untreated or acute gallbladder disease
Setmelanotide *Melanocortin-4 receptor agonist*	BBS, or POMC, PCKS1, or LEPR deficiency, or Bardet-Biedl Syndrome	12.5-25.6%	- Injection site reactions - Skin darkening - Nausea - Vomiting - Abdominal pain - Diarrhea - Adverse sexual reactions	- None

(Continued)

TABLE 17-5 • FDA-Approved medications for the treatment of obesity (*Continued*)

Drug *Mechanism of action*	Additional conditions to consider	Average TBWL*	Side effects	Contraindications
Tirzepatide *GLP-1 and GIP agonist*	Type 2 Diabetes CVD	15-20.9%	- Nausea - Vomiting - Diarrhea - Constipation - HA - Injection site reaction	- Personal or family history of MEN 2 of medullary thyroid cancer - Pancreatitis

5-HT, 5-hydroxytryptamine; BBS, Bardet-Biedl syndrome; BP, blood pressure; CVD, cardiovascular disease; DA, dopamine agonist; GIP, glucose-dependent insulinotropic polypeptide; GABA, gamma-aminobutyric acid; GLP-1, glucagon-like peptide 1; HA, headache; HR, heart rate; LEPR, leptin receptor; MAOI, monoamine oxidase inhibitor; MEN 2, multiple endocrine neoplasia type 2; NE, norepinephrine; PCKS1, proprotein convertase subtilisin/kexin type 1; POMC, proopiomelanocortin; SR, sustained release; TBW, total body weight.

TABLE 17-6 • Surgical therapies for obesity

Procedure	Description	Total body weight loss
Adjustable Gastric Band	Silicone band secured around top part of stomach	15–25%
Vertical Sleeve Gastrectomy	Surgical stapler used to remove 80% of stomach	20–25%
Roux-en-Y Gastric Bypass	Creation of small stomach pouch. Larger part of stomach as well as duodenum are bypassed via creation of roux limb (jejunum attached to gastric pouch). The duodenum is then attached to the distal roux limb.	30–35%
Biliopancreatic Diversion with Duodenal Switch	A gastric sleeve is created. The duodenum is then separated from the sleeve and part of the jejunum is pulled up and connected to the gastric sleeve, bypassing roughly 75% of the small intestine.	35–45%

gastrectomy is the most commonly performed procedure since 2013.[13,27] New guidelines recommend MBS for individuals with a BMI of ≥ 35 kg/m² or ≥30 kg/m² with associated comorbidities, including obstructive sleep apnea, diabetes, hypertension, or fatty liver disease.[28]

Nutritional counseling and education are essential pre- and postoperatively as changes in nutrient handling and micronutrient deficiencies may occur.[3] The adjustable gastric band is the least invasive surgical procedure (15–25% predicted body weight loss) and has little risk of nutritional complications, while the most invasive surgical intervention, the biliopancreatic diversion with duodenal switch (35–45% predicted body weight loss) is associated with multiple nutritional and gastrointestinal complications related to its malabsorption effects. Lifelong nutrition supplementation is required following all of these interventions. Table 17-7 lists postoperative nutrition supplementation and repletion requirements.[3,29]

● INDIVIDUALIZED INTERVENTIONS

In obesity care, it is essential to appreciate the great individual variation in treatment response. Although it may be easier to assess response to pharmacological and surgical interventions, this approach needs to be more appreciated when delivering medical nutrition therapy. One size does not indeed fit all.

TABLE 17-7 • Postoperative nutrient deficiencies

Nutrient	Postoperative prevalence	Deficiency symptoms	Recommended daily allowance	Supplementation	Repletion
Vitamin A	8–11% after RYGB 70% after BPD-DS	Skin hyperkeratinization Night blindness Loss of taste	Men: 900 mcg (3000 IU) Women: 700 mcg (2,300 IU)	LAGB: 5,000 IU daily RYGB or SG: 5,000–10,000 IU daily BPD-DS: 10,000 IU daily	Without corneal changes: 10,000–25,000 IU orally daily for 1–2 weeks or until clinical improvement With corneal changes: 50,000–100,000 daily IM for 3 days followed by 50,000IU IM daily for 2 weeks
Vitamin D	25–80%	Muscle Pain Tetany Hypocalcemia Metabolic Bone Disease	600 IU Pregnancy, lactation, over 70 years of age: 800 IU	3,000 IU vitamin D 3 daily from all source to maintain 25-OH level of greater than 30 ng/mL	3,000–6,000 IU of D3 daily

TABLE 17-7 • Postoperative nutrient deficiencies (*Continued*)

Nutrient	Postoperative prevalence	Deficiency symptoms	Recommended daily allowance	Supplementation	Repletion
Vitamin B1	1–49%	Extremity Tingling Confusion Gait ataxia Edema Vomiting	1.5 mg	Greater than 12 mg daily, preferably 50–100 mg daily from a B complex supplement	100 mg orally 2 or 3 times per day until symptoms resolve
Vitamin B12	33% after RYGB 4-20% after SG	Macrocytic anemia Neuropathy Depression Mild pancytopenia	2.4 mcg	Oral dose 350–1,000 mcg daily OR 1000 mcg IM or SQ monthly or by nasal spray	1,000 mcg daily until normal level, then resume maintenance dose
Folate	Up to 65% after RYGB 18% after SG	Neural tube defects Macrocytic anemia Mild pancytopenia	400 mcg	400–800 mcg daily from multivitamin Women of child-bearing age: 800-1,000 mcg daily Should NOT exceed 1 mg per day	1,000 mcg daily orally until normal level, then resume maintenance dose
Iron	LAGB: 14% SG: < 18% RYGB: 20–55% BPD-DS: 13–62%	Pica Anemia Impaired learning	Men 19 and older, Women 51 and older: 8 mg Women 19–50, 18 mg	Males, post-menopausal women, and patients without anemia: 18 mg from a multivitamin Menstruating women and men or women who underwent RYGB, SG, BPD-DS: Greater than 45 to 60 mg of elemental iron from all sources	150–300 mg orally 2–3 times daily
Calcium	1.9% after RYGB 9.3% after SG 10% after BPD-DS	Secondary hypoparathyroidism Bone disease	1,000–1,200 mg	RYGB, SG, or LAGB: 1,200–1,500 mg daily in divided doses BPD-DS: 1,800–2,400 mg daily in divided doses	Same as supplementation
Zinc	70% after BPD-DS 40% after RYGB 19% after SG 34% after LAGB	Impotence Impaired immune function Growth retardation	Women: 8 mg Men: 11 mg	BPD-DS: 16–22 mg RYGB: 8–22 mg SG or LAGB: 8–11 mg Maintain ratio 8–15 mg of zinc per 1 mg of copper	Optimal repletion dose unknown
Copper	90% after BPD-DS 10–20% after RYGB	Neutropenia Ataxia Anemia	900 mcg	BPD-DS or RYGB: 2 mg daily SG or LAGB: 1 mg daily Maintain ratio 8–15 mg of zinc per 1 mg of copper	Mild to moderate deficiency: 3-8mg copper orally until normal level Severe deficiency: 2–4 mg intravenous copper for 6 days or until symptoms resolve
Selenium	14–22% after RYGB and BPD-DS	Cardiomyopathy Mood disorder Macrocytosis Impaired immune function Skeletal muscle dysfunction	55 mcg	Unknown but likely more than 100 mcg per day	2 mcg per kilogram per day in patients who develop cardiomyopathy

BPD-DS, biliopancreatic diversion with duodenal switch; IM, intramuscular; IU, international units; LAGB, laparoscopic gastric band; RYGB, Roux-en-Y gastric bypass; SG, sleeve gastrectomy; SQ, subcutaneous.
Modified from Kushner RF, Herron DM, Herrington H. Bariatric surgery: Postoperative nutritional management. *UpToDate*. Accessed January 9, 2023. https://www.uptodate.com/contents/bariatric-surgery-postoperative-nutritional-management?search=nutrient%20deficiencies%20bariatric%20surgery&source=search_result&selectedTitle=1~150&usage_type=default&display_rank=1.

The chronicity of obesity requires a continuous treatment model; one will likely include several trials of a combination of interventions before finding the one that leads to an effective response.

We need to treat obesity like other chronic diseases, appreciating the lack of response a specific diet, an exercise plan, a medication, or even a surgical intervention, is not necessarily a failure of the patient or a result of poor adherence, rather may be a failure of the therapy itself.

Most lifestyle approaches are only transiently effective, producing modest weight loss results; however, certain individuals may have a dramatic response. Although the obesogenic environment driving sedentary behavior and consumption of energy dense foods can easily be identified, it is critical to appreciate existing biological barriers to an individual treatment response. More specifically, contributions may come from the strong biological response to weight loss (i.e., reduced energy expenditure and increased hunger and reduced satiety) that promotes weight regain or the complex nature of appetite regulation and eating behaviors that may drive a reduce adherence to a lifestyle modification. Figure 17-2 demonstrates the differences in historical and modern perceptions of obesity through the lenses of lifestyle modifications and assessment/management.

A review on evidence-based weight loss interventions concluded that current treatments for obesity, including lifestyle modifications, produce a weight loss of 5–7% on average.[30]

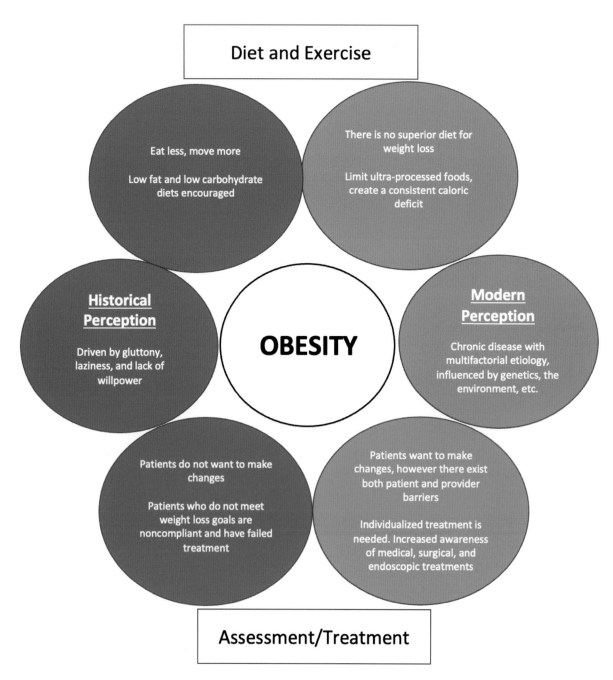

FIGURE 17-2 • Historical (in blue) vs. modern (in orange) views of obesity

Despite persistent investigation, a superior dietary approach to weight loss has not been identified. The current medications approved by the U.S. FDA for long-term obesity management are not as effective as surgery, adding an average of 5% to weight loss via lifestyle modifications.[30] There is marked variability in the amount of weight lost among all of the available treatments, highlighting the need for an individualized approach to management.

As such, a patient should not be placed at fault when there is lack of weight loss in response to an intervention or if there is weight gain/plateau following a period of loss. Individuals will respond to a single intervention with varying degrees of weight loss. These points are exemplified by participants involved in the LOOK AHEAD study and the DPP Outcomes Study (DPPOS). At the end of the first year of the LOOK AHEAD trial, individuals in the top 90th percentile had lost almost over 18% of their baseline body weight compared to those in the bottom 10th percentile having lost < 1%. DDPOS data reveals weight regain beginning 1 year following initial weight loss, with an ultimate 1–2 kg difference relative to the placebo group from years 5–10.[30] The existing landmark studies suggest maximum weight loss within the first 3–6 months following initiation of a dietary intervention.[3] This time frame can be used as a benchmark to guide nutrition therapy and gauge intervention efficacy in the clinical setting.

Several studies in humans have shown differences in the gut bacteria profiles between lean individuals and those with obesity.[31] Altered gut flora has thus been proposed as a potential driver for obesity. Moreover, changes in gut microbiota composition to reflect that of lean individuals have been observed in patients with obesity who lose weight after dieting or Roux-en-Y gastric bypass. However, there is no strong evidence in humans to suggest causality when it comes to obesity-associated changes in gut microbiota composition and the development of obesity. While several studies suggest that the secretion of gut hormones involved in hunger and satiety cues in humans are affected by an individual's gut microbiota, further research of these interactions is warranted in order to determine their pathological implications and therapeutic potential. Studies investigating individualized therapy based on patient genotype and microbiome profile are underway (see Chapter 8, "Precision Nutrition").

TAKE-HOME POINTS

1. The goal of obesity management should be to improve patient health by preventing and treating psychological, physical, and metabolic complications associated with obesity

2. Identification of individual barriers to obesity care (e.g., psychological, biological, and environmental) in the absence of blaming the patient is a healthy part of the management of obesity in the primary care setting.

3. Clinical decisions regarding interventions should be based on the assessment of patient risk and burden of weight-associated complications.

4. Appreciate the variation of individual response to obesity interventions.

5. Weight stigma towards individuals with obesity has significant physical and mental health implications. Healthcare providers are a common source of this. It is thus critical to acknowledge and educate health care providers and the public about the impact of weight stigma and obesity on mental and physical health.

6. Obesity is a chronic disease requiring a continuous treatment model.

CASE STUDY ANSWERS

1. BMI does not distinguish weight derived from muscle versus fat. It also does not identify fat distribution, which is an important determinant of metabolic health. Additionally, BMI cutoffs vary by country.

2. There are multiple factors that could potentially be contributing to this patient's weight gain. Her fatigue and recent weight gain could be due to hypothyroidism or untreated obstructive sleep apnea (patient is hypertensive on exam). She also experiences frequent circadian disruption by taking on night shifts as a nurse. She is also taking medications that can induce weight gain, including citalopram and the Depo-Provera injection. Her dietary habits of skipping breakfast, snacking on processed foods, and eating a majority of her calories in the evening are also likely contributing. In addition, apart from walking at work, she lives a relatively sedentary lifestyle.

3. Given the patient's elevated blood pressure, BMI, and fatigue, she is at risk for obstructive sleep apnea and should be initially screened via the STOP-BANG questionnaire. If this indicates risk for obstructive sleep apnea, a sleep study should be ordered. Additionally, the patient already has two criteria for metabolic syndrome (blood pressure ≥ 130/85 and waist circumference > 35 inches) and should undergo further testing for this with a lipid panel and fasting glucose. The fasting glucose will also help screen for presence of diabetes.

(Continued)

CASE STUDY ANSWERS *(Continued)*

4. As she has no established associated complications and has only had one weight loss attempt in the past, her initial intervention should mainly focus on lifestyle modification including diet and physical activity changes. Start by asking what the patient sees as important to her for own health. Other useful questions are often "What have you tried in the past? What has worked for you? What changes do you feel you would like to make for your health?" Patient-centered solutions are more likely to be maintained. Any of the potential contributors above (in answer b) can be targeted first; a first success will lead to a positive change and more self-efficacy for further positive changes. You should help the patient to set a SMART goal for her to promote consistency. You could also counsel her on habits including substituting day shifts instead of night shifts in order to ensure better regulation of her circadian cycle. You could offer a medication at this time as an adjunct to lifestyle modifications as she meets criteria for initiation of an obesity medication (BMI $\geq$ 30 or $\geq$ 27 kg/m^2 with an obesity-related co-morbidity, such as T2DM, hypertension, dyslipidemia, and sleep apnea).

5. Tell her that there has been no identification in the literature of a superior diet when it comes to weight loss. Obesity interventions much be individualized for the patient. She is unlikely to remain consistent with a diet that she does not find sustainable and from which she experiences adverse side effects and is more likely to lose weight following habits to which she can adhere. Initial discussion to achieve this should include the shared development of SMART goals. It is also important to encourage her and provide reassurance that she is not a failure for stopping her previous diet.

6. Tell her that while individuals typically start seeing weight loss results within 3–6 months (ideally not at a higher rate than 2 pounds lost per week), response to an intervention varies greatly from person to person. If she does not attain a weight loss of < 5% within this time period, consideration can be taken to switch to another dietary approach or trial a medication. Additionally, it should be emphasized that results are not only measured by changes in the number on the scale, but also via other methods including improvements in sleep quality, the way clothes fit, body measurements and composition, physical endurance, and mental health.

7. Reassure the patient. Given metabolic adaptations including decreased energy expenditure with restricted caloric intake, remaining at a stable weight rather than gaining is a marker of intervention efficacy. At this point, weight maintenance should be the goal if her health status has improved (i.e., improvement in lipids/glucose, less fatigue, better mood). If further weight loss is desired, intervention should be intensified. If she was not started on a medication during her first visit with you, she can be started on one during this visit to help with weight loss in conjunction with sustained dietary modifications and active lifestyle. If she was already on a medication, increases in dosage or switching to a different type of medication can be trialed. She does not meet criteria for bariatric surgery (BMI of $\geq$40 kg/m^2 or $\geq$35 kg/m^2 with associated comorbidities, including obstructive sleep apnea, diabetes, hypertension, or fatty liver disease).

REFERENCES

1. Aronne LJ. Classification of obesity and assessment of obesity-related health risks. *Obes Res.* 2002;10(S12):105S-115S.

2. Kuk JL, Ardern CI, Church TS, et al. Edmonton obesity staging system: association with weight history and mortality risk. *Appl Physiol Nutr Metab.* 2011;36(4):570-576.

3. Gossmann M, Butsch WS, Jastreboff AM. Treating the chronic disease of obesity. *Med Clin North Am.* 2021;105(6):983-1016.

4. Bessell E, Markovic TP, Fuller NR. How to provide a structured clinical assessment of a patient with overweight or obesity. *Diabetes Obes Metab.* 2021;23(S1):36-49.

5. Theilade S, Christensen MB, Vilsbøll T, Knop FK. An overview of obesity mechanisms in humans: endocrine regulation of food intake, eating behaviour and common determinants of body weight. *Diabetes Obes Metab.* 2021;23(Suppl 1):17-35.

6. Richard D. Cognitive and autonomic determinants of energy homeostasis in obesity. *Nat Rev Endocrinol.* 2015;11(8):489-501.

7. Keesey RE, Hirvonen MD. Obesity: common symptom of diverse gene-based metabolic dysregulations body weight set-points: determination and adjustment 1. *J Nutr.* 1997;127:1875-1883.

8. Rosenbaum M, Kissileff HR, Mayer LES, Hirsch J, Leibel RL. Energy intake in weight-reduced humans. *Brain Res.* 2010; 1350:95.

9. Hall KD. Energy compensation and metabolic adaptation: "The Biggest Loser" study reinterpreted. *Obesity.* 2022;30(1):11-13.

10. Loos RJF, Yeo GSH. The genetics of obesity: from discovery to biology. *Nat Rev Genet.* 2022;23(2):120-133.

11. Longo VD, Panda S. Fasting, circadian rhythms, and time restricted feeding in healthy lifespan. *Cell Metab.* 2016;23(6):1048-1059.

12. Grundy SM, Cleeman JI, Daniels SR, et al. Diagnosis and management of the metabolic syndrome: an American Heart

Association/National Heart, Lung, and Blood Institute scientific statement. *Circulation*. 2005;112(17):2735-2752.

13. Bray GA, Heisel WE, Afshin A, et al. The science of obesity management: an endocrine society scientific statement. *Endocr Rev*. 2018;39(2):79-132.

14. Kaplan LM, Golden A, Jinnett K, et al. Perceptions of barriers to effective obesity care: results from the national ACTION study. *Obesity*. 2018;26(1):61-69.

15. Puhl RM, Heuer CA. The stigma of obesity: a review and update. *Obesity*. 2009;17(5):941-964.

16. Hall KD, Ayuketah A, Brychta R, et al. Ultra-processed diets cause excess calorie intake and weight gain: an inpatient randomized controlled trial of ad libitum food intake. *Cell Metab*. 2019;30(1):67-77.e3.

17. De Souza RJ, Bray GA, Carey VJ, et al. Effects of 4 weight-loss diets differing in fat, protein, and carbohydrate on fat mass, lean mass, visceral adipose tissue, and hepatic fat: results from the POUNDS LOST trial. *Am J Clin Nutr*. 2012;95(3):614-625.

18. Dansinger ML, Gleason JA, Griffith JL, Selker HP, Schaefer EJ. Comparison of the atkins, ornish, weight watchers, and zone diets for weight loss and heart disease risk reduction: a randomized trial. *JAMA*. 2005;293(1):43-53.

19. Gardner CD, Trepanowski JF, Gobbo LCD, et al. Effect of low-fat vs. low-carbohydrate diet on 12-month weight loss in overweight adults and the association with genotype pattern or insulin secretion: the DIETFITS randomized clinical trial. *JAMA*. 2018;319(7):667-679.

20. Patikorn C, Roubal K, Veettil SK, et al. Intermittent fasting and obesity-related health outcomes: an umbrella review of meta-analyses of randomized clinical trials. *JAMA Netw Open*. 2021;4(12):e2139558-e2139558.

21. Varady KA, Allister CA, Roohk DJ, Hellerstein MK. Improvements in body fat distribution and circulating adiponectin by alternate-day fasting versus calorie restriction. *J Nutr Biochem*. 2010;21(3):188-195.

22. Ravussin E, Beyl RA, Poggiogalle E, Hsia DS, Peterson CM. Early time-restricted feeding reduces appetite and increases fat oxidation but does not affect energy expenditure in humans. *Obesity (Silver Spring)*. 2019;27(8):1244-1254.

23. Diet Review: Ketogenic Diet for Weight Loss. The Nutrition Source | Harvard T.H. Chan School of Public Health. Accessed August 13, 2022. Available at: https://www.hsph.harvard.edu/nutritionsource/healthy-weight/diet-reviews/ketogenic-diet/.

24. Diewald L, Scott Kahan, MD, MPH-ABCDEF Approach to Obesity Management COPE WEBINAR SERIES FOR HEALTH PROFESSIONALS Obesity Treatment, Beyond the Guidelines: A Structured "A-B-C-D-E-F" Framework for Primary Care Practice. Published online 2020. Accessed August 13, 2022. Available at: www.villanova.edu/COPE.

25. Novo Nordisk. *Rethink Your Obesity Discussions*.

26. Batterham RL, Cummings DE. Mechanisms of diabetes improvement following bariatric/metabolic surgery. *Diabetes Care*. 2016;39(6):893-901.

27. Clapp B, Ponce J, DeMaria E, et al. American Society for Metabolic and Bariatric Surgery 2020 estimate of metabolic and bariatric procedures performed in the United States. *Surg Obes Relat Dis*. 2022;18(9):1134-1140.

28. Eisenberg D, Shikora SA, Aarts E, et al. American Society for Metabolic and Bariatric Surgery (ASMBS) and International Federation for the Surgery of Obesity and Metabolic Disorders (IFSO): indications for metabolic and bariatric surgery. *Surg Obes Relat Dis*. 2022;18(12):1345-1356.

29. Bariatric surgery: Postoperative nutritional management - UpToDate. Accessed January 9, 2023. Available at: https://www.uptodate.com/contents/bariatric-surgery-postoperative-nutritional-management?search=nutrient%20deficiencies%20bariatric%20surgery&source=search_result&selectedTitle=1~150&usage_type=default&display_rank=1.

30. Bray GA, Ryan DH. Evidence-based weight loss interventions: individualized treatment options to maximize patient outcomes. *Diabetes Obes Metab*. 2021;23(S1):50-62.

31. Castaner O, Goday A, Park YM, et al. The gut microbiome profile in obesity: a systematic review. *Int J Endocrinol*. 2018:2018:4095789.

chapter 18

Diabetes Mellitus

Allison Kimball, MD / Caitlin Colling, MD / Stacey L. Nelson, MS, RDN

Chapter Outline

CASE STUDY 1

A 60-year-old male with type 2 diabetes and hypertension presents to clinic for a follow-up appointment. His BMI is 28.4 kg/m² (overweight category), and his HbA1c is 8.3% (goal < 7%) on metformin monotherapy. He lives a relatively sedentary lifestyle. He says that he follows a "meat and potatoes" diet (red meat, chicken, white rice, potatoes). He drinks fruit juice and full-fat milk on occasion. He would prefer not to add any additional medications and inquires if he can make lifestyle changes to improve his glycemic control.

1. What dietary recommendations would you make?
2. How would you counsel him about weight loss?

CASE STUDY 2

A healthy 17-year-old female is hospitalized for nausea/vomiting, and she thinks she has lost weight over the preceding month despite eating more than usual. Her admission weight is 60 kg and BMI is 22.7 kg/m². She is found to have diabetes ketoacidosis and is diagnosed with type 1 diabetes. Following treatment and resolution of the ketoacidosis, she and her parents meet with the physician, diabetes nurse educator, and registered dietician to learn about diabetes management.

1. In addition to basal insulin, she is prescribed rapid-acting insulin using an insulin-to-carbohydrate ratio of 1:16. What does this mean?
   A. 1 unit insulin is expected to lower blood glucose by 16 mg/dL.

B. 1 unit insulin should be administered for every 16 grams of carbohydrate.
C. 16 units insulin is administered per gram carbohydrate.

2. Which of the following elements affect postprandial glucose excursion (choose all that apply)?
   A. Total carbohydrate content
   B. Whether the source of carbohydrate is liquid or solid (e.g., fruit juice vs. whole fruit)
   C. Protein content
   D. Fat content
   E. Fiber content

DEFINITIONS

Diabetes mellitus is a group of metabolic diseases characterized by hyperglycemia resulting from defects in insulin secretion, insulin action, or both. Diabetes can be classified into several different categories, the most common of which are type 1 diabetes, type 2 diabetes, and gestational diabetes. Type 1 diabetes results from autoimmune destruction of the pancreatic beta cells, causing complete insulin deficiency. Type 2 diabetes is characterized by relative insulin deficiency, which results from a combination of longstanding insulin resistance and eventually inadequate insulin production to overcome the persistent insulin resistance. The initial predominant mechanism underlying type 2 diabetes is insulin resistance, which is often present for years before the diabetes diagnosis; over time, pancreatic beta cell dysfunction leading to impaired insulin secretion can also occur. Gestational diabetes refers to diabetes diagnosed in the second or third trimester of pregnancy that was not present prior to pregnancy. It results from the imbalance between insulin secretion and insulin resistance, this time putatively due to increases in levels of hormones produced by the placenta on top of preexisting insulin resistance or limited insulin secretion adaptability. It does not exclude the possibility that unrecognized glucose intolerance may have preceded or begun concomitantly with the pregnancy.

The diagnosis of diabetes mellitus is made by a fasting plasma glucose ≥ 126 mg/dL; plasma glucose ≥ 200 mg/dL 2 hours after a 75-gram oral glucose load (oral glucose tolerance test); hemoglobin A1c $\geq 6.5\%$; or random plasma glucose level ≥ 200 mg/dL with associated symptoms of hyperglycemia, such as polyuria and polydipsia. Two abnormal tests are needed to confirm the diagnosis of diabetes.

The World Health Organization, the American College of Obstetricians and Gynecologists[1] and the American Diabetes Association (ADA)[2] are among the organizations that have published guidelines on the screening and diagnosis of diabetes in pregnancy. Gestational diabetes can be diagnosed using oral glucose tolerance tests (over 2 hours or 3 hours), following a two-step or a one-step strategy usually at the end of the second trimester (24–28 weeks of gestation), and the various organizations have suggested different cut-off glucose values and number of values above certain thresholds. The ADA guidelines are shown in Box 18-1.

BASIC EPIDEMIOLOGY

While diabetes is treatable and rarely acutely fatal, its treatment and complications have major impacts on the quality of life of patients, and life expectancy is shortened. Diabetes is the seventh-leading cause of death in the United States. The prevalence of both type 1 diabetes and type 2 diabetes has increased over the last two decades. In the United States in 2022, 37 million people (1 in 9) have type 2 diabetes (of which 8.5 million are undiagnosed), and 1.6 million have type 1 diabetes. In addition, 96 million adults in the United States (just over 1 in 3) have prediabetes.

Gestational diabetes affects 5–10% of all pregnancies in the United States,[3] and the International Diabetes Federation (IDF) declared in 2019 that 1 in 6 births were affected by gestational diabetes. The prevalence of gestational diabetes in the United States has also been increasing steadily from 47.6 to 63.5 per 1,000 live births from 2011 to 2019. Rates increased in all racial and ethnic subgroups, with individuals from Asian Indian descent demonstrating the highest gestational diabetes rate (129.1 per 1,000 live births).[4]

Age-adjusted data for 2018–2019 from the CDC indicate that the prevalence of diagnosed type 2 diabetes was highest among American Indians and Alaska Natives, followed by non-Hispanic blacks, people of Hispanic origin, non-Hispanic Asians, and non-Hispanic whites. These differences are at least in part due to factors such as education level, socioeconomic status, and other social factors. According to the CDC, 13.4% of adults with less than a high school education had diagnosed diabetes versus 9.2% of those with a high school education and 7.1% of those with more than a high school education. Adults

---

BOX 18-1

American Diabetes Association guidelines for the diagnosis of gestational diabetes

One-step strategy

75-gram oral glucose tolerance test with plasma glucose measurement at 1 and 2 hours (performed after overnight fast or at least 8 hours).

Diagnosis of gestational diabetes is made if any of the following plasma glucose levels are met or exceeded:

- Fasting: 92 mg/dL
- 1 hour: 180 mg/dL
- 2 hour: 153 mg/dL

Two-step strategy

Step 1: 50-gram oral glucose loading test (nonfasting) with plasma glucose measurement at 1 hour. If plasma glucose level 1 hour after load is ≥ 130, proceed to 100-gram oral glucose tolerance test.

Step 2: 100-gram oral glucose tolerance test performed when fasting with plasma glucose levels measured fasting and at 1, 2, and 3 hours during oral glucose tolerance test. Gestational diabetes is diagnosed if at least two of the following four plasma glucose levels are met or exceeded:

- Fasting: 95 mg/dL
- 1 hour: 180 mg/dL
- 2 hour: 155 mg/dL
- 3 hour: 140 mg/dL

with a family income below the federal poverty level had the highest prevalence of diabetes. Importantly, socioeconomic status affects access to healthy food, ability to participate in physical activity, and healthcare access and utilization, among other social determinants of health, all of which play a major role in the risk for overweight/obesity and the risk for type 2 diabetes.

In addition to overweight or obesity and physical inactivity, risk factors for the development of type 2 diabetes include older age, high waist-to-hip ratio, family history of type 2 diabetes, and history of gestational diabetes. Additionally, people who consume sugary-sweetened beverages (SSB) regularly (one to two cans per day or more) have a 26% greater risk of developing type 2 diabetes, and the effect of SSB consumption on diabetes risk is even greater in young adults.[5] SSB refers to any beverage with added sugar or other sweeteners (high fructose corn syrup, sucrose, fruit juice concentrates, and more). In the United States, these beverages are the single largest source of calories and added sugar.[6] Intake of high-fructose corn syrup and concentrated sweets (as well as overweight/obesity) are also risk factors for non-alcoholic fatty liver disease, which is associated with the development of type 2 diabetes. Many patients with type 2 diabetes have a cluster of abnormalities called metabolic syndrome, which includes visceral obesity, hypertension, dyslipidemia (low level of high-density lipoprotein, high level of triglycerides), and increased risk for cardiovascular disease. Metabolic syndrome often precedes the diagnosis of type 2 diabetes by many years, in parallel to insulin resistance. Whether insulin resistance causes the non-glycemic components of the syndrome, or whether visceral obesity directly induces the other components, is still a matter of debate.

Prediabetes is a laboratory finding that identifies individuals at high risk for developing diabetes. It can be classified as impaired fasting glucose (fasting plasma glucose 100–125 mg/dL), impaired glucose tolerance (plasma glucose 140–199 mg/dL two hours after a 75-gram oral glucose load), or both. Making the diagnosis of prediabetes allows lifestyle (and sometimes pharmacologic) intervention before diabetes has developed, thus lowering the risk of progression to diabetes. Due to the strong evidence for effectiveness of preventative measures and potential benefits of early treatment, the U.S. Preventive Services Task Force recommends screening for prediabetes and type 2 diabetes in adults aged 35–70 years with overweight or obesity.

RELEVANT PATHOPHYSIOLOGY

Glucose Homeostasis and Insulin Action

Insulin plays a key role in the regulation of glucose homeostasis, which reflects the balance between glucose intake from ingested carbohydrates, glucose uptake and utilization by peripheral tissues, and glucose production from and storage in the liver (Figure 18-1).[7]

Glucose-induced stimulation of insulin release by the pancreatic beta cells leads to glucose uptake into insulin-sensitive tissues, such as muscle and adipose tissue; suppression of glucose production by the liver through inhibition of glycogenolysis and gluconeogenesis; and suppression of lipolysis and protein catabolism. This process works to maintain a normal plasma glucose level after ingesting carbohydrates. Overall, the effects of insulin are anabolic and promote the synthesis of carbohydrates, lipids, and protein (Figure 18-2).[8] The pancreas releases insulin continuously (to suppress hepatic glucose output and prevent ketogenesis between meals and overnight) and releases a bolus of insulin prandially in response to a rise in blood glucose after eating, which promotes glucose utilization.

In a fasting state, insulin production decreases and levels of counterregulatory hormones, the most important of which is glucagon, rise. These hormonal changes cause several processes to ensue, including increased glycogenolysis, gluconeogenesis, and lipolysis, which work to prevent hypoglycemia as normal physiologic regulation.

Diabetes occurs due to a deficiency of insulin, either absolute (type 1 diabetes) or relative (type 2 diabetes). Relative

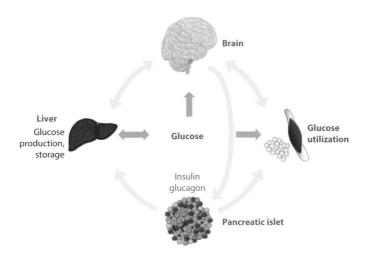

FIGURE 18-1 • Glucose homeostasis involves the pancreas, liver, and peripheral tissues.
(Reproduced with permission from Loscalzo J, Fauci A, Kasper D, Hauser S, Longo D, Jameson JL. Diabetes mellitus: diagnosis, classification, and pathophysiology. In *Harrison's Principles of Internal Medicine*. 21st ed. New York, NY: McGraw Hill; 2022.)

Metabolic effects	Insulin stimulates	Insulin inhibits
Carbohydrate metabolism	Glucose transport in adipose tissue and muscle Rate of glycolysis in muscle and adipose tissue Glycogen synthesis in adipose tissue, muscle, and liver	Glycogen breakdown in muscle and liver Rate of glycogenolysis and gluconeogenesis in the liver
Lipid metabolism	Fatty acid and triacylglycerol synthesis in tissues Uptake of triglycerides from the blood into adipose tissue and muscle Rate of cholesterol synthesis in the liver	Lipolysis in adipose tissue, lowering the plasma fatty acid level Fatty acid oxidation in muscle and liver Ketogenesis
Protein metabolism	Amino acid transport into tissues Protein synthesis in muscle, adipose tissue, liver, and other tissues	Protein degradation in muscle Urea formation

FIGURE 18-2 • Effects of insulin on carbohydrate, fat, and protein metabolism.
(Reproduced with permission from Molina P. Endocrine pancreas. In: *Endocrine Physiology.* 5th ed. New York, NY: McGraw Hill; 2018.)

deficiency of insulin means that there is not enough insulin to meet demands. Regardless of the underlying cause of diabetes, chronic hyperglycemia resulting from insulin deficiency will increase the risk for microvascular complications (e.g., nephropathy, retinopathy) and cardiovascular disease if hyperglycemia is inadequately controlled.

Effect of Carbohydrates on Glycemia

Carbohydrate intake is the primary dietary driver of postprandial hyperglycemia in all types of diabetes and frequently observable in prediabetes. Foods containing carbohydrates with various proportions of sugars, starches, and fiber have a wide range of effects on glycemia. Whole grains and vegetables, which are high in fiber, result in an extended rise and fall of blood glucose, while refined sugar and white bread result in a rapid rise and fall in blood glucose. SSB and juices, which are absorbed very quickly, result in a *very* rapid rise and fall in blood glucose. The total number of carbohydrates (grams) in a meal has a significant effect on the degree of postprandial hyperglycemia; however, the protein and/or fat content of the meal may change how quickly carbohydrates are absorbed and the overall glycemic postprandial excursion.

● NUTRITION AND LIFESTYLE INTERVENTIONS AS PRIMARY PREVENTION FOR TYPE 2 DIABETES

As food quantity and quality has a significant impact on blood glucose levels, body weight, and progression from prediabetes to type 2 diabetes, there have been multiple studies examining nutrition interventions for the prevention of type 2 diabetes. These studies have demonstrated that lifestyle interventions can improve glucose tolerance and prevent progression from prediabetes to type 2 diabetes. Table 18-1 summarizes the results of several landmark trials of lifestyle interventions for the prevention of type 2 diabetes. In all trials, the lifestyle intervention

included a diet and physical activity component aimed at weight loss and increasing activity levels. In follow-up ranging from 1 to 6 years, the risk reduction for the development of type 2 diabetes with lifestyle versus control ranged from 33% to 77% in individuals with impaired glucose tolerance (only one trial included individuals with impaired fasting glucose). A meta-analysis found that compared with usual care, diet and physical activity promotion programs significantly reduced type 2 diabetes incidence (risk ratio [RR], 0.59 [95% CI, 0.52 to 0.66]), with the beneficial effects of the intervention programs persisting for years after study completion.[11,18-21] In the Diabetes Prevention Trial (DPP) conducted in U.S. multi-ethnic populations, which demonstrated that intensive lifestyle intervention could reduce the risk of incident type 2 diabetes by 58% over 3 years, the two major goals were to achieve and maintain a minimum of 7% weight loss and 150 minutes of physical activity per week similar in intensity to brisk walking. In the DPP lifestyle intervention, dietary counseling included a reduction of total dietary fat and calories,[11] but other dietary approaches have been shown effective if they lead to weight loss and are sustainable over time (see Table 18-1). Notably, the DPP has been adapted for implementation in a variety of settings and populations, with modifications to accommodate various social and culture factors, with robust results.[22] Some of the settings studied include YMCAs, churches, primary care practices, medically underserved communities, and other countries.[23]

Nearly all type 2 diabetes prevention trials examined the effect of a combination of dietary changes and exercise with the goal of some weight loss. Of note, the amount of weight loss aimed at and achieved by participants is usually modest, ranging from 5% to 10% on average; thus, we should encourage our patients that these weight loss goals are achievable for many people. There are limited data about the efficacy of dietary changes alone (without weight loss). Studies examining the effects of two Mediterranean diets versus a low-fat control diet on cardiovascular outcomes in adults at high

TABLE 18-1 • Summary of landmark trials of lifestyle interventions for the prevention of type 2 diabetes.

Study	Country	N, characteristics	Study duration	Risk reduction of T2D with lifestyle versus control	Dietary goals	Changes in diet when available	Physical activity goals/changes
Da Qing IGT and Diabetes Study[9]	China	In total, 577; all had IGT; 33 health care clinics; 133 in control; 130 in diet; 141 in exercise; 126 in diet + exercise	6 yrs	Diet 33%; exercise 47%; diet + exercise 38%	Weight reduction in overweight; calorie restriction	58–60% of total energy in carb; 11% protein; 25–27% fat; total calories decrease 100–240 kcal	Increase, e.g., walking
Finnish Diabetes Prevention Study (FDPS)[10]	Finland	In total, 522; IGT; five centers; 265 in intervention; 257 in control	3.2 yrs; median 4	In total, 58%, weight loss; difference 3.5 and 2.6 kg after 1 and 3 yrs, respectively.	Weight reduction >5%; reduce total and SFA; increase dietary fiber	3 yr results: energy reduction 204 kcal; 3% increase in total energy from carb; 5% reduction total energy from fat; saturate fat reduce 3% of total energy; fiber increase 2 g/1,000 kcal	4 h/wk, sedentary people at yr 3: 17% vs. 29% for intervention and control groups, respectively
The Diabetes Prevention Program (DPP)[11]	USA	In total, 3234; IGT; 27 centers; 1082 in placebo, 1073 in metformin; 1079 in lifestyle	2.8 yrs	Lifestyle 58%; Metformin 31%; weight loss at yr 1: −5.6 vs. −0.1 kg for intervention vs. control, respectively.	NCEP Step 1; weight loss goal 7%	Energy intake reduction 450 vs. 249 kcal and fat intake reduction 6.6 vs. 0.8 of total energy for intervention and control, respectively.	150 min/wk
Japanese trial in IGT males[12]	Japan	In total, 458 IGT; 356 in control, 102 in intervention, OGTT (100 g glucose dose)	4 yrs	Incidence of T2D 3.0% vs. 9.3%; risk reduction 67.4%; weight loss −2.18 kg	BMI goal 22 kg/m²; increase vegetables; reduce food intake by 10%; fat < 50 g/d; alcohol restriction	Not reported	30–40 min walking/d
The Indian Diabetes Prevention Programme (IDPP-1)[13]	India	In total, 531; IGT; 133 in lifestyle; 133 in metformin; 129 in lifestyle-plus-metformin; 136 in control	30 months	Lifestyle 28.5%; Metformin 26.4%; lifestyle-plus-Metformin 28.2%; no change in body weight	Reduce total calories, refined CHO, fat and sugar; increase high fiber-rich foods	Dietary adherence increased in Intervention groups	Walking 30 min a day

(Continued)

TABLE 18-1 · Summary of landmark trials of lifestyle interventions for the prevention of type 2 diabetes. *(Continued)*

Study	Country	N, characteristics	Study duration	Risk reduction of T2D with lifestyle versus control	Dietary goals	Changes in diet when available	Physical activity goals/changes
Lifestyle intervention on metabolic syndrome[14]	Italy	In total, 375 with dysmetabolism; 169 in intervention; 166 in control; focus on metabolic syndrome	1 yr	Risk reduction for T2D 77%, (OR 0.23; 95% CI 0.06–0.85) at year 1.	General recommendations to lose weight, decrease SFA, and increase PUFA and fiber	Body weight minus 0.75 vs. plus 1.63 kg; total calories minus 74.6 vs. 43.7 kcal; fat reduced 2.6% total energy; saturated fat reduced 2.0%; carb increased 2%; protein increased 1.7%; NS for control	Increase
European Diabetes Prevention Study (EDIPS-Newcastle)[15]	UK	In total, 102; IGT; 51 in intervention and control, respectively	3 yrs	Diabetes incidence 5% vs. 11, 1% yr. body weight change −2.5 kg	Like in FDPS, decrease fat and SFA; increase fiber; body weight reduction	Not reported	Like in FDPS
Lifestyle Modification and Prevention of Type 2 Diabetes in Overweight Japanese With IFG Levels[16]	Japan	641 overweight adults with IFG; 311 in intervention; 330 in control	3 yrs	Diabetes incidence 12.2% vs. 16.%, adjusted HR 0.56 (95% CI 0.36-0.87); 12 mo: 32% of intervention and 15% control with ≥ 5% weight loss	Reduce total energy intake; limit fat intake at 20% to 25% of total energy intake and carbohydrate intake at 55% to 60% of total energy intake; target 5% weight loss	% with reduction in total energy intake ≥ 5%: 57% vs. 49%	Increase physical activity to 200 kcal/d; participants set own goals; common goal 10,000 steps per day

Adapted from Uusitupa M, Khan TA, Viguiliouk E, et al. Prevention of type 2 diabetes by lifestyle changes: a systematic review and meta-analysis. *Nutrients.* 2019;11(11).[17]

cardiovascular risk found a reduced risk of type 2 diabetes development at 3 years of follow-up with both Mediterranean diets compared to the control diet with no difference in weight change between the groups.[24,25] The success of diabetes prevention programs has led to dissemination nationally across the United States; providers refer patients to programs locally or regionally, which can be found on the CDC website. Diabetes prevention programs have been adapted to various settings using less intensive and more scalable interventions with similar results.[23]

NUTRITION AS THERAPY FOR TYPE 1 DIABETES

As patients with type 1 diabetes have absolute insulin deficiency, they must be treated pharmacologically with insulin. In the absence of insulin, the body is in a catabolic state; protein and adipose tissue are broken down to yield amino acids and glycerol for gluconeogenesis as well as free fatty acids that are converted to ketone bodies and can accumulate to cause ketoacidosis. This explains why the usual presentation of new-onset type 1 diabetes is diabetic ketoacidosis, often preceded by unexplained weight loss.

Diet is a critical component in the treatment of type 1 diabetes as the aim of insulin therapy is to maintain near-normal glucose levels, and the appropriate administration of insulin with carbohydrates is fundamental to glycemic control. Bolus insulin (as described below) is intended to cover the carbohydrates an individual is about to consume with a meal or a snack.

Principles of Medical Nutrition Therapy (MNT) for Individuals with Type 1 Diabetes

Highlighting the importance of nutrition in type 1 diabetes care, it is recommended that all patients with type 1 diabetes receive medical nutrition therapy (MNT), which is an evidence-based application of the nutrition care process provided by a registered dietitian nutritionist. The goals of MNT are to promote and support healthful eating patterns; address individual nutrition needs based on personal and cultural preferences, health literacy and numeracy, and food access; maintain the pleasure of eating by providing nonjudgmental messaging; and provide an individual with practical tools to develop healthy eating patterns.[26] MNT recognizes that a "one-size-fits-all" approach to eating is unrealistic and instead tailors recommendations to the individual. Components of MNT are assessment, nutritional diagnosis, interventions, and monitoring with ongoing follow-up. In randomized trials of individuals with type 1 diabetes, individualized MNT has contributed to a decrease in HbA1c of 1.0% to 1.9% at 6 months that was maintained at 12 months.[27]

A major challenge for patients with type 1 diabetes is determining what to eat and to estimate the carbohydrate content of meals. Skill training promoting dietary freedom was demonstrated to significantly improve HbA1c (mean improvement of 1%) and quality of life at 6 months in 169 individuals with type 1 diabetes and inadequate glycemic control. The skills course

taught participants to dose insulin by matching it to desired carbohydrate intake on a meal-by-meal basis.[28]

The optimal macronutrient composition of the diet in patients with type 1 diabetes is unknown. As such, dietary recommendations are customized to a patient's ability and lifestyle. The increasing use of continuous glucose monitors (CGMs) in patients with type 1 diabetes has allowed the close monitoring of glycemic responses to various foods and facilitated individualization of diet and insulin doses.

Management of Insulin Dosing and Carbohydrates in Type 1 Diabetes

Patients with type 1 diabetes are commonly prescribed a basal-bolus insulin therapy, as this regimen best mimics physiologic insulin release. The basal insulin is a long-acting insulin taken once per day, intended to maintain normal blood glucose while fasting, while the bolus insulin refers to a rapid-acting insulin taken at mealtimes and snacks to counteract postprandial hyperglycemia (Figure 18-3).

Most patients with type 1 diabetes require about 50% of their total daily insulin as basal insulin and 50% as prandial insulin (split across meals and snacks). This "basal-bolus" regimen can be achieved with injection of two types of insulin (long-acting and rapid-acting) or with continuous infusion of rapid-acting insulin via pump therapy. Pump therapy usually allows more flexibility in lifestyle and facilitates frequent prandial boluses for meals and snacks along the day. When integrated with a CGM, the "closed-loop" pump systems can offer adaptative algorithms to eating and activity patterns, but they still optimally require the individual with diabetes to actively inform the system to deliver a bolus for carbohydrate intake.

The prandial insulin (by pump or injection) is often dosed using an insulin-to-carbohydrate ratio (ICR), which represents the grams of carbohydrate that are covered (or utilized) by 1 unit of insulin. The ICR is based on insulin sensitivity, which varies across individuals (largely determined by body mass index), can vary according to time of day, and is affected by factors such as physical activity and use of certain medications (for example, corticosteroids). The ICR is determined by a diabetes provider upon review of the patient's fingerstick blood glucose values or continuous glucose monitor tracings and total insulin requirements. For example, insulin resistant patients may require an ICR of 1 to 6 (1 unit insulin for every 6 grams of carbohydrate), while insulin sensitive patients may require an ICR of 1 to 12. Patients calculate how much rapid-acting insulin to administer at each meal based on their ICR and the number of total carbohydrates they plan to eat (this includes sugar, starch, and fiber) (Table 18-2).

In addition to nutrition labels, there are many tools and apps available to assist with carbohydrate counting (for example, the U.S. Department of Agriculture's Food Composition Database has nutrition information for thousands of foods).[29] Rapid-acting insulin starts working about 15 minutes after injection (or pump bolus), reaches peak effect in about 1 hour, and continues to work for 2 to 4 hours. Due to the onset time of 15 minutes, patients are advised to take their rapid-acting insulin dose

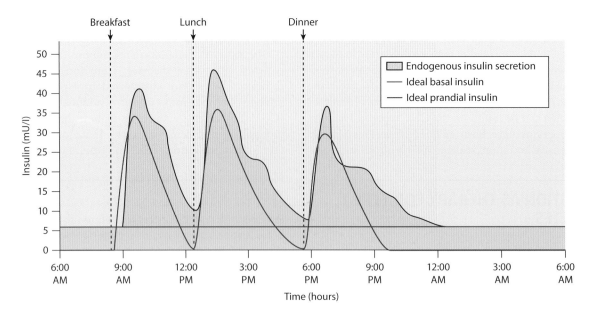

FIGURE 18-3 • Representation of basal and prandial insulin dosing.
(Reproduced with permission from Tintinalli JE, Ma OJ, Yealy DM, et al. Type 1 diabetes mellitus. In: *Tintinalli's Emergency Medicine: A Comprehensive Study Guide*. 9th ed. New York, NY: McGraw Hill; 2019.)

Food	Carbohydrates	Insulin dose using ICR of 1:6 (grams carbohydrates divided by ICR)	Insulin dose using ICR of 1:12 (grams carbohydrates divided by ICR)
Medium-sized navel orange or 1 cup 2% fat milk	12 gm	2 units	1 unit
1 slice whole grain (100% whole wheat) bread	21 gm	3.5 units[a]	1.75 units[a]
1 cup oatmeal squares cereal	44 gm	7.3 units[a]	3.6 units[a]

TABLE 18-2 • Carbohydrate content of selected foods and insulin dose using insulin-to-carbohydrate ratio (ICR)

[a]Rapid-acting insulin injections by pen or vial can only be administered in 1-unit (or sometimes 0.5-unit) increments, so the dose may need to be rounded up or down. In contrast, pump systems can deliver very precise insulin dosage amount (usually to the 0.1 unit).

15 minutes prior to eating. It is important to note that a meal high in protein and fat may change how quickly carbohydrates are absorbed, which may impact blood glucose levels and timing of insulin administration. For example, adding peanut butter (low-carbohydrate, high-fat) to bread results in a lower rise in blood sugar compared to eating bread alone. In contrast, SSB or juices are absorbed very rapidly, often much quicker than can be matched by the rapid-insulin injection or bolus, even if administered 15 minutes before. In general liquid-form carbohydrates

are absorbed and raise blood glucose faster than their full-form food origin (for example apple juice versus one full apple), and the liquid form often represents a larger amount of carbohydrates (for example 12 oz of orange juice is the equivalent of 6 medium oranges). Thus, recommendations are to limit SSB/juice intake, except to treat hypoglycemia (in which case the rapid absorption is the desired effect) (see Box 18-2).

Overall, in addition to the carbohydrate total content, people with type 1 diabetes need to pay attention to the form of

BOX 18-2

Treatment of Hypoglycemia ("15-15 Rule")

If blood glucose < 70 mg/dL, consume 15 grams of fast-acting carbohydrate to raise blood glucose and check it after 15 minutes. If it is still < 70 mg/dL, have another serving. Repeat these steps until blood glucose is at least 70 mg/dL.

Examples:
- 4 ounces (1/2 cup) of juice or regular soda (not diet)
- 1 tablespoon of sugar, honey, or corn syrup
- 3–4 glucose tablets or 1 tube glucose gel
- Hard candies, jellybeans, or gumdrops (see nutrition label for how much to eat).

the food (liquid or food), the fiber content, and the fat and protein content of the food they consume, and they often need to adjust the insulin dose or delivery timing/mode at every meal.

NUTRITION AS THERAPY FOR TYPE 2 DIABETES

Diet is a critical behavioral aspect of type 2 diabetes treatment and is a key component in the comprehensive care of patients with type 2 diabetes. As in type 1 diabetes, MNT is recommended for all individuals with type 2 diabetes. It is recommended that MNT involve a series of 3 to 6 encounters with a registered dietician lasting 45 to 90 minutes within 6 months and ideally should begin at the time of diagnosis. In individuals with type 2 diabetes and overweight/obesity, the individualized eating plan should result in an energy deficit to help achieve moderate weight loss goals.[30]

In patients with newly diagnosed type 2 diabetes, randomized trials of MNT have demonstrated HbA1c reductions of 2%; in patients with a longer duration of type 2 diabetes, HbA1c reduction was found to be 1%.[31–33] The Look AHEAD trial, which examined whether an intensive lifestyle intervention for weight loss would decrease cardiovascular morbidity and mortality in patients with type 2 diabetes, found that weight loss (8.6% vs. 0.7% at 1 years; 6.0% vs. 3.5% at median 9.6 years of follow-up) and HbA1c reduction were greater in the intervention than control group. In addition, 11.5% of participants in the intervention group compared to 2% in the control group achieved at least partial diabetes remission.[34] Although the Look AHEAD study did not find that the intensive lifestyle intervention reduced the rate of cardiovascular events, the participants in the lifestyle intervention arm required fewer medications for their glycemic control and blood pressure management.

Studies of a variety of eating plans have demonstrated efficacy in achieving weight loss over 1–2 years in patients with type 2 diabetes. Structured low-calorie meal plans with meal replacements, Mediterranean diet, vegetarian or vegan, very low-fat, DASH, and low-carbohydrate meals plans have been studied and shown to be effective.[30] There is limited data on the efficacy of intermittent fasting on outcomes in patients with type 2 diabetes. A recent study of individuals with obesity found that time-restricted eating with calorie restriction was not more beneficial with regard to reduction in body weight, body fat, or metabolic risk factors compared to daily calorie restriction alone.[35] No one dietary plan has been shown to be superior, and professional organizations emphasize the importance of providing individualized meal plan guidance that considers the health status, personal preferences, and abilities of the patient.

No ideal mix of macronutrients has been identified for patients with type 2 diabetes, and it is recommended that macronutrient proportions be individualized.[36] As the glycemic response to foods containing carbohydrates varies greatly, the quality of carbohydrates is an important component of an individualized eating plan. While there has been interest in using glycemic index (a system of assigning a number to

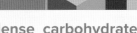

Examples of nutrient-dense carbohydrate sources

- Legumes (beans, peas, lentils)
- Steel cut or old-fashioned oats
- Fruits such as apples, blueberries, and strawberries

carbohydrate-containing foods according to how much each food increases blood glucose) and glycemic load (similar to glycemic index but also accounts for the grams of carbohydrate in a serving) in the dietary management of type 2 diabetes, reviews of the literature did not find a significant impact on HbA1c. It is recommended that SSB be replaced with water as much as possible, which means avoiding sodas and other beverages that may contain sugar, including coffee (if sugar is added), iced tea, energy drinks, and fruit juices. It is recommended that individuals focus on nutrient-dense carbohydrate sources that are high in fiber and minimally processed (see Box 18-3).

A meta-analysis found that high-protein eating plans (25–32% vs. 15–20% of total energy) resulted in 0.5% greater HbA1c improvement and 2 kg greater weight loss than eating plans containing a lower proportion of protein. No optimal amount of dietary fat for treatment of type 2 diabetes has been reported, however it is recommended that the percent of total calories from saturated fats be limited in the optic to reduce risk of cardiovascular diseases that are common complications in people with diabetes (see also Chapter 20, "Cardiovascular Disease"). Reduction of saturated fats to less than 10% of calories is recommended by replacing saturated fats with monounsaturated and polyunsaturated fatty acids. No specific herbal or nonherbal supplements are recommended for patients with diabetes without underlying deficiencies. Nutritional recommendations for adults with diabetes are summarized in Figure 18-4.

NUTRITION AS THERAPY FOR GESTATIONAL DIABETES

Gestational diabetes management begins with non-pharmacologic treatments such as dietary modification, exercise, monitoring of blood glucose, and maternal weight gain management. Many professional organizations (ADA, Endocrine Society, ACOG) recommend MNT by a registered dietitian and exercise as the initial treatment of gestational diabetes. Depending on the population, studies suggest that 70–85% of women diagnosed with gestational diabetes can be managed with dietary and lifestyle modifications alone.[37]

The goals for MNT in pregnancy affected by gestational diabetes should be to improve glycemic control while meeting energy and nutrient needs while also supporting appropriate gestational weight gain to optimize both perinatal and fetal outcomes. Box 18-4 lists the blood glucose targets recommended by the Fifth International Workshop-Conference on Gestational Diabetes Mellitus.[38]

General dietary guidelines

- Vegetable, fruits, whole grains, legumes, low-fat dairy products and food higher in fiber and lower in glycemic content; optimal diet composition and eating pattens are not known

Fat in diet (optimal % of diet is not known; should be individualized)

- Mediterranean-style diet rich in monounsaturated and polyunsaturated fatty acids
- Minimal or no trans fat consumption

Carbohydrate in diet (optimal % of diet is not known; should be individualized)

- Monitor carbohydrate intake in regard to calories and set limits for meals to reduce postprandial glycemia
- Avoid fructose- and sucrose-containing beverages and minimize consumption of foods with added sugar that may displace healthier, more nutrient-dense food choices and elevate postprandial glycemia
- Estimate grams of carbohydrate in diet for flexible insulin dosing (type 1 DM and insulin-dependent type 2 DM)
- Consider using glycemic index to predict how consumption of a particular food may affect blood glucose

Protein in diet (optimal % of diet is not known; should be individualized)

Other components

- Reduced-calorie and nonnutritive sweeteners may be useful
- Routine supplements of vitamins, antioxidants, or trace elements not supported by evidence
- Sodium intake as advised for general population

FIGURE 18-4 • Nutritional recommendations for adults with diabetes. (Reproduced with permission from Loscalzo J, Fauci A, Kasper D, Hauser S, Longo D, Jameson JL. Diabetes mellitus: management and therapies. In *Harrison's Principles of Internal Medicine*, 21 ed. New York: McGraw Hill; 2022.)

According to the Academy of Nutrition and Dietetics Evidenced Based Practice Guidelines for Gestational Diabetes,[39] the calorie prescription and meal plan should be tailored to the individual as there is no definitive research that identifies a specific optimal calorie intake for women with gestational diabetes or suggests that their calorie needs are different from those of pregnant women without gestational diabetes. The Dietary Reference Intakes for all pregnant women, including those with gestational diabetes, recommends a minimum of 175 g carbohydrate, a minimum of 71 g/protein (or 1.1 g/kg/day) and 28 g fiber. The amount and type of carbohydrate should be individualized based on nutrition assessment, treatment goals, blood glucose response, and patient needs. The distribution of meals and snacks should be individualized as well based on blood glucose levels, physical activity, and medication, if any, and adjusted as needed. Three meals and two or more snacks daily help to distribute carbohydrate intake and reduce postprandial blood glucose elevations.

Unless contraindicated, women with gestational diabetes should be encouraged to engage in a goal to achieve daily moderate exercise of 30 minutes or more per day at least 5 days/week (or 150 minutes/week). In addition to a healthy diet, exercise can help improve blood glucose control and achieve weight gain recommendations. Both aerobic exercise and non-weight-bearing exercise (e.g., stretching, swimming, and yoga) have been shown to lower blood glucose levels in women with gestational diabetes.

● SUMMARY: CLINICAL PRACTICE GUIDELINES

In 2019, the ADA released a consensus report on nutrition therapy for adults with diabetes or prediabetes. The aim of the consensus was to provide professionals "with evidence-based guidance about individualizing nutrition therapy for adults with diabetes or prediabetes."[26] Nutrition counseling should aim towards improving glycemic targets, achieving weight goals, and improving cardiovascular risk factors. It is recommended that all adults with type 1 or type 2 diabetes be referred to MNT at diagnosis and as needed throughout life and that all adults with prediabetes and overweight/obesity be referred to an intensive lifestyle intervention program that includes individualized goal-setting components.

The ADA guidelines highlight that a variety of eating patterns are acceptable for diabetes management and that health care providers should focus on key factors that are common among the different patterns: (1) emphasize nonstarchy vegetables; (2) minimize added sugars and refined grains; and (3) choose whole foods over highly processed foods. In patients with type 2 diabetes, 5% weight loss is recommended to achieve clinical benefit; 15% weight loss should be targeted when feasible and safe to achieve optimal outcomes. The ADA uses the Diabetes Plate Method to create healthy meals composed of vegetables, protein, and carbohydrates (Figure 18-5).

BOX 18-4

Glucose Targets in Gestational Diabetes Mellitus

- Fasting glucose < 95 mg/dL (5.3 mmol/L) and either
- One-hour postprandial glucose < 140 mg/dL (7.8 mmol/L) or
- Two-hour postprandial glucose < 120 mg/dL (6.7 mmol/L)

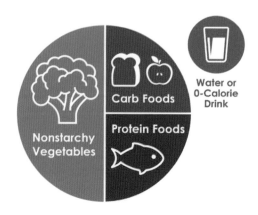

FIGURE 18-5 • Diabetes plate method. (Reproduced from American Diabetes Association. https://diabetes.org/healthy-living/recipes-nutrition/eating-well)

THREE TAKE-HOME POINTS

1. Diabetes mellitus is a group of metabolic diseases characterized by hyperglycemia resulting from defects in insulin secretion, insulin action, or both. Diabetes is the seventh-leading cause of death in the United States. The disease disproportionately affects American Indians, Alaska Natives, non-Hispanic blacks, and people of Hispanic origin. Patients with type 1 diabetes have absolute insulin deficiency and are treated pharmacologically with insulin. The predominant mechanism underlying type 2 diabetes is insulin resistance.

2. It is recommended that adults with overweight/obesity at high risk of type 2 diabetes be referred to an intensive lifestyle behavior change program with a goal to achieve and maintain 7% loss of initial body weight and at least 150 minutes/week of moderate intensity physical activity (such as brisk walking). Studies of a variety of eating plans have demonstrated efficacy in achieving weight loss over 1–2 years. As such, various eating patterns can be considered to prevent diabetes in individuals with prediabetes, and recommendations should be tailored to address individual nutrition needs based on personal and cultural preferences, health literacy and numeracy, and food access.

3. Medical nutrition therapy (MNT) is recommended for all individuals with type 1 and type 2 diabetes, has been proven to reduce HbA1c, and is fundamental in the overall diabetes management plan. MNT is the primary treatment for gestational diabetes and is sufficient to achieve adequate blood glucose control in the majority of pregnancies affected by gestational diabetes. MNT is an evidence-based application of the nutrition care process provided by a registered dietitian nutritionist. Essential components of MNT are assessment, nutrition diagnosis, interventions (e.g., education and counseling), and monitoring with ongoing follow-up to support long-term lifestyle changes, evaluate outcomes, and modify interventions as needed.

CASE STUDY 1 ANSWERS

1. Dietary counseling would be provided using a patient-centered approach. After understanding the patient's goals, specific recommendations for this patient could include: choose non-starchy vegetables and whole grains instead of potatoes and refined grains, choose whole fruits in lieu of fruit juice, and switch to low-fat dairy products. Additional general recommendations could include: avoid all sugar-sweetened beverages; minimize added sugar; choose whole foods over processed foods; consider replacing red meat with nuts, legumes, poultry, and fish; and choose healthful polyunsaturated fats (sunflower oil, salmon, walnuts, soybeans) and monounsaturated fats (olive oil, avocado, almonds) in place of saturated fats, trans fats, and refined carbohydrates and sugar wherever possible (Mediterranean-style diet). Although it is not a guarantee, some patients are able to reduce or stop using diabetes medication after making healthy lifestyle changes.

2. At least 5% weight loss is recommended for patients with type 2 diabetes and overweight/obesity (can target up to 15% weight loss if feasible and safe). In addition to diet change, he could be referred to an intensive lifestyle behavior change program and should be advised to gradually increase physical activity to at least 150 minutes per week of moderate intensity activity. Dietary changes and increased physical activity have independent benefits for diabetes, so even if he does not achieve his goal weight loss, he will gain health benefits from increased physical activity.

CASE STUDY 2 ANSWERS

1. B

2. A, B, C, D, E

Foods containing carbohydrates with various proportions of sugars, starches, and fiber have a wide range of effects on glycemia. Foods high in fiber, such as legumes and fruits, result in an extended rise and fall of blood glucose, while refined sugar results in a rapid rise and fall in blood glucose. SSB and juices, which are absorbed very quickly, result in a very rapid rise and fall in blood glucose. The total number of carbohydrates (grams) in a meal has a significant effect on the degree of postprandial hyperglycemia, however the protein and/or fat content of the meal may change how quickly carbohydrates are absorbed and the overall glycemic postprandial excursion.

REFERENCES

1. ACOG Practice Bulletin No. 190: Gestational diabetes mellitus. *Obstet Gynecol*. 2018;131(2):e49-e64.

2. American Diabetes Association. Classification and diagnosis of diabetes: standards of medical care in diabetes-2021. *Diabetes Care*. 2021;44(Suppl 1):S15-S33.

3. Prevention CfDCa. National Diabetes Statistics Report. Available at: https://www.cdc.gov/diabetes/data/statistics-report/index.html. Accessed July 1, 2022.

4. Shah NS, Wang MC, Freaney PM, et al. Trends in gestational diabetes at first live birth by race and ethnicity in the US, 2011-2019. *JAMA*. 2021;326(7):660-669.

5. Malik VS, Popkin BM, Bray GA, Després JP, Willett WC, Hu FB. Sugar-sweetened beverages and risk of metabolic syndrome and type 2 diabetes: a meta-analysis. *Diabetes Care*. 2010;33(11):2477-2483.

6. Hu FB, Malik VS. Sugar-sweetened beverages and risk of obesity and type 2 diabetes: epidemiologic evidence. *Physiol Behav*. 2010;100(1):47-54.

7. Loscalzo J FA, Kasper D, Hauser S, Longo D, Jameson J. Diabetes Mellitus: Diagnosis, Classification, and Pathophysiology. In *Harrison's Principles of Internal Medicine*, 21 ed. McGraw Hill; 2022.

8. Molina PE. *Endocrine Pancreas*. In Endocrine Physiology, 5 ed. McGraw Hill; 2018.

9. Pan XR, Li GW, Hu YH, et al. Effects of diet and exercise in preventing NIDDM in people with impaired glucose tolerance: the Da Qing IGT and Diabetes Study. *Diabetes Care*. 1997;20(4):537-544.

10. Tuomilehto J, Lindström J, Eriksson JG, et al. Prevention of type 2 diabetes mellitus by changes in lifestyle among subjects with impaired glucose tolerance. *N Engl J Med*. 2001;344(18):1343-1350.

11. Diabetes Prevention Program Research Group; Knowler WC, Barrett-Connor E, Fowler SE, et al. Reduction in the incidence of type 2 diabetes with lifestyle intervention or metformin. *N Engl J Med*. 2002;346(6):393-403.

12. Kosaka K, Noda M, Kuzuya T. Prevention of type 2 diabetes by lifestyle intervention: a Japanese trial in IGT males. *Diabetes Res Clin Prac*. 2005;67(2):152-162.

13. Ramachandran A, Snehalatha C, Mary S, et al. The Indian Diabetes Prevention Programme shows that lifestyle modification and metformin prevent type 2 diabetes in Asian Indian subjects with impaired glucose tolerance (IDPP-1). *Diabetologia*. 2006;49(2):289-297.

14. Bo S, Ciccone G, Baldi C, et al. Effectiveness of a lifestyle intervention on metabolic syndrome. A randomized controlled trial. *J Gen Intern Med*. 2007;22(12):1695-1703.

15. Penn L, White M, Oldroyd J, Walker M, Alberti KG, Mathers JC. Prevention of type 2 diabetes in adults with impaired glucose tolerance: the European Diabetes Prevention RCT in Newcastle upon Tyne, UK. *BMC Public Health*. 2009;9:1-14.

16. Saito T, Watanabe M, Nishida J, et al. Lifestyle modification and prevention of type 2 diabetes in overweight Japanese with impaired fasting glucose levels: a randomized controlled trial. *Arch Intern Med*. 2011;171(15):1352-1360.

17. Uusitupa M, Khan TA, Viguiliouk E, et al. Prevention of Type 2 diabetes by lifestyle changes: a systematic review and meta-analysis. *Nutrients*. 2019;11(11):2611.

18. Balk EM, Earley A, Raman G, Avendano EA, Pittas AG, Remington PL. Combined diet and physical activity promotion programs to prevent type 2 diabetes among persons at increased risk: a systematic review for the community preventive services task force. *Ann Intern Med*. 2015;163(6):437-451.

19. Li G, Zhang P, Wang J, et al. The long-term effect of lifestyle interventions to prevent diabetes in the China Da Qing Diabetes Prevention Study: a 20-year follow-up study. *Lancet*. 2008;371(9626):1783-1789.

20. Perreault L, Pan Q, Mather KJ, et al. Effect of regression from prediabetes to normal glucose regulation on long-term reduction in diabetes risk: results from the diabetes prevention program outcomes study. *Lancet*. 2012;379(9833):2243-2251.

21. Knowler WC, Fowler SE, Hamman RF, et al. 10-year follow-up of diabetes incidence and weight loss in the diabetes prevention program outcomes study. *Lancet*. 2009;374(9702):1677-1686.

22. Neamah HH, Sebert Kuhlmann AK, Tabak RG. Effectiveness of program modification strategies of the diabetes prevention program: a systematic review. *Diabetes Edu*. 2016;42(2):153-165.

23. Johnson M, Jones R, Freeman C, et al. Can diabetes prevention programmes be translated effectively into real-world settings and still deliver improved outcomes? A synthesis of evidence. *Diabet Med: a journal of the British Diabetic Association*. 2013;30(1):3-15.

24. Estruch R, Ros E, Salas-Salvadó J, et al. Primary prevention of cardiovascular disease with a mediterranean diet supplemented with extra-virgin olive oil or nuts. *N Engl J Med*. 2018;378(25):e34.

25. Salas-Salvadó J, Bulló M, Babio N, et al. Reduction in the incidence of type 2 diabetes with the mediterranean diet: results of the PREDIMED-Reus nutrition intervention randomized trial. *Diabetes Care*. 2011;34(1):14-19.

26. Evert AB, Dennison M, Gardner CD, et al. Nutrition therapy for adults with diabetes or prediabetes: a consensus report. *Diabetes Care*. 2019;42(5):731-754.

27. Franz MJ, MacLeod J, Evert A, et al. Academy of Nutrition and Dietetics Nutrition Practice Guideline for Type 1 and Type 2 Diabetes in Adults: systematic review of evidence for medical nutrition therapy effectiveness and recommendations for integration into the nutrition care process. *J Acad Nutr Diet*. 2017;117(10):1659-1679.

28. Group DS. Training in flexible, intensive insulin management to enable dietary freedom in people with type 1 diabetes: dose adjustment for normal eating (DAFNE) randomised controlled trial. *BMJ*. 2002;325(7367):746.

29. American Diabetes Association. *Carb counting and diabetes*. Available at: https://www.diabetes.org/healthy-living/recipes-nutrition/understanding-carbs/carb-counting-and-diabetes. Accessed July 1, 2022.

30. Draznin B, Aroda VR, Bakris G, et al. 5. Facilitating behavior change and well-being to improve health outcomes: standards of medical care in diabetes-2022. *Diabetes Care*. 2022;45(Suppl 1):S60-S82.

31. UK Prospective Diabetes Study 7: response of fasting plasma glucose to diet therapy in newly presenting type II diabetic patients, UKPDS Group. *Metabolism*. 1990;39(9):905-912.

32. Andrews RC, Cooper AR, Montgomery AA, et al. Diet or diet plus physical activity versus usual care in patients with newly diagnosed type 2 diabetes: the Early ACTID randomised controlled trial. *Lancet*. 2011;378(9786):129-139.

33. Coppell KJ, Kataoka M, Williams SM, Chisholm AW, Vorgers SM, Mann JI. Nutritional intervention in patients with type 2 diabetes who are hyperglycaemic despite optimised drug treatment—Lifestyle Over and Above Drugs in Diabetes (LOADD) study: randomised controlled trial. *BMJ.* 2010;341:c3337.

34. Gregg EW, Chen H, Wagenknecht LE, et al. Association of an intensive lifestyle intervention with remission of type 2 diabetes. *JAMA.* 2012;308(23):2489-2496.

35. Liu D, Zhang H. Calorie restriction with or without time-restricted eating in weight loss. Reply. *N Engl J Med.* 2022;387(3):281.

36. Wheeler ML, Dunbar SA, Jaacks LM, et al. Macronutrients, food groups, and eating patterns in the management of diabetes: a systematic review of the literature, 2010. *Diabetes Care.* 2012;35(2):434-445.

37. Johns EC, Denison FC, Norman JE, Reynolds RM. Gestational diabetes mellitus: mechanisms, treatment, and complications. *Trends Endocrinol Metab: TEM.* 2018;29(11):743-754.

38. Metzger BE, Buchanan TA, Coustan DR, et al. Summary and recommendations of the Fifth International Workshop-Conference on Gestational Diabetes Mellitus. *Diabetes Care.* 2007;30(Suppl 2):S251-S260.

39. Duarte-Gardea MO, Gonzales-Pacheco DM, Reader DM, et al. Academy of Nutrition and Dietetics Gestational Diabetes Evidence-Based Nutrition Practice Guideline. *J Acad Nutr Diet.* 2018;118(9):1719-1742.

chapter 19

Stroke and Hypertension

Aleksandra Pikula, MD, DipABPN, DipABLM / Chetan P. Phadke, BPhT, DRPT, PHD / Andrée LeRoy, MD FAAPMR, DipABLM / Elizabeth Pegg Frates, MD FACLM DipABLM

Chapter Outline

CASE STUDY 1: ISCHEMIC STROKE

A 56-year-old-woman presents with acute language deficits and a right (R) sided weakness. On clinical examination, she has an elevated blood pressure (systolic blood pressure [SBP] 145 mm Hg and diastolic blood pressure [DBP] 85 mm Hg). A head computer tomography (CT)/CT angiography (CTA) confirms left middle cerebral artery occlusion and left internal carotid artery atherosclerosis. She was treated with endovascular therapy, and her language deficits improved, but she remained moderately weak on the R side.

On the review of lifestyle habits, the patient reports that she works night shifts. She does not smoke and does not drink alcohol. Her diet consists mostly of processed food from the local stores (pastries, cured meat, yogurts, grilled chicken, pizza, fried fish, or some pre-made salads). She usually drinks three cups of coffee with artificial sweeteners to help her stay awake during the day. She does not participate in any specific exercise programs, but she walks daily.

1. What are the risk factors contributing to this patient's ischemic stroke?

2. What dietary changes would you recommend to this patient to prevent a second stroke?

CASE STUDY 2: HEMORRHAGIC STROKE

A 61-year-old-man with a history of poorly controlled hypertension (HTN), was recently admitted with R thalamic intracranial hemorrhage (ICH). On the day of the admission, he was found to be confused with severe L sided hemiplegia. Over time, he improved and was transferred to rehabilitation. The stroke workup also revealed that he has a small intracranial aneurysm.

In addition, the patient reported poor compliance with prescribed medications for hypertension (diagnosed 5 years before). He has been a heavy smoker for over three decades but denied any illicit drug use. He is a manager at the local bank, which he described as a very stressful job and a major reason for his need

to drink alcohol to relax. He reports drinking a six pack of beer a night and sometimes more on the weekends. He lives alone and was never interested in cooking. He buys food mostly on the go (sandwiches, pasta, soups, snacks), and eats at his desk for lunch, and in front of the TV/streaming screen in the evenings, which includes snacking on things such as chips, crackers, pretzels, and popcorn.

1. What are the risk factors contributing to this patient's uncontrolled HTN?
2. List dietary interventions or adjustments the patient can follow to optimize the outcomes of uncontrolled hypertension.

INTRODUCTION

Strokes are emerging as a major global public health challenge. A mostly heterogeneous condition, stroke can be caused by a wide range of disease processes and pathological mechanisms. More importantly, 10 potentially modifiable risk factors are collectively linked to ~ 90% of the population attributable risk of stroke in each major region of the world, among different race-ethnic groups, in both sexes, and at all ages.[1] Among all the factors, *hypertension (HTN)* is the single most important modifiable risk factor for all cerebrovascular diseases [ischemic stroke (IS), intracerebral hemorrhage (ICH), and vascular cognitive impairment (VCI)], while an unhealthy *diet* is among the 10 factors as well. Therefore, the importance of nutrition, as an evidence-based approach for prevention of both hypertension and stroke, cannot be overemphasized. In this chapter, we will specifically focus on **nutrition** as a modifiable lifestyle factor and how it contributes to the risk of hypertension and stroke.

STROKE: EPIDEMIOLOGY, TYPES, AND RISK FACTORS

From 1990 to 2019, the absolute number of incident strokes increased by 70%, prevalent strokes by 85%, and deaths from stroke by 43%, with 12 million new cases of stroke, and 6.5 million deaths worldwide from stroke.[2] While the overall mortality rates have decreased as a result of improvements in stroke detection and highly advanced acute stroke management in an area of the world with access to this type of care, there has been a worrisome ~ 25% increase in the incidence of stroke among younger adults over the past decade.[3] This is partially explained by the higher burden of traditional risk factors (including hypertension) among younger population; all likely as a result of introduction of the modern lifestyle in the last few decades.[4] Therefore, prevention is *the most* effective strategy for reducing the health and economic consequences of cerebrovascular diseases and its risk factors, and of all strategies,

dietary modification is one key approach to reduce incidence of stroke, and to prevent hypertension or control blood pressure in affected individuals.

Definition of Stroke

Stroke is a clinically defined syndrome with an acute focal neurological deficit attributed to vascular injury, which could be manifested as an infarction or hemorrhage within the central nervous system and is primarily confirmed by neuroimaging.[5,6] Most strokes are ischemic (85%), predominantly caused as a result of vessel occlusion from the embolus or thrombus due to (a) small vessel arteriosclerosis (lacunar strokes), (b) cardioembolic source (intracardiac thrombus, valve disease, atrial fibrillation, etc.), (c) large artery athero-thrombo-embolism (secondary to athero plaques or dissections), and (d) other determined (hypercoagulable state, inflammatory conditions, patent foramen ovale, monogenic conditions, etc.) or (e) other undetermined causes. Approximately 15% of strokes are the result of intracerebral hemorrhage, which can be (a) deep (basal ganglia, brainstem), cerebellar or lobar, and usually results from a vessel rupture due to deep perforator arteriopathies (hypertensive arteriosclerosis), or (b) lobar hemorrhages, mainly caused by cerebral amyloid angiopathy or arteriolosclerosis. A minority (15–20%) of all ICHs are caused by vessel ruptures due to macrovascular lesions (vascular malformations, aneurysms, cavernomas), venous sinus thrombosis, or other rarer conditions, mostly observed in younger patients (< 50 years).

Major Risks for Stroke

Cerebrovascular diseases are linked to various nonmodifiable and modifiable risk factors, such as diabetes mellitus, dyslipidemia, metabolic syndrome, obesity, atrial fibrillation (AFib), smoking, excessive alcohol use, and environmental risks such as diet, passive smoking, stress, and air pollution, but *hypertension* is the single most important modifiable risk factor for all.[1,2]

HYPERTENSION: EPIDEMIOLOGY AND RISK FACTORS[7]

As an independent medical condition and as a major risk factor for cerebrovascular and cardiovascular diseases, hypertension is a growing epidemic around the globe. Hypertension is the leading cause of death; with 10.4 million deaths per year. Currently, there are ~ 116 million people (1 in 2) with hypertension in the USA, but given its asymptomatic nature, people are often unaware of this diagnosis.[8] Hypertension is a well-established major risk factor for many other conditions in addition to stroke, including coronary artery disease, end-stage renal disease, peripheral vascular disease, retinopathy, and sexual dysfunction, and all interlinked to vascular damage.

Definition of Hypertension

In 2017, the ACC and the American Heart Association (AHA) lowered the blood pressures (BP) thresholds, and defined hypertension as BP at or above 130/80 mm Hg, and a normal BP as below 120/80 mm Hg[9] recorded on two or more occasions (https://www.nhlbi.nih.gov/health/high-blood-pressure/diagnosis). Figure 19-1 outlines hypertension classifications and recommended management approaches.[10]

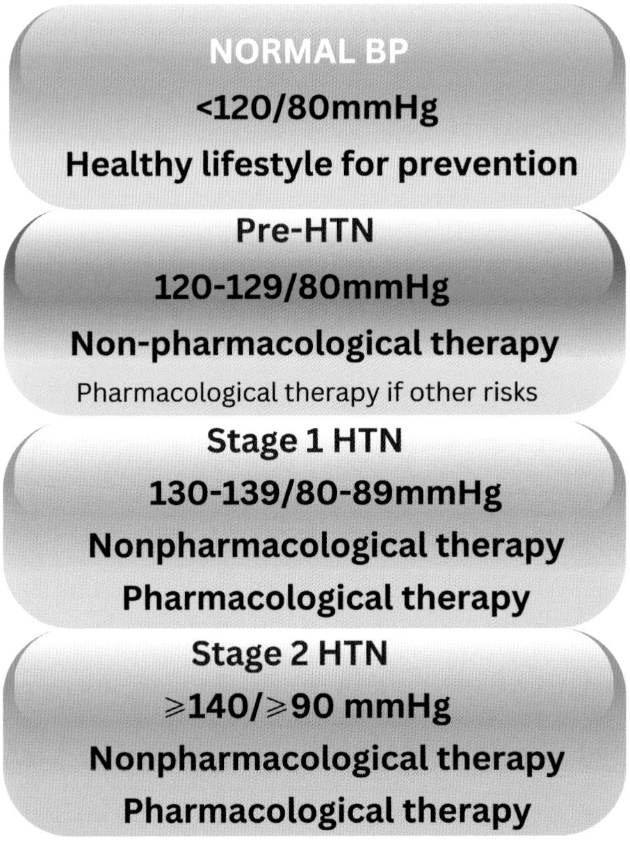

NORMAL BP
<120/80mmHg
Healthy lifestyle for prevention

Pre-HTN
120-129/80mmHg
Non-pharmacological therapy
Pharmacological therapy if other risks

Stage 1 HTN
130-139/80-89mmHg
Nonpharmacological therapy
Pharmacological therapy

Stage 2 HTN
≥140/≥90 mmHg
Nonpharmacological therapy
Pharmacological therapy

FIGURE 19-1 • Hypertension classifications and recommended management
BP, blood pressure; HTN, hypertension.

Risks for Hypertension

Although the causes of hypertension are complex and multifactorial, there is clear evidence that unbalanced dietary habits (consumption of high sodium, low potassium, and limited fruit and vegetable intake), physical inactivity, smoking, and excess alcohol consumption are major contributors to the development of hypertension and its complications.[9] A dietary pattern based on a frequent and high consumption of red and processed meats (high in sodium/saturated fat); fried food (high in sodium/saturated fat); refined grains (high in sugar); soft drinks and sweets; and low in fruits, vegetables, whole grains and omega-3 fatty acids have been associated with both hypertension and stroke.[11,12]

Given the interlinked risks for hypertension and stroke via dietary choices, in the following sections, we will illustrate the importance of nutrition through risk mechanisms and in prevention and management of both.[11,13]

HYPERTENSION AND STROKE— INTERLINKED RISK MECHANISMS

Since the 1950s, numerous population-based studies confirmed a strong correlation between hypertension and all stroke types.[9] In a large meta-analysis, the risk of stroke increased with increasing blood pressure, even with the pre-hypertension BP range. Lowering blood pressure to < 130 mm Hg in patients with hypertension[14] had been recommended for the primary and secondary stroke prevention to reduce the risk of first-ever stroke and prevent recurrent stroke.[9,12,14,15] But what are the pathophysiological mechanisms that would link the risks between hypertension and stroke? Among many, endothelial injury and atherosclerotic cascade, platelet activation and aggregation, as well as cardiometabolic changes, are described in more detail. Figure 19-2 depicts mechanistic links between hypertension and stroke.

Endothelial Injury and Atherosclerosis

Inflammation, oxidative stress and elevated blood pressure can all result in endothelial damage. A chronic exposure to elevated blood pressure increases the intraluminal pressure through sheer pressure in arteries leading to arterial endothelial injury that subsequently led to a cascade of pathophysiological progressive processes (remodeling, lipid infiltration, further inflammation), which can happen across the vascular tree (from aorta to small vessels in the brain). Atherosclerosis, if left uncorrected, can continue to advance from early stages where inflammatory cells migrate into the endothelial layer of the arterial wall and to mid-to late stage with a *scar formation or fibrotic cap and its rupture.*[16]

There are a number of factors that contribute individually and in combination to the atherosclerotic progression, such as insulin resistance, hyperglycemia, type 2 diabetes, hyperlipidemia, lack of physical exercise and overnutrition (including highly processed foods),[16] smoking, alcohol, stress, and inadequate sleep.[17] As mentioned, dietary patterns (especially transfat and high sodium intake) have been described to play a

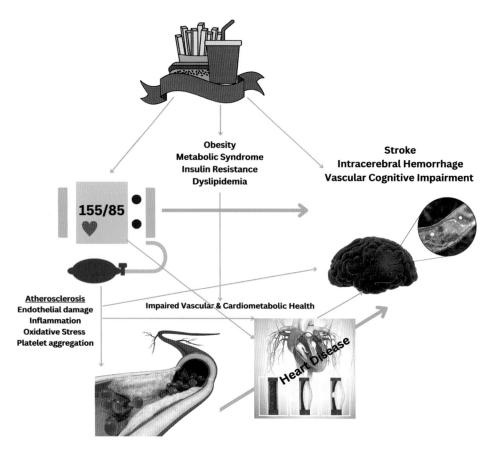

FIGURE 19-2 • The mechanistic links between hypertension and stroke 155/85 is the blood pressure (mm Hg).

major role in the progression of atherosclerotic plaques, hence closely linked to all the related consequences of its progression.

Platelet Activation and Aggregation

These play an integral role in endothelial hemostasis and thrombosis, and if endothelial homeostasis is challenged by chronic high BP, platelet activations can be accelerated as a result. Nutrients have a potential role in modifying endothelial dysfunction and progression of atherosclerosis, particularly through platelet function.[18] Foods with low glycemic index, garlic, dark chocolate, omega-3 PUFA, tomato juice (randomized controlled trials) and purple grape juice, and red wine (nonrandomized controlled feeding studies) all reduce platelet aggregation, while sugary and energy drinks have been shown to increase platelet aggregation.[18]

Cardiometabolic Changes

Eating a diet low in vegetables, fruits, and whole grains poses a risk for not only endothelial damage but chronic inflammation. Eating excessive protein and high amounts of unhealthy fat instead of fiber rich foods may lead to oxidative stress.[19] More importantly, poor eating habits have been associated with both, poor cardiometabolic health and AFib.[20] Ultimately, such diets (low fiber/high unhealthy fat) have also been associated with higher risk of coronary artery disease (see Chapter 20,

"Cardiovascular Disease"), which by itself has been linked to Afib, and stroke risk.[20]

⬤ HYPERTENSION AND STROKE PREVENTION AND MANAGEMENT— DIETARY PATTERNS

Lifestyle modifications[17,21] are fundamental initial steps in the prevention and treatment of hypertension and stroke. These strategies include a reduction in sodium intake, favoring healthy fats (and avoiding saturated and trans-fat), reduction in alcohol use, maintenance of healthy body weight, optimized physical activity (e.g., leisure, moderate, or vigorous), sleep hygiene and stress reduction through various methods (e.g., walking, meditation, or yoga). While the best results are achieved with implementation of all lifestyle strategies together, herein we focus on the evidence of the dietary patterns in prevention and management of hypertension and stroke. The existing randomized controlled trial (RCT) evidence suggests that some dietary patterns (Table 19-1) such as the Dietary Approaches to Stop Hypertension (DASH) diet, the Mediterranean diet, and the Nordic diet are highly beneficial for BP reduction and stroke prevention. Higher adherence to these dietary patterns had been also linked to ~30% lower risk of stroke and cardiovascular diseases.[9]

TABLE 19-1 • Recommended dietary patterns for prevention of hypertension and stroke			
Food/drink intake	Dash diet	Mediterranean diet	Nordic diet
Fruits	High	High	High (wild berries)
Vegetables	High	High	High
Whole grains	Moderate	High	Moderate
Nuts	Moderate	Moderate	Moderate
Dairy	Moderate	Low to moderate	Low-fat dairy
Fats	Low	Moderate (olive oil)	Moderate (rapeseed oil)
Proteins	Poultry, fish	Fish, legumes, poultry	Fish, legumes
Red meat	Low	Low or no intake	Limited
Sweets (food/drinks)	Low	Minimal or none	Minimal
Alcohol	-	Moderate red wine	-

The DASH diet has been consistently endorsed by major health organizations [e.g., AHA, U.S. guidelines for treatment of high BP] as the most effective diet for controlling BP and treating hypertension. In 1997, the first DASH clinical trial (a controlled feeding trial) evaluated the effects of 3 different dietary patterns (controlled diet, fruits/vegetables diet, and combination diet) on BP levels over 8 weeks in 459 adults with SBP of < 160 mm Hg and DBP of 80–95 mm Hg.[22] The control diet consisted of a 7-day menu cycle with 21 meals at four calorie levels (1,600, 2,100, 2,600, and 3,100 kcal) and was identical at all centers, using the same brands of a given food, typical of the diets of a substantial number of Americans with higher content of fat-based food (meat) and less fruits and vegetables (on average one to two servings a day of each). The fruits/vegetables diet was geared to provide potassium and magnesium close to the 75th percentile of U.S. consumption and allowed more fruits and vegetables, but fewer snacks/sweets than the control diet; but this diet was similar to the control diet for rest of the allowed food items. The most effective "combination" diet, now termed the DASH diet, was based on a combination of high intake of fruits and vegetables (on average four to five servings a day, respectively), moderate intake of low-fat dairy products; it included whole grains, poultry, fish, and nuts; and was low in fats, red meat, sweets, and sugar-containing beverages. This diet was rich in potassium, magnesium, calcium, and fiber and was low in sodium, total fat, saturated fat, and cholesterol, but also slightly high in proteins. Among all participants, the DASH diet significantly lowered both SBP and DBP levels by a means of 5.5/3.0 mm Hg, compared to controls (controlled diet). BP-lowering effects of this diet were also rapid and visible in only 2 weeks of use, while changes in BP were even greater in participants with higher baseline BP or BMI. This was true for all subgroups (women, men, African Americans, non–African Americans, hypertensive, and non-hypertensive participants). Moreover, the combination of the DASH diet with additional reduction of dietary sodium, had even greater BP reduction (~11 mm Hg[9]) in an RCT.[23] Comparing the effects on blood pressure of three levels of sodium intake in two diets among adults with blood pressure > 120/80 mm Hg, including those with stage 1 HTN (SBP 140 to 159 mm Hg or DBP of

90 to 95 mm Hg). The three sodium levels were defined as high (a target of 150 mmol = 3,450 mg per day for an energy intake of 2,100 kcal, reflecting typical consumption in the United States in 1997), intermediate (a target of 2,300 mg per day, reflecting the upper limit of the national recommendations in 1997), and low (a target of 1,150 mg, reflecting a level that was hypothesized might produce an additional lowering of blood pressure) which was the one showing the greatest benefit on reduction of BP.

The Mediterranean Diet (MD) is a general term for dietary pattern (see also Chapter 20, "Cardiovascular Disease"), or rather lifestyle practiced in several regions close to the Mediterranean Sea. The diet itself has some similarities with the DASH Diet, such as high intake of fruits and vegetables, whole grains, legumes, and nuts, but is much more oriented to low intake of red meat, minimal intake of sweets, and no sugary drinks. Among the particularities, the MD includes a high intake of olive oil, seafood, and moderate amount of red wine, while the DASH diet focuses on adjustments and elimination of certain food items to achieve lower sodium intake, more dairy (nonfat or low fat), and allows higher intake of red meat. Inevitably, both diets have a higher intake of fibers and unsaturated fats and reduced intake of simple carbohydrates and saturated fats. A meta-analysis of three short-term randomized trials found that the effect of MD on BP was modest with SBP mean difference −3.02 mm Hg (95% confidence interval (CI): −3.47 to −2.58).[24] However, in a large randomized clinical trial, the Prevención con Dieta Mediterránea,[35] MD combined with supplemental food items (either extra-virgin olive oil or mixed nuts) reduced the risk of stroke. Importantly, the implementation of the MD in 772 subjects (55–80 years) who were at high risk for cardiovascular disease by other parameters, resulted in SBP reduction of 7.1 mm Hg, indicating higher impact of a healthy diet on BP reduction in patients with a higher burden of the risk factors.[9,12,24]

Both the DASH diet and MD rely on high intake of fruits and vegetables, equally rich in minerals, vitamins, and fibers. The combination of those nutrients plays an important role in reducing BP via several mechanisms, hence reducing the risk for stroke as a consequence. Specifically, the DASH diet used

2,300 mg of sodium a day and lowering sodium to 1,500 mg a day reduced BP even more.[23] Now, the AHA guidelines recommend sodium intake to < 2,400 mg/day, while further reduction to < 1,500 mg/day may be associated with even greater BP reduction, and lower stroke risk.[12,25]

In contrast, MD is high in fruits, vegetables, nuts, and unsaturated oils, but a number of food components such as higher levels of potassium (legumes, potato, chard, tomato), higher serum concentrations of lutein (from green veggies), and beta-cryptoxanthin (from yellow to orange fruits/veggies) have also been shown to improve endothelial function in a dose-dependent way.[9,13,24]

The Nordic Diet is mainly consumed in Nordic countries. It consists of foods of Nordic origin such as whole grains, rapeseed oil, wild berries, fruits, vegetables, fish, nuts, and low-fat dairy products. In the SYSDIET RCT sub-study (n = 37),[26] the Nordic diet when compared with a control diet (lower in dietary fiber and higher in dietary saturated fat) maintained for 12 weeks decreased 24-hour ambulatory BP in subjects with metabolic syndrome during weight-stable condition. Since the 24-hour urine sodium and potassium levels were unchanged, the authors proposed a potential effect of Nordic wild berries on the changes in BP. Interestingly, moderate consumption of berries,[27] which are packed with polyphenols, had contributed to the BP-lowering effect, and the Nordic diets that typically include these fruits. Fruits like purple grapes and certain berries, with high concentrations of flavonols, anthocyanins, and procyanidins in addition to polyphenols had been found to be effective in reducing cardiovascular risk, especially through lowering BP and optimizing vascular function.[26,27] Importantly, higher adherence to the Nordic diet[26,27] was also associated with higher reduction in stroke risk, but mostly ischemic (with a large vessel disease pattern), while the protective association was not true to hemorrhagic stroke.

● NOVEL MECHANISMS IN NUTRITION FOR HYPERTENSION

Microbiome Dysfunction

In more recent years, the role of nutritional therapy on HTN through addressing microbiome dysfunction has been a focus of many studies. Gut microbiome diversity and balance can be disrupted due to number of reasons, and this altered balance is often referred to as dysbiosis that has been associated with HTN.[28,29] Dietary approaches to restore this microbiome balance can be categorized into two: prebiotics and probiotics. Prebiotics are a group of nutrients (usually resistant starches) that feed our gut microbiome[30] and thus, support in restoring the balance of gut microbiome. Prebiotic rich foods include a variety of common whole grains, vegetables, and fruits (such as asparagus, garlic, onions, wheat, bananas, tomato, barley, soybean, peas, and beans).[30] Thus, an approach for promotion of microbiome restoration could be to advocate a diet rich in prebiotic rich foods and minimizing processed foods. Probiotics are a group of foods that contain microorganisms, such as bacteria similar to the beneficial bacteria that are native

to the human gut. Benefits of probiotic foods can be derived by consuming fermented foods found in different cultures (e.g., yogurt, buttermilk, tempeh) or consuming probiotic supplements that are packed with probiotic bacteria. Though not comprehensive, there is evidence indicating fermented foods can have a beneficial effect on hypertension and general well-being. However, since controlling the probiotic dose in supplement form is far easier, probiotic supplements have been well-studied in the literature. A recent meta-analysis of RCTs of probiotic treatment approaches for HTN found a modest but significant benefit of probiotics on lowering both systolic and diastolic blood pressure.[31] This study included a variety of approaches to deliver probiotics including probiotic-fortified foods in the form of bread, juice, milk, cheese, and probiotics packed into a tablet, powder, and capsule.[31]

Salt Sensitivity

Salt sensitivity is a physiological trait defined as an increased blood pressure sensitivity to salt consumption. Although there are no diagnostic tests available to determine if a person has this particular sensitivity, it is more common among women, elderly, African Americans, and those with insulin resistance and chronic renal disease.[32,33] The mechanism underlying this sensitivity has not been fully elucidated; however, it is an exploration that a patient can undertake by reducing their sodium intake to see if their BP lowers when all other factors including medications are unchanged.

Sugar Sensitivity

Hyperglycemia and hyperinsulinemia are both related to endothelial damage which results in increased arterial resistance and can thus promote development of HTN if left uncorrected.[16] In addition, hyperinsulinemia can promote sodium reabsorption and high blood glucose concentrations can increase arterial fluid volume both resulting in HTN.[16] Reducing sugar in a diet as an intervention can thus address the mechanism that leads to HTN. Sugar is frequently consumed in the form of liquids such as fruit juices and sweetened carbonated and energy drinks. Sugar-sweetened beverage intake causes immediate impairment in microvascular function[34] and is also associated with higher HTN rates, and consequently reduction in sugar sweetened beverages is critical for managing HTN.

● SPECIFICS ON NUTRITION IN STROKE PREVENTION

The relationship between nutrition and stroke is very complex because dietary patterns and specific food groups can affect almost all modifiable stroke risk factors, including HTN, but also diabetes, hyperlipidemia, and many others.[11] Importantly, Prevención con Dieta Mediterránea is one of the rare RCT that tested a dietary intervention and followed participants long enough to collect data on strokes incidence: they show that a healthy diet such as the Mediterranean-style diet[35] provides a protective effect against strokes (combined ischemic and hemorrhagic). Figure 19-3 outlines dietary

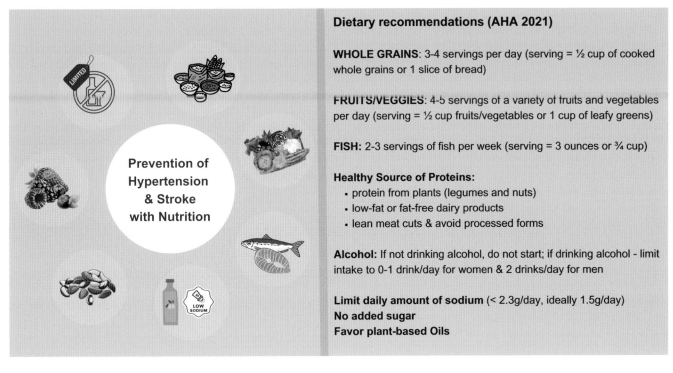

FIGURE 19-3 • Nutrition for prevention and management of hypertension and stroke[9,10,14,21] AHA, American Heart Association.

recommendations for prevention and management of hypertension and stroke. Observational studies suggest that in addition to the above-mentioned dietary patterns, other nutrients (dietary sodium and potassium, monounsaturated fat, long-chain omega-3 polyunsaturated fatty acids [PUFA}, and dietary fiber), and foods such as chocolate, fruits, vegetables, fish, tea, coffee, and nuts) may be beneficial against stroke,[11,21,25] while some like red meat and excess alcohol consumptions are not. The beneficial effect of nutrition in stroke prevention is likely mediated by the interlinked effect of overall dietary patterns and combination of food choices, and not one particular food. While such observations are not yet confirmed in clinical trials, the plausible effect of macro and micronutrient benefits on stroke pathophysiology is explained in more details and should be considered for prevention (primary and secondary) based on the current recommendations.

Micronutrients for Stroke Prevention

Sodium Excess intake of sodium (see common sources in Table 19-2) promotes water retention in the bloodstream, subsequently causing extra volume of blood to stiffen and narrow blood vessels, requiring the heart to work harder to maintain blood flow.[11] This eventually can lead to HTN and an increased risk of heart disease and stroke. So, a reduction of just 5 mm Hg in SBP was associated with ~15% reduction in stroke-related mortality. An umbrella review of 15 prospective cohort studies ($n = 942,140$) and 31 controlled trials ($n = 4,414$) across various cardiovascular disease (CVD) outcomes observed that the DASH dietary pattern was associated with ~20% reduction in

incidence of stroke, as well as with a healthy effect on regulation of blood lipid levels, glycemic control, and body weight reduction.[36] For common sources of sodium in the American Diet, see Table 19-2.

Potassium As a mineral, potassium counteracts sodium, and it lowers blood pressure. In a large meta-analysis, including observational studies totaling up to 333,250 participants,

TABLE 19-2 • Common sources (contributing to 40%) of sodium in the standard north american diet	
Adults >18 years age	**Children 6-18 years age**
Breads	Breads
Burritos (and tacos)	Cheese
Cheese	Chicken/poultry
Chicken	Cold cuts and cured meats
Cold cuts and cured meats	Mexican mixed dishes (American style)
Eggs	Milk
Pizza	Sandwiches
Sandwiches	Soups
Savoury snacks (chips, crackers, popcorn, pretzels)	Savoury snacks (chips, crackers, popcorn, pretzels)
Soups	

Created by authors based information from Centers for Disease Control and Prevention (CDC) website: https://www.cdc.gov/salt/index.htm

followed for up to at least 4 years (range 5–19 years) in whom 10,659 incident stroke events were observed,[37] higher intake of dietary potassium was associated with 20% reduced stroke incidence.[9] Thus, it is recommended to consume a healthy number of foods high in potassium (avocado, pomegranate, bananas, sweet potato, and others) to achieve current recommendation of potassium to meet > 4.7 g/day,[12] unless there are medical contra-indications to high potassium intake. As per the DASH or MD diet recommendations, four to five portions of vegetables or fruits a day, can provide ~ 3 g/day.[9]

Monounsaturated and Polyunsaturated Fats A large meta-analysis of observational studies showed that the effect of highest versus lowest dietary intake of monounsaturated fat (including olive oil) and in a subsequent study that higher long chain n-3 PUFA intake from seafood sources were associated with lower risk of stroke.[11,12,25] Therefore, recommending food rich in (a) monounsaturated such as olive, canola, or safflower oil and (b) polyunsaturated fatty acids such as fatty fish (salmon, trout, sardines), walnuts, chia seeds, or tofu is prudent for prevention of stroke risk.[11,12,21]

Whole Grains In a large systematic review of the prospective observation studies eating higher intake of at least three servings of whole grains has been shown to decrease stroke by ~20%.[38,39] However, less than 5% of American adults meet this recommendation. Apart from fibers, the micronutrients found in the whole kernel (wheat, rye, brown rice, quinoa, bulgur), such as vitamin B complex, vitamin E, magnesium, and selenium, are individually observed to be associated with lower risk of stroke.[21]

Fruits and Vegetables In a large meta-analysis of observational studies totaling ~ 2 million people from 95 studies, consumption of 10 servings of fruits and vegetables was associated with moderate stroke reduction.[12,25] The protective association consumption of fruits and vegetables and stroke was attributed to protective effect of the citrus fruits, apples/pears, and leafy vegetables, and all in the linear dose-response relationship, with risk of stroke decrease by 32% and 11% for every 200 g per day increment in fruit and vegetables consumption, respectively.[12] As with all other healthy food items, the protective effect of fruit and vegetables is likely achieved through numerous interlinked mechanisms leading to maintenance of healthy blood pressure, cholesterol, and sugar levels, hence, less HTN, dyslipidemia and T2DM. It is now recommended to eat a wide variety of fruit and vegetables to meet adequate essential nutrients and phytonutrients. All forms of fruits and vegetables (fresh, frozen, canned, and dried) can be incorporated in healthy dietary patterns. Importantly, frozen fruits and vegetables have a longer shelf-life than fresh forms, are ready-to-use, have similar nutrient content, and may have a lower price.[11]

Vitamins and Antioxidants There is no evidence to support the use of vitamins and antioxidant supplements for prevention of stroke.[12]

Fish As a key component of the Mediterranean-style diet, fish is a great source of healthy fat, a long-chain omega-3 fatty acid that has been inversely associated with cerebrovascular disease risk.[12,25] Moderate-quality evidence suggested that each 100-g/d increment in fish consumption was associated with approximately a 15% lower risk of stroke (RR 0.86; 95% CI: 0.75, 0.99[25]) in observational studies. If well sourced, nonfried fish like salmon, sardines, herrings, and other fatty fish, should be consumed two to three times per week as per current recommendations for stroke and cardiovascular prevention.[11,12]

Chocolate In a meta-analysis of 23 observational studies,[40] the most appropriate dose of chocolate consumption for reducing risk of cardiovascular disease was 45 g per week (RR 0.89; 95%CI 0.85 to 0.93). A reduction in stroke risk of 3.5% was observed with each increase in chocolate intake of 20 g, with the highest benefits seen for intake of 45 g of chocolate a week (~ 1 square of chocolate per day = 1 chocolate bar per week).

Tea and Coffee In a publication from UK Biobank cohort,[41] drinking 2 to 3 cups of coffee or 2 to 3 cups of tea per day (compared to no coffee/tea) was significantly associated with a 32% (hazard ratio [HR] 0.68, 95%CI, 0.59 to 0.79) lower risk of stroke and with a 48% (HR 0.52, 95%CI, 0.32 to 0.83) lower risk of poststroke dementia.

Nuts Daily intake of tree nuts consumption, as part of the Mediterranean-style dietary pattern, showed evidence of a reduction in stroke events in individuals with high cardiovascular risk (HR, 0.60 [95% CI, 0.45–0.80][12]) in one of the arm of Prevención con Dieta Mediterránea (PREDIMED) trial.

Dairy Products Although the association between dairy and stroke risk is not entirely clear, adding low to moderate consumption of low-fat or fat-free dairy products, as seen in the DASH, Mediterranean and Nordic diets, is tolerable and can be safely consumed to ensure sufficient protein intake as well as control of hypertension and high cholesterol.[12,21,25]

Alcohol In the USA, it has been estimated that alcohol may account for close to 10% of the population burden of HTN (higher in men than in women).[9] Alcohol has been associated with both ischemic and hemorrhagic stroke, often in a U-shaped pattern in observational studies. Compared with no alcohol consumption, having 1–2 drinks per day was associated with a roughly 10% lower risk for ischemic stroke, while consumption of both 2–4 drinks per day and > 4 drinks per day was associated with an 8% and 14% greater risk, respectively. Having > 4 drinks/day was associated with a 67% and 82% greater risk for intracerebral hemorrhage (ICH) and subarachnoid hemorrhage.[12,25] For this reason, assessing and addressing the amount of alcohol patients drink can be one of the most important interventions a physician does in the clinic. Patients with substance use disorders require the guidance of a specialist trained in addiction medicine who has expertise in the area. Using behavior change techniques and motivational interviewing, as reviewed in Chapter 26, is useful for those in primary care seeking to assist patients and refer them to these specialists.

Red Meat Results from observational studies meta-analysis[42] indicate that consumption of total red meat (> 3.5 ounces/day) and even smaller amounts of processed meat is associated with 13–20% increased risk of total stroke and ischemic stroke, respectively.[12,25] Processed meat such as bacon, sausage, hot dogs, pepperoni, and salami are high in salt, saturated fat, and cholesterol, which may contribute to atherosclerosis.[11] Therefore, the AHA recommendations currently limit red meat consumption (processed or not).

● SPECIAL NUTRITION CONSIDERATIONS AFTER A STROKE

After a person experiences a stroke, adequate nutrition is an essential part of recovery and secondary stroke prevention.[21] Thus, dietary counseling poststroke should focus on dietary patterns similar to the ones described for primary prevention of stroke (DASH, MD, Nordic). However, there are specific considerations to keep in mind.

Dietary Challenges with Dysphagia

Dysphagia is highly prevalent following stroke with estimates ranging 30%–65% of individuals.[43] Complications associated with dysphagia poststroke include pneumonia, malnutrition, dehydration, and poorer long-term outcome.[44] Most stroke patients recover from dysphagia within the first 4 weeks, although 15% of patients may develop long-term swallowing difficulties, and as such would require diet modifications. Modifying the consistency of solid food and/or liquid is a mainstay of compensatory intervention for patients with dysphagia. The goal of diet modification is to improve the safety and/or ease of oral consumption and thus maintain safe and adequate oral intake of food/liquid.[44]

Food and Medication Interactions

Warfarin is an anticoagulant commonly used for stroke prevention in patients with atrial fibrillation[45]. It works by decreasing vitamin K and as such reducing clotting factor production, hence thinning the blood. Almost all leafy dark greens, grapefruit juice, cranberry juice, and alcohol are rich in vitamin K. So, it is very important to advise patients and caregivers about consistent daily amount of such food and drinks intake to be able to maintain the warfarin levels. This does not mean to eliminate these foods, but rather to make sure the amount of vitamin K intake is constant from day to day. Otherwise, too much vitamin K would counteract the effect of warfarin and anticoagulation would be hard to achieve. Adequate intake of vitamin K for men and women older than 19 years is 120 mcg and 90 mcg, respectively. For example, a cup of uncooked spinach contains 145 mcg of vitamin K, but a cup of cooked broccoli can contain 220 mcg of vitamin K.[46,47] Daily supplementation with low oral dose vitamin K increases stability of anticoagulation for people who have variable intake of vitamin K food items, and this recommendation has been included in some guidelines. More recently, a set of novel oral anticoagulants (NOACs) have been approved specifically for thromboembolism prophylaxis in patients with atrial fibrillation. The NOACs have not been as broadly researched, but they do not require close monitoring of vitamin K.[46]

Hypertension control carries the highest benefit in reducing stroke burden on a population level. *Angiotensin-converting enzyme inhibitors (ace inhibitor)* like lisinopril can result in elevations in potassium levels so it is recommended to limit potassium intake (avocado, pomegranate, bananas, sweet potato, dates) while taking an ace inhibitor.[48] *Diuretics such as hydrochlorothiazide, and furosemide* lower BP by helping the body eliminate sodium and water through the urine and can both lead to losses in potassium. So, it is important to optimize this with adequate potassium-rich food.

Statins, which are HMG CoA reductase inhibitors, inhibit the production of cholesterol, and are often used for stroke prevention. However, concomitant consumption of larger quantities of grapefruit juice with certain statins, simvastatin, lorvastatin, and atorvastatin, can potentiate the effect of statins and increase the risk of side effects, whereas other statins such as pravastatin, rosuvastatin, and fluvastatin have little to no interaction with grapefruit juice.

THREE TAKE-HOME POINTS

1. HTN, as a major risk factor for stroke, is preventable or manageable by lifestyle approaches, including dietary choices characterized by low sodium, higher potassium, as well as being physically active, avoiding smoking, and limiting alcohol.
2. The main approach to nutrition in HTN and stroke prevention is to focus on dietary patterns that are rich in vegetable, fruits, whole grains, nuts, legumes, plant-based oils, fish, and low in processed foods, or added sodium and sugars.
3. Physicians and other healthcare play a critical role in providing education and motivation in the process of learning what dietary patterns and food choices could help prevent and treat HTN, hence prevent stroke and cardiovascular disease.

CASE STUDY 1 ANSWERS

1.

- Women in their 50s (perimenopause/menopausal life stage) are at a higher risk for acquiring vascular risk factors, especially due to hormonal changes and loss of vasoprotective effect of estrogen, which drops substantially during menopause.

- High blood pressure in women during this life stage has a higher effect on stroke risk compared to men of the same age.

- Night shift work increases risks for several conditions, including sleep and mood disturbances, obesity, and less physical activity, hence, can contribute to risks for all cardiovascular and cerebrovascular disease. (More information on sleep and physical activity in Chapter 31.)

- Processed food of any type is high in sodium, sugar, and unhealthy fat, all of which are associated with a variety of health risks, including hypertension and stroke.

- Poor intake of fibers, fruits, and vegetables, as well as low intake of fish are associated with higher risk of both hypertension and stroke.

2. Dietary recommendations would be focused on how to replace unhealthy food choices with healthy food choices (Table 19-1) by:

- Replacing pastries with a whole grain bread or morning oats (no added sugar)

- Replacing cured meat with occasional sardines or cooked lean meat.

- Replacing fried fish with cooked or baked lean meat or fatty fish (two to three times/week)

- Increasing intake of fresh whole and plant-based food choices instead of processed food would optimize an overall fiber and micronutrients (vitamins and minerals) intake and daily requirements.

- Preparing food with little or no salt and avoiding store-bought sauces and dressing (packed with additional sodium).

- Special recommendations would be based on the medical management in cases of dysphagia or medication interactions (page 191).

CASE STUDY 2 ANSWERS

1.

- Apart from the stress that is not discussed in this chapter, excess alcohol use is a major contributing factors for uncontrolled hypertension in men. (Stress is discussed in Chapter 31.)

- Processed food, savory snacks, and food from restaurants/stores are high in sodium and unhealthy fat and low in potassium.

- Poor compliance with medical management

2. The most important intervention is to stop drinking and this would require some behavioral therapy

- Education on nutrition and hypertension with specifics on dietary patterns (Table 19-1)

- Smoking cessation is recommended for hypertension and stroke prevention, as it increases the risk for both.

REFERENCES

1. O'Donnell MJ, Chin SL, Rangarajan S, et al. Global and regional effects of potentially modifiable risk factors associated with acute stroke in 32 countries (INTERSTROKE): a case-control study. *Lancet*. 2016;388(10046):761-775.

2. Collaborators GBDS. Global, regional, and national burden of stroke and its risk factors, 1990-2019: a systematic analysis for the global burden of disease study 2019. *Lancet Neurol*. Oct 2021;20(10): 795-820.

3. Ekker MS, Verhoeven JI, Vaartjes I, van Nieuwenhuizen KM, Klijn CJM, de Leeuw FE. Stroke incidence in young adults according to age, subtype, sex, and time trends. *Neurology*. May 21 2019;92(21):e2444-e2454.

4. George MG, Tong X, Bowman BA. Prevalence of cardiovascular risk factors and strokes in younger adults. *JAMA Neurol*. Jun 1 2017;74(6):695-703.

5. Adams HP Jr., Bendixen BH, Kappelle LJ, et al. Classification of subtype of acute ischemic stroke. Definitions for use in a multicenter clinical trial. TOAST. Trial of Org 10172 in acute stroke treatment. *Stroke*. Jan 1993;24(1):35-41.

6. Krafft PR, Bailey EL, Lekic T, et al. Etiology of stroke and choice of models. *Int J Stroke*. Jul 2012;7(5):398-406.

7. Mills KT, Bundy JD, Kelly TN, et al. Global disparities of hypertension prevalence and control: a systematic analysis of population-based studies from 90 countries. *Circulation*. Aug 9 2016;134(6):441-450.

8. (CDC) CfDCaP. Hypertension Cascade: Hypertension Prevalence, Treatment and Control Estimates Among US Adults Aged 18 Years and Older Applying the Criteria From the American College of Cardiology and American Heart Association's 2017 Hypertension Guideline—NHANES 2017–2020. 2023. Available at: https://millionhearts.hhs.gov/data-reports/hypertension-prevalence.html.

9. Whelton PK, Carey RM, Aronow WS, et al. 2017 ACC/AHA/AAPA/ABC/ACPM/AGS/APhA/ASH/ASPC/NMA/PCNA Guideline for the prevention, detection, evaluation, and management of high blood pressure in adults: a report of the American College of Cardiology/American Heart Association Task Force on Clinical Practice Guidelines. *Hypertension*. Jun 2018;71(6):e13-e115.

10. Collaborators GBDRF. Global, regional, and national comparative risk assessment of 84 behavioural, environmental and occupational, and metabolic risks or clusters of risks for 195 countries and territories, 1990-2017: a systematic analysis for the global burden of disease study 2017. *Lancet*. Nov 10 2018;392(10159):1923-1994.

11. Lichtenstein AH, Appel LJ, Vadiveloo M, et al. 2021 Dietary guidance to improve cardiovascular health: a scientific statement from the American Heart Association. *Circulation*. Dec 7 2021;144(23):e472-e487.

12. Kleindorfer DO, Towfighi A, Chaturvedi S, et al. 2021 Guideline for the prevention of stroke in patients with stroke and transient ischemic attack: a guideline from the American Heart Association/American Stroke Association. *Stroke*. Jul 2021;52(7):e364-e467.

13. Cara KC, Goldman DM, Kollman BK, Amato SS, Tull MD, Karlsen MC. Commonalities among dietary recommendations from 2010 to 2021 clinical practice guidelines: a meta-epidemiological study from the American College of Lifestyle Medicine. *Adv Nutr*. May 2023;14(3):500-515.

14. Ettehad D, Emdin CA, Kiran A, et al. Blood pressure lowering for prevention of cardiovascular disease and death: a systematic review and meta-analysis. *Lancet*. Mar 5 2016;387(10022):957-967.

15. Meschia JF, Bushnell C, Boden-Albala B, et al. Guidelines for the primary prevention of stroke: a statement for healthcare professionals from the American Heart Association/American Stroke Association. *Stroke*. Dec 2014;45(12):3754-3832.

16. Bornfeldt Karin E, Tabas I. Insulin resistance, hyperglycemia, and atherosclerosis. *Cell Metab*. 2011;14(5):575-585.

17. Lloyd-Jones DM, Allen NB, Anderson CAM, et al. Life's essential 8: updating and enhancing the American Heart Association's Construct of Cardiovascular Health: a presidential advisory from the American Heart Association. *Circulation*. Aug 2 2022;146(5):e18-e43.

18. McEwen BJ. The influence of diet and nutrients on platelet function. *Semin Thromb Hemost*. Mar 2014;40(2):214-226.

19. Tan BL, Norhaizan ME, Liew WP. Nutrients and oxidative stress: friend or foe? *Oxid Med Cell Longev*. 2018;2018:9719584. doi:10.1155/2018/9719584.

20. Chung MK, Eckhardt LL, Chen LY, et al. Lifestyle and risk factor modification for reduction of atrial fibrillation: a scientific statement from the American Heart Association. *Circulation*. Apr 21 2020;141(16):e750-e772.

21. Phadke CP, Schwartz J, Vuagnat H, Philippou E. The ABCs for nutrition poststroke: an evidence-based practice guide for rehabilitation professionals. *Arch Phys Med Rehabil*. Oct 2018;99(10):2125-2127.

22. Appel LJ, Moore TJ, Obarzanek E, et al. A clinical trial of the effects of dietary patterns on blood pressure. DASH Collaborative Research Group. *N Engl J Med*. Apr 17 1997;336(16):1117-1124.

23. Sacks FM, Svetkey LP, Vollmer WM, et al. Effects on blood pressure of reduced dietary sodium and the Dietary Approaches to Stop Hypertension (DASH) diet. DASH-Sodium Collaborative Research Group. *N Engl J Med*. Jan 4 2001;344(1):3-10.

24. Ndanuko RN, Tapsell LC, Charlton KE, Neale EP, Batterham MJ. Dietary patterns and blood pressure in adults: a systematic review and meta-analysis of randomized controlled trials. *Adv Nutr*. Jan 2016;7(1):76-89.

25. Lakkur S, Judd SE. Diet and stroke: recent evidence supporting a mediterranean-style diet and food in the primary prevention of stroke. *Stroke*. Jul 2015;46(7):2007-2011.

26. Brader L, Uusitupa M, Dragsted LO, Hermansen K. Effects of an isocaloric healthy nordic diet on ambulatory blood pressure in metabolic syndrome: a randomized SYSDIET sub-study. *Eur J Clin Nutr*. Jan 2014;68(1):57-63.

27. Erlund I, Koli R, Alfthan G, et al. Favorable effects of berry consumption on platelet function, blood pressure, and HDL cholesterol. *Am J Clin Nutr*. Feb 2008;87(2):323-331.

28. Avery EG, Bartolomaeus H, Maifeld A, et al. The gut microbiome in hypertension: recent advances and future perspectives. *Circ Res*. Apr 2 2021;128(7):934-950.

29. Bien J, Palagani V, Bozko P. The intestinal microbiota dysbiosis and clostridium difficile infection: is there a relationship with inflammatory bowel disease? *Therap Adv Gastroenterol*. Jan 2013;6(1):53-68.

30. Davani-Davari D, Negahdaripour M, Karimzadeh I, et al. Prebiotics: definition, types, sources, mechanisms, and clinical applications. *Foods*. Mar 9 2019;8(3):92.

31. Chi C, Li C, Wu D, et al. Effects of probiotics on patients with hypertension: a systematic review and meta-analysis. *Curr Hypertens Rep*. 2020;22(5):33.

32. Balafa O, Kalaitzidis RG. Salt sensitivity and hypertension. *J Hum Hypertens*. Mar 2021;35(3):184-192.

33. Barris CT, Faulkner JL, Belin de Chantemele EJ. Salt sensitivity of blood pressure in women. *Hypertension*. Feb 2023;80(2):268-278.

34. Hirshman E, Crecelius AR. Acute consumption of a sugar-sweetened beverage impairs microvascular function in midwestern hispanic males. *Human Nutrition & Metabolism*. 2021;26:200129. https://doi.org/10.1016/j.hnm.2021.200129.

35. Estruch R, Ros E, Salas-Salvado J, et al. Retraction and republication: primary prevention of cardiovascular disease with a mediterranean diet. *N Engl J Med*. 2013;368:1279-90. *N Engl J Med*. Jun 21 2018;378(25):2441-2442.

36. Chiavaroli L, Viguiliouk E, Nishi SK, et al. DASH dietary pattern and cardiometabolic outcomes: an umbrella review of systematic reviews and meta-analyses. *Nutrients*. Feb 5 2019;11(2):338.

37. D'Elia L, Iannotta C, Sabino P, Ippolito R. Potassium-rich diet and risk of stroke: updated meta-analysis. *Nutr Metab Cardiovasc Dis*. Jun 2014;24(6):585-587.

38. Aune D, Keum N, Giovannucci E, et al. Whole grain consumption and risk of cardiovascular disease, cancer, and all cause and cause specific mortality: systematic review and dose-response meta-analysis of prospective studies. *BMJ*. Jun 14 2016;353:i2716.

39. Juan J, Liu G, Willett WC, Hu FB, Rexrode KM, Sun Q. Whole grain consumption and risk of ischemic stroke: results from 2 prospective cohort studies. *Stroke*. Dec 2017;48(12):3203-3209.

40. Yuan S, Li X, Jin Y, Lu J. Chocolate consumption and risk of coronary heart disease, stroke, and diabetes: a meta-analysis of prospective studies. *Nutrients*. Jul 2 2017;9(7):688.

41. Zhang Y, Yang H, Li S, Li WD, Wang Y. Consumption of coffee and tea and risk of developing stroke, dementia, and poststroke dementia: a cohort study in the UK Biobank. *PLoS Med*. Nov 2021;18(11):e1003830.

42. Yang C, Pan L, Sun C, Xi Y, Wang L, Li D. Red meat consumption and the risk of stroke: a dose-response meta-analysis of prospective cohort studies. *J Stroke Cerebrovasc Dis*. May 2016; 25(5):1177-1186.

43. Arnold M, Liesirova K, Broeg-Morvay A, et al. Dysphagia in acute stroke: incidence, burden and impact on clinical outcome. *PLoS One*. 2016;11(2):e0148424.

44. Sura L, Madhavan A, Carnaby G, Crary MA. Dysphagia in the elderly: management and nutritional considerations. *Clin Interv Aging*. 2012;7:287-298.

45. Association AH. Medication interactions: food, supplements and other drugs. American Heart Association 2023. Available at: https://www.heart.org/en/health-topics/consumer-healthcare/medication-information/medication-interactions-food-supplements-and-other-drugs.

46. Blog PHaV. The Truth About Blood Thinners, Leafy Greens, And Vitamin K 2022. Available at: https://www.pennmedicine.org/updates/blogs/heart-and-vascular-blog/2015/june/consistency-not-avoidance-the-truth-about-blood-thinners-leafy-greens-and-vitamin-k.

47. Kampouraki E, Kamali F. Dietary implications for patients receiving long-term oral anticoagulation therapy for treatment and prevention of thromboembolic disease. *Expert Rev Clin Pharmacol*. Aug 2017;10(8):789-797.

48. Esenwa C, Gutierrez J. Secondary stroke prevention: challenges and solutions. *Vasc Health Risk Manag*. 2015;11:437-450.

chapter 20

Cardiovascular Disease

Alaina Bever, PhD / Francine K. Welty, MD, PHD

Chapter Outline

CASE STUDY 1

A 35-year-old woman presents to primary practice for a well visit. She recently lost 25 pounds (BMI from 27.5 kg/m² to 23.2 kg/m²) using a low-carbohydrate diet that a friend recommended to her. However, she is concerned because her LDL-C has increased from 82 mg/dL to 100 mg/dL since her last visit. She wants to continue restricting carbohydrates because she is feeling much better since making this dietary change; however, she is willing to make changes to other parts of her diet if it would improve her long-term risk of cardiovascular disease.

1. Should your patient be concerned about the change in her LDL-C? Are there other parameters that you could measure to give her a better idea of how future lifestyle changes are impacting her cardiovascular risk?

2. What dietary recommendations would you give to this patient to minimize her long-term risk of CHD?

You are counseling a 72-year-old man with a history of CHD. His BMI is 32.4 kg/m², LDL-C 125 mg/dL, HDL-C 52 mg/dL, TG 83 mg/dL. When you inquire about his diet, he tells you that his LDL-C has decreased since he started taking a statin and he plans to adhere to his treatment, so he does not need to worry about diet.

1. Is your patient correct that diet does not influence CHD risk beyond the effects of pharmacologic lipid-lowering treatment? What would you tell him about the different ways that diet influences CHD prevention?

   After explaining some of the ways that diet is involved in secondary CHD prevention, your patient is interested in discussing diet. He tells you that he has very particular eating preferences: for most

meals he cooks white rice or noodles with stir-fried chicken, pork, or beef and snacks on commercial sweetened iced tea, commercial crackers, and dried fruit. He says that he would be willing to make some changes but wants to stick to familiar foods. He is not yet ready to meet with a dietician and asks you if you could suggest just a few changes that he can start with.

2. What two or three suggestions might you make to this patient with regards to dietary changes?

3. Your patient forgot to mention that he does not like the taste of fish, and he is curious if there is any benefit to taking marine omega-3 fatty acid supplements. What would you tell him?

INTRODUCTION AND DEFINITIONS

Cardiovascular disease (CVD) refers to all disorders affecting the heart or blood vessels, including coronary heart disease (CHD) and cerebrovascular disease (Figure 20-1). The pathophysiology and prevention of cerebrovascular disease (conditions that affect the blood vessels of the brain) is covered in Chapter 19 ("Stroke and Hypertension"), and this chapter will focus primarily on CHD, the leading cause of CVD mortality worldwide. CHD prevention is usually designated as either primary or secondary, with primary prevention referring to the prevention of disease onset in either low- or high-risk individuals and secondary prevention referring to

the prevention of cardiac events and mortality in individuals with prevalent CHD. As with other noncommunicable diseases, the development of CHD is a chronic, incremental process influenced by modifiable risk factors throughout the life course.

This chapter begins with an overview of the global epidemiology of CHD, followed by a summary of key pathology relevant to diet, including lipid disorders, hypertension, chronic glycemia and insulin resistance, and inflammation. The rest of the chapter is devoted to the role of diet in the primary and secondary prevention of CHD, highlighting landmark trials and other evidence for the role of dietary components and patterns in CHD development and prevention.

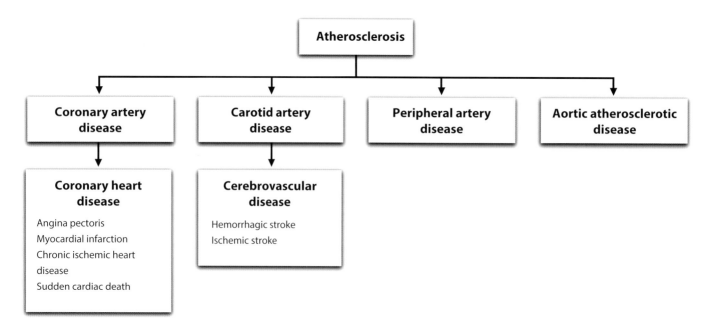

FIGURE 20-1 • Common cardiovascular diseases resulting from atherosclerosis. Coronary artery disease, carotid artery disease, peripheral artery disease, aortic atherosclerotic disease, and resulting complications all originate from atherosclerosis. Coronary artery disease and carotid artery disease are the leading causes of mortality worldwide. (Created by Bever A. for *Nutrition Essentials*.)

DISEASE BURDEN

CVD is the leading cause of death in high-income countries and worldwide, with CHD and cerebrovascular disease accounting for 16% and 11% of all global deaths in 2019, respectively. The CHD mortality rate in the United States (US) peaked in the 1960s and has been declining ever since, a trend that is attributed to the identification of key risk factors (e.g., hypertension, cigarette smoking, dyslipidemia) and improved medical care. Conversely, trends in CHD mortality in low- and middle-income countries are less favorable, thought to be due in large part to changes in physical activity, diet, alcohol consumption, and cigarette use. Poor quality diet is one of the leading risk factors contributing to CHD incidence and mortality. Given the high global incidence of CHD and its significantly preventable nature, dietary modification for primary and secondary prevention of CHD has the potential for monumental impact on individual patients and population health.

RELEVANT PATHOPHYSIOLOGY

Atherosclerosis is a chronic, inflammatory process of the arterial wall. The earliest stage of atherosclerosis is thought to begin with endothelial cell injury and dysfunction, resulting in increased endothelial permeability and the migration of apolipoprotein (apo) B particles into the arterial wall. The accumulation and oxidation of trapped apoB particles attracts monocytes and macrophages (foam cells), which together constitute the earliest stage of an atherosclerotic lesion, called a fatty streak. As fatty streaks progress to intermediate and advanced lesions, they recruit smooth muscle cells and eventually form a fibrous cap. Figure 20-2 illustrates the progression of atherosclerosis. Individuals with advanced atherosclerosis may present with angina when these plaques enlarge to the point that blood flow to the myocardium is reduced; frequently, however, the first indication of severe coronary artery disease is acute thrombosis resulting in myocardial infarction.

Although symptoms of CHD do not usually manifest until the sixth decade of life, the development of atherosclerosis starts at birth, which calls attention to the importance of primary prevention across the life course and partially explains why many of the dietary recommendations related to CHD prevention are common to the dietary recommendations for the general population starting early in life (see Chapter 5, "Nutrition Through the Life Span"). Diet influences CHD outcomes via effects on endothelial dysfunction, chronic inflammation, lipoprotein metabolism, and, in cases of late primary or secondary prevention, atherosclerotic plaque stability. In the following sections, we briefly summarize physiologic risk factors involved in the development of atherosclerosis and CHD as pertains to diet.

Lipid Disorders

The accumulation of apoB particles, or lipoproteins that carry apoB, in the arterial wall is central to the initiation and progression of atherosclerosis and is primarily influenced by the concentration of apoB particles in circulation. ApoB particles include chylomicrons, very-low-density lipoproteins (VLDL), intermediate-density lipoproteins (IDL), and low-density lipoproteins (LDL), each of which contains a single molecule of apoB and variable amounts of cholesterol ester and triglyceride (Figure 20-3). Because the number of LDL particles in circulation is many-fold greater than other apoB particles due to the substantially longer plasma residence time of LDL, and each LDL particle contains a single apoB molecule, apoB concentration can be used as a surrogate measure of LDL particle count (LDL-P). ApoB is more commonly reported in research studies than LDL-P, and in clinical practice, apoB assays are more widely available and better standardized than LDL-P assays.

LDL-cholesterol (LDL-C) is a measure of the total cholesterol ester concentration contained in all LDL particles in circulation. In most individuals, LDL-C is strongly correlated with LDL-P and apoB; however, because LDLs vary in density and amount of cholesterol ester being carried, LDL-C is not always a reliable measure of LDL particle concentration. When there is discordance between the two measures (e.g., LDL-C indicates low or moderate risk while apoB indicates high risk for a particular individual), apoB is a better predictor of CHD risk than LDL-C. Discordance between LDL-C and apoB is more common among women and individuals with insulin resistance or hypertriglyceridemia.

Although apoB particle concentration is perhaps the most well-established lipid-related risk factor for atherosclerosis and CHD, there are several other measures that may contribute to CHD risk beyond the effects of apoB alone. Elevated lipoprotein(a) (Lp(a)), a variant of LDL with an additional apolipoprotein called apo(a), has been shown to confer additional CHD risk beyond apoB. Lp(a) is strongly determined by the *LPA* gene locus, thus it is less likely than apoB to be directly modified in response to dietary changes; nonetheless, elevated Lp(a) can help to identify individuals for whom the importance of modifying all other CHD risk factors, including diet, is even more critical. It has been posited that apoB particle size, in addition to concentration, determines atherogenicity because small, cholesterol-depleted apoB particles may be able to enter the arterial wall more easily; whether particle size adds additional information to apoB in determining CHD risk is not well-established. Finally, apoA-I is the main apolipoprotein carried by high-density lipoprotein (HDL) particles, and there is some evidence to suggest that the ratio of apoB to apoA-I is an even better predictor of CHD risk than apoB alone. However, the mechanistic role of apoA-I in CHD is less well understood than the role of apoB, as evidenced by the failure of pharmaceutical therapies that successfully increased plasma HDL-C and apoA-I but did not impact CHD risk. Thus, while apoA-I particles are likely to be involved in cardiovascular health, subspecies heterogeneity that is not yet well-understood indicates that interventions that increase apoA-I are not certain to improve CHD outcomes.

In many studies, lipid measures are used as a substitute for outcomes of interest (e.g., CHD incidence and mortality), and as

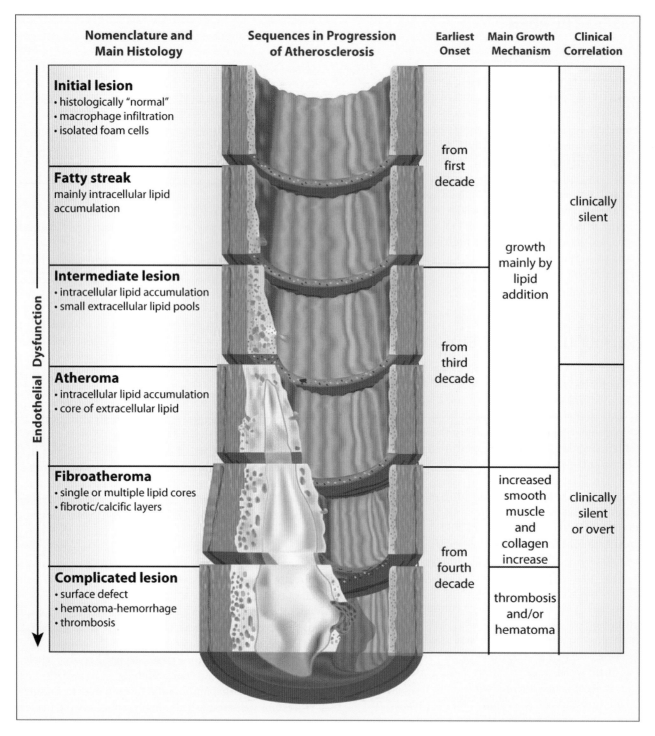

FIGURE 20-2 • Progression of atherosclerosis. Although typically clinically silent until midlife or later, atherosclerosis is a chronic condition that begins as early as childhood, progressing incrementally throughout the life course. (Reproduced with permission from Houston CM. New concepts in cardiovascular disease. *J Restor Med*. 2013;2:36.)

such, it is crucial to be able to distinguish lipoproteins that play a causal role in CHD from those that are proxies for cardiometabolic health but do not consistently translate to changes in CHD risk when altered via intervention. For example, the conventional model of the cholesterol in LDL as "bad cholesterol" and the cholesterol in HDL as "good cholesterol" that has been prominent for many years is now understood to be an oversimplification of how

lipoproteins relate to human health and has even contributed to incorrect conclusions regarding the effects of both dietary and pharmaceutical interventions on CHD outcomes. Plasma triglyceride concentration (TG) is another measure associated with CHD risk, but this association appears to be largely mediated by increased apoB particle synthesis resulting from elevated hepatic TG. Nevertheless, most clinical laboratory lipid profile reports

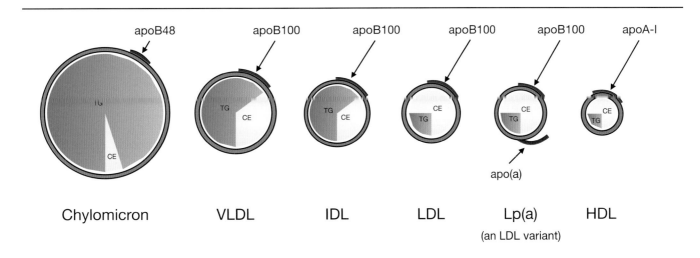

FIGURE 20-3 • Major lipoproteins. Major lipoproteins are depicted with typical fraction of triglyceride and cholesterol ester carried, major apolipoproteins, and relative size. Because LDL has a significantly longer plasma residence time compared to the other apoB containing particles, it typically accounts for > 90% of apoB in plasma and apoB is considered a proxy for LDL particle count. apoB48 is carried by lipoproteins originating in the small intestine, and apoB100 is carried by lipoproteins originating in the liver. *Abbreviations:* apo, apolipoprotein; CE, cholesterol ester; HDL, high-density lipoprotein; IDL, intermediate density lipoprotein; Lp(a), lipoprotein(a); LDL, low-density lipoprotein; TG, triglyceride; VLDL, very-low-density lipoprotein. (Adapted from figure by Sniderman, AD. Apolipoprotein B particles and cardiovascular disease: a narrative review. *JAMA Cardiol.* 2019 Dec 1;4(12):1287-1295. doi: 10.1001/jamacardio.2019.3780. https://pubmed.ncbi.nlm.nih.gov/31642874/.)

include HDL-C, LDL-C (calculated from measured total cholesterol, HDL-C, and TG), non-HDL cholesterol (calculated from measured total cholesterol and HDL-C), and TG. Thus, clinicians still frequently refer to these measures to make clinical decisions. In the sections that follow, we describe the effects of dietary factors on apoB and Lp(a) whenever available, and include less specific markers including apoA-I, LDL-C, HDL-C, and TG for context. The different lipid measures and relation to CHD are summarized in Table 20-1.

Hypertension (See also Chapter 19)

Hypertension most likely contributes to the development of atherosclerosis and plaque vulnerability by increasing physical stress on the arterial wall. Both systolic and diastolic blood pressures are independently associated with increased risk of CHD. Despite its significant contribution to CHD risk, the cause of hypertension in most individuals is not well understood. Observational studies have revealed that in addition to family history, hypertension is associated with body mass index (BMI), physical activity, cigarette smoking, alcohol consumption, and diet, leading to its classification as a modifiable risk factor and a candidate target for dietary intervention. See Chapter 19 ("Stroke and Hypertension") for more details on dietary interventions influencing blood pressure.

Diabetes, Chronic Hyperglycemia, and Insulin Resistance (See also Chapter 18, "Diabetes Mellitus")

Both type 1 and type 2 diabetes are significant risk factors for CHD and have been hypothesized to induce atherosclerosis through mechanisms related to chronic hyperglycemia and insulin resistance. Hyperglycemia promotes endothelial cell dysfunction, atherogenic modification of apoB particles, and systemic inflammation; insulin resistance additionally contributes to hypertension, hyperuricemia, and hepatic TG synthesis and promotes the secretion of apoB particles while impairing apoB particle clearance. The significant prevalence of prediabetes and diabetes in the US and worldwide warrants attention to dietary factors related to insulin resistance and glycemic control.

Inflammation

A series of observational studies published in the 1990s demonstrated that individuals with elevated C-reactive protein (CRP) and other markers of inflammation were at increased risk of CHD; the association between CRP and CHD was present even among individuals who appeared otherwise healthy and was independent of cigarette smoking, lipids, and other CHD risk factors. Since then, randomized controlled trials (RCTs) have demonstrated that pharmacologic interventions to selectively reduce inflammation among individuals with prevalent CHD already treated with lipid-lowering drugs resulted in a reduction of the primary endpoint of combined cardiovascular mortality, myocardial infarction, ischemic stroke, and urgent coronary revascularization. Inflammation is now understood to be a central component of both atherosclerosis and subsequent cardiac events; inflammatory markers, particularly CRP, serve as additional surrogate endpoints to evaluate the effects of dietary interventions on CHD risk.

TABLE 20-1 • Lipid definitions in the context of laboratory reports and relation to CHD				
Lipid measure	Full name	Definition	Direction and strength of association with CHD risk	Relevance to CHD and major dietary components
TG	Triglyceride	Triglycerides within all lipoproteins in plasma	↑	TG is elevated in patients with insulin-resistant metabolic syndrome; TG is associated with apoB and apoB/LDL-C discordance (elevated apoB and low LDL-C), as seen in the context of a low-fat, high-carbohydrate diet
TC	Total cholesterol	Cholesterol within all lipoprotein in plasma	↑	Early metric used to predict CHD risk before lipoproteins were well understood, poor predictor of CHD relative to other lipid measures
LDL-C	Low-density lipoprotein cholesterol	Cholesterol within all LDLs in plasma	↑	Early metric used to predict CHD risk before the importance of particle number was well understood; relatively poor predictor of CHD compared to ApoB or LDL-P, although still widely used as a metric of CHD risk because commonly measured in clinical laboratories; elevated with total fat and particularly saturated fatty acid and trans fatty acid consumption
LDL-P	Low-density lipoprotein particle count	Number of LDL particles in plasma	↑↑	Current theory posits that particle number is the most relevant metric predictive of lipoprotein entry into arterial intima and development of atherosclerosis
ApoB	Apolipoprotein B	Concentration of all apoB particles in plasma	↑↑	Can be used as a proxy for LDL-P (apoB assay more widely available), based on assumption that > 90% of apoB particles in plasma are LDL; significantly better predictor of CHD risk than other lipid measures
Non-HDL-C	Non-high-density-lipoprotein cholesterol	Cholesterol within all apoB particles (VLDL, IDL, LDL) in plasma	↑	Used as a proxy for LDL-P, slightly weaker correlation with LDL-P compared to apoB, often reported in lipid profile report from clinical laboratories
LDL particle size	Low-density lipoprotein particle size		↓ (Larger particle size associated with decreased CHD risk)	Although LDL particle size does not directly influence the likelihood of entering the arterial intima, an individual with smaller particles requires a higher number of particles to carry the same amount of lipid, increasing the LDL particle count
Lp(a)	Lipoprotein(a)		↑	LDL variant and independent risk factor for CHD after accounting for other lipid parameters including apoB; appears to be less influenced by modifiable risk factors than other lipids; utility in identifying high-risk individuals who will benefit from optimizing other lipid parameters
HDL-C	High-density lipoprotein cholesterol	Cholesterol within all HDLs in plasma	↓	Reduced in patients with insulin-resistant metabolic syndrome; elevated with omega-3 polyunsaturated fatty acid and saturated fatty acid consumption; decreased with trans fatty acid consumption
HDL-P	High-density lipoprotein particle count	Number of HDL particles in plasma	↓↓	HDL particle count, potentially the most powerful predictor of CHD risk in combination with LDL-P (LDL-P:HDL-P ratio), although the mechanistic role of HDL in CHD is not well-understood
ApoA-I	Apolipoprotein A-I	Concentration of all apoA-I particles in plasma	↓↓	Used as a proxy for HDL-P, potentially the most powerful predictor of CHD risk in combination with apoB (apoA-I:apoB ratio, a proxy for LDL-P:HDL-P ratio)

Created by Bever A for *Nutrition Essentials.*

Key:

↓ decreased risk

↓↓ stronger decreased risk

↑ increased risk

↑↑ stronger increased risk

Overweight and Obesity (See also Chapter 17, "Overweight and Obesity")

Obesity has long been understood to be a significant risk factor for CHD, both due to its association with and independent of other risk factors. A detailed description of dietary approaches in the prevention and management of excess adiposity can be found in Chapter 17; the focus of this chapter is on dietary interventions that promote cardiovascular health independent of changes in weight. Although dietary interventions that prevent weight gain are largely consistent with dietary recommendations for the prevention of CHD, there is some controversy regarding the use of a low-carbohydrate for weight loss, which can sometimes involve high intake of saturated fat. We address this topic in the section regarding carbohydrate intake and CHD.

● MEDITERRANEAN-STYLE DIET IN THE PRIMARY AND SECONDARY PREVENTION OF CVD

Two of the most successful diet RCTs for the primary and secondary prevention of CVD or CHD both used a Mediterranean-style diet as the intervention (Box 20-1). The first of these studies, the Lyon Diet Heart Study, was initiated in 1988 with the enrollment of 605 men and women with prevalent CHD in Lyon, France. Participants were randomized and instructed to follow the experimental Mediterranean-style diet or to follow a "prudent" diet (control arm).[1] After a mean follow-up of 4 years, individuals in the Mediterranean diet arm had 77% decreased risk of the primary outcome of combined cardiac death and nonfatal acute myocardial infarction compared to the control group (hazard ratio (HR), 0.23; 95% confidence

---

BOX 20-1

Definition of Mediterranean-Style Diet

A Mediterranean-style diet, also called the Mediterranean diet, is a dietary pattern inspired by the traditional foods consumed in parts of Greece, Italy, and Spain. Its origins stem from the work of Ancel Keys, who published findings in the mid-20th century remarking on the low rate of CHD in these areas of the Mediterranean compared to Northern Europe and the United States. Features of a Mediterranean-style diet include the following:
- Abundant consumption of vegetables, fruits, legumes, olive oil, nuts, and seeds
- Moderate consumption of fish, white meats, bread, cheese, and yogurt
- Minimal consumption of red and processed meats, cream, butter, sugar-sweetened beverages, pastries, and other commercial or highly processed foods
- Wine as the primary source of alcohol (if any)

In the Lyon Diet Study, canola oil and canola-based margarine containing 5% omega-3 alpha-linolenic acid were also recommended and supplied to the Mediterranean diet intervention arm. In the PREDIMED trial, one Mediterranean diet arm was provided with olive oil, and the other Mediterranean diet arm was provided with nuts (both in ample supply).

Because both the Lyon Diet and PREDIMED RCTs compared a Mediterranean-style diet to a healthy diet (as "control" arm) with overlapping features—minimal consumption of red meat, dairy, and processed foods and abundant intake of fruits, vegetables, and whole grains—the reduction in CHD observed in these trials is thought to be driven by unique aspects of a Mediterranean-style diet such as the emphasis on olive oil, nuts, seeds, and fatty fish.

Based on self-reported intake, individuals in the Mediterranean diet arm of the Lyon study consumed less meat, butter, and cream and more fruit, vegetables, legumes, bread, fish, and margarine compared to the control group; in terms of nutrients, the Mediterranean diet arm consumed less total fat, saturated fat, cholesterol, and omega-6 fatty acids and more fiber, monounsaturated fat, and omega-3 fatty acids compared to the control group. Individuals in the Mediterranean diet arms of the PREDIMED study reported consuming more legumes, fish, nuts, and virgin olive oil compared to the control group; on average, self-reported intake of other food groups, including whole grains, fruits, vegetables, meat, alcohol, and dairy products, were not significantly different. In terms of nutrients, the PREDIMED Mediterranean diet arms reported higher intake of total fat, omega-6 linoleic acid, omega-3 alpha-linolenic acid, marine omega-3 fatty acids, and fiber and lower intake of carbohydrates and protein compared to control arm; percent energy from saturated fat and cholesterol were not significantly different.

One drawback of the Mediterranean diet is that it was inspired by and designed to be appealing to individuals living in Europe and North America. Interestingly, Ancel Keys considered that the traditional diets of Japan, Korea, and Taiwan were likely to have similar health benefits to those of the Mediterranean, however, he concluded that East Asian dietary patterns were too unfamiliar to Americans to be accepted in the United States. As a result, there are aspects of traditional cuisines around the world that may have unique benefits in the prevention of CHD that have never been formally evaluated. In this chapter, we often use the name "Mediterranean-style diet" in place of "Mediterranean Diet" to emphasize that many health-promoting effects of the Mediterranean diet are transferable.

interval (CI), 0.11–0.48). Strikingly, there were no significant differences in BMI, systolic or diastolic blood pressure, LDL-C, HDL-C, TG, apoB, apoA-I, Lp(a), glycated hemoglobin, uric acid, or leukocyte count in the Mediterranean diet group compared to the control group during the first year of the trial or at the end of year two of follow-up.

The second major dietary intervention study to demonstrate the efficacy of a Mediterranean-style diet is the *Prevención con Dieta Mediterránea* (Prevention with Mediterranean Diet, PREDIMED) trial. Starting in 2003, 7,447 individuals with high CVD risk but no history of CVD and living in Spain were randomized to one of three diets: a Mediterranean-style diet supplemented with extra virgin olive oil (EVOO), a Mediterranean-style diet supplemented with mixed tree nuts, or a low-fat diet consistent with the 2000 American Heart Association (AHA) dietary guidelines (control arm).[2,3] After a median 5 years of follow-up, individuals in the combined Mediterranean diet groups had 30% decreased risk of the primary endpoint of combined myocardial infarction, stroke, or death from cardiovascular causes compared to the control group (HR, 0.70; 95% CI, 0.55–0.89). There were no differences in the primary endpoint between the Mediterranean diet groups supplemented with EVOO or mixed nuts; only the Mediterranean diet with EVOO group had significantly lower average apoB and higher average apoA-I compared to the control group, only the Mediterranean diet with mixed nuts group had lower prevalence of hypertension compared to the control group, and both Mediterranean diet groups reduced hypertriglyceridemia and abdominal obesity compared to the control group. Of note, the original PREDIMED results were withdrawn due to deviations from the randomization protocol, however, the results were reanalyzed and published again after corrections with the same conclusions.

Both the Lyon Diet Heart Study and PREDIMED achieved great success in demonstrating the effectiveness of a Mediterranean-style diet in the primary and secondary prevention of CVD and CHD. Additional review of individual nutrients and foods in relation to CHD has the potential to expand upon our current understanding of how a Mediterranean-style diet protects against CVD incidence and mortality, and to facilitate the successful translation of a Mediterranean-style diet to a broader population with varying underlying risk profile as well as differing personal and cultural food preferences.

● INDIVIDUAL NUTRIENTS, FOODS, AND BEVERAGES RELATED TO CVD

Total Dietary Fat

Due to observed associations of high plasma cholesterol with CHD and the presence of cholesterol-rich plaques found in the arteries of deceased CHD patients, there was early interest in the role of dietary fat as a causal agent in atherosclerosis. Several observational studies published during the 1990s showed no association between low-fat diet and CHD events

or mortality, and RCTs showed that although a low-fat diet resulted in decreased plasma LDL-C, it also caused decreased HDL-C and increased TG and fasting insulin.[4-6] In 2006, the results of the Women's Health Initiative Dietary Modification Trial demonstrated that a low-fat diet had no effect on the incidence of nonfatal myocardial infarction, CHD death, or total cardiovascular disease among a diverse study population of 48,835 postmenopausal women in the United States.[7] In this trial, participants in the experimental diet group were instructed to reduce total fat intake from a baseline of > 30% to 20% of total energy intake, replacing fat with vegetables, fruits, and whole grains; the control group received a copy of the Dietary Guidelines for Americans without any specific dietary counseling.

In addition to providing convincing evidence that a low-fat diet does not protect against CHD, the results of the Women's Health Initiative trial highlighted the importance of considering cardiometabolic markers in aggregate and the limitations of LDL-C as a marker of CHD risk. At year one of follow-up, the low-fat diet arm had significantly more substantial decreases in BMI and waist circumference and trended towards more substantial decreases in LDL-C compared to the control group, however, the low-fat diet arm also trended towards more significant increases in TG, Lp(a), and LDL-P compared to the control group, markers that are now understood to be critical to the development of CHD.[8] It is now almost unanimously accepted that a "simply" low-fat diet does not decrease risk of CHD, whereas the type of fatty acids consumed influences cardiometabolic health, as described in the following sections.

Types of Dietary Fat

Dietary fatty acids and fatty acid metabolism are introduced in Chapter 1 ("Macronutrient Metabolism"). The major categories of dietary fatty acids relevant to CVD are saturated fatty acids, monounsaturated fatty acids, polyunsaturated fatty acids, and trans fatty acids (Figure 20-4). Polyunsaturated fatty acids are further classified as omega-3 or omega-6 fatty acids, two groups that may have distinct implications for health. Although each of these categories is further comprised of a variety of different fatty acids, most studies use these categories based on the assumption that there are shared properties among the fatty acids in each group.

Saturated fat was first implicated in the development of CHD around the 1950s, when a large ecological study called the Seven Countries Study demonstrated that select countries with the highest rates of CHD also had an average diet high in saturated fat, whereas select countries with the lowest rates of CHD had an average diet low in saturated fat.[9,10] A series of RCTs in the 1960s, 1970s, and 1980s aimed to answer the question of whether replacing dietary saturated fat with polyunsaturated fat reduced the incidence of CVD and CVD mortality. The results of these studies were inconsistent, with one meta-analysis concluding that the RCTs that replaced saturated fat with sources of mixed omega-3 and omega-6 fatty acids (e.g., soybean oil, fatty fish) demonstrated reduced CHD mortality, whereas RCTs that replaced

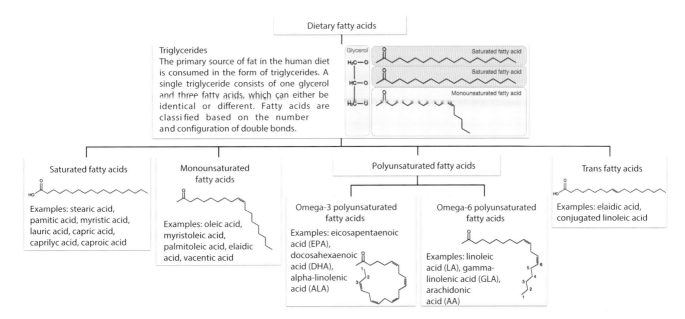

FIGURE 20-4 • Major categories of dietary fatty acids. The major categories of dietary fatty acids relevant to CHD are saturated fatty acids, monounsaturated fatty acids, polyunsaturated fatty acids, and trans fatty acids. Polyunsaturated fatty acids are further classified as omega-3 and omega-6 fatty acids. Most studies of fatty acids use these categories based on the assumption that there are shared properties among the individual fatty acids in each group. (Created by Bever A. for *Nutrition Essentials.*)

saturated fat with sources of almost 100% omega-6 fatty acids (e.g., safflower oil, corn oil), resulted in increased CHD mortality; this is consistent with findings of the Lyon Diet Heart Study and PREDIMED study, both of which recommended a mixture of unsaturated fatty acids, including omega-3, in the Mediterranean diet arm.[11]

Observational studies have relatively consistently demonstrated a reduction in CHD incidence and mortality in substitution analyses modeling the effects of increased general polyunsaturated fat acid in place of saturated fat, and several short-term controlled studies have shown an increase in apoB when polyunsaturated fat is replaced with saturated fat.[12–15] Conversely, the effects of replacing saturated fat with monounsaturated fat or carbohydrates in observational substitution analyses have been less consistent. To add further nuance, in some observational studies, the association of saturated fat with CHD depended on the food source of saturated fat, with saturated fat from red and processed meats, pastries, processed foods, and butter associated with increased CHD risk and saturated fat from yogurt, cheese, and fish associated with decreased CHD risk.[16,17] The current AHA guidelines recommend no more than 10% of total calories from saturated fat, and there is no compelling evidence that reducing saturated fatty acid significantly below 10% (about 20 g/day on a 2,000 calorie diet) has additional benefits for CHD; the reported saturated fatty acid consumption in the experimental arms of the PREDIMED and Lyon studies was about 8–10% of total energy.

With regards to unsaturated fatty acids, both monounsaturated fatty acid and omega-3 fatty acids are widely regarded as having a protective effect on CHD based on their prominence in Mediterranean-style diets, particularly in the intervention diets of both the Lyon and PREDIMED studies. In observational studies, high compared to low consumption of plant omega-3 fatty acids (alpha-linolenic acid) or fatty fish (a source of omega-3 fatty acids eicosatetraenoic acid (EPA) and docosahexaenoic acid (DHA)) was inversely associated with CHD.[18,19] It has been postulated that high intake of omega-6 fatty acids or a high omega-6:omega-3 ratio in the diet contributes to inflammation and LDL oxidation. Omega-3 and omega-6 fatty acids are typically found together in unprocessed foods; some of the foods highest in omega-6:omega-3 ratio are safflower oil, corn oil, and cottonseed oil, which tend to be found in highly processed and fried foods.

A final fatty acid that unmistakably contributes to CHD is trans fatty acid. While small amounts of trans fat are found in nature as a product of intestinal microbes of ruminant species, most trans fat in the human diet is sourced from the partial hydrogenation of vegetable oils, a manufacturing technique designed to extend the shelf life of food products made with vegetable oils. Controlled feeding trials and prospective cohort studies consistently show a detrimental effect on lipoprotein markers and CHD risk when trans fatty acid is substituted for any other macronutrient.[20] In 2015, the U.S. Food and Drug Administration (FDA) declared that commercial trans fat is unsafe; however, due to some exceptions, trans fatty acid may still be found in small amounts in manufactured foods in the United States. The World Health Organization called for the global elimination of commercial trans fatty acid in 2018; unfortunately, many nations around the world lack any policy on commercial trans fatty acid and it continues to be a cause of CHD morbidity and mortality worldwide. There is no evidence

TABLE 20-2 • Different example food sources of fatty acids in comparison to the average fatty acid composition of the mediterranean-style diets consumed in the PREDIMED trial and lyon diet heart study

	Omega-3 polyunsaturated fatty acid		Omega-6 polyunsaturated fatty acid	Monounsaturated fatty acid	Saturated fatty acid	Trans fatty acid
	ALA	EPA + DHA (marine)				
Sample Mediterranean-style diet, based on 2,000 kcal/day	1.6 g/day	1 g/day	14 g/day	45 g/day	20 g/day	0 g/day
Extra virgin olive oil, 1 oz (2 T)	0.2 g	0.0 g	2.4 g	19.4 g	4.3 g	0.0 g
Canola oil, 1 oz (2 T)	2.1 g	0.0 g	5.0 g	17.5 g	1.8 g	0.0 g
Avocado oil, 1 oz (2 T)	0.3 g	0.0 g	3.5 g	19.8 g	3.2 g	0.0 g
Walnuts, 1 oz	2.5 g	0.0 g	5.1 g	2.5 g	1.7 g	0.0 g
Flaxseed meal, 1 oz	5.4 g	0.0 g	1.5 g	1.7 g	0.9 g	0.0 g
Mackerel, 3 oz	0.0 g	2.0 g	0.0 g	4.7 g	2.8 g	0.0 g
Sardines, 3 oz	0.1 g	1.2 g	0.2 g	4.1 g	2.3 g	0.0 g
Cheddar cheese, 1 oz	0.0 g	0.0 g	0.2 g	2.1 g	5.4 g	0.0 g
Whole milk Greek-style yogurt, 3 oz	0.0 g	0.0 g	0.1 g	0.7 g	2.0 g	0.0 g
Chicken thigh (no skin), 3 oz	0.1 g	0.0 g	1.3 g	2.9 g	2.0 g	0.0 g
Egg, 1 large (50 g)	0.0 g	0.0 g	0.6 g	2.0 g	1.6 g	0.0 g
Butter, 1 oz (2 T)	0.1 g	0.0 g	0.5 g	17.5 g	12.8 g	0.0 g
Pork bacon, 3 oz	0.2 g	0.0 g	4.5 g	13.4 g	10.7 g	0.2 g
Commercially produced cookies, 3 oz	0.2 g	0.0 g	2.0 g	2.0 g	13.7 g	0.4 g

ALA, alpha-linolenic acid; DHA, docosahexaenoic acid; EPA, eicosapentaenoic acid; PREDIMED, Prevention with Mediterranean Diet.
Created by Bever A for *Nutrition Essentials*.

that ruminant (natural occurring) trans fat is associated with CHD.

The fatty acid compositions of different example foods are shown in Table 20-2.

Dietary Cholesterol

As with total fat, dietary cholesterol was presumed to play a major role in the development of CHD based on the finding of cholesterol-rich lipoproteins in atherosclerotic lesions. Most observational studies to date investigating the association of egg intake (a primary source of cholesterol) and CVD incidence and mortality have been null, except for a handful of studies showing that egg consumption is associated with increased incidence of CVD among individuals with diabetes.[21] Controlled feeding studies have shown that dietary cholesterol results in increased LDL-C and HDL-C; without information on additional markers, it is difficult to draw any conclusions from these findings. Given that eggs are rich in nutrients such as iron, choline,

and vitamin D, eggs and other cholesterol-containing foods can be consumed in moderation as part of a heart-healthy diet, especially for individuals who do not consume meat products.

Total Carbohydrate

The effect of carbohydrate restriction on CHD has proven to be a controversial topic. Although observational studies have shown no consistent association between carbohydrate intake and CHD, a handful of short-term (5–12 months) RCTs have shown that low-carbohydrate diets have favorable effects on BMI, systolic and diastolic blood pressure, Lp(a), and LDL particle size compared to healthy moderate- or high-carbohydrate diets, even when saturated fat consumption increased and among individuals with and without diabetes.[22–25] Although these data are promising and warrant follow-up, short-term data on CHD risk factors does not always translate to favorable long-term effects on CHD morbidity and mortality.

Patients may report improvements in weight and blood glucose management by adhering to a low- or very-low-carbohydrate diet, raising questions about whether a diet that both results in weight loss and is high in saturated fat is net beneficial for CHD. The short answer is that we do not have enough data to answer this question, however, a low-carbohydrate diet in which most of the fat comes from quality sources of polyunsaturated fatty acid and monounsaturated fatty acid is unlikely to be harmful and can be recommended to patients who prefer to follow a low-carbohydrate dietary pattern. In general, a diet with similar carbohydrate content as the Mediterranean-style diets shown to have CHD benefits in RCTs (40–50% energy from carbohydrates sourced from fruits, vegetables, whole grains, nuts, and legumes) is the best supported guideline to date.

Refined Starches and Added Sugars

Like fatty acids, carbohydrates are a heterogenous group of nutrients with different implications for cardiovascular health. Consumption of refined starches (typically grains from which the bran and germ have been removed, such as flour or white rice) and added sugars (sucrose or fructose added during the processing of foods) is likely to contribute to CHD risk, particularly among individuals with diabetes or prediabetes. In observational studies, added sugar consumption was associated with increased risk of CHD; of individual sugar-containing foods, sugar-sweetened beverages were the most consistently associated with increased CHD.[26,27] Limited evidence from small controlled feeding studies suggests that very high consumption of fructose (~25% of daily energy intake) and hypercaloric fructose consumption, relative to glucose consumption, increases apoB and TG, providing a potential mechanism that needs to be confirmed with longer trials and more reasonable fructose consumption.

Refined starches have a high glycemic index and may contribute to increased risk of CHD among individuals with diabetes for whom glycemic control has been linked to CHD. RCTs show that a low glycemic dietary pattern reduces hemoglobin A1C (HbA1c), glucose, apoB, and CRP among individuals with type I or type II diabetes. In most observational studies among healthy individuals, high vs. low refined grain intake or glycemic load was associated with slightly increased CHD.[28,29] Added sugars and refined grains were discouraged as part of the Mediterranean-style diet intervention in the Lyon Diet Heart Study and are often found in processed foods that also contain high amounts of saturated fat and trans fat; as such, it is advisable that all individuals, and especially those managing diabetes, minimize refined starch and added sugar consumption. See Chapter 18 for more details on dietary and lifestyle approaches to reduce insulin resistance and hyperglycemia in individuals with prediabetes and diabetes.

Of note, there is no evidence that the naturally occurring fructose in fruit and fruit juice contribute to CHD risk factors, incidence, or mortality. Daily consumption of fruit was a key recommendation in the Lyon Diet Heart Study Mediterranean-style diet, and a number of mechanisms could explain the cardiovascular benefits of fruit, such as fiber and polyphenol content. While fruit juice has not been shown to be associated with CHD in observational studies, it should be consumed in moderation given the high fructose content, especially in people with prediabetes and diabetes (see Chapter 18) and in young children (see Chapter 5). Dried fruit, like fruit juice, should be eaten in moderation due to a more concentrated fructose content relative to fresh and frozen fruit.

Fiber

Dietary fiber intake from a variety of sources has been associated with a significantly lower risk of CHD in observational cohort studies, potentially due to beneficial effects on glycemic control.[30] Examples of food sources of fiber include whole grains, legumes, fruits, vegetables, seeds, and nuts. Meta-analyses of RCTs reported a reduction of LDL-C, TG, CRP, HbA1c, and fasting insulin and glucose with consumption of any dietary fiber (from food or supplement) and a reduction of LDL-C and apoB with consumption of psyllium fiber.[31,32] Despite showing consistent favorable effects of fiber on CHD risk factors, none of these studies had CHD events as primary outcomes.

Alcohol

The association between alcohol and CHD, as with many of the aforementioned dietary factors, is complicated. Most meta-analyses of observational studies show a J-shaped association of alcohol with CHD, with the nadir for CHD mortality at 32 g/day (or about two U.S. standard drinks) for men and 11 g/day (about one U.S. standard drink) for women.[33] Observational studies on type of alcohol have been more consistent in showing a J-shaped association for wine consumption than for beer.[34] Wine as the primary source of alcohol was recommended in both experimental (Mediterranean diet) arms of the PREDIMED trial. Red wine and beer both contain a number of polyphenolic compounds that may confer anti-inflammatory properties, although a cardioprotective effect specific to the polyphenols in wine or beer has not been definitively shown. In a handful of RCTs, moderate alcohol consumption has been shown to increase apoA-I and decrease apoB, Lp(a), fasting insulin, and HbA1c.

Due to the potential for significant confounding by health factors that influence an individual's decision to abstain from alcohol, the observed benefit of light alcohol consumption compared to no alcohol consumption should be interpreted with caution. In contrast to the above, several meta-analyses of observational studies have concluded that any amount of alcohol is associated with increased risk of CHD.[35] Due to the complex behavioral component of alcohol consumption, the AHA recommends drinking in moderation, if at all, and recommends that individuals do not start drinking based on the purported health benefits.

Marine Omega-3 Fatty Acid Supplements

Two specific omega-3 fatty acids found in marine food sources appear to be uniquely beneficial for secondary CHD prevention: EPA and DHA. The meta-analyzed results of over a dozen RCTs suggest that marine omega-3 supplementation is associated with significantly lower risk of myocardial infarction and CHD mortality among individuals with prevalent CHD.[36] The trials had a mean treatment duration of 5 years and used varying doses and combinations of EPA and DHA or EPA alone; the magnitude of effect appears to increase with dose, which may explain why several of the studies found no significant CHD risk reduction with low or moderate doses of marine omega-3 supplement.

One of the largest and most recent RCTs, the Reduction of Cardiovascular Events with Icosapent Ethyl–Intervention Trial (REDUCE-IT) trial, showed a 25% reduction in combined fatal and non-fatal CHD with 4,000 mg/d EPA alone (with the majority of participants having documented prior CAD); the results of this trial have been called into question because the control group received a mineral oil that may have in fact increased inflammation and CHD. However, the meta-analyzed results of RCTs of marine omega-3 supplement still showed a protective effect, albeit weaker, on myocardial infarction and CHD death after excluding the REDUCE-IT trial or excluding open-label trials and trials with smaller sample size, lower dose, and shorter follow-up duration. In RCTs, marine omega-3 fatty acids reduced TG, apoB, systolic and diastolic blood pressure, and CRP.[37] Although there is currently no clinical consensus about the use of marine omega-3 supplements in the secondary prevention of CHD, EPA was recently approved for certain high-risk patients in conjunction with lipid-lowering therapy, and it is probable that omega-3 supplements reduce the risk of CHD at a sufficient dose.

A summary of the nutrients and foods discussed in this section in relation to CHD are summarized in Tables 20-3 and 20-4.

● AMERICAN HEART ASSOCIATION AND DIETARY GUIDELINES FOR AMERICANS

Most of the recommendations included in the 2020–2025 Dietary Guidelines for Americans (DGA) are in line with the principles that we have outlined over the course of this chapter. The most recent DGA and the recent AHA recommendations focused more on overall dietary patterns than individual aspects of the diet, recognizing that people eat foods and few individuals can recognize type of fat or carbohydrates in their daily dietary choices. The DGA recommend a Mediterranean-style diet since it has been shown to lower CHD and total mortality in long-term RCTs, in addition to other potential health benefits (see Chapter 6). Of note, most of the principles of a Mediterranean-style diet are transferable to dietary patterns based on non-Western traditions and varying personal preferences. As providers, it may be beneficial to discuss principles of a Mediterranean-style diet without using the term *Mediterranean* to avoid ostracizing patients from non-Western cultural backgrounds. The Mediterranean-style diet has never been compared to other traditional dietary patterns, which may offer unique benefits for cardiovascular health that have yet to be studied.

● CONCLUSION

Given the high rate of CHD and CVD in the United States and around the world, a vast majority of the population would benefit to adopt a dietary pattern that promotes cardiovascular health and is shown to reduce risk of CHD (as primary or secondary prevention). Unprocessed sources of plant monounsaturated fatty acid and plant and marine omega-3 fatty acids, including olive oil, fatty fish, nuts, and seeds, are the cornerstone of a heart healthy diet, as has been demonstrated by two major RCTs. The inclusion of a diverse mixture of vegetables, fruits, and legumes is also very likely to play a role in the promotion of cardiovascular health. Dairy, eggs, and poultry can be part of a balanced diet when enjoyed in moderation, and fermented dairy products (yogurt, kefir, cheese) may even have a beneficial effect on cardiovascular health. Consumption of refined starches and added sugars, which are abundant in commercial snack and dessert items, has the potential to increase CHD risk, particularly for individuals with insulin resistance, and offers very little in terms of nutritional quality. Although there is not strong evidence that a low- or very-low-carbohydrate diet reduces CVD risk compared to a moderate carbohydrate diet, reduced carbohydrate intake is unlikely to be detrimental when consumed as part of a diet that includes plant and marine foods as the primary sources of fat and limited processed foods. Ultra-processed foods, especially sugar sweetened beverages and foods containing refined grains and/or commercial trans fats, are very likely to increase risk of CHD without providing other nutritional benefits and should be avoided (these include processed meat and commercial snacks). EPA supplements have been approved for secondary prevention in conjunction with pharmacologic lipid-lowering treatment, and although the effects of these supplements are not conclusive, they are likely to reduce CHD. Clinicians have the potential to make a significant impact on CHD morbidity and mortality by discussing these principles of a heart healthy diet with patients of all ages.

TABLE 20-3 • Summary of individual diet components in relation to CHD based on observational studies and randomized controlled trials

Dietary component	Observational studies	Randomized controlled trials		Key results	Strength of evidence (very low, low, moderate, high)
	CHD incidence or mortality	Biomarkers of cardiometabolic health	CHD incidence or mortality		
NUTRIENTS					
Low-fat diet	**High vs. low total fat** CHD incidence ↔ CHD mortality ↔	**Low-fat diet compared to a moderate- or high-fat diet[a]** LDL-C ↓ HDL-C ↓ TG ↑ Fasting glucose ↑↓ SBP ↑↓ DBP ↑↓	**Total fat reduced from 30% to 20% of total energy** Nonfatal myocardial infarction ↔ CHD mortality ↔	In meta-analyzed observational cohort studies and one large, randomized controlled trial among post-menopausal women there was consistently no effect of low-fat as compared to moderate- or high-fat diet on risk of CHD event and mortality.	High
Saturated fatty acids	**High vs. low SFA** ↔ CHD incidence ↔ CHD mortality **Carbohydrate → SFA** ↓ CHD incidence ↔ CHD mortality **PUFA → SFA** ↑ CHD incidence ↑ CHD mortality	**MUFA or PUFA → SFA** apoB ↑ apoA-I ↔ LDL-C ↑ HDL-C ↑ TG ↔	**SFA → Combination of omega-3 and omega-6 PUFA** CHD mortality ↓	In meta-analyzed observational cohort studies, the replacement of SFA with PUFA resulted in decreased CHD whereas replacement of SFA with carbohydrate resulted in no change or increased CHD risk. In a few randomized-controlled trials with moderate potential for bias, replacing SFA with combined omega-3 and omega-6 PUFA decreased CHD mortality. The effects of SFA may further depend on the food source, with some observational studies showing that SFAs from red meat, butter, cream, and processed foods are harmful whereas SFAs from vegetable, fermented dairy, fish, and poultry are not.	Moderate
Omega-3 fatty acid	**High vs. low plant source omega-3 fatty acid (ALA)** CHD incidence ↓ CHD mortality ↓ **High vs. low marine source omega-3 fatty acid (DHA, DPA, and EPA)** CHD mortality ↓	**EPA and/or DHA supplementation** apoB ↓[b] apoA-I ↔[b] LDL-C ↑[b] HDL-C ↑[b] VLDL-C ↓[b] Non-HDL-C ↓[b] TG ↓[b] HbA1c ↔[c] Fasting insulin ↔[c] SBP ↓[b] DBP ↓ CRP ↓	**EPA and/or DHA supplementation** Total CHD ↓ CHD mortality ↓	In observational studies, plant and marine sources of omega-3 fatty acids were consistently associated with decreased risk of CHD incidence or mortality. In randomized trials, marine omega-3 supplementation was associated with favorable changes to CVD risk factors, most notably TG. Although randomized trials of marine omega-3 supplements have not consistently shown a reduction in CHD, the meta-analyzed results show a protective effect of marine omega-3 supplements, even after excluding the controversial REDUCE-IT trial.	High

(Continued)

TABLE 20-3 • Summary of individual diet components in relation to CHD based on observational studies and randomized controlled trials (*Continued*)

Dietary component	Observational studies — CHD incidence or mortality	Randomized controlled trials — Biomarkers of cardiometabolic health	Randomized controlled trials — CHD incidence or mortality	Key results	Strength of evidence (very low, low, moderate, high)
Trans fatty acids (industrial)	**High vs. low TFA** CHD event ↑ CHD mortality ↑	**SFA → TFA** apoB ↑ apoA-I ↓ apoB:apoA-I ↑ Lp(a) ↑ LDL-C ↔ HDL-C ↓ TG ↔ **MUFA → TFA** apoB ↑ apoA-I ↓ apoB:apoA-I ↑ Lp(a) ↑ LDL-C ↑ HDL-C ↓ TG ↑ **PUFA → TFA** apoB ↑ apoA-I ↓ apoB:apoA-I ↑ Lp(a) ↑ LDL-C ↔ HDL-C ↓ TG ↔	∅	In meta-analyzed observational cohort studies, high compared to low TFA consumption was consistently associated with increased risk of CHD. In randomized controlled trials, the substitution of TFA for any other fatty acid was associated with detrimental changes in cardiovascular risk profile.	High
Low-carbohydrate diet	**Low vs. high total carbohydrate** CVD incidence[d] ↓ CVD mortality[d] ↔	**Low-carbohydrate compared to moderate- or high-carbohydrate diet**[a] Lp(a)[e] ↓ LDL-C ↓ HDL-C ↑ TG ↓ HbA1c[c] ↓ SBP ↔ DBP ↔ CRP[c] ↔	∅	In meta-analyzed observational cohort studies, a low-carbohydrate diet was sometimes associated with decreased CHD incidence and often had no effect on CHD. Meta-analyzed randomized controlled trials of CHD biomarkers provide some evidence of protective effects of a low-carbohydrate diet on CHD risk, however, almost all of these trials were in the context of weight loss and do not provide evidence of a direct effect of low-carbohydrate diet on CHD independent of changes in fat mass. Additional trials are warranted to determine if there are benefits to reducing carbohydrate intake in the context of an otherwise healthy diet (i.e., high in fiber, omega-3 PUFA, and MUFA) in terms of CHD incidence and mortality, particularly among individuals with prediabetes or diabetes.	Very low

TABLE 20-3 • Summary of individual diet components in relation to CHD based on observational studies and randomized controlled trials (*Continued*)

Dietary component	Observational studies	Randomized controlled trials		Key results	Strength of evidence (very low, low, moderate, high)
	CHD incidence or mortality	Biomarkers of cardiometabolic health	CHD incidence or mortality		
Low glycemic load	**Low vs. high glycemic load** CHD incidence ↓	**Low glycemic load or index diet compared to usual diet**[c] apoB ↓ LDL-C ↓ HDL-C ↔ TG ↓ HbA1c ↔ Fasting insulin ↔ Fasting glucose ↓ SBP ↓ DBP ↔ CRP ↓	Ø	In observational studies, low glycemic load was usually associated with decreased incidence of CHD. Among individuals with type 1 or type 2 diabetes, randomized trials consistently showed favorable changes to different CVD biomarkers when usual diet was replaced with low glycemic load or index diet. It is very likely that replacing high glycemic foods with low glycemic foods reduces risk of CHD.	Moderate
Added sugar	**High vs. low added sugar intake** CHD incidence ↑ **10–14.9% vs. < 10% energy from added sugar** CHD incidence ↔ **15% vs. < 10% energy from added sugar** CHD incidence ↑	Ø	Ø	In observational studies, higher intake of added sugars, particularly when >15% of total energy, was associated with increased risk of CHD. Although evidence is limited to a few observational studies, the lack of nutritional benefits of added sugars and the tendency for added sugars to be present in highly processed foods also containing SFA and TFA warrants their limitation.	Low
Fiber	**High vs. low fiber** CHD incidence ↓ CHD mortality ↓	**Any dietary fiber (food or supplement), compared to no fiber**[c] LDL-C ↓ HDL-C ↑ TG ↓ HbA1c ↓ Fasting insulin ↓ Fasting glucose ↓ SBP ↔ DBP ↔ CRP ↓	Ø	In meta-analyzed observational cohort studies, fiber was consistently associated with decreased CHD, and in meta-analyzed randomized controlled trials, fiber intake had favorable effects on markers of CHD risk. There is no strong evidence that this effect is specific to any one type of fiber or to fiber from food sources or supplement.	Moderate

(Continued)

TABLE 20-3 • Summary of individual diet components in relation to CHD based on observational studies and randomized controlled trials (*Continued*)

Dietary component	Observational studies CHD incidence or mortality	Randomized controlled trials Biomarkers of cardiometabolic health	Randomized controlled trials CHD incidence or mortality	Key results	Strength of evidence (very low, low, moderate, high)
		Psyllium fiber supplement compared to supplement containing no fiber, low fiber, or another type of fiber apoB ↓ LDL-C ↓			
Alcohol	↑↓ CHD incidence ↑↓ CHD mortality	**Alcohol intake up to 60 g/day compared to no or low alcohol intake** ApoB^e ↑↓ ApoA-I ↑ Lp(a)^e ↓ LDL-C ↑↓ HDL-C ↑ HbA1c ↓ Fasting insulin ↓ Fasting glucose ↔	∅	The results of many meta-analyzed observational studies provide conflicting results regarding the effects of alcohol consumption on CHD incidence and mortality. The results of short-term randomized trials suggest a potential beneficial effect of moderate alcohol consumption on various markers of CHD, particularly HDL-C.	Low

Abbreviations: ALA, alpha-linolenic acid; apoA-I, apolipoprotein A-I; apoB, apolipoprotein B; CHD, coronary heart disease; CRP, C-reactive protein; CVD, cardiovascular disease; DBP, diastolic blood pressure; DHA, docosahexaenoic acid; DPA, docosapentaenoic acid; EPA, eicosapentaenoic acid; HbA1c, hemoglobin A1c; HDL-C, high-density lipoprotein cholesterol; LDL-C, low-density lipoprotein cholesterol; Lp(a), lipoprotein(a); MUFA, monounsaturated fatty acid; PUFA, polyunsaturated fatty acid; REDUCE-IT, Reduction of Cardiovascular Events with Icosapent Ethyl–Intervention Trial; SBP, systolic blood pressure; SFA, saturated fatty acid; TFA, trans fatty acid; TG, triglyceride.

^{a}Includes studies not controlled for differences in weight loss between comparison diets

^{b}Among individuals with hypertriglyceridemia

^{c}Among individuals with prediabetes or diabetes

^{d}Insufficient data on CHD-specific outcomes

^{e}Based on only a limited number of studies

Key:

↓ Decreased (CHD incidence, or level of biomarker) in the majority of studies

↑ Increased (CHD incidence, or level of biomarker) in the majority of studies

→ Indicates that the first dietary component is replaced with the second

↔ No net effect in either direction in the majority of studies

↑↓ Conflicting results

∅ Insufficient data

Created by Bever A for *Nutrition Essentials*.

TABLE 20-4 • Association of high vs. low consumption of individual food groups with CHD incidence among individuals without CHD at baseline, based on meta-analysis of observational cohort studies

Food group	Direction of effect on CHD incidence
Legumes	↓
Nuts	↓
Fish	↓
Fruit	↓
Vegetables	↓
Whole grains	↓
Dairy	↔
Eggs	↔
Red meat	↑
Processed meat	↑
Refined grains	↑
Sugar-sweetened beverages	↑

Key:
↓ Decreased (CHD incidence) in the majority of studies
↑ Increased (CHD incidence) in the majority of studies
↔ No net effect in either direction in the majority of studies
Created by Bever A for *Nutrition Essentials.*

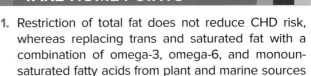

TAKE-HOME POINTS

1. Restriction of total fat does not reduce CHD risk, whereas replacing trans and saturated fat with a combination of omega-3, omega-6, and monoun-saturated fatty acids from plant and marine sources has been shown to reduce both CHD incidence and mortality.
2. Adherence to a relatively low-glycemic load diet consisting of whole grains, legumes, fruits, and vegetables in place of refined starches has car-diometabolic benefits and is particularly important to reducing CHD risk among individuals with pre-diabetes or diabetes.
3. Avoiding added sugars and ultra-processed foods, especially sugar-sweetened beverages, is a straightforward action to reduce CHD risk.
4. A Mediterranean-style dietary pattern has been shown to reduce CHD incidence and mortality in the setting of primary and secondary prevention in large RCTs.

CASE STUDY 1 ANSWERS

1. LDL-C is generally correlated with CHD; however, LDL-C is known to increase when total dietary fat consumption increases and this change does not necessarily correspond to increased CHD risk. You may consider measuring this patient's apoB to get a better idea of her risk and create a baseline to compare to future visits. Monitoring her HbA1c and CRP could also give you an idea of her overall CHD risk, although for a healthy 35-year-old without symptoms of diabetes, the additional labs are prob-ably unnecessary. Her systolic and diastolic blood pressures, which are likely to have decreased based on her recent weight loss, are another met-ric you can use to assess her CHD risk over time. Importantly, you might want to discuss the sustain-ability of her dietary choices, as restrictive diets are often difficult to maintain in the long term.

2. The amount of total fat or carbohydrate in the diet is one of the least important factors in deter-mining CHD risk, and most of the principles of a Mediterranean-style diet, which is shown to reduce CHD risk, can be adapted to a patient's preference for a very-low, low-, or moderate-carbohydrate diet. Some principles that may be particularly relevant to a patient who is restricting carbohydrates include the following:

- Because she is consuming a high percent energy from fat, it is even more important to choose high-quality sources of plant and marine fats for the majority of dietary fat. Sources include olive oil, canola oil, fatty fish, nuts, and seeds.
- If possible within the guidelines of her diet, consuming non-starchy vegetables, legumes, and fruit are likely to be beneficial based on the nutrient and fiber content. She would benefit from aiming to fill her carbohydrate quota with these nutrient-dense foods.
- She is most likely already minimizing sugar-sweetened beverages and refined starches due to the high carbohydrate content of these foods; other foods to minimize for general CHD prevention include red and processed meats, cream, and butter.
- Fish, white meats, cheese, and yogurt are part of a Mediterranean-style diet and are relatively low-carbohydrate foods that can be consumed in moderate amounts.

CASE STUDY 2 ANSWERS

1. Although LDLs play a central role in the development of atherosclerosis and CHD, there are many other factors involved. In the Lyon Diet Heart Study, a protective effect of the Mediterranean-style diet was observed even in the absence of changes to average lipid biomarkers in the treatment arm. Although it is excellent and significant that your patient is serious about adhering to pharmacologic treatment, there are many additional benefits he can gain from a healthy diet. Some possible ways that diet may influence secondary CHD prevention beyond lipid disorders include via the prevention or lessening of insulin resistance, inflammation, hypertension, and fat mass, which translate to beneficial effects on endothelial function, the progression of atherosclerosis, and, in cases of late primary or secondary prevention, atherosclerotic plaque stability.

2. Although a Mediterranean-style diet is the only dietary pattern shown to prevent CHD in RCTs, it sounds like this patient is not ready to overhaul his entire eating pattern and presenting him with a specific diet may be overwhelming or discouraging. Some potential suggestions you could make that are in line with both the principles of a Mediterranean-style diet and his current preferences include:

   - Use high-quality virgin olive oil or canola oil when stir-frying (as olive oil has a relatively low smoke point, canola oil is a better choice for high-heat cooking).
   - Depending on his preferences, replace the pork and beef in his stir fry with fish or tofu while using the same flavors, or, of his current options, choose chicken more often.
   - Consider whether the stir fry sauces he is currently using contain added sugars, and, if so, if there are low-sugar options available or if he could make a similar substitute himself. Most sauces are also high in sodium, which contribute to higher blood pressure, so overall it might be wise to advise him trying to use sauces in moderation.
   - Replace his current selection of noodles and white rice with whole-grain noodles and/or whole-grain rice (brown rice).
   - Add vegetables (fresh or frozen), legumes (e.g., edamame), and/or nuts and seeds (e.g., peanuts, sesame seeds, cashews) to his stir fry for additional fiber and other nutrients.
   - Replace his current dried fruit snacks with fresh or frozen fruit.
   - Decrease the sweetness of his iced tea by either buying versions with less sugar, or making iced tea at home so he can control the sugar content.
   - Replace his current commercial crackers with unprocessed snack items (e.g., dry roasted mixed nuts), or, as an alternative, look for commercial crackers with minimal added sugar, saturated fat, and trans fat.

3. Although not definitive, there is good quality evidence that use of marine omega-3 fatty acid supplements reduces CHD incidence and mortality in the setting of secondary prevention, with little risk of harm (there is a small increased risk of atrial fibrillation associated with marine omega-3 fatty acid use).

REFERENCES

1. de Lorgeril M, Renaud S, Salen P, et al. Mediterranean alpha-linolenic acid-rich diet in secondary prevention of coronary heart disease. *Lancet.* 1994;343(8911):1454-1459.

2. Estruch R, Ros E, Salas-Salvadó J, et al. Primary prevention of cardiovascular disease with a Mediterranean diet supplemented with extra-virgin olive oil or nuts. *N Engl J Med.* 2018;378(25):e34. doi:10.1056/NEJMoa1800389.

3. Krauss RM, Eckel RH, Howard B, et al. AHA dietary guidelines. *Circulation.* 2000;102(18):2284-2299.

4. Jeppesen J, Schaaf P, Jones C, Zhou MY, Chen YD, Reaven GM. Effects of low-fat, high-carbohydrate diets on risk factors for ischemic heart disease in postmenopausal women. *Am J Clin Nutr.* 1997;65(4):1027-1033.

5. Marckmann P, Sandström B, Jespersen J. Low-fat, high-fiber diet favorably affects several independent risk markers of ischemic heart disease: observations on blood lipids, coagulation, and fibrinolysis from a trial of middle-aged Danes. *Am J Clin Nutr.* 1994;59(4):935-939.

6. Skeaff CM, Miller J. Dietary fat and coronary heart disease: summary of evidence from prospective cohort and randomised controlled trials. *Ann Nutr Metab.* 2009;55(1-3):173-201.

7. Howard BV, Van Horn L, Hsia J, et al. Low-fat dietary pattern and risk of cardiovascular disease. The women's health initiative randomized controlled dietary modification trial. *JAMA.* 2006;295(6):655-666.

8. Howard BV, Curb JD, Eaton CB, et al. Low-fat dietary pattern and lipoprotein risk factors: the women's health initiative dietary modification trial. *Am J Clin Nutr.* 2010;91(4):860-874.

9. Keys A. Seven countries: a multivariate analysis of death and coronary heart disease. In: *Seven Countries.* Harvard University Press; 2013. doi:10.4159/harvard.9780674497887.

10. le Riche H. Dietary fat, essential fatty acids and coronary heart disease. *Can Med Assoc J.* 1956;74(8):644-645.

11. Ramsden CE, Zamora D, Leelarthaepin B, et al. Use of dietary linoleic acid for secondary prevention of coronary heart disease and death: evaluation of recovered data from the Sydney diet heart study and updated meta-analysis. *BMJ.* 2013;346(feb04 3): e8707-e8707.

12. Bergeron N, Chiu S, Williams PT, King SM, Krauss RM. Effects of red meat, white meat, and nonmeat protein sources on atherogenic lipoprotein measures in the context of low compared with high saturated fat intake: a randomized controlled trial. *Am J Clin Nutr.* 2019 Jul 1;110(1):24-33.

13. Drouin-Chartier JP, Tremblay AJ, Lépine MC, Lemelin V, Lamarche B, Couture P. Substitution of dietary ω-6 polyunsaturated fatty acids for saturated fatty acids decreases LDL apolipoprotein B-100 production rate in men with dyslipidemia associated with insulin resistance: a randomized controlled trial. *Am J Clin Nutr.* 2018;107(1):26-34.

14. Demacker PNM, Reijnen IGM, Katan MB, Stuyt PMJ, Stalenhoef AFH. Increased removal of remnants of triglyceride-rich lipoproteins on a diet rich in polyunsaturated fatty acids. *Eur J Clin Invest.* 1991;21(2):197-203.

15. Bergeron N, Havel RJ. Influence of diets rich in saturated and omega-6 polyunsaturated fatty acids on the postprandial responses of apolipoproteins B-48, B-100, E, and lipids in triglyceride-rich lipoproteins. *Arterioscler Thromb Vasc Biol.* 1995;15(12):2111-2121.

16. Steur M, Johnson L, Sharp SJ, et al. Dietary fatty acids, macronutrient substitutions, food sources and incidence of coronary heart disease: findings from the EPIC-CVD Case-Cohort Study Across Nine European Countries. *J Am Heart Assoc.* 2021;10(23):e019814.

17. Guasch-Ferré M, Babio N, Martínez-González MA, et al. Dietary fat intake and risk of cardiovascular disease and all-cause mortality in a population at high risk of cardiovascular disease1. *Am J Clin Nutr.* 2015;102(6):1563-1573.

18. Naghshi S, Sadeghi O, Willett WC, Esmaillzadeh A. Dietary intake of total, animal, and plant proteins and risk of all cause, cardiovascular, and cancer mortality: systematic review and dose-response meta-analysis of prospective cohort studies. *BMJ.* 2020;370:m2412.

19. Giosuè A, Calabrese I, Lupoli R, Riccardi G, Vaccaro O, Vitale M. Relations between the consumption of fatty or lean fish and risk of cardiovascular disease and all-cause mortality: a systematic review and meta-analysis. *Adv Nutr.* 2022;13(5):1554-1565.

20. Mozaffarian D, Clarke R. Quantitative effects on cardiovascular risk factors and coronary heart disease risk of replacing partially hydrogenated vegetable oils with other fats and oils. *Eur J Clin Nutr.* 2009;63(2):S22-S33.

21. Shin JY, Xun P, Nakamura Y, He K. Egg consumption in relation to risk of cardiovascular disease and diabetes: a systematic review and meta-analysis. *Am J Clin Nutr.* 2013;98(1):146-159.

22. Gardner CD, Kiazand A, Alhassan S, et al. Comparison of the Atkins, Zone, Ornish, and LEARN diets for change in weight and related risk factors among overweight premenopausal women: the A TO Z weight loss study: a randomized trial. *JAMA.* 2007;297(9):969-977.

23. Gardner CD, Trepanowski JF, Del Gobbo LC, et al. Effect of low-fat vs. low-carbohydrate diet on 12-month weight loss in overweight adults and the association with genotype pattern or insulin secretion: the DIETFITS randomized clinical trial. *JAMA.* 2018;319(7):667-679.

24. Ebbeling CB, Knapp A, Johnson A, et al. Effects of a low-carbohydrate diet on insulin-resistant dyslipoproteinemia-a randomized controlled feeding trial. *Am J Clin Nutr.* 2022;115(1):154-162.

25. Davis NJ, Tomuta N, Schechter C, et al. Comparative study of the effects of a 1-year dietary intervention of a low-carbohydrate diet versus a low-fat diet on weight and glycemic control in type 2 diabetes. *Diabetes Care.* 2009;32(7):1147-1152.

26. Yang B, Glenn AJ, Liu Q, et al. Added sugar, sugar-sweetened beverages, and artificially sweetened beverages and risk of cardiovascular disease: findings from the women's health initiative and a network meta-analysis of prospective studies. *Nutrients.* 2022;14(20):4226.

27. Sun T, Zhang Y, Ding L, Zhang Y, Li T, Li Q. The relationship between major food sources of fructose and cardiovascular outcomes: a systematic review and dose-response meta-analysis of prospective studies. *Adv Nutr.* 2023;14(2):256-269.

28. Hu H, Zhao Y, Feng Y, et al. Consumption of whole grains and refined grains and associated risk of cardiovascular disease events and all-cause mortality: a systematic review and dose-response meta-analysis of prospective cohort studies. *Am J Clin Nutr.* 2023;117(1):149-159.

29. Li Y, Hruby A, Bernstein AM, et al. Saturated fats compared with unsaturated fats and sources of carbohydrates in relation to risk of coronary heart disease: a prospective cohort study. *J Am Coll Cardiol.* 2015;66(14):1538-1548.

30. Liu L, Wang S, Liu J. Fiber consumption and all-cause, cardiovascular, and cancer mortalities: a systematic review and meta-analysis of cohort studies. *Mol Nutr Food Res.* 2015;59(1):139-146.

31. Cicero AFG, Fogacci F, Veronesi M, et al. A randomized Placebo-controlled clinical trial to evaluate the medium-term effects of oat fibers on human health: the Beta-Glucan Effects on Lipid Profile, Glycemia and inTestinal Health (BELT) study. *Nutrients.* 2020;12(3):686.

32. Jovanovski E, Yashpal S, Komishon A, et al. Effect of psyllium (Plantago ovata) fiber on LDL cholesterol and alternative lipid targets, non-HDL cholesterol and apolipoprotein B: a systematic review and meta-analysis of randomized controlled trials. *Am J Clin Nutr.* 2018;108(5):922-932.

33. Roerecke M. Alcohol's impact on the cardiovascular system. *Nutrients.* 2021;13(10):3419.

34. Costanzo S, Di Castelnuovo A, Donati MB, Iacoviello L, de Gaetano G. Wine, beer or spirit drinking in relation to fatal and non-fatal cardiovascular events: a meta-analysis. *Eur J Epidemiol.* 2011;26(11):833-850.

35. Hoek AG, van Oort S, Mukamal KJ, Beulens JWJ. Alcohol consumption and cardiovascular disease risk: placing new data in context. *Curr Atheroscler Rep.* 2022;24(1):51-59.

36. Hu Y, Hu FB, Manson JE. Marine omega-3 supplementation and cardiovascular disease: an updated meta-analysis of 13 randomized controlled trials involving 127 477 participants. *J Am Heart Assoc.* 2019;8(19):e013543.

37. Yang Y, Deng W, Wang Y, et al. The effect of omega-3 fatty acids and its combination with statins on lipid profile in patients with hypertriglyceridemia: a systematic review and meta-analysis of randomized controlled trials. *Front Nutr.* 2022;9:1039056.

chapter 21

Renal Disease

Lea Borgi, MD, MMSc / Jad Mitri, MD / Armida Lefranc Torres, MD

Chapter Outline

CASE STUDY

A 60-year-old patient with diabetes and hypertension was recently diagnosed with chronic kidney disease (CKD) stage 3b. She is asking you, as her physician, what she should eat.

1. She knows to restrict carbohydrates to control blood glucose, but she read on the internet that she must eat less protein. What would you say?

2. She also heard about being careful to eat potassium. Is that true? What foods contain high amount of potassium?

3. She then progresses to end-stage renal disease (ESRD) and is wondering if she needs to eat differently.

INTRODUCTION

In this chapter, we will give an overview of nutrition in CKD patients. We will first define CKD and outline the criteria used to diagnose CKD. We will then review the dietary factors associated with the risk of developing CKD in the general population, and the recommended diet in patients with kidney disease to try and slow down the progression of CKD to ESRD. We will then go over the dietary changes required of ESRD patients who are now on dialysis or have received a transplant.

Finally, we will address the dietary modifications needed in patients with kidney stones to prevent formation of new stones.

DIAGNOSTIC CRITERIA OF CKD AND STAGES

CKD is diagnosed when one of the following persists for more than three months: the estimated glomerular filtration rate (eGFR) is below 60 mL/min/1.73 m^2, albuminuria of 30 mg or more in 24 hours, or markers of kidney disease such as hematuria.[1] eGFR is calculated using serum creatinine or cystatin C. Like creatinine, cystatin C is freely filtered; however, it is independent of gender, age or muscle mass.[2] Using cystatin C to calculate eGFR has been shown to have a stronger association between the kidneys' filtration rate and ESRD and deaths.[3]

KDOQI Definition and Staging of CKD

According to the National Kidney Foundation's (NKF) Kidney Disease Outcomes Quality (KDOQI), CKD is confirmed when there is kidney damage documented through biologic/radiologic markers or pathologic evidence, or an eGFR< 60 ml/min/1.73 m², or both for 3 months or more.[4]

Stage 1 kidney disease is defined by a normal Egfr (≥ 90 mL/min/1.73 m²) and the presence of kidney damage by biological (such as hematuria or proteinuria) or radiological markers (polycystic kidney disease on imaging). In stage 2 kidney disease, there is a mild decrease of the eGFR and the presence of kidney damage. Stages 3, 4, and 5 CKD is confirmed irrespective of kidney damage as the eGFR is below < 60 mL/min/1.73 m².

CKD staging helps healthcare professionals apply guidelines in clinical practice, advise patients on how to slow down CKD progression and, ultimately, prepare patients for renal replacement therapy (RRT) if CKD progresses to stage 5.

Once CKD is diagnosed, eGFR alone is not a strong predictor of CKD progression to end-stage kidney disease. The presence and degree of albuminuria plays an important role in CKD prognosis, cardiovascular disease, and mortality.[5] Therefore, classifying CKD based on eGFR and albuminuria helps identify patients who need closer monitoring and higher level of care (Figure 21-1). For example, a patient with an eGFR of 50 mL/min/1.73 m² and albuminuria of 400 mg has a higher risk of disease progression and complications than a patient with an eGFR of 35 mL/min/1.73 m² and no albuminuria.

● INCIDENCE AND PROGRESSION OF KIDNEY DISEASE

Dietary Risk Factors Associated with Incident and Progressive Kidney Disease

Dietary Acid Load A high dietary acid load has been linked with an increased risk of CKD and CKD progression to ESRD.[6] Dietary acid load represents the balance between acid-producing and base-producing foods. Foods are classified depending on their potential renal acid load (PRAL), which estimates the approximate production of acid by the diet or food.[6] Examples of different food PRALs are depicted in Figure 21-2.

The typical "Western" diet, characterized by low fruits and vegetables, high salt, processed foods, and sugar, has a high net endogenous acid production. The potential mechanisms by which a high dietary acid load leads to CKD include: (1) activation of the renin-angiotensin system, (2) an increase in endothelin-1 leading to endothelial dysfunction, (3) complement pathway activation, and (4) an increase in ammonium excretion by the kidneys to prevent acidosis.

The chronic increased workload by the kidneys to maintain a normal serum bicarbonate and prevent acidosis has been

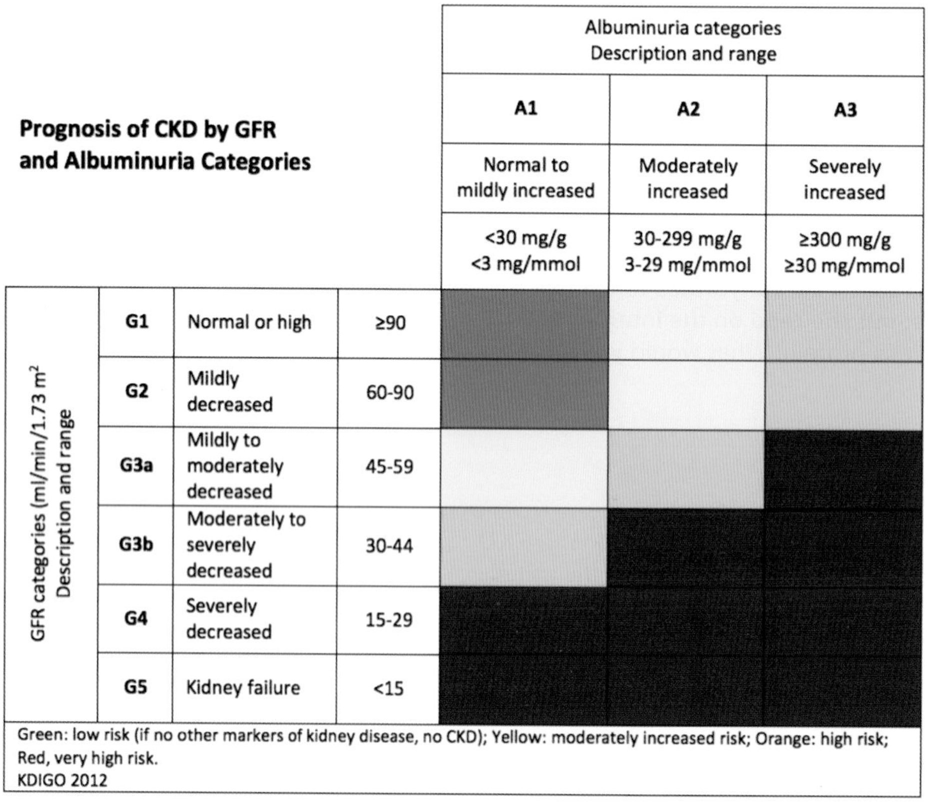

Prognosis of CKD by GFR and Albuminuria Categories

				Albuminuria categories Description and range		
				A1	**A2**	**A3**
				Normal to mildly increased	Moderately increased	Severely increased
				<30 mg/g <3 mg/mmol	30-299 mg/g 3-29 mg/mmol	≥300 mg/g ≥30 mg/mmol
GFR categories (ml/min/1.73 m² Description and range	G1	Normal or high	≥90			
	G2	Mildly decreased	60-90			
	G3a	Mildly to moderately decreased	45-59			
	G3b	Moderately to severely decreased	30-44			
	G4	Severely decreased	15-29			
	G5	Kidney failure	<15			

Green: low risk (if no other markers of kidney disease, no CKD); Yellow: moderately increased risk; Orange: high risk; Red, very high risk.
KDIGO 2012

FIGURE 21-1 • Prognosis of CKD by GFR and albuminuria.[1]
(**Source:** Levin A, Stevens PE. Summary of KDIGO 2012 CKD Guideline: behind the scenes, need for guidance, and a framework for moving forward. *Kidney Int.* 2014;85(1):49-61.)

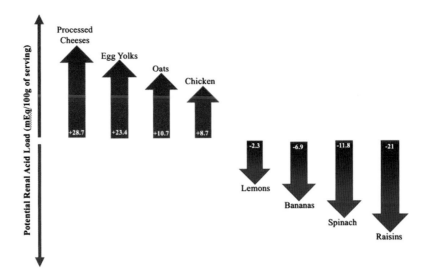

FIGURE 21-2 • Estimated acid-producing potential of selected foods. Potential renal acid load (PRAL) of selected food items (per 100-g serving).

associated with continuous tubular injury leading to CKD, and, ultimately, to ESRD.[7]

Macro and Micronutrients

Protein The typical "Western" diet contains approximately twice the daily recommended protein intake of 0.8 grams per kilogram of body weight. A high protein intake has been associated with repeated episodes of hyperfiltration (an increase in eGFR) through activation of endocrine mediators dilating the afferent arteriole and altering the tubulo-glomerular feedback. While hyperfiltration due to a high protein intake is not fully understood, the continuous distention of the glomerular capillaries leads to mesangial expansion, interstitial fibrosis and kidney injury as represented in Figure 21-3.[8] In patients with CKD 3–5, a continued high-protein diet will accelerate the loss of nephrons through glomerular hyperfiltration and lead to progression of CKD to ESRD.

Because red and processed meat are associated with higher nitrogen waste production and the metabolism of L-carnitine

by gut microbiome to trimethylamine *N*-oxide (TMAO).[9] patients who consume high amount of animal protein in their diet have a higher risk of developing CKD and ESRD as compared to patients who consume mostly plant-based protein. Indeed, several observational studies have shown a higher risk of CKD incidence and progression with animal protein intake, especially red and processed meat with a hazard ratio of 1.4 (1.15–1.71, p < 0.01) when comparing higher and lower quartiles of red meat intake.[10]

Additionally, a diet high in animal protein produces high amounts of advanced glycation end-products (AGE), molecules promoting inflammation and oxidative stress throughout the kidney, and apoptosis of the podocytes leading to albuminuria and subsequently kidney injury.[11] AGEs, TMAO (an intestinal metabolic toxin), and uremic toxins such as p-cresyl sulfate are all associated with progression of kidney disease to ESRD.[9]

Sodium The Dietary Guidelines for Americans as well as the American Heart Association recommend less than 2,300 mg of sodium per day in the general population, and less than 1,500 mg per day for individuals with high blood pressure. Most populations, including Americans, consume 3,000 to 5,000 mg of sodium per day; more than twice the amount recommended in general.[12]

As per the Centers for Disease Control (CDC), the main sources of sodium in the North American diet are breads, rolls, pizza, cold cuts, and soups (commercially made). In the United States, more than 70% of consumed sodium comes from processed foods and restaurant/take-out foods.

Sodium is directly and indirectly related to kidney injury and progression of kidney disease to ESRD, indirectly through high blood pressure leading to endothelial dysfunction, vascular injury, and ultimately kidney disease and CKD progression.[13] Furthermore, high sodium directly affects the kidneys and their vascular systems independently of blood pressure.

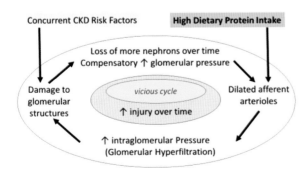

FIGURE 21-3 • Effect of high dietary protein intake on kidney.[8] (**Source:** Jee Ko G, Obi Y, Tortorici AR, Kalantar-Zadeh K. Dietary protein intake and chronic kidney disease. *Curr Opin Clin Nutr Metab Care.* 2017;20(1):77-85.)

This is believed to occur through the breakdown of oxidative species, increasing the production of nitric oxide and TGF β1, leading to glomerular vascular injury, proteinuria, and glomerular sclerosis.[13]

A meta-analysis of randomized controlled trials (RCTs) and prospective cohort studies of a low-salt diet in CKD found that consuming a sodium-restricted diet led to a 28% decrease in adverse renal outcomes, defined as any of the following (1) more than 50% decline in eGFR during follow-up, (2) doubling of serum creatinine, or (3) end-stage renal disease.[13]

Phosphorus High dietary phosphorus intake has been associated with high serum phosphorus level in patients with CKD, leading to progression on their disease to ESRD.[14] High-protein foods from animal sources are usually also high in phosphorus (e.g., meats, cheeses, eggs). The bioavailability of phosphorus however differs based on its source; organic phosphorus is naturally present in plant and animal-based foods, while inorganic phosphorus is found in added to foods as phosphates. Phosphorus additives are used as texture and taste preservatives, leavening agents and others; they are highly bioavailable with more than 90–100% absorbed in the intestinal tract. In contrast, only 40–60% of organic (food-based) phosphorus is absorbed. Plant-based phosphorus is the least bioavailable due to the absence of phytase in humans. Because phosphorus is found as phytate in plants, the inability to degrade this form of phosphorus makes is less absorbable.

Dietary Patterns As described above, a typical "Western" dietary pattern, high in salt, red and processed meat, is associated with an increased risk of incident and progressive CKD. In a meta-analysis of 17 observational studies comprising of about 150,000 participants, the Western-type dietary pattern, characterized by high intakes of red and processed meats, refined grains, sweets, high-fat foods, was associated with an increased risk of CKD (OR = 1.86; CI: 1.21, 2.86; P = 0.005).[15]

In recent years, there has been a trend towards more plant-based or plant-forward diets. Because these diets can still be high in saturated fats, processed foods, and refined sugar,

plant-based indices have been developed to assess the healthiness of these diets. For example, as depicted in Table 21-1, in a healthy plant-based diet index, higher intakes of whole grains, fruits, vegetables, nuts, legumes, tea, and coffee receive a positive score, while refined grains, potatoes, fruit juices, sugar-sweetened and artificially sweetened beverages, sweets, desserts, and all animal foods receive a negative score. Therefore, if an individual's diet is mostly oatmeal with blueberries or raspberries for breakfast; quinoa, broccoli/cauliflower or carrots, and chickpeas for lunch; tofu or lentils with spaghetti squash for dinner and almonds/coffee or a chocolate chip cookie as snacks, their diet would score high on the healthy plant-based diet index because all the consumed foods receive a positive score, except the chocolate chip cookie, which receives a negative score.

For the less healthy plant-based index, aside from all animal foods, the scoring is reversed; the less healthy plant-based foods receive a positive score while the healthy plant-based foods receive a negative score.[16] In the Atherosclerosis Risk in Communities (ARIC) study, a prospective cohort study of ~15,000 participants, diets are classified in four different categories: overall plant-based diet index, healthy plant-based diet index, less healthy plant-based diet index, and provegetarian diet index. Participants with high scores on a healthy plant-based diet had lower risk of developing CKD (HR comparing quintile 5 versus quintile 1 [HRQ5 versus Q1], 0.86; 95% confidence interval [95% CI], 0.78 to 0.96; P for trend = 0.001). In contrast, consuming a less healthy plant-based diet was linked to a higher risk of CKD (HRQ5 versus Q1, 1.11; 95% CI, 1.01 to 1.21; P for trend = 0.04).[16]

Dietary Recommendations for Patients with CKD

Medical Nutrition Therapy In the 2020 guideline update in nutrition in CKD, medical nutrition therapy (MNT) is recommended for patients with CKD stages 3–5.[17] Registered dietitians (RDs) and nephrologists would provide individualized recommendations based on patients' comorbid conditions. After assessing a patient's nutritional status,

Food groups	Examples	Healthy plant-based diet index	Less healthy plant-based diet index
Whole grains	Oatmeal, quinoa, brown rice	Positive	Reverse
Fruits	Apples, pears, bananas	Positive	Reverse
Vegetables	Carrots, spinach, tomatoes, cauliflower, sweet potatoes	Positive	Reverse
Nuts	Peanut butter, almonds	Positive	Reverse
Potatoes	Chips, mashed or baked potatoes, French fries	Reverse	Positive
Fruits juices	Orange juice, apple juice	Reverse	Positive
Sugar-sweetened and artificially sweetened beverages	Coke, diet Coke, fruit-flavored punch	Reverse	Positive
Animal foods	Butter, dairy, eggs, chicken, beef and others	Reverse	Reverse

TABLE 21-1 • Example of a plant-based diet score

reviewing laboratory results such as electrolytes, serum phosphorus, inflammatory biomarkers, and others, the multidisciplinary team uses behavioral approaches, meal planning, and continuous support throughout disease progression into different CKD stages. It is important for healthcare professionals to tailor individual and culturally appropriate dietary recommendations.

Protein The guidelines were updated in 2020 to differentiate protein restriction between CKD patients with and without diabetes; for CKD 3-5 patients not on dialysis and without diabetes, the guidelines recommend a low-protein diet at 0.55–0.6 grams/kg/day or a very low protein diet of 0.28–0.43 gm/kg/day with keto-acids analogues supplements, usually of essential amino acids. For CKD 3-5 patients with diabetes, the protein recommendation is higher at 0.6–0.8 grams/kg/day. The guidelines do not comment on the type of protein, probably because of the lack of randomized controlled diets comparing animal and plant-based proteins on CKD progression and complications in CKD patients. However, following the Dietary Guidelines for Americans, healthcare professionals should recommend lean meats and plant-based protein instead of processed and red meat.[17]

Dietary Pattern While current evidence did not show any eGFR changes associated with a Mediterranean diet, it has been shown to result in an improved lipid panel. As such, the guidelines do recommend a Mediterranean-style dietary pattern for CKD 1-5 patients, given other demonstrated benefits on cardiovascular factors and CVD events (see Chapter 20, "Cardiovascular Disease"). In accordance with the Mediterranean-style dietary pattern, panel experts advise for an increase in fruits and vegetables in patients with CKD 1-4 patients; Mediterranean-style dietary pattern trials assessing blood pressure and body weight changes in CKD patients did not include CKD 5 or dialysis patients.[17]

Sodium, Potassium, and Phosphorus In the 2020 KDOQI guidelines, expert recommend consuming less than 2.3 g sodium intake per day in CKD 1-5 and dialysis patients.[17] The guidelines do not give specific recommendations for dietary potassium and phosphorus daily intake in CKD and dialysis patients. Instead, adjustments of dietary intakes are encouraged to maintain normal levels of potassium ($\leq$ 5.0 mEq/L) and phosphorus ($\leq$ 4.5 mg/dL).

In Fouque et al.'s comprehensive review in 2017, the authors did recommend 4.7 g/day dietary potassium intake for CKD 1-3 patients, unless episodes of hyperkalemia (serum potassium level above 5.0–5.5 mEq/L) occur often, and/or patients with consistent severe hyperkalemia (serum potassium level above 6.5 mEq/L).[18] For CKD 4-5 and dialysis patients, the recommended dietary potassium intake per day is less than 3 g. Furthermore, the review suggests consuming less than 800 mg of dietary phosphorus per day in CKD 1-5 and dialysis patients.[18]

There is insufficient evidence to advise on phosphorus sources, but the guidelines do recommend counseling patients on the different bioavailability of the different sources (animal, plant or added phosphorus). While potassium binders such as patiromer and sodium zirconium cyclosilicate have been more widely prescribed in hyperkalemic CKD patients regardless of CKD stage, no trial has assessed the liberalization of dietary potassium on serum potassium levels in patients on a potassium binder.[19]

Finally, because dietary restrictions can be discouraging to patients and potentially lead to poor quality of life, as described in Kalantar-Zadeh's review, "Dietary Restrictions in Dialysis Patients: Is There Anything Left to Eat?", educating CKD and dialysis patients on their dietary choices might lead to better and long-term results. Table 21-2 provides several suggestions on how to discuss dietary restrictions with CKD and dialysis patients.[20]

Relevant Nutrition Studies in Nephrology—Table 21-3

Nutrition for Patients Receiving Renal Replacement Therapy (RRT) When CKD progresses to ESRD, patients have the option between hemodialysis (in-center or home-based), peritoneal dialysis, transplantation (if eligible), or conservative management.

Regardless of the choice of RRT, patients should be closely followed by a registered dietitian, and monitored for Protein Energy Wasting (PEW).[21] PEW refers to the ongoing protein and energy in advanced CKD and ESRD patients. Because of inadequate intake, muscles are catabolized to provide energy, leading to protein malnutrition.

The prevalence of PEW ranges from 28–54% in CKD patients requiring dialysis. Anorexia develops in patients with inadequate dialysis, chronic inflammation or depression. Effective dialysis treatments to remove uremic toxins, continued dietary assessments and counseling, removal of temporary dialysis catheters to reduce chronic systemic inflammation are important measures to treat and prevent PEW.[21]

Dialysis In patients on hemodialysis (HD) and peritoneal dialysis (PD), the recommended protein intake is 1.0–1.2 g/kg per day.[20] The increase in protein requirement from CKD to dialysis is in the setting of increased energy needs, chronic inflammation and ongoing dialysis-related protein losses.

Transplantation Immediately post kidney transplant (up to 4 weeks postop), it is recommended that patients consume 1.3–2 gm/kg/d of protein to avoid post-op muscle loss and enhance wound healing.[17] There is insufficient evidence for long-term protein intake requirements in stable kidney transplant recipients. The current recommendations are not to exceed the Recommended Dietary Allowance (RDA) of protein at 0.7–0.8 gm/kg/d.

Nutrition and Kidney Stones

In a recent analysis of 10,521 participants in National Health and Nutrition Examination Survey (NHANES) from 2015 to 2018, the prevalence of kidney stones was 11%.[22] They have a recurrence rate of almost 50% at 10 years, and, if large enough,

TABLE 21-2 • Dietary recommendations for patients on dialysis			
	CKD 3-5*	Dialysis	Helpful tips

Protein (g/kg/d)	• Non-diabetic Patients
	   ◦ 0.55–0.6 or 0.28–0.43 + supplements
	• Diabetic Patients
	   ◦ 0.6–0.8
		1.0–1.2	• 3 oz of poultry, meat and fish is about the size of the palm of one's hand
			• Include plant-based proteins such as chickpeas, tofu, beans
			• For dialysis patients, high protein snacks in between meals such as nuts, protein shakes and bars are encouraged

Sodium (g/d)	< 2.3	< 2.3	• Check Nutrition Facts Label and pick low sodium foods (≤ 140 mg per serving) • Avoid take-out and restaurant foods • Remove salt-shaker from the dining table
Potassium (mg/d)	Maintain normal serum potassium levels by modifying dietary intake		• Check Nutrition Facts Label and pick low potassium foods (< 200 mg per serving) • Soak high potassium vegetables (such as potatoes) in water for a few hours before cooking • Kidney.org has a detailed food list of high and low potassium foods
Phosphorus (mg/d)	Maintain normal serum potassium levels by modifying dietary intake		• Avoid phosphate additives by checking a food's ingredient list for "PHOS" (such as calcium phosphate, phosphoric acid) • What you drink might also have phosphates so check the ingredient list as well (examples: cola and energy drinks, fruit punch, powdered mixes)

*CKD 3-5: Chronic Kidney disease stages 3 to 5.

can lead to obstruction and repeated insults to the kidneys, predisposing patients to CKD.

Calcium oxalate and calcium phosphate stones comprise the majority (about 80%) of all kidney stones, followed by uric acid, struvite, and cystine stones.[22]

Diet is an important component in the pathophysiology of kidney stones. Some nutrients may favor supersaturation of the urine with stone-forming salt, thus modifying the urine pH and increasing the risk of stone formation. Therefore, one of the first intervention to prevent recurrent stone formation is through dietary modification. Stone analysis helps identify the type of kidney stone and possibly the presence of metabolic disturbances (hypercalciuria, hypocitraturia, hyperoxaluria, and hyperuricosuria).[23] Once this information is available to the treating physician, specific nutritional measures are addressed with the patient.

Relevant dietary measures for the prevention of kidney stones are:[23]

• Fluid: adequate fluid intake is the first recommendation that can be made to any patient with kidney stones, even before knowing the type of stone. A high fluid intake of about 2.5 L per day or more will dilute the urine and decrease the concentration of lithogenic components and eliminating crystals. Water without electrolytes or additives is usually recommended as the drink of choice.

• Protein/fruits and vegetable balance: high dietary acid load has been found to be associated with increased stone formation. As described in the previous section on "Dietary Acid Load," meats and cheeses are acid producing whether fruits and vegetables are base producing foods.

• Oxalate: a high urinary oxalate is a primary risk factor for the formation of calcium oxalate stones. Because oxalate is present in a wide variety of foods, reviewing a patient's dietary intake would help identify sources of high oxalate intake. Limiting oxalate-rich foods such as spinach, almonds, beets and others decreases the risk of stone recurrent by decreasing hyperoxaluria.

• Calcium: while increased urinary calcium excretion could precipitate calcium stone formation, it is only recommended that calcium intake be balanced (1,000–1,200 mg/day), not reduced. Calcium restriction predisposes to bone loss and increases intestinal absorption of unbound oxalate, thus subsequently increase oxaluria.

• Sodium: increased salt intake leads to expansion of extracellular volume in turn increasing calcium excretion through the inhibition of renal tubular calcium reabsorption. Limiting sodium intake decreases urinary calcium excretion, decreasing stone formation.

● CONCLUSION

Nutrition in patients with kidney disease is based on the stage of the disease and whether they are on dialysis or not.

TABLE 21-3 · Relevant nutrition studies in nephrology

	Study	Study type	Sample size	Diet or intervention	eGFR$	Findings	Comments
Protein (g/kg/d)	Klahr et al. Study 1[24]	RCT*	585	1.3 vs. 0.6	CKD[ε] 3-4	No eGFR differences between groups	Only 3% of CKD due to IDDM[η]
	Klahr et al. Study 2[24]		255	0.6 vs. 0.3 + KA[φ]	CKD 4-5	Slight slower decline in the very low protein group + supplements	
	Jhee et al.[25]	Prospective	9,226	Quintiles of protein intake	≥ 60	A higher protein intake (~ > 1.7 gm/kg/d) leads rapid decline of kidney function	CKD patients excluded
	Cianciaruso et al.[26]	RCT	423	0.8 vs. 0.55	CKD 4-5	No differences on dialysis initiation or death	No PEW**
	Garneata et al.[27]	RCT	207	0.6 vs. vegetarian 0.3 + KA	< 30	Less patients started dialysis in the vegetarian very low protein diet	Patients with diabetes were excluded
Phosphorus	Kestenbaum et al.[28]	Retrospective	6,730	NA	< 60	Phosphorus > 3.5 mg/dL linked to increased risk of death	Patients mostly men, white and older
	Block et al.[29]	Observational	40,538	NA	Hemodialysis	Phosphorus > 5.0 mg/dL linked to increased risk of death	Observational study Peritoneal dialysis patients not included
	Sullivan et al.[30]	RCT	279	Education to avoid foods with additives and fast foods vs. usual care	Hemodialysis	- Slight improvement of phosphorus levels in education arm - Increased reading of nutrition facts labels	Short follow-up of 3 months
Acid load	Rebholz et al.[6]	Prospective	15,055	NA	60	Increased risk of incident CKD with increasing quartiles of dietary acid load	Serum bicarbonate levels not available
	Goraya et al.[31]	RCT	108	Fruits and vegetables vs. bicarbonate supplementation vs. usual care	30-59 + serum bicarbonate level between 22-24 mmol/L	Decreased eGFR decline in the fruits/vegetables group or bicarbonate supplementation compared to usual care	Excluded patients with eGFR ⩽ 30

[φ]KA, KetoAnalogues.
*RCT, randomized controlled trial.
$eGFR is estimated Glomerular Filtration Rate in mL/min/1.73 m²
[ε]CKD: Chronic Kidney Disease
[η]IDDM: Insulin Dependent Diabetes Mellitus
**PEW: protein energy wasting.

SEVERAL TAKE-HOME POINTS

1. For patients with an eGFR > 60 mL/min/1.73 m² at risk for CKD (such as patients with diabetes and/or hypertension), advise for a healthy dietary pattern incorporating lean meats, plant-based proteins, and fruits and vegetables.

2. Dietary restrictions in CKD 3-5 patients not on dialysis should be individualized based on the patient's laboratory data and dietary preferences.

3. Protein restriction is recommended in CKD 3-5 patients, while an increase in protein intake is encouraged in dialysis patients.

4. When asking a patient to modify their diet or restrict certain foods, real-life food examples are helpful.

5. In patients with kidney stones, increasing fluid intake to ≥ 2.5 L per day is recommended regardless of the type of stone.

CASE STUDY ANSWERS

1. Protein restriction is recommended in CKD patients, however, because she has diabetes, guideline recommendations are to achieve a protein intake of 0.6–0.8 g/kg/d which is higher than in CKD 3b patients without diabetes (e.g., 0.55-0.6 g/kg/d or 0.28–0.43 g/kg/d with keto-acids analogues supplements).

2. If her serum potassium level is above 5.0–5.5 mE/L, then going over the patient's usual dietary intake is helpful to see if she already consumes high-potassium foods (for example, eats a banana with her cereals every morning; or potatoes every dinner).

3. If she opts to start dialysis, then yes, she now needs to eat more protein (aiming for 1.0–1.2 g/kg/d when on dialysis). Additionally, she should avoid foods with phosphate additives by reading the ingredient list near the Nutrition Facts Label.

REFERENCES

1. Levin A, Stevens PE. Summary of KDIGO 2012 CKD guideline: behind the scenes, need for guidance, and a framework for moving forward, *Kidney Int*. 2014;85(1):49-61.

2. Inker LA, Eneanya ND, Coresh J, et al. New creatinine- and cystatin C-based equations to estimate GFR without race. *N Engl J Med*. 2021;385(19):1737-1749.

3. Gutiérrez OM, Sang Y, Grams ME, et al. Association of estimated GFR calculated using race-free equations with kidney failure and mortality by black vs. non-black race. *JAMA*. 2022;327(23):2306-2316.

4. Levey AS, Coresh J, Balk E, et al. National Kidney Foundation practice guidelines for chronic kidney disease: evaluation, classification, and stratification. *Ann Intern Med*. 2003;139(2):137-147.

5. Chronic Kidney Disease Prognosis Consortium; Matsushita K, van der Velde M, et al. Association of estimated glomerular filtration rate and albuminuria with all-cause and cardiovascular mortality in general population cohorts: a collaborative meta-analysis. *Lancet*. 2010;375(9731):2073-2081.

6. Rebholz CM, Coresh J, Grams ME, et al. Dietary acid load and incident chronic kidney disease: results from the ARIC study. *Am J Nephrol*. 2015;42(6):427-435.

7. Raphael KL. Metabolic acidosis in CKD: core curriculum 2019. *Am J Kidney Dis*. 2019;74(2):263-275.

8. Jee Ko G, Obi Y, Tortorici AR, Kalantar-Zadeh K. Dietary protein intake and chronic kidney disease. *Curr Opin Clin Nutr Metab Care*. 2017;20(1):77-85.

9. Moraes C, Fouque D, Amaral ACF, Mafra D. Trimethylamine N-oxide from gut microbiota in chronic kidney disease patients: focus on diet. *J Ren Nutr*. 2015;25(6):459-465.

10. Lew QJ, Jafar TH, Koh HW, et al. Red meat intake and risk of ESRD. *J Am Soc Nephrol*. 2017;28(1):304-312.

11. Bettiga A, Fiorio F, Di Marco F, et al. The modern Western diet rich in advanced glycation end-products (AGEs): an overview of its impact on obesity and early progression of renal pathology. *Nutrients*. 2019;11(8):1748.

12. Mente A, O'donnell M, Yusuf S. Sodium intake and health: what should we recommend based on the current evidence? *Nutrients*. 2021;13(9):3232.

13. Shi H, Su X, Li C, Guo W, Wang L. Original research: effect of a low-salt diet on chronic kidney disease outcomes: a systematic review and meta-analysis. *BMJ Open*. 2022;12(1):e050843.

14. Chang AR Anderson C. Dietary phosphorus intake and the kidney. *Annu Rev Nutr*. 2017;37:321-346.

15. He LQ, Wu XH, Huang YQ, Zhang XY, Shu L. Dietary patterns and chronic kidney disease risk: a systematic review and updated meta-analysis of observational studies. *Nutr J*. 2021;20(1):4.

16. Kim H, Caulfield LE, Garcia-Larsen V, et al. Plant-based diets and incident CKD and kidney function. *Clin J Am Soc Nephr*. 2019;14(5):682-691.

17. K/DOQI clinical practice guidelines for chronic kidney disease: evaluation, classification, and stratification - PubMed. Available at: https://pubmed.ncbi.nlm.nih.gov/11904577/. accessed Mar. 5, 2023.

18. Kalantar-Zadeh K Fouque D. Nutritional management of chronic kidney disease. *N Engl J Med*. 2017;377(18):1765-1776.

19. Natale P, Palmer SC, Ruospo M, Saglimbene VM, Strippoli GFM. Potassium binders for chronic hyperkalaemia in people with chronic kidney disease. *Cochrane Database Syst Rev*. 2020;6(6):CD013165.

20. Kalantar-Zadeh K, Tortorici AR, Chen JL, et al. Dietary restrictions in dialysis patients: is there anything left to eat? *Semin Dial.* 2015;28(2):159-168.

21. Koppe L, Fouque D, Kalantar-Zadeh K. Kidney cachexia or protein-energy wasting in chronic kidney disease: facts and numbers. *J Cachexia Sarcopenia Muscle.* 2019;10(3):479-484.

22. Hill AJ, Basourakos SP, Lewicki P, et al. Incidence of kidney stones in the United States: the continuous national health and nutrition examination survey. *J Urol.* 2022;207(4):851-856.

23. Siener R. Nutrition and kidney stone disease. *Nutrients.* 2021;13(6). doi:10.3390/NU13061917.

24. Klahr S, Levey AS, Beck GJ, et al. The effects of dietary protein restriction and blood-pressure control on the progression of chronic renal disease. Modification of Diet in Renal Disease Study Group. *N Engl J Med.* 1994;330(13):877-884.

25. Jhee JH, Kee YK, Park S, et al. High-protein diet with renal hyperfiltration is associated with rapid decline rate of renal function: a community-based prospective cohort study. *Nephrol Dial Transplant.* 2020;35(1):98-106.

26. Cianciaruso B, Pota A, Bellizzi V, et al. Effect of a low- versus moderate-protein diet on progression of CKD: follow-up of a randomized controlled trial. *Am J Kidney Dis.* 2009;54(6):1052-1061.

27. Garneata L, Stancu A, Dragomir D, Stefan G, Mircescu G. Ketoanalogue-supplemented vegetarian very low–protein diet and CKD progression. *J Am Soc Neph.* 2016;27(7):2164-2176.

28. Kestenbaum B, Sampson JN, Rudser KD, et al. Serum phosphate levels and mortality risk among people with chronic kidney disease. *J Am Soc Nephrol.* 2005;16(2):520-528.

29. Block GA, Klassen PS, Lazarus JM, Ofsthun N, Lowrie EG, Chertow GM. Mineral metabolism, mortality, and morbidity in maintenance hemodialysis. *J Am Soc Nephrol.* 2004;15(8):2208-2218.

30. Sullivan C., et al. Effect of food additives on hyperphosphatemia among patients with end-stage renal disease: a randomized controlled trial. *JAMA.* 2009;301(6):629-635.

31. Goraya N, Munoz-Maldonado Y, Simoni J, Wesson DE. Fruit and vegetable treatment of chronic kidney disease-related metabolic acidosis reduces cardiovascular risk better than sodium bicarbonate. *Am J Nephrol.* 2019;49(6):438-448.

chapter 22

Cancer

Amy Comander, MD, DipABLM / Carol Sullivan, MS, RD, CSO, LDN / Nigel Brockton, PHD

Chapter Outline

CASE STUDY

A 45-year-old woman presents to clinic to see you, her new primary care physician. She reports that she has not seen a doctor in the past 2 years given the COVID19 pandemic. She acknowledges that she has been feeling tired, and she notes intermittent lightheadedness. On exam, she appears pale, and she is tachycardic. The patient reports that she has been having intermittent rectal bleeding, which she attributes to a prior history of hemorrhoids. On review of her family history, the patient notes that her father was diagnosed with colon cancer in his early 50s. You inquire as to whether she has had a screening colonoscopy, and she recalls that her father advised her to do this, but she deferred this test due to the pandemic, and her busy schedule.

Given her family history and her symptoms, you recommend laboratory evaluation as the next step. Laboratory data reveals that the patient has a hemoglobin of 8.6 and a hematocrit of 28. Her iron studies reveal a ferritin of 10, iron level of 10, and TIBC of 480. You recommend that the patient start taking oral iron supplementation, and you arrange for her to have a colonoscopy the following week.

Her colonoscopy reveals a circumferential mass in the mid-ascending colon, 10 cm proximal to the cecum. The mass is biopsied, and pathology reveals a moderately differentiated adenocarcinoma. Further laboratory testing revealed a CEA level of 4.5.

Your patient is referred to a colorectal surgeon. She undergoes a right colectomy. Pathology reveals an adenocarcinoma of the ascending colon with focal mucinous features. The tumor measures 4.4 cm in greatest dimension, and is noted to be T3, which means that it invades through the muscularis propria into the peri-colorectal tissues. Small vessel invasion is absent. Large vessel invasion is present. Intramural venous invasion is present without extramural venous invasion. Mismatch repair proteins are intact. Twenty-two regional lymph nodes are removed, all of which are negative for malignancy.

Your patient recovers well from her surgery. She sees a medical oncologist who discusses with her the potential role of adjuvant chemotherapy treatment. The oncologist reviews with your patient that the role of adjuvant chemotherapy for Stage II colorectal cancer is controversial, but given her young age, the role of chemotherapy treatment certainly merits consideration. Your patient has many questions for you. "Doc, I am nervous about getting chemotherapy.- How can I remain healthy during treatment? Is there anything I can change about my lifestyle to improve my health moving forward?"

1. There is an increasing incidence of colorectal cancer that is being diagnosed in younger patients. What type of diet pattern may increase risk for colorectal cancer?

2. If this patient were to proceed with chemotherapy treatment, how would she benefit from a nutrition consultation during chemotherapy?

3. After your patient completes her chemotherapy treatment and is followed in clinic, what type of dietary advice would you give her?

Definition of Terms:

Carcinogenesis: The process of transformation from normal cell to the malignant state.

Cancer risk reduction: This concept may be defined as the actions an individual can take to lower risk for development of cancer. These actions may include maintaining a healthy lifestyle, avoiding exposure to known carcinogens, or by receiving vaccinations that can lower risk for the development of cancer.

Cancer survivorship: Experts from the National Cancer Institute define cancer survivorship as "the focus on the health and well-being of a person with a diagnosis of cancer, from the time of initial diagnosis, throughout treatment, and until the end of life."[1] Survivorship care involves addressing the physical, mental, emotional, social, and financial effects of cancer, which begin at diagnosis and continue through treatment and beyond.

OVERVIEW OF THE BURDEN OF DISEASE

Cancer is the second leading cause of death in both men and women in the United States, and a major public health problem worldwide.[2] Men have a slightly higher lifetime probability for receiving a cancer diagnosis (40.2%) as compared with women (38.5%). This difference reflects numerous factors that can increase risk for cancer, including exposure to cancer-causing environmental factors, and other biologic exposures.[2] In 2023, an estimated 609,802 people in the United States will die from cancer.[3] In 2023, breast cancer is the most commonly diagnosed cancer in women, followed by lung cancer and colorectal cancer. For men, in 2023, prostate cancer is the most commonly diagnosed cancer, followed by lung cancer and colorectal cancer.[3] In men, the leading cause of cancer-related deaths are from cancers of the lung, prostate, and colorectum. In women, the leading cause of cancer-related deaths are from cancers of the lung, breast, and colorectum.

The number of cancer survivors living in the United States continues to increase each year. There were 16.9 million cancer survivors living in the United States in 2019, and this number is expected to surpass 22 million by 2030.[2] This increase in the population of cancer survivors is due to many factors, including increased cancer incidence rates due to the aging of the population, advances in early detection, as well as advances in treatment.[2] In men, those with a diagnosis of prostate cancer, melanoma, and colorectal cancer represent the largest number of cancer survivors.[2] In women, those with a diagnosis of breast cancer, uterine corpus cancer, and thyroid cancer represent the largest number of cancer survivors.

Prior to reviewing the relationship between dietary factors and cancer risk, we will provide an overview of carcinogenesis.

THE COMPLEX PATHOPHYSIOLOGY OF CANCER

Cancer is characterized by the uncontrolled growth of cells and, critically, the ability of those cells to invade adjacent and distant tissues. Progressive growth of cancer cells in adjacent and distant tissues can compromise the function of those tissues, potentially leading to death. Carcinogenesis was originally hypothesized to occur through a stepwise process of *initiation promotion and progression/metastasis*.[4] Carcinogenesis was tied, at least implicitly to the Knudson "two-hit hypothesis" whereby accumulated mutations could be tolerated if only one allele was mutated but a second "hit" could stop a critical function in a tumor suppressor gene or activate an oncogene. However, the modern definition of cancer may be described as the "hallmarks of cancer,"[5] which refers to the multistep process by which normal cells evolve to form a tumor. The "hallmarks of cancer" were originally proposed in 2000 by Hanahan and Weinberg, who noted that neoplastic cells were capable of proliferative signaling, evading growth suppressors, resisting cell death, enabling replicative immortality, inducing angiogenesis, and activating invasion and metastasis. These "hallmarks" were updated and expanded in 2011[6] to include two emerging hallmarks: (1) reprogramming of energy metabolism and (2) evading immune destruction. Furthermore, the authors consider genome instability and inflammation as enabling characteristics. Subsequently, other researchers have sought to refine the definitions and interpretations of the hallmarks so that they remain aligned with our rapidly evolving knowledge and insights.

In the original publication by Hanahan and Weinberg,[5] it is repeatedly stated that the acquisition of each hallmark is accomplished through the successive accumulation of genetic changes in critical genes that encode key regulators of the pathways involved in the respective hallmarks. However, the last two decades have witnessed an increasing appreciation that the functional acquisition of each hallmark may be accomplished independent of gene mutations. Nongenetic changes, such as functional regulation through signal transduction, or epigenetics, can constitutively activate or deactivate pathways that control the hallmarks. Subsequently, such changes can facilitate the emergence of malignancy, or premalignant precursor lesions, which retain the potential to progress to malignancy with the acquisition of the critical hallmark of invasion and metastasis-the fundamental feature that defines malignancy.[7]

As we continue to learn more about these hallmarks of cancer, as well as the role of epigenetics, researchers are interested in undestanding the role of modifiable factors which may influence cancer risk. In this chapter, we will focus on the role of dietary factors that may affect cancer risk, and a patient's health during the course of their treatment and beyond.

MODIFIABLE FACTORS AND CANCER RISK

In the United States, the most important modifiable cancer risk factors include avoiding use of tobacco products, staying at a healthy body weight throughout life, eating a healthy diet, and staying physically active.[8] These lifestyle factors are also associated with a lower risk for development of cardiovascular disease and diabetes.[9] It is estimated that at least 18% of all cancers diagnosed in the United States are related to excess body weight, physical inactivity, excessive alcohol use, and/or poor nutrition.[8] Thus, government and non-profit health organizations, such as the American Cancer Society (ACS) and World Cancer Research Fund/American Institute of Cancer Research (WCRF/AICR) have made specific recommendations to target these behaviors, with the goal to reduce the cancer burden in the United States, and worldwide.[10,11]

The current recommendations for cancer prevention are shown below (Figure 22-1).[11] These recommendations result from the Continuous Update Project conducted by WCRF/AICR. This comprehensive process includes systematic reviews and meta-analyses of all relevant lifestyle exposures and judgments of the strength of evidence by an Expert Panel. Recommendations are only made for factors for which the evidence is judged to be strong (Convincing or Probable) by the CUP Expert Panel.[11] The WCRF/AICR Cancer Prevention Recommendations are consistent with several of other organizations, including the ACS guidelines, the U.S. Department of Health and Human Services Dietary Guidelines for Americans (DGA), as well as the dietary recommendations for prevention and management of cardiovascular disease and diabetes.

Over time, these guidelines have changed to reflect the evolving scientific evidence that has shifted to a focus on the concept of dietary patterns, rather than a reductionist approach, which focuses on specific nutrients. The focus on dietary patterns is also more consistent with *how* people actually eat.[10]

NUTRITION AND CANCER RISK REDUCTION

The most comprehensive analyses of the published literature relating diet, nutrition (including body fatness, usually marked by BMI) and physical activity to cancer risk are those conducted as part of the Continuous Update Project (CUP) of the WCRF/AICR.[11] The CUP conducts systematic literature reviews, and meta-analyses according to a prescribed method developed as part of the 2007 2nd WCRF/AICR Expert Report Food, Nutrition, Physical Activity, and the Prevention of Cancer: a Global Perspective.[11] These data are then judged by an independent expert panel who draw conclusions based on modified Bradford-Hill criteria. The criteria for judgment include several domains of the overall evidence, including the size and consistency of the effect, the presence of a graded relationship ("dose–response"), the amount and quality of data (e.g., correction for known confounders), the presence of evidence for biological plausibility in humans and correction for potential bias or confounding. The full criteria are found in the WCRF report.[12] Based on these judgements, the panel makes recommendations. Recommendations are generally only based on evidence of causality that is regarded as strong (predefined categories of causality of "convincing" or "probable"). Other evidence is generally regarded as too limited as a basis for recommendations. The full systematic literature reviews, as well as a summary of the conclusions and recommendations is

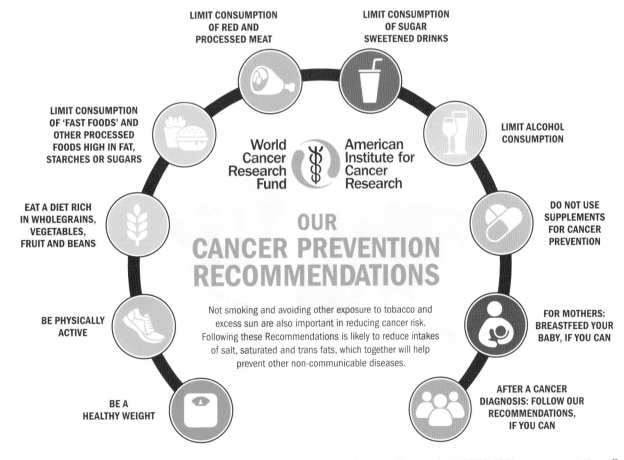

FIGURE 22-1 • World Cancer Research Fund/American Institute of Cancer Research (WCRF/AICR) recommendations.[12]

published as part of the WCRF/AICR 3rd Expert Report Diet, Nutrition, Physical Activity and Cancer: a Global Perspective.[11]

Each of the 10 Cancer Prevention Recommendations is based on strong evidence, according to the judgments of the CUP Expert Panel. However, not all strong evidence results in a specific recommendation. The 10 recommendations are intended to address the most important aspects of lifestyle that impact cancer risk. The recommendations are also intended to function as a package rather than an emphasis on individual recommendations. The recommendations are presented below with a brief explanation and the supporting evidence summarized. The first two recommendations address body weight and physical activity, and are then followed by five recommendations that address aspects of diet and nutrition.

1. **Maintain a healthy weight.** *Keep your weight within the healthy range and avoid weight gain in adult life. Avoid weight gain (measured as body weight or waist circumference) throughout adulthood.* This recommendation is based on abundant evidence that overweight and obesity are linked to higher cancer risk for at least 12 types of cancer (see Figures 22-2 and 22-3).

2. **Be physically active.** *Be physically active as part of everyday life—walk more and sit less. Be at least moderately physically active and follow or exceed national guidelines. Limit sedentary habits.* The strongest evidence for a direct effect of physical activity on cancer risk is for colorectal, endometrial and breast cancer (both pre-menopausal and post-menopausal) (see Figures 22-4 and 22-5).

3. **Eat a diet rich in whole grains, vegetables, fruits, and beans.** *Make whole grains, vegetables, fruits, and pulses (legumes) such as beans and lentils a major part of your usual daily diet. Consume a diet that provides at least 30 g/day of fiber from food sources. Include in more meals foods containing whole grains, non-starchy vegetables, fruits, and*

pulses (legumes) such as beans and lentils. Eat a diet high in all types of plant foods including at least five portions or servings (at least 400 g or 15 oz in total) of a variety of nonstarchy vegetables and fruits every day. If you eat starchy roots and tubers as staple foods, eat nonstarchy vegetables, fruit, and pulses (legumes) regularly too if possible.

The direct evidence supporting the impact of diets rich in whole grains, vegetables, fruits, and beans comes from both aggregated impacts on a collection of cancer sites, particularly upper aerodigestive cancers for fruit and vegetables, but also the impact of specific components such as fiber and whole grains on colorectal cancer, the second most common cancer in men and women in America (Figure 22-6).

4. **Limit consumption of "fast foods" and other processed foods high in fat, starches, or sugars.** *Limiting these foods helps control calorie intake and maintain a healthy weight. Limit consumption of processed foods high in fat, starches, or sugars—including fast foods; many prepared dishes, snacks, bakery foods and desserts, and confectionery (candy).*

The direct research evidence linking consumption of "fast foods" and other processed foods with cancer incidence is relatively limited. However, there is strong evidence that these foods contribute to weight gain, overweight and obesity.[11] Consequently, since overweight and obesity are such strong risk factors for cancer, this recommendation provides guidance to limit consumption of these foods.

5. **Limit consumption of red and processed meat.** *Eat no more than moderate amounts of red meat, such as beef, pork, and lamb. Eat little, if any, processed meat. If you eat red meat, limit consumption to no more than about three portions per week. Three portions are equivalent to about 350 to 500 g (about 12 to 18 oz) cooked weight of red meat.*

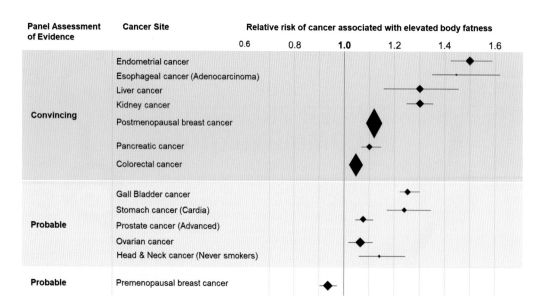

FIGURE 22-2 • Summary of meta-analyses results and continuous update project expert panel evidence conclusions for the impact of body mass index on cancer risk (per 5 kg/m²).[13]

BODY FATNESS AND WEIGHT GAIN AND THE RISK OF CANCER

WCRF/AICR GRADING		DECREASES RISK		INCREASES RISK	
		Exposure	Cancer site	Exposure	Cancer site
STRONG EVIDENCE	**Convincing**			Adult body fatness	Oesophagus (adenocarcinoma) 2016[1]
					Pancreas 2012[1]
					Liver 2015[2]
					Colorectum 2017[1]
					Breast (postmenopause) 2017[1,3]
					Endometrium 2013[4,5]
					Kidney 2015[1]
				Adult weight gain	Breast (postmenopause) 2017[3]
	Probable	Adult body fatness	Breast (premenopause) 2017[1,3]	Adult body fatness	Mouth, pharynx and larynx 2018[1]
		Body fatness in young adulthood	Breast (premenopause) 2017[3,6]		Stomach (cardia) 2016[2]
					Gallbladder 2015[2,7]
			Breast (postmenopause) 2017[3,6]		Ovary 2014[2,5,8]
					Prostate (advanced) 2014[1,9]
LIMITED EVIDENCE	**Limited – suggestive**			Adult body fatness	Cervix (BMI ≥ 29 kg/m²) 2017[2,5]
STRONG EVIDENCE	**Substantial effect on risk unlikely**	None identified			

1. Conclusions for adult body fatness and cancers of the following types were based on evidence marked by body mass index (BMI), waist circumference and waist-hip ratio: mouth, pharynx and larynx; oesophagus (adenocarcinoma); pancreas; colorectum; breast (pre and postmenopause); prostate (advanced); and kidney.

2. Conclusions for adult body fatness and cancers of the following types were based on evidence marked by BMI: stomach (cardia), gallbladder, liver, ovary and cervix (BMI ≥ 29 kg/m²).

3. Evidence for the link between body fatness, weight gain and breast cancer is presented separately for the risk of pre and postmenopausal breast cancer because of the well-established effect modification by menopausal status.

4. The conclusion for adult body fatness and endometrial cancer was based on evidence marked by BMI (including BMI at age 18 to 25 years), weight gain, waist circumference and waist-hip ratio.

5. There is no evidence of effect modification by menopausal status for body fatness and the risk of endometrial, ovarian or cervical cancer so the evidence for all women (irrespective of menopausal status) is presented together.

6. Evidence for body fatness in young adulthood and breast cancer (pre and postmenopause) comes from women aged about 18 to 30 years and includes evidence marked by BMI.

7. Adult body fatness may act indirectly, through gallstones, or directly, either after gallstone formation or in their absence, to cause gallbladder cancer. It is not yet possible to separate these effects.

8. The effect of adult body fatness on the risk of ovarian cancer may vary according to tumour type, menopausal hormone therapy use and menopausal status.

9. The effect of adult body fatness on the risk of prostate cancer was observed in advanced, high-grade and fatal prostate cancers.

FIGURE 22-3 • Body fatness and weight gain and the risk of cancer: A summary matrix.[13]

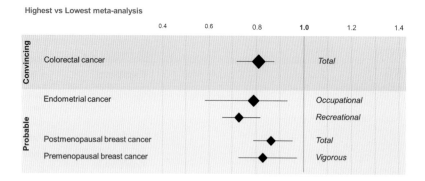

FIGURE 22-4 • Summary of meta-analyses results and continuous update project expert panel evidence conclusions for the impact of physical activity on cancer risk.[13]

PHYSICAL ACTIVITY AND THE RISK OF CANCER

WCRF/AICR GRADING		DECREASES RISK		INCREASES RISK	
		Exposure	Cancer site	Exposure	Cancer site
STRONG EVIDENCE	**Convincing**	**Physical activity**[1]	**Colorectum (colon) 2017**[2]		
	Probable	**Physical activity**[1]	**Breast (postmenopause) 2017**[3]		
			Endometrium 2013		
		Vigorous-intensity physical activity	**Breast (premenopause) 2017**[3]		
			Breast (postmenopause) 2017[3]		
LIMITED EVIDENCE	**Limited – suggestive**	Physical activity[1]	Oesophagus 2016[4]	Sedentary behaviours	Endometrium 2013[5]
			Lung 2017		
			Liver 2015		
			Breast (premenopause) 2017[3]		
STRONG EVIDENCE	**Substantial effect on risk unlikely**	None identified			

1 The exposure of physical activity includes evidence for all types of activity and all intensity levels.

2 The evidence for physical activity and colorectum is for colon cancer only – no conclusion was drawn for rectal cancer.

3 In addition to physical activity, there was sufficient evidence for the Panel to make a separate judgement for vigorous-intensity physical activity and breast cancer (pre and postmenopause).

4 The evidence for physical activity and oesophageal cancer includes unspecified, adenocarcinoma and squamous cell carcinoma.

5 The evidence for sedentary behaviours and endometrial cancer was marked by sitting time.

FIGURE 22-5 • Physical activity and the risk of cancer: A summary matrix.[13]

WHOLEGRAINS, VEGETABLES AND FRUIT AND THE RISK OF CANCER

WCRF/AICR GRADING		DECREASES RISK		INCREASES RISK	
		Exposure	Cancer site	Exposure	Cancer site
STRONG EVIDENCE	Convincing			Aflatoxins	Liver 2015[1]
	Probable	Wholegrains	Colorectum 2017	Foods preserved by salting (including preserved non-starchy vegetables)	Stomach 2016[2]
		Foods containing dietary fibre	Colorectum 2017[3]		
		Non-starchy vegetables and fruit (aggregated)	Aerodigestive cancer and some other cancers (aggregated)[4]		
STRONG EVIDENCE	Substantial effect on risk unlikely	Beta-carotene: Prostate 2014[16]			

1 The evidence for aflatoxins and liver cancer relates to foods that may be contaminated with aflatoxins and includes cereals (grains) as well as pulses (legumes), seeds, nuts and some vegetables and fruit. The studies reported on elevated levels of biomarkers of aflatoxin exposure.

2 For preserved non-starchy vegetables and stomach cancer, there is no separate conclusion. The evidence was included in 'foods preserved by salting', which assessed the evidence for salt-preserved vegetables, salt-preserved fish and salt-preserved foods. The term 'foods preserved by salting' refers mainly to high-salt foods and salt-preserved foods, including pickled vegetables and salted or dried fish, as traditionally prepared in East Asia.

3 The evidence for foods containing dietary fibre and colorectal cancer includes both foods that naturally contain fibre and foods that have had fibre added.

4 The Panel notes that while the evidence for links between individual cancers and non-starchy vegetables or fruit is limited, the pattern of association is consistent and in the same direction, and overall the evidence is more persuasive of a protective effect: greater consumption of non-starchy vegetables or fruit probably protects against a number of aerodigestive cancers.

16 The evidence for beta-carotene and prostate cancer is derived from studies on dietary intake and serum or plasma levels, as well as studies on supplement use (20, 30 and 50 milligrams per day).

FIGURE 22-6 • Whole grains, vegetables, and fruit and the risk of cancer: A strong evidence summary matrix.[13] (This material has been reproduced from the World Cancer Research Fund/American Institute for Cancer Research. *Diet, Nutrition, Physical Activity and Cancer: a Global Perspective. Continuous Update Project Expert Report 2018.* Available at dietandcancerreport.org.)

There is strong evidence that regular excessive consumption of red meat and even small amounts of processed meats increases the risk of colorectal cancer (Figure 22-7). The dose-response meta-analyses conducted by for the WCRF/AICR CUP illustrate the levels at which consumption of these foods significantly impact cancer risk. Lower amounts of red meat do not significantly increase cancer risk, so the recommendation is to limit consumption. However, the impact of processed meats is evident even at very low daily intakes so more stringent advice recommends eating very little or any.

6. **Limit consumption of sugar-sweetened drinks.** *Drink mostly water and unsweetened drinks. Do not consume sugar-sweetened drinks.* Similarly to the recommendation on fast and processed foods, the direct research evidence linking consumption of sugar-sweetened beverages with cancer incidence is relatively limited. However, there is strong evidence that consuming these drinks contribute to weight gain, overweight and obesity.[11] Consequently, since having overweight and obesity are such strong risk factors for cancer, this recommendation provides guidance to limit consumption of these drinks.[13]

7. **Limit alcohol consumption.** *For cancer prevention, it's best not to drink alcohol.*

The consumption of alcoholic beverages increases the risk of six types of cancer (Figures 22-8 and 22-9). Importantly, the cancer risk is similar for all types of alcoholic drink despite the common misconception that wine, particularly red wine, may be beneficial. There does not seem to have a lower boundary of "safe" amount of alcohol

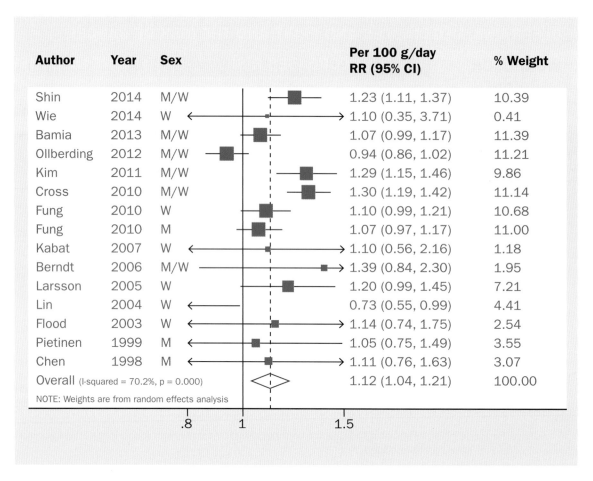

Author	Year	Sex	Per 100 g/day RR (95% CI)	% Weight
Shin	2014	M/W	1.23 (1.11, 1.37)	10.39
Wie	2014	W	1.10 (0.35, 3.71)	0.41
Bamia	2013	M/W	1.07 (0.99, 1.17)	11.39
Ollberding	2012	M/W	0.94 (0.86, 1.02)	11.21
Kim	2011	M/W	1.29 (1.15, 1.46)	9.86
Cross	2010	M/W	1.30 (1.19, 1.42)	11.14
Fung	2010	W	1.10 (0.99, 1.21)	10.68
Fung	2010	M	1.07 (0.97, 1.17)	11.00
Kabat	2007	W	1.10 (0.56, 2.16)	1.18
Berndt	2006	M/W	1.39 (0.84, 2.30)	1.95
Larsson	2005	W	1.20 (0.99, 1.45)	7.21
Lin	2004	W	0.73 (0.55, 0.99)	4.41
Flood	2003	W	1.14 (0.74, 1.75)	2.54
Pietinen	1999	M	1.05 (0.75, 1.49)	3.55
Chen	1998	M	1.11 (0.76, 1.63)	3.07
Overall (I-squared = 70.2%, p = 0.000)			1.12 (1.04, 1.21)	100.00

NOTE: Weights are from random effects analysis

.8   1   1.5

FIGURE 22-7 • Does-response meta-analysis of red and processed meat and colorectal cancer per 100 grams per day.[40]

intake for the risk of cancer, in contrast to the association between alcohol intake and CVD that follows a J-shape curve in many long-term observational studies (see Chapter 20, "Cardiovascular Disease").

8. **Do not use supplements for cancer prevention.** *Aim to meet nutritional needs through diet alone. High-dose dietary supplements are not recommended for cancer prevention.*

Dietary supplement us is common in individuals without cancer and approximately 30–40% of cancer patients use dietary supplements.[14] While there is strong evidence that calcium supplements can reduce colorectal cancer risk, the overall advice to not use supplements for cancer prevention is based on the absence of benefit and the potential deleterious effects on other cancers.[15] In individuals diagnosed with cancer, the potential for disadvantageous interactions of dietary supplements with treatment are a further reason to advise against using these products.[16] It should be noted that there are legitimate reasons to take dietary supplements but these products are not recommended for cancer prevention or during cancer treatment (see also Chapter 7, "Herbs and Dietary Supplements").

9. **For mothers: breastfeed your baby, if you can.** *Breastfeeding is good for both mother and baby. This recommendation aligns with the advice of the WHO, which* recommends infants are exclusively breastfed for 6 months, and then up to 2 years of age or beyond alongside appropriate complementary foods.

10. **After a cancer diagnosis: follow our recommendations, if you can.** *Check with your health professional about what is right for you. All cancer survivors should receive nutritional care and guidance on physical activity from trained professionals. Unless otherwise advised, and if you can, all cancer survivors are advised to follow the Cancer Prevention Recommendations as far as possible after the acute stage of treatment.*

As reviewed in the prior section, the WCRF/AICR expert panel has concluded that an eating pattern including regular consumption non-starchy fruits and vegetables is associated with a reduced risk for development of cancer. A Western diet pattern has been associated with increased risk of several adverse health outcomes, including cancer. Using a nationally representative sample of U.S. adults from NHANES reveals more than 80,000 new cancer cases were estimated to be associated with poor diet among U.S. adults in 2015.[17] A number of studies have demonstrated that among individuals who follow the AICR/WCRF recommendations noted below, there is a lower risk of cancer. For example, in a study of 54,000 men and women in Sweden, those individuals who adhered the most to the recommendations noted above had a substantially lower

ALCOHOLIC DRINKS AND THE RISK OF CANCER

WCRF/AICR GRADING		DECREASES RISK		INCREASES RISK	
		Exposure	Cancer site	Exposure	Cancer site
STRONG EVIDENCE	Convincing			Alcoholic drinks[1]	Mouth, pharynx and larynx 2018 Oesophagus (*squamous cell carcinoma*) 2016 Liver 2015[2] Colorectum 2017[3] Breast (postmenopause) 2017[4]
	Probable	Alcoholic drinks	Kidney 2015[5]	Alcoholic drinks	Stomach 2016[2] Breast (premenopause) 2017[4]
LIMITED EVIDENCE	Limited – suggestive			Alcoholic drinks	Lung 2017 Pancreas 2012[2] Skin (*basal cell carcinoma* and malignant *melanoma*) 2017
STRONG EVIDENCE	Substantial effect on risk unlikely		None identified		

1 Alcoholic drinks include beers, wines, spirits, fermented milks, mead and cider. The consumption of alcoholic drinks is graded by the International Agency for Research on Cancer as carcinogenic to humans (Group 1)[3].

2 The conclusions for alcoholic drinks and cancers of the liver, stomach and pancreas were based on evidence for alcohol intakes above approximately 45 grams of ethanol per day (about three drinks a day). No conclusions were possible for these cancers based on intakes below 45 grams of ethanol per day.

3 The conclusion for alcoholic drinks and colorectal cancer was based on alcohol intakes above approximately 30 grams of ethanol per day (about two drinks a day). No conclusion was possible based on intakes below 30 grams of ethanol per day.

4 No threshold level of alcohol intake was identified in the evidence for alcoholic drinks and breast cancer (pre and postmenopause).

5 The conclusion for alcoholic drinks and kidney cancer was based on alcohol intakes up to approximately 30 grams of ethanol per day (about two drinks a day). There was insufficient evidence to draw a conclusion for intakes above 30 grams of ethanol per day.

FIGURE 22-8 • Alcoholic drinks and the risk of cancer: A summary matrix.[11]
(This material has been reproduced from the World Cancer Research Fund/American Institute for Cancer Research. *Diet, Nutrition, Physical Activity and Cancer: a Global Perspective. Continuous Update Project Expert Report 2018*. Available at dietandcancerreport.org.)

risk of total cancer.[18] A predominantly plant-based diet consisting of whole grains, vegetables, fruits, and pulses (legumes) has consistently been shown to be associated with a lower risk of cancer, obesity, and other noncommunicable diseases.[19] As reviewed above, the WCRF/AICR expert panel has concluded that an eating pattern including regular consumption non-starchy fruits and vegetables is protective of cancer.

NUTRITION DURING THE COURSE OF CANCER TREATMENT, AND BEYOND

Both childhood and adult cancer survivors experience numerous short-term, as well as long-term side effects from cancer treatment, and thus lifestyle factors, such as nutrition play an important role in recovery, quality of life, and in some cases,

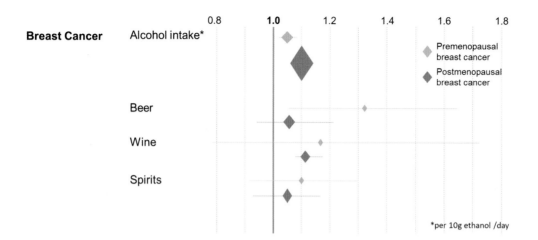

FIGURE 22-9 • Summary of meta-analysis results for the association between ethanol intake from different types of alcoholic beverage on breast cancer risk.[11]
(This material has been reproduced from the World Cancer Research Fund/American Institute for Cancer Research. *Diet, Nutrition, Physical Activity and Cancer: a Global Perspective. Continuous Update Project Expert Report 2018.* Available at dietandcancerreport.org.)

outcome from cancer. Due to advances in treatment and early detection, the number of cancer survivors living in the United States continues to increase each year, and this number is expected to surpass 22 million by 2030.[2] Two leading causes of death in cancer survivors include development of a subsequent primary cancer, as well as cardiovascular disease. The National Comprehensive Cancer Network Clinical Practice Guidelines in Oncology (NCCN Guidelines) for Survivorship, provide recommendations for screening, evaluation, and treatment to guide healthcare professionals who provide care for cancer survivors.[20] Key aspects of survivorship care include (1) screening for a new primary cancer, (2) monitoring for recurrence of disease, (3) screening for cardiovascular disease, and (4) counseling regarding *healthy lifestyle behaviors* which may reduce the risk of subsequent cancers, as well as cardiovascular disease.

Recent studies show that less than half of cancer survivors discuss the importance of nutrition, physical activity, tobacco cessation, and other lifestyle changes with their physician.[21] This is unfortunate, since evidence from both experimental and observational studies suggests that addressing modifiable risk factors, such as dietary habits, may also have implications for reducing risk of cancer recurrence and improving overall survival. Observational studies suggest that cancer survivors who follow a healthy dietary pattern, and avoid obesity after completion of cancer treatment, have improved long-term survival.[21,22] As outlined above, to improve long-term health, cancer survivors are encouraged to follow similar guidelines for a healthy eating pattern as recommended for cancer risk reduction (WCRF/AICR).[22] Cancer survivors thus derive great benefit from dietary assessment and counseling from the time of diagnosis, during treatment, and through long-term follow-up.

Nutritional counseling is particularly important for individuals undergoing cancer treatment, who need assistance with management of treatment-related side effects, including nausea, vomiting, and poor appetite. Nutritional assessment is indicated to address nutritional deficiencies, to help patients preserve muscle mass, and address problems that may occur as a result of a cancer diagnosis, or during treatment. In particular, nutritional assessment is key for evaluation of cancer-related malnutrition, cachexia, and sarcopenia.

CANCER-RELATED MALNUTRITION AND CACHEXIA

Individuals undergoing cancer treatment may experience a number of potential complications related to their disease, or the treatment itself. The importance of addressing malnutrition, cachexia, and sarcopenia will be reviewed below.

Malnutrition

In the oncology setting, malnutrition is generally considered the presence of undernutrition and changes in body composition that are due to the cancer itself, or because of the cancer treatment. Malnutrition studies evaluating tolerance to chemotherapy in patients with different types of advanced cancer demonstrate that patients with sarcopenia, weight loss, or low body mass are at risk for increased chemotherapy toxicities and are at risk for receiving less treatment than those who are not undernourished.[23] Studies have attempted to differentiate between cancer types that result in increased resting energy expenditure. Patients with pancreatic, gastric, bile duct, kidney, adrenal, non-small-cell lung and head and neck cancers are considered hypermetabolic, and at higher risk for malnutrition.[23]

Additionally, anorexia and weight loss are very distressing to patients with cancer and their caregivers often creating tension within the family unit. Ideally, a patient experiencing these issues should be referred to a board-certified oncology registered dietitian (RD) who is uniquely trained to support the patient's needs throughout the course of treatment. In the

United States, the ratio of RDs to patients in cancer centers is 1:2,308 and they are often absent from community cancer centers[24]; therefore, oncologists and MDs should be aware of the existing updated clinical nutrition guidelines and interventions in this population.

Cachexia and Sarcopenia

Malnutrition may or may not be associated with cachexia. Cancer cachexia is a metabolic syndrome driven by inflammation and reduced oral intake characterized by negative protein and energy balance.[25] Up to 80% of patients with advanced cancer may be diagnosed with cachexia.[25] Cancer cachexia is most prevalent in individuals with a diagnosis of gastric, pancreatic, esophageal, head and neck, lung, colorectal, and prostate cancer,[25] and may contribute to mortality in individuals with cancer. Tumor burden contributes to systemic inflammation promoting lipolysis, proteolysis, increased resting energy expenditure, insulin resistance, and decreased appetite, characterized by negative protein and energy balance.[25] Cytokines may directly influence the activity of hypothalamic centers thereby altering appetite and metabolic rate. The degree and persistence of inflammation may result in reduction of lean body mass and cause functional impairment and decreased quality of life.[25]

The second condition that puts individuals with cancer at increased risk for loss of muscle mass is sarcopenia occurring in 40–50% of patients with newly diagnosed cancer compared to about 15% in healthy individuals of a similar age.[26] Sarcopenia is associated with poor performance status, toxicity from chemotherapy, and shorter time of tumor control. Sarcopenia and cachexia can be present in any BMI, and often goes unnoticed in patients who present with a higher BMI.

Management of Malnutrition and Cachexia

In 2020, the American Society of Clinical Oncology (ASCO) outlined guidelines for the management of cancer cachexia.[27] The guidelines report limited evidence for use of pharmacotherapy. Dietary counseling, with or without oral nutrition supplements, which have been shown to improve body weight in some trials are recommended. All patients benefit from screening to assess the risk of malnutrition on entry to oncology services.

A key component in management and prevention of malnutrition and cachexia lies in managing complex symptoms that negatively affect food intake, digestion, absorption, utilization of nutrients, and overall nutrition status.[28] Many of these symptoms can be prevented or minimized when identified early and managed effectively through patient and caregiver education, behavior modification, and appropriate pharmacotherapy.

Specialized Nutrition Support in Cancer Patients

Evidence is inconclusive as to whether specialized nutrition support, as enteral nutrition (EN) or parenteral nutrition (PN), stimulates tumor growth or causes cancer progression.[29] Most of the data are from animal studies and human outcomes data do not show that PN contributes to tumor growth.[28] EN may be vital for those with head and neck cancer, esophageal cancer, gastric cancer, and other gastrointestinal malignancies where the patient may experience significant dysphagia, esophageal obstruction, gastric outlet obstruction or significant gastroparesis.[28] EN is the preferred route of nutrition support over PN in this population.

There is a lack of high-quality data to help guide clinicians choosing candidates for PN in the oncology setting. Patients who cannot obtain their nutrition enterally, have an acceptable quality of life and would die of malnutrition prior to progression of their cancer are considered appropriate candidates for PN. Oncology-specific indications for PN include multiple clinical scenarios where the gastrointestinal tract cannot be used for enteral nutrition including paralytic or postoperative ileus, malignant bowel obstruction, high output distal GI fistula, inability to tolerate EN for > 7 days, large-volume diarrhea, or high-output ostomies refractory to medication management.[28]

● AREAS OF INTEREST IN NUTRITION AND CANCER

Soy Intake and Cancer Risk

The soy isoflavones genistein and daidzein are classified as phytoestrogens, and they can bind to estrogen receptors. This fact alone has raised concerns that soy foods raise estrogen levels and therefore can cause estrogen dependent cancer. Studies in rodents have suggested genistein alone increases the growth of estrogen receptor positive breast cancer cells and promoted breast cancer growth; however, further research has revealed that rats and mice metabolize phytoestrogens differently than humans.[30] The binding of soy isoflavones to beta rather than alpha forms of estrogen receptors may be cancer protective, but this is an area that needs further study.[31]

Observational studies in humans suggest that soy may be protective against some types of cancer. In Asia, where moderate levels of soy are consumed, soy consumption is associated with the lower risk of breast cancer.[32] However, broader research suggests that the hormone protective effect of soy may come from consumption in childhood and adolescence.[33] In a large, population-based, prospective cohort study assessing soy intake and breast cancer risk, the researchers reported that women who consistently consumed a high amount of soy foods during adolescence and adulthood had a reduced risk of breast cancer.[33]

Gut Microbiome

An exciting area of research is the study of the role of the gut microbiome in the development and progression of chronic diseases, including cancer. Since our case at the beginning of this chapter focused on a patient with colon cancer, we highlighted here a recent study that reported an association between diet quality and microbiome composition in human colonic mucosa, and the potential role in development of colon cancer.[34] The researchers found that a "high-quality" diet, associated with fruits, vegetables, and whole grains, was associated with more potentially beneficial gut bacteria, whereas a "low-quality" diet was associated with more potentially harmful gut bacteria, such as *Fusobacterium nucleatum*, a bacteria that has been shown to induce a proinflammatory immune response, and has been associated with colorectal cancer. Given that our diet plays a key role in determining the gut microbial makeup, and the gut microbiome can mediate nutrient uptake, metabolism, and the body's immune response, it is of interest to explore the gut microbiome's role in modulating disease risk. Further research may provide insight into how modification of the gut microbiome may reduce the risk of chronic diseases, including cancer.[34]

Time-Restricted Feeding

Intermittent fasting, or time-restricted feeding (TRF), are approaches that have been used for weight loss, and these practices have been studied with regard to cancer development.[35] A number of studies in animal models have shown that daily caloric restriction, or alternate day fasting reduces the development of spontaneous tumors.[36] These approaches have also been shown in animal models to suppress the growth of induced tumors, and increase sensitivity to cancer treatment, such as chemotherapy and radiation therapy.[37] Proposed mechanisms of the benefit of TRF for cancer cells are felt to be through (1) impairment of metabolism and (2) inhibition of growth. There are ongoing trials evaluating the role of intermittent fasting in patients with cancer, to determine if there is benefit for this intervention in reducing the risk of cancer recurrence in humans.[35]

Ketogenic Diet and Cancer

The popularization of the ketogenic diet (KD), combined with some evidence for the diet as potential adjuvant therapy to some brain cancers,[38] has made this diet a popular for patients with all cancer types. However, the effectiveness of the KD as an adjuvant therapy in antitumor treatment remains controversial. The KD is a very low carbohydrate, moderate protein, high fat diet; the standard macronutrient composition of the KD is 90% fat, 6% protein, and 4% carbohydrate, with a ratio of 4 grams of fat to every 1 gram of protein plus carbohydrate. Typically, the KD limits carbohydrates to less than 50 grams of carbohydrate per day, and meals are usually comprised of oils, butter, meats, full fat cheeses, heavy cream, some nuts and seeds, and limited amounts of nonstarchy vegetables. The KD's potential as adjuvant treatment to standard chemotherapy and radiotherapy is due to cancer cells deriving their energy source of ATP through glycolysis regardless of oxygen availability, instead of oxidative phosphorylation the cell's normal aerobic cycle.[39] This observation, known as the Warburg effect, has led to the theory that changing the energy source from glucose to ketone bodies can induce oxidative stress within the cancer cell, causing apoptosis. At present, evidence for the KD in terms of benefit for cancer patients is limited to case reports and feasibility studies. Clinical evidence from RCTs is lacking and long-term epidemiologic evidence does not exist. Furthermore, before starting the diet, patients should be screened for metabolic conditions where initiation of the diet could be contraindicated, including carnitine deficiency, carnitine palmitoytransferase I or II deficiency, beta-oxidation defects, and pyruvate carboxylase deficiency. Patients may choose to initiate the KD on their own thinking it is "just a diet" when in fact the strict and modified KD are metabolic therapies that require assessment for potential contraindications from the medical team.

THREE TAKE-HOME POINTS

1. In the United States, the most important modifiable cancer risk factors include avoiding use of tobacco products, staying at a healthy body weight throughout life, eating a healthy diet, and staying physically active.
2. A predominantly plant-based diet consisting of whole grains, vegetables, fruits, and pulses (legumes) has consistently been associated with a lower risk of cancer, obesity, and other noncommunicable diseases.
3. Observational studies suggest that cancer survivors who follow a healthy dietary pattern, and avoid obesity after completion of cancer treatment, have improved long-term survival.

CASE STUDY ANSWERS

1. The rates of overall incidence of colorectal cancer are declining, but rates are increasing by 1.5% per year in adults younger than 50 years. The explanation for rising incidence since the mid-1990s in younger adults in the United States and several other high-income countries is unknown, but likely relates to lifestyle factors. There is strong evidence that physical activity; whole-grain consumption; and consumption of foods containing fiber, dairy products, and calcium supplements are associated with lower colorectal cancer risk (Figure 20-10). Conversely, consumption of red and processed meat, consumption of alcoholic beverages, and excess body fatness are associated with greater colorectal cancer risk.

2. Nutritional counseling is particularly important for individuals undergoing cancer treatment, who need assistance with management of treatment-related side effects, including nausea, vomiting, and poor appetite. Nutritional assessment is indicated to address nutritional deficiencies, to help patients preserve muscle mass (reduce risk

(Continued)

CASE STUDY ANSWERS *(Continued)*

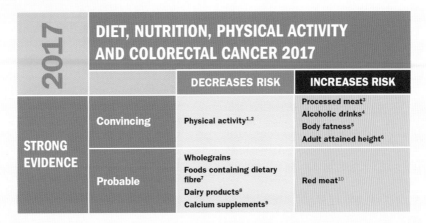

2017	DIET, NUTRITION, PHYSICAL ACTIVITY AND COLORECTAL CANCER 2017		DECREASES RISK	INCREASES RISK
STRONG EVIDENCE	Convincing		Physical activity[1,2]	Processed meat[3] Alcoholic drinks[4] Body fatness[5] Adult attained height[6]
	Probable		Wholegrains Foods containing dietary fibre[7] Dairy products[8] Calcium supplements[9]	Red meat[10]

FIGURE 22-10 • Diet, nutrition, physical activity, and colorectal cancer risk.[40]
(This material has been reproduced from the World Cancer Research Fund/American Institute for Cancer Research. *Diet, Nutrition, Physical Activity and Cancer: a Global Perspective. Continuous Update Project Expert Report 2018.* Available at dietandcancerreport.org.)

of sarcopenia), and address other symptoms that may occur as a result of a cancer diagnosis, or during treatment. The goal of the nutrition consultation is to ensure the patient is able to maintain body weight and lean mass and improve quality of life, and ultimately outcome from cancer.

3. Data suggests that cancer survivors who follow a healthy dietary pattern have improved long-term survival.[22] As outlined above, in order to improve long-term health, cancer survivors are encouraged to follow similar guidelines for a healthy eating pattern, and for physical activity, as recommended for cancer risk reduction (WCRF/AICR). Cancer survivors thus derive great benefit from dietary assessment and counseling from the time of diagnosis, during treatment, and through long-term follow-up.[22]

REFERENCES

1. National Cancer Institute. *NCI Dictionary of cancer terms.* https://www.cancer.gov/publications/dictionaries/cancer-terms/def/survivorship.

2. Miller KD, Nogueira L, Devasia T, et al. Cancer treatment and survivorship statistics. 2022;*CA Cancer J Clin.* 2022;72(5):409-436.

3. Siegel RL, Miller KD, Wagle NS, Jemal A. Cancer statistics, 2023. *CA Cancer J Clin.* 2023;73(1):17-48.

4. Berenblum I, Shubik P. An experimental study of the initiating state of carcinogenesis, and a re-examination of the somatic cell mutation theory of cancer. *Br J Cancer.* 1949;3(1):109-118.

5. Hanahan D, Weinberg RA. The hallmarks of cancer. *Cell.* 2000;100(1):57-70.

6. Hanahan D, Weinberg RA. Hallmarks of cancer: the next generation. *Cell.* 2011;144(5):646-674.

7. Lazebnik Y. What are the hallmarks of cancer? *Nat Rev Cancer.* 2010;10(4):232-233.

8. Islami F, Goding Sauer A, Miller KD, et al. Proportion and number of cancer cases and deaths attributable to potentially modifiable risk factors in the United States. *CA Cancer J Clin.* 2018;68(1):31-54.

9. Nyberg ST, Singh-Manoux A, Pentti J, et al. Association of healthy lifestyle with years lived without major chronic diseases. *JAMA Intern Med.* 2020;180(5):760-768.

10. Rock CL, Thomson C, Gansler T, et al. American Cancer Society guideline for diet and physical activity for cancer prevention. *CA Cancer J Clin.* 2020;70(4):245-271.

11. World Cancer Research Fund/American Institute for Cancer Research. Diet, Nutrition, Physical Activity and Cancer: A Global Perspective. Continuous Update Project Expert Report. 2018.

12. World Cancer Research Fund / American Institute for Cancer Research. Food, Nutrition, Physical Activity, and the Prevention of Cancer: A Global Perspective. Washington DC: AICR; 2007.

13. Energy Balance and Body Fatness. The Continuous Update Project. 2020; Available at: https://www.aicr.org/research/the-continuous-update-project/energy-balance-and-body-fatness/.

14. Tank M, Franz K, Cereda E, Norman K. Dietary supplement use in ambulatory cancer patients: a survey on prevalence, motivation and attitudes. *J Cancer Res Clin Oncol.* 2021;147(7):1917-1925.

15. Yeung KS, Gubili J, Mao JJ. Herb-drug interactions in cancer care. *Oncology (Williston Park).* 2018;32(10):516-520.

16. Ambrosone CB, Zirpoli GR, Hutson AD, et al. Dietary supplement use during chemotherapy and survival outcomes of patients with breast cancer enrolled in a cooperative group clinical trial (SWOG S0221). *J Clin Oncol.* 2020;38(8):804-814.

17. Zhang FF, Cudhea F, Shan Z, et al. Preventable cancer burden associated with poor diet in the United States. *JNCI Cancer Spectr.* 2019;3(2):pkz034.

18. Kaluza J, Harris HR, Hakansson N, Wolk A. Adherence to the WCRF/AICR 2018 recommendations for cancer prevention and risk of cancer: prospective cohort studies of men and women. *Br J Cancer*. 2020;122(10):1562-1570.

19. Boeing H, Bechthold A, Bub A, et al. Critical review: vegetables and fruit in the prevention of chronic diseases. *Eur J Nutr*. 2012;51(6):637-663.

20. Denlinger CS, Sanft T, Moslehi JJ, et al. NCCN guidelines insights: survivorship, version 2.2020. *J Natl Compr Canc Netw*. 2020;18(8):1016-1023.

21. Ligibel JA, Pierce LJ, Bender CM, et al. Attention to diet, exercise, and weight in oncology care: results of an American Society of Clinical Oncology National Patient Survey. *Cancer*. 2022;128(14):2817-2825.

22. Rock CL, Thomson CA, Sullivan KR, et al. American Cancer Society nutrition and physical activity guideline for cancer survivors. *CA Cancer J Clin*. 2022;72(3):230-262.

23. Bossi P, Delrio P, Mascheroni A, Zanetti M. The spectrum of malnutrition/cachexia/sarcopenia in oncology according to different cancer types and settings: a narrative review. *Nutrients*. 2021;13(6):1980.

24. Trujillo EB, Claghorn K, Dixon SW, et al. Inadequate nutrition coverage in outpatient cancer centers: results of a national survey. *J Oncol*. 2019;2019:7462940.

25. Fearon K, Strasser F, Anker SD, et al. Definition and classification of cancer cachexia: an international consensus. *Lancet Oncol*. 2011;12(5):489-495.

26. Prado CM, Cushen SJ, Orsso CE, Ryan AM. Sarcopenia and cachexia in the era of obesity: clinical and nutritional impact. *Proc Nutr Soc*. 2016;75(2):188-198.

27. Roeland EJ, Bohlke K, Baracos VE, et al. Management of cancer cachexia: ASCO guideline. *J Clin Oncol*. 2020;38(21):2438-2453.

28. Arends J, Bachmann P, Baracos V, et al. ESPEN guidelines on nutrition in cancer patients. *Clin Nutr*. 2017;36(1):11-48.

29. Bossola M, Pacelli F, Rosa F, Tortorelli A, Doglietto GB. Does nutrition support stimulate tumor growth in humans? *Nutr Clin Pract*. 2011;26(2):174-180.

30. Setchell KD, Brown NM, Zhao X, et al. Soy isoflavone phase II metabolism differs between rodents and humans: implications for the effect on breast cancer risk. *Am J Clin Nutr*. 2011;94(5):1284-1294.

31. Spagnuolo C, Russo GL, Orhan IE, et al. Genistein and cancer: current status, challenges, and future directions. *Adv Nutr*. 2015;6(4):408-419.

32. Chen M, Rao Y, Zheng Y, et al. Association between soy isoflavone intake and breast cancer risk for pre- and post-menopausal women: a meta-analysis of epidemiological studies. *PLoS One*. 2014;9(2):e89288.

33. Lee SA, Shu XO, Li H, et al. Adolescent and adult soy food intake and breast cancer risk: results from the Shanghai women's health study. *Am J Clin Nutr*. 2009;89(6):1920-1926.

34. Liu Y, Ajami NJ, El-Serag HB, et al. Dietary quality and the colonic mucosa-associated gut microbiome in humans. *Am J Clin Nutr*. 2019;110(3):701-712.

35. de Cabo R, Mattson MP. Effects of intermittent fasting on health, aging, and disease. *N Engl J Med*. 2019;381(26):2541-2551.

36. Mattison JA, Colman RJ, Beasley TM, et al. Caloric restriction improves health and survival of rhesus monkeys. *Nat Commun*. 2017;8:14063.

37. Martinez-Outschoorn UE, Peiris-Pages M, Pestell RG, Sotgia F, Lisanti MP. Cancer metabolism: a therapeutic perspective. *Nat Rev Clin Oncol*. 2017;14(1):11-31.

38. Winter SF, Loebel F, Dietrich J. Role of ketogenic metabolic therapy in malignant glioma: a systematic review. *Crit Rev Oncol Hematol*. 2017;112:41-58.

39. Weber DD, Aminzadeh-Gohari S, Tulipan J, Catalano L, Feichtinger RG, Kofler B. Ketogenic diet in the treatment of cancer—Where do we stand? *Mol Metab*. 2020;33:102-121.

40. Colorectal Cancer. *The Continuous Update Project*. 2020.

Dementia

Uma Naidoo, MD / John D. Matthews, MD, MSc

Chapter Outline

CASE STUDY

Alexandra is a 25-year-old woman who works at Staples as a cashier. She is worried about her brain health because her grandmother was diagnosed with dementia at the age of 72. Alexandra forgot where she put her keys at work and started remembering how her grandmother would search for things for hours. Since Alexandra's grandmother lived with her family, Alexandra knows how challenging dementia is on many levels. For this reason, Alexandra really wants to be proactive and prevent dementia for herself. She exercises about a half an hour a day 5 days a week and tries to get 7 hours of sleep a night. But, with regard to food, she is confused as to what is healthy for her brain.

1. The patient asks if there are foods she can eat that will help prevent dementia. How do you respond?
2. What foods are known to be healthy for the brain and backed by research?
3. What foods are unhealthy for the brain?

● ALZHEIMER'S PATHOPHYSIOLOGY

Alzheimer's disease (AD) is a neurodegenerative disease manifested by the accumulation of β-amyloid plaques and neurofibrillary tangles.[1] The degenerative process generally begins in the medial temporal lobes and spreads to other lobes as the disorder progresses.

Genetics and midlife medical conditions contribute to the development of AD. Gut microbiota dysbiosis, metabolic syndrome, obesity, type 2 diabetes, and hypertension are among the best-studied risk factors for the development of AD.[2] Elevated inflammatory markers have been shown to be present in each of these risk factors. In a meta-analysis of cytokines in AD,

Swardfager et al.[3] showed elevated blood concentrations of interleukin-1β (IL-1β), interleukin-6 (IL-6), and tumor necrosis factor-alpha (TNF-α) in AD. Other studies have also shown the presence of inflammatory cytokines in affected areas of the brains of AD patients.[4] In general, there appears to be a bidirectional relationship between peripheral and central nervous system (CNS) immune cell activation.[5] Chronic peripheral inflammation produced by the release of cytokines from macrophages has been shown to produce chronic central nervous system (CNS) inflammation by the activation and release of cytokines by CNS microglia and astrocytes. Peripherally produced IL-1β, IL-6, and TNF-α cross the blood brain barrier (BBB), thus providing a mechanism for the development of neurodegenerative diseases from metabolic disorders.[6] Also, Aβ aggregates in the CNS can activate microglia, resulting in CNS-induced inflammation in AD.[7] Thus, there are both peripheral and CNS contributing factors for neuroinflammation in AD.

LINK BETWEEN GUT MICROBIOTA AND BRAIN HEALTH

There is a link between gut microbiota and brain health. This relationship is bidirectional and referred to as the gut-brain axis. The gut microbiota are diverse and dynamic and include bacteria, viruses, protozoa, fungi, and archaea, primarily located in the ileum and colon.[8] The gut microbiota influence brain functioning via metabolites released into the circulation that regulate blood brain barrier (BBB) permeability and brain functioning, thus regulating behavior, mood, and cognition.[9] These metabolites include many neurotransmitters found in the brain including serotonin, dopamine, gamma aminobutyric acid (GABA), glutamate, and acetylcholine. Also, the short chain fatty acids (SCFA) acetate, propionate, and butyrate, are products of health-promoting microbiota, which not only maintain the integrity of the gut mucosal lining but also are transported to the brain via the systemic circulation to promote the integrity of the BBB and impact neuron function by binding to SCFA receptors in the brain. There is evidence that there is an optimal balance of these three SCFAs that establish gut and brain health. To achieve optimal homeostasis of gut and brain functioning, there is a required diversity and number of specific species of microbiota.

Microbiota dysbiosis occurs when the number and/or diversity of beneficial microbes is not present in the gut. For example, *Lactobacillus* and *Bifidobacterium* genera have been shown to be beneficial to gut health by promoting tight epithelial cell junctions in the gut lining, which prevents leakage of inflammation-producing toxins into the systemic circulation, thus protecting the person from a variety of potential inflammatory and metabolic diseases throughout the body, including the brain. Alternatively, an over-abundance (dysbiosis) of Clostridium in the gut microbiome contributes to increased gut lining permeability resulting in a "leaky gut" and the spread of pro-inflammatory metabolites both peripherally and in the CNS.

In the absence of dysbiosis, microbiota and their metabolites provide protection from the development of a variety of common age-related diseases, including neurodegenerative diseases like AD. Ho et al.[10] demonstrated that SCFA increase resilience against the development of AD by reducing misfolding of β-amyloid. In addition, experimental models have shown that SCFA have neuroactive properties promoting improved cognition.[11]

APPROACHES TO PROMOTE HEALTHY MICROBIOTA

Approaches that have been shown to promote a healthy microbiota include probiotics, prebiotics, nutrients, and specific diets.[2] Probiotics are nonpathogenic, live microorganisms that can used to supplement the health-promoting gut microbiota when taken in adequate amounts. Typical probiotic supplements include *Lactobacillus, Bifidobacterium, Lactococcus,* and several more. Examples of food sources include plain dairy or non-dairy yogurt. Probiotics have been shown to have a positive effect on mood and cognition in humans; these probiotics are referred to as psychobiotics.[12] A limited number of human studies suggest that probiotics may provide benefit in improving cognition in AD. Leblhuber et al.[13] reported improvement in Mini Mental Status Exam (MMSE) scores in patients with AD following treatment with a probiotic containing a combination of *Bifidobacteria* and *Lactobacilli* species. MMSE scores have been shown to improve in a small number of randomized, double-blinded, placebo-controlled trials with supplements containing *Bifidobacteria* and *Lactobacilli* species.[14,15] The underlying mechanisms for the impact of probiotics on AD are unclear; however, inflammation is found in the brains of patients with AD, and probiotics have been shown to reduce serum inflammatory markers.[15] Sarkar et al.[16] suggest that probiotics and manipulations of the gut microbiota might be an approach to promote a healthier balance between pro-inflammatory and anti-inflammatory cytokines, thus providing neuroprotection by maintaining gut lining and BBB integrity.

Prebiotics are nondigestible substances that are consumed by health-promoting microbiota that produce metabolites like SCFA, which, in part, promote gut and brain health, as noted above. Prebiotics are "food" for the health-promoting microbiota. Examples of prebiotics include resistant starches, fructooligosaccharides (FOS), galactooligosaccharides (GOS), and polysaccharides starches. The Mediterranean diet, for example, includes prebiotic food components including fiber and resistant starches like oligopolysaccharides. Food examples of prebiotics include leeks, leafy greens, onions, garlic, oats, bananas, and asparagus. Of clinical interest, preclinical studies have shown that FOS and GOS promote the growth of the beneficial species, *Bifidobacteria*, which is associated with a reduction of anxiety-like behaviors, reduction of the stress response, and increased engagement in social interactions.[17,18] Studies in humans are few in number and inconclusive. In a study of healthy human subjects, GOS intake showed a reduction in the stress response as measured by morning salivary cortisol levels; however, there is an absence of randomized controlled studies in psychiatric disorders, including Alzheimer's disease.[19] Studies are in process to assess the benefit of combining prebiotics and probiotics.

Midlife obesity has been shown to be another potential risk factor for the development of AD. In an 18-year follow-up study of non-demented adults, an elevated body mass index (BMI) predicted the development of AD.[20] Obesity is a risk factor for metabolic syndrome and is associated with other metabolic syndrome risk factors including elevated lipids, hypertension, and insulin resistance. The common denominator for all of these risk factors is chronic inflammation. Obesity alone can increase the risk for insulin resistance, hypertension, and hypercholesterolemia, all of which have been associated with AD. Hypertrophied abdominal adipocytes contribute to chronic low-grade inflammation by secreting increased levels of pro-inflammatory cytokines. Tumor necrosis factor-alpha (TNF-α) in particular, promotes insulin resistance by activating serine kinases that phosphorylate the IRS1 (insulin receptor substrate 1), thus impairing the function of insulin.[21]

Glucose utilization and energy metabolism are regulated by insulin and insulin-like growth factor in the CNS and peripherally as well. CNS insulin resistance has been shown to reduce amyloid clearance, resulting in amyloid accumulation in the brain and impaired cognitive functioning.[22] Normally, insulin has a beneficial role in cognitive functioning; however, patients with AD demonstrate impaired insulin signaling. Potential preventative approaches targeting insulin resistance could include diets like the Mediterranean diet supplemented with foods containing omega-3 fatty acids, flavonoids, and curcumin.[22]

Hypertension that begins in mid-life is another a risk factor for both vascular dementia and AD.[23] AD and vascular dementia often co-occur. In the Honolulu-Asian Study, a longitudinal study of 26 years involving 3,065 Japanese-American men, subjects with the apolipoprotein E€4 allele and elevated blood pressure (≥ 160 mm Hg) developed significantly greater cognitive decline compared with hypertensive subjects without the allele.[24]

EPIGENETICS

Epigenetics is becoming a new approach to understanding complex diseases like AD. AD is, in part, a genetic neurodegenerative disorder and, like all genetic disorders, environmental factors play a role in gene expression and can influence whether a given disorder becomes manifest. DNA methylation, histone modifications, and microRNAs are three epigenetic mechanisms that have been studied in AD.[25] DNA methylation refers to the addition of methyl groups to the DNA molecule. Promoter regions along the DNA sequence facilitate RNA transcription and these promoter regions include multiple cytosine-phosphate-guanine nucleotide (CpG) pairings. Methylation of these CpG sites in promoter regions suppress gene expression by blocking the enzymes necessary for transcription, or mRNA synthesis.

Histone modification via acetylation and methylation is also important in determining whether genes associated with the development of AD are active or inactive. Histones are proteins that form an organizing structure for DNA and promote the process of transcription to produce mRNA. Chromatin units provide a structure for DNA to wrap around a core of histone proteins. Each core histone protein has an outward-facing tail of amino acids including lysine. Acetylation and methylation of lysine residues of specific histone proteins change the configuration of chromatin units, thus increasing or decreasing specific gene exposure in the service of gene expression. Acetylation of specific lysine sites on the histone tail produces a state of chromatin activation, whereas deacetylation on the histone tails renders chromatin inactive.

More recently, microRNAs have been found to be a third group of epigenetic modulators of gene expression in AD. MicroRNAs are nonprotein coding RNA molecules consisting of approximately 20 nucleotide bases with the capacity to bind to complementary mRNA sites to regulate the production of proteins. Thus, microRNAs regulate translation, whereas DNA methylation and chromatin modulation regulate transcription. MicroRNAs are typically inhibitors of gene expression at specific mRNA regions.

These epigenetic processes—DNA methylation, histone modification, and dysregulation of microRNA—provide mechanisms by which environmental risk factors promote neuropsychiatric disorders like AD. There is now evidence that dietary components and nutrients can turn on or off genes without changing the DNA sequence via these three epigenetic mechanisms in AD. Many AD risk-reducing factors, including several vitamins (vitamins A, B, C, D, and E), omega-3 fatty acids, resveratrol, curcumin, and adherence to the Mediterranean diet, have their effects, in part, via these epigenetics mechanisms.[26]

In summarizing the pathophysiology section, it is important to acknowledge the controversy that has arisen over original research in Alzheimer's disease now being questioned as fraudulent.[27] This is where an integrative approach, as we are outlining in this chapter, includes nutrition and lifestyle factors become key to helping with treatment in such conditions.

NUTRITIONAL ASPECTS OF DEMENTIA

A Personal Anecdote from the Author

Dementia is an illness that touches all our lives, whether in a loved one, a patient or through someone we know. Like cancer it is pervasive and consuming for a family member, caregivers, friends, and treaters. Early in my career I met Marina, a wildly brilliant 60-year-old professor who came to see me about her anxiety. It was in March, as she was struggling with anxiety about preparing her taxes, when I first noticed that she seemed to be fading away. The effect was subtle; it wasn't as if she just came in one day without the ability to remember. But slowly, week after week, I saw an ever-so-slightly vacant look on her face, a tremor so subtle that I couldn't tell if it came from having too much coffee and slips of the tongue so minor that I would have ignored them had I not noticed the other signs. It was a sad situation at a very formative stage of my career and it felt helpless. Thinking back, I wish I understood more about the gut brain connection and the power of the microbiome, and how eating certain foods can help lower neuroinflammation.

DEMENTIA CLASSIFICATIONS

In the DSM-5 TR, dementias are classified under Neurocognitive Disorders which may include Alzheimer's disease, frontotemporal degeneration, Lewy body disease, vascular disease, traumatic brain injury, substance/medication use, HIV infection, prion disease, Parkinson's disease, Huntington's disease, other medical conditions, multiple etiologies, and unspecified etiology. These categories are broad and clinically need more exploration when interviewing a patient.

Let's look at the burden of this disease: Alzheimer's is the nation's most expensive disease with the cost of Alzheimer's and other dementias to the U.S. economy is $355 billion, in health care, long-term care, and hospice. Many are concerned that Alzheimer's will eventually bankrupt Medicaid. The expected cost of Alzheimer's is projected to reach $1.1 trillion by 2050. The costs for care far exceed other terminal illness such as cancer and heart disease. The average total cost of care for a person with dementia over the last 5 years of their life is $287,038.

Basic Epidemiology:[28]

- Every 65 seconds, someone in the USA is diagnosed with Alzheimer's disease
- An estimated 6 million Americans today live with Alzheimer's disease.
- Alzheimer's begins to develop in the brain 20–30 years before diagnosis.
- 2/3 of those diagnosed are women.
- 2/3 of Alzheimer's caregivers are also women.
- A woman in her 60s is twice as likely to develop Alzheimer's over the course of her lifetime than breast cancer.
- After 60, a woman has a 1 in 5 chance of developing Alzheimer's.
- By 2060, approximately 13.8 million brains in the United States will be living with Alzheimer's, and millions more family members and friends will suffer alongside those diagnosed.
- Alzheimer's disease is still 100% fatal. There is no treatment or cure. Of the top 10 causes of death in America, it is the only disease without any effective drug or course of action.
- If a member of your family has Alzheimer's, that does not necessarily mean you will develop Alzheimer's.
- And the opposite is also true: if it does not run in your family, you are still at risk.
- Healthy habits can prevent or slow the symptoms of Alzheimer's disease.

1. Nutrition
2. Exercise
3. Lifestyle changes

⬤ NUTRITION AS PRIMARY PREVENTION FOR DEMENTIA

Diet is a significant lifestyle factor that is now impacting most major diseases.[29] From cardiology to cognition, longevity, or metabolic diseases, how we eat is a powerful tool to help reduce the burden of disease. Americans tend to eat a Western diet or so-called "SAD" (Standard American Diet) high in very sugary foods, fast foods, processed, ultra-processed junk foods, artificial sweeteners, and unhealthy fats. Any move away from this dietary pattern can begin to impact health changes. Ultimately, the goal is to support habit change over time and encourage patients that lifestyle changes are a marathon and not a sprint.

The MIND diet (**M**editerranean-DASH **I**ntervention for **N**eurodegenerative **D**elay) has been shown to be effective at reversing and protecting against cognitive decline and Alzheimer's disease. As the name hints, the MIND diet is a combination of two diets, the Mediterranean diet and the DASH diet.[30] Features of this diet are that it is low in saturated fats and high in healthy oils, with red meat eaten infrequently. DASH stands for **D**ietary **A**pproaches to **S**top **H**ypertension. It typically includes 5 daily servings of vegetables, 5 servings of fruit, about 7 servings of carbohydrates, 2 servings of low-fat dairy products, 2 or fewer servings of lean meat products, and nuts and seeds two to three times per week.[31]

Earlier studies of these individual diets had shown that each of these diets had demonstrated some protection over cognitive decline. However, in 2015, the late Martha Clare Morris and her colleagues researched and developed the MIND diet as a powerful combination of the two for long-term brain health.[30] Based on previous research, they put together a list of diet components that were either positive or negative for cognition. They named 10 brain-healthy food groups: green leafy vegetables, other vegetables (like peppers, carrots, and broccoli), nuts, berries, beans, whole grains, seafood, poultry, olive oil, and wine. They also named five unhealthy food groups: red meats, butter and margarine, cheese, pastries and sweets, and fried or fast food. See Table 23-1 for optimal mind score servings of the 10 brain-healthy food groups.

Each of these components was assigned a MIND diet score, which allowed researchers to quantify how well participants were following the diet. Since Morris's initial study, there have been several other studies that support her findings and show how the MIND diet affects individual diseases. In 2019, another research group found that the MIND diet was more likely to prevent progression to Alzheimer's disease over 12 years.[32] Another study found that the MIND diet was associated with a reduced incidence and delayed progression of Parkinsonism in old age.[33]

There is also a body of research being done with plant-based diets and their impact on cognition. While results suggest that a plant-based diet is related to better cognition, especially through improved executive control, researchers feel that future work should also examine underlying potential mechanisms such as reduced inflammation.[34]

Work done in the Blue Zones® should also be mentioned here. This began as a National Geographic expedition, led by Dan Buettner. What began as an expedition to uncover the secrets of longevity, evolved into the discovery of the five places around the world (Sardinia, Okinawa, Ikaria, Loma Linda, Nicoya) where people consistently live over 100 years old, which then became known as the Blue Zones®.[35] They uncovered nine evidence-based habits among the world's centenarians that are believed to slow this aging process. It's important to include these to emphasize the importance of a holistic and integrated approach to care.

- Sense of purpose: "why I wake up in the morning"
- Moving naturally in your environment (spending time walking everyday)
- Downshift (taking time to relax and destress each day)
- 80% rule (eating until you are 80% full)
- Plant slant (eating plenty of vegetables, fruits, whole grains, nuts, seeds, and legumes)

TABLE 23-1 • Mind diet "good" foods and their optimal mind score serving sizes	
Green leafy vegetables (kale, collards, greens, spinach, lettuce/tossed salad)	6 or more servings per week
Other vegetables (green/red peppers, squash, carrots, broccoli, celery, potatoes, peas or lima beans, potatoes, tomatoes, tomato sauce, string beans, beets, corn, zucchini/summer squash/eggplant)	1 or more servings per day
Berries (strawberries, blueberries, raspberries, blackberries)	2 or more servings per week
Nuts	5 or more servings per week
Olive oil	Use olive oil as your primary oil
Whole grains	3 or more servings per day
Fish (not fried, particularly high-omega-3 fish such as salmon)	1 or more meals per week
Beans (beans, lentils, soybeans)	More than 3 meals per week
Poultry (chicken or turkey)	2 or more meals per week
Wine	1 glass per day (it's important to note that 1 glass of wine per day resulted in a higher MIND score than any more or less)

Adapted from Morris MC, Tangney CC, Wang Y, et al. MIND diet slows cognitive decline with aging. *Alzheimer's & Dementia*. 2015;11(9): 1015-1022. doi:10.1016/j.jalz.2015.04.011.

- Wine at 5 (enjoying one or two drinks of wine with meals)
- Belong (participating in faith-based activities and communities)
- Loved ones (prioritizing your loved ones and making sure young and old family members are cared for)
- Right tribe (spending time with people engaging in healthy behaviors)

The Blue Zones incorporates many of the six pillars of lifestyle medicine (nutrition, exercise, sleep, social connection, stress reduction, and elimination or moderation of risky substances). The interaction of these six pillars is discussed in Chapter 31.

CLINICAL PRACTICE GUIDELINES (RELATED TO NUTRITION-BASED PREVENTION)

While many clinicians are not leading with dietary changes as an intervention and this is not yet a gold standard, it is critical for us to see the value in dietary changes being added to how we evaluate patients moving forward. Here is a six-step guide to follow when working with patients.

The first step is to ask about nutrition as part of other lifestyle questions.

1. Explore nutrition, dietary patterns, eating habits.
2. Ask about movement (e.g., exercise, dance, Zumba, walking)
3. Mindfulness (e.g., meditation practice, affirmations, breath work)
4. Hydration; encouraging water as the basis

5. Sleep hygiene
6. Stress reduction

FOODS TO ADD INTO A DIET FOR BETTER COGNITION HEALTH

1. Encourage a balance of foods without excluding food groups unless there is a confirmed allergy, food sensitivity, or intolerance
2. General guidelines: Focus on

   a. Fiber-rich foods like vegetables, fruit, beans nuts, seeds, healthy whole grains. The colors of plant foods (vegetables and fruit) bring rich plant polyphenols with vitamins, minerals and fiber, and biodiversity to the gut.

   b. Healthy fats from e.g., olive oil, avocadoes and avocado oil, wild salmon

   c. Clean sources of protein: if possible grass-fed meats, pasture raised chicken, grass-fed milk, cage-free eggs, wild caught salmon, organic non-GMO tofu, tempeh. (We fully acknowledge that not everyone has economic, social, or other access to the same quality of foods. Working to consume less highly processed foods is the goal.)

   d. Emphasize healthy whole foods and fewer processed, ultra-processed junk foods becomes critical. An example is: "eat the apple, skip the apple juice." Explaining the removal of fiber in store bought juices and the addition of sugars.

   e. Limit soda, artificially sweetened foods, fast foods, junk foods, processed and ultra-processed foods, processed vegetable and seed oils (e.g., corn, soy)

THREE TAKE-HOME POINTS

1. Dementia is not a disease of the elderly anymore, as small undetectable changes occur in our brain life-long. If we persist in eating poorly these microscopic changes can evolve into pathology that presents as cognitive changes. We should therefore be discussing nutrition with all our patients.

2. Nutrition is a powerful lever of change to lower neuroinflammation in the brain and body. Using the guidelines above helps patients make better choices toward any improvement away from the Standard American Diet (SAD).

3. Work with a patient to start with small simple changes they can easily incorporate such as

- a plant-rich diet: simply adding more vegetables to every meal.
- Stepping back from one unhealthy habit and replacing it with a better option e.g., blueberry fruited yogurt which may contain 6 teaspoons of added sugar in exchange for plain grass-fed milk whole yogurt, fresh or frozen blueberries, and a sprinkle of cinnamon for sweetness.

4. We in the healthcare profession need to move forward the food as medicine movement to effect change in the clinical care of our patients and improve health outcomes.

CASE STUDY ANSWERS

1. Fending off neuroinflammation is something we can each do with our daily diet by adjusting to including more healthy whole foods. These would include using the MIND diet, which contains healthy dietary principles based on extensive research by the late Martha Claire Morris PhD and her team. Eat green leafy vegetables, colorful vegetables, berries, nuts, olive oil, whole grains, fish, beans, and poultry.

2.
   - Healthy fats: olive oil, avocadoes, nuts (hazelnuts, macadamia nuts), seeds (flax, hemp, chia)
   - Plant-rich foods: colorful vegetables, fruit, beans, legumes, whole grains (also great sources of fiber)
   - Reminder: Ten brain-healthy food groups: green leafy vegetables, other vegetables (like peppers, carrots, and broccoli), nuts, berries, beans, whole grains, seafood, poultry, olive oil, and wine.

3. A reliance on only eating components of the Western diet:
   - Foods high in saturated fats (fried foods) and high-GI carbs (white bread, white rice, potatoes, pasta, and anything else made from refined flour).
   - Trans fats, hydrogenated fats found in shelf-stable baked goods and cookies and in processed and ultra-processed foods. Added/refined sugars and high fructose corn syrup; even found in savory foods (store bought pasta sauce; salad dressings; ketchup for example)
   - Processed vegetable oils (e.g., corn, soy)

   Reminder: Five unhealthy food groups: red meats, butter and margarine, cheese, pastries and sweets, and fried or fast food.

REFERENCES

1. He Z, Guo JL, McBride JD, et al. Amyloid-β plaques enhance Alzheimer's brain tau-seeded pathologies by facilitating neuritic plaque tau aggregation. *Nat Med*. 2018;24(1):29-38.

2. Martins LB, Malheiros Silveira AL, Teixeira AL. The link between nutrition and Alzheimer's disease: from prevention to treatment. *Neurodegener Dis Manag*. 2021;11(2):155-166.

3. Swardfager W, Lanctôt K, Rothenburg L, Wong A, Cappell J, Herrmann N. A meta-analysis of cytokines in Alzheimer's disease. *Biol Psychiatry*. 2010;68(10):930-941.

4. Perry VH, Nicoll JA, Holmes C. Microglia in neurodegenerative disease. *Nat Rev Neurol*. 2010;6(4):193-201.

5. Ferreira ST, Clarke JR, Bomfim TR, De Felice FG. Inflammation, defective insulin signaling, and neuronal dysfunction in Alzheimer's disease. *Alzheimers Dement (N Y)*. 2014;10(1):S76-S83.

6. Banks WA. Blood-brain barrier transport of cytokines: a mechanism for neuropathology. *Curr Pharm Des*. 2005;11(8):973-984.

7. Combs CK. Inflammation and microglia actions in Alzheimer's disease. *J Neuroimmune Pharmacol*. 2009;4(4):380-388.

8. Harach T, Marungruang N, Dutilleul N, et al. Reduction of Alzheimer's disease beta-amyloid pathology in the absence of gut microbiota. *arXiv preprint arXiv*:1509.02273. 2015 Sep 8.

9. Hoyles L, Snelling T, Umlai UK, et al. Microbiome–host systems interactions: protective effects of propionate upon the blood–brain barrier. *Microbiome*. 2018;6(1):1-3.

10. Ho L, Ono K, Tsuji M, Mazzola P, Singh R, Pasinetti GM. Protective roles of intestinal microbiota derived short chain fatty acids in Alzheimer's disease-type beta-amyloid neuropathological mechanisms. *Expert Rev Neurother*. 2018;18(1):83-90.

11. Silva YP, Bernardi A, Frozza RL. The role of short-chain fatty acids from gut microbiota in gut-brain communication. *Front Endocrinol*. 2020;11:25.

12. Dinan TG, Stanton C, Cryan JF. Psychobiotics: a novel class of psychotropic. *Biol Psychiatry*. 2013;74(10):720-726.

13. Leblhuber F, Steiner K, Schuetz B, Fuchs D, Gostner JM. Probiotic supplementation in patients with Alzheimer's dementia – an explorative intervention study. *Curr Alzheimer Res*. 2018;15(12):1106-1113.

14. Akbari E, Asemi Z, Daneshvar Kakhaki R, et al. Effect of probiotic supplementation on cognitive function and metabolic status in Alzheimer's disease: a randomized, double-blind and controlled trial. *Front Aging Neurosci*. 2016;8:256.

15. Tamtaji OR, Heidari-Soureshjani R, Mirhosseini N, et al. Probiotic and selenium co-supplementation, and the effects on clinical, metabolic and genetic status in Alzheimer's disease: a randomized, double-blind, controlled trial. *Clin Nutr*. 2019;38(6):2569-2575.

16. Sarkar A, Lehto SM, Harty S, Dinan TG, Cryan JF, Burnet PW. Psychobiotics and the manipulation of bacteria–gut–brain signals. *Trends Neurosci*. 2016;39(11):763-781.

17. Savignac HM, Corona G, Mills H, et al. Prebiotic feeding elevates central brain derived neurotrophic factor, N-methyl-D-aspartate receptor subunits and D-serine. *Neurochem Int*. 2013;63(8):756-764.

18. Burokas A, Arboleya S, Moloney RD, et al. Targeting the microbiota-gut-brain axis: prebiotics have anxiolytic and antidepressant-like effects and reverse the impact of chronic stress in mice. *Biol Psychiatry*. 2017;82(7):472-487.

19. Schmidt K, Cowen PJ, Harmer CJ, Tzortzis G, Errington S, Burnet PW. Prebiotic intake reduces the waking cortisol response and alters emotional bias in healthy volunteers. *Psychopharmacology*. 2015;232(10):1793-1801.

20. Pedditizi E, Peters R, Beckett N. The risk of overweight/obesity in mid-life and late life for the development of dementia: a systematic review and meta-analysis of longitudinal studies. *Age Ageing*. 2016;45(1):14-21.

21. Marcelin G, Silveira AL, Martins LB, Ferreira AV, Clément K. Deciphering the cellular interplays underlying obesity-induced adipose tissue fibrosis. *J Clini Invest*. 2019;129(10):4032-4040.

22. Talbot K. Brain insulin resistance in Alzheimer's disease and its potential treatment with GLP-1 analogs. *Neurodegener Dis Manag*. 2014;4(1):31-40.

23. Sierra C. Hypertension and the risk of dementia. *Front Cardiovasc Med*. 2020;7:5.

24. Peila R, White LR, Petrovich H, et al. Joint effect of the APOE gene and midlife systolic blood pressure on late-life cognitive impairment: the Honolulu-Asia aging study. *Stroke*. 2001;32(12):2882-2889.

25. Balazs R. Epigenetic mechanisms in Alzheimer's disease. *Degener Neurol Neuromuscul Dis*. 2014;4:85-102.

26. Athanasopoulos D, Karagiannis G, Tsolaki M. Recent findings in Alzheimer disease and nutrition focusing on epigenetics. *Adv Nutr*. 2016;7(5):917-927.

27. Piller, C. Science, Vol 377, Issue 6604, Page 358 July 2022.

28. 2021 Alzheimer's disease facts and figures. *Alzheimers Dement*. 2021 Mar;17(3):327-406.

29. The US Burden of Disease Collaborators. The State of US Health, 1990-2016: burden of diseases, injuries, and risk factors among US states. *JAMA*. 2018;319(14):1444-1472.

30. Morris MC, Tangney CC, Wang Y, Sacks FM, Bennett DA, Aggarwal NT. MIND diet associated with reduced incidence of Alzheimer's disease. *Alzheimers Dement*. 2015 Sep;11(9):1007-1014.

31. Challa HJ, Tadi P, Uppaluri KR. *DASH Diet (Dietary Approaches to Stop Hypertension)*. [updated May 15, 2019]. In: StatPearls.

32. Hosking DE, Eramudugolla R, Cherbuin N, Anstey KJ. MIND not Mediterranean diet related to 12-year incidence of cognitive impairment in an Australian longitudinal cohort study. *Alzheimers Dement*. 2019 Apr;15(4):581-589.

33. Agarwal P, Wang Y, Buchman AS, Holland TM, Bennett DA, Morris MC. MIND diet associated with reduced incidence and delayed progression of Parkinsonism in old age. *J Nutr Health Aging*. 2018;22(10):1211-1215.

34. Ramey MM, Shields GS, Yonelinas AP. Markers of a plant-based diet relate to memory and executive function in older adults. *Nutr Neurosci*. 2022 Feb;25(2):276-285.

35. Buettner D, Skemp S. Blue zones: lessons from the world's longest lived. *Am J Lifestyle Med*. 2016 Jul 7;10(5):318-321.

chapter 24

Depression and Anxiety

Uma Naidoo, MD / Connor Hatfield, BSc

Chapter Outline

CASE STUDY

Tamira is a 33-year-old woman with a history of depression who comes to her annual visit feeling down. Tamira also reports feeling fatigued and foggy during the afternoon. She is not taking any medications, currently. In the past about 4 years ago, she was on Prozac for 2 years. You inquire about the patient's diet. You learn that she is very busy at work where she is a chief financial officer of a company that is going public soon. Tamira only has time for fast food at the cafeteria at work and frozen meals for dinner. Since she is single, she does not feel the need to sit at the dinner table. Instead, she eats in front of the television watching her favorite shows. She skips breakfast every morning to make it to work on time. Her stress levels are high.

1. **What are three suggestions you can make to help Tamira use food to enhance her mood?**

2. **Which diet shows an association with a reduced risk of depression in research studies?**
   A. Depression Diet
   B. FODMAP Diet
   C. Mediterranean Diet
   D. SAD Diet

3. **Dietary fiber is important for people with anxiety. True or False?**

INTRODUCTION

Within medicine and health care, we often discuss nutrition in the context of physical health: diabetes, heart disease, cancer, and a myriad of other physical ailments have clear connections to our daily diets. More recently, however, researchers have begun exploring the relationship between nutrition and our thoughts, feelings, and emotions. The link between food and mental health may seem obscure or unlikely to some, but virtually everyone has experienced the mood-altering effects of food at some point: the sugar high after consuming sweets (and the associated crash shortly after), the burst of energy after consuming caffeine, and/or the clean, energized feeling after eating a healthy, well-balanced meal. These examples likely don't shock you and may even seem insignificant. However, as we'll discuss throughout this chapter, food does have a tremendous, lasting impact on our moods, well beyond momentary rises or dips in energy. We will see that our diet can dramatically influence our risk of developing two of the most common and costly diseases plaguing modern society: depression and anxiety.

DSM-5 DIAGNOSTIC CRITERIA OF MAJOR DEPRESSIVE DISORDER

Please review the full criteria in the DSM-V-TR.[1]

DSM-5 DIAGNOSTIC CRITERIA OF GENERALIZED ANXIETY DISORDER

Please review the full criteria in the DSM-V-TR.[1]

BASIC EPIDEMIOLOGY OF DEPRESSION IN RELATION TO NUTRITIONAL PATTERNS

Nutritional research is notoriously difficult to conduct, given the practical and ethical challenges of controlling the dietary intake of a sufficiently large participant population, along with numerous potential confounding factors. However, there are a significant number of longitudinal studies, including one randomized controlled trial, evaluating dietary patterns and their associated risk of depression.[2] The dietary pattern with the most substantial evidence backing its efficacy in reducing the risk of depression is the Mediterranean diet. The Mediterranean diet entails:[3]

- High consumption of extra virgin olive oil, vegetables (especially leafy green vegetables), whole grains, nuts, fruits, and legumes
- Moderate consumption of fish and poultry, dairy, and red wine
- Low consumption of red meat, eggs, and sweets

The PREDIMED study, conducted by Sánchez-Villegas and colleagues in 2013, was a large, randomized controlled-trial that evaluated the effectiveness of a Mediterranean diet for reducing the risk of depression.[4] The study yielded promising (but inconclusive) results regarding the efficacy of the Mediterranean diet in reducing future incidence of clinical depression. The study was composed of three groups:

1. A control group advised to follow a low-fat diet consistent with American Heart Association guidelines[5]
2. An experimental group advised to follow a Mediterranean diet supplemented with extra-virgin olive oil
3. An experimental group advised to follow a Mediterranean diet supplemented with mixed tree nuts

When analyzed together, the two Mediterranean diet groups had a lower relative risk (RR) of depression (RR = 0.85; 95% CI 0.64, 1.13) compared to controls, but the reduction was not statistically significant. However, additional evidence for the potential efficacy of the Mediterranean diet in reducing depression risk comes from two large observational cohort studies: one following 10,094 participants for a median of 4.4 years[6] and the other following 3,502 participants for a median of 7.2 years.[7] Both studies reported an inverse association between consumption of a "Mediterranean-type diet" and the incidence of depression. Notably, the former study found that the more closely a participant adhered to a "Mediterranean-type diet, the greater the reduction in depression risk.[6]

On the opposite end of the spectrum, a 2014 systematic review by Rahe and colleagues reported that "Western dietary patterns may be associated with higher odds of depression".[8] The Western diet or Standard American Diet (SAD) is generally defined as being high in ultra-processed foods, refined sugars, and processed red meats while being low in the consumption of vegetables, fruits, whole grains, and other foods that are characteristic of the Mediterranean diet. In essence, the Western diet is the opposite of the Mediterranean diet.

BASIC EPIDEMIOLOGY OF ANXIETY IN RELATION TO NUTRITIONAL PATTERNS

The nutritional epidemiology of anxiety is similar to that of depression. Dietary patterns that emphasize "vegetables, fruit, limited sugar and refined grains, and greater consumption of minimally processed foods" (such as the Mediterranean diet) are associated with lower anxiety, while diets high in refined carbohydrates, processed meats, and other ultra-processed foods are potentially associated with a greater incidence of anxiety.[9,10]

THE ROLE OF NUTRITION IN THE PATHOPHYSIOLOGY OF DEPRESSION

Depression is an extraordinarily complex and heterogeneous disease with a wide range of biopsychosocial causes that may underlie its development.[11] From the biological perspective, one factor that may cause or contribute to depressive symptoms is a nutritional deficiency.

B Vitamins (B1, B6, B9, and B12)

The B vitamins (particularly, B1, B6, B9, and B12) are critical to brain health and proper brain function. In the context of depression, the two most important are vitamin B9 (folate) and vitamin B12.[12] Folate contributes to hippocampal neurogenesis (growth of new neurons) and may play a role in serotonin synthesis, suggesting two potential mechanisms for inducing depressive symptoms: folate-deficient patients may experience a loss of hippocampal neurons and/or have low serotonin levels, both of which are associated with depression.[13,14] Notably, the functions of folate and vitamin B12 are highly interconnected, as a deficiency of vitamin B12 will result in a deficiency of folate.[15] This transitive deficiency may then set the stage for the development of depressive symptoms. Clinical evidence supporting the link between folate deficiency and depression comes from a 2009 study by Alpert and Fava, which reported that "depressive symptoms are the most common neuropsychiatric manifestation of folate deficiency".[16]

Deficiencies in vitamin B1 (thiamine) and vitamin B6 (pyridoxine) may also contribute to the development of depression, as each vitamin is key to the production of mood-regulating neurotransmitters.[12,17] Both vitamins are essential to serotonin synthesis, and pyridoxine also plays a critical role in dopamine and gamma-aminobutyric acid (GABA) synthesis.[17]

It is important to note that a 2022 systematic review by Moncrieff and colleagues called the serotonin theory of depression into question.[18] After analyzing the evidence of seventeen studies, the researchers concluded that there was "no consistent evidence of there being an association between serotonin and depression, and no support for the hypothesis that depression is caused by lowered serotonin activity or concentrations".[18] As a result, any mechanisms that allegedly ameliorate depressive symptoms by raising serotonin levels must be carefully reconsidered.

Foods rich in these critical B vitamins include legumes, citrus fruits, bananas, avocados, leafy green and cruciferous vegetables, asparagus, nuts and seeds, and fish and shellfish.[12] Vitamin B12 is found primarily in animal products (meat, eggs, dairy, etc.), so vegans and other plant-based patients may want to speak to their doctor about taking a vitamin B12 supplement if needed.

Vitamin A

Vitamin A is also essential to proper brain function, as it plays a role in the growth and adaptation of neurons.[12,19] Similar to vitamin B12, vitamin A deficiency may lead to the atrophy of particular brain regions (such as the hippocampus), resulting in maladaptive changes to the body's stress response.[20] The hippocampus is critical to learning and memory, so hippocampal atrophy caused by a vitamin A deficiency may impair the affected individual's ability to learn new coping strategies for their stress.[12] Importantly, a 2007 study by Bremner and McCaffery reported that excess levels of retinoic acid (a vitamin A metabolite) have been associated with depression and suicidality.[12,21] However, this association was observed in patients treated with an isomer of retinoic acid for acne—the amount of dietary vitamin A one would have to consume to reach these levels is far greater than is typical of a well-balanced diet.[12,21]

Spinach, kale, sweet potatoes, fish, carrots, and black-eyed peas are all excellent dietary sources of vitamin A.

Vitamin C

Vitamin C plays a role in the regulation of neurotransmitter synthesis, particularly for dopamine, norepinephrine, epinephrine, and possibly serotonin.[22] Additionally, multiple observational studies have found an association between low vitamin C levels and depression.[12,23]

Some vitamin C rich foods are citrus fruits, kiwi, red bell peppers, and green veggies like broccoli, Brussels sprouts, parsley, and thyme.

Vitamin D

There are currently three proposed mechanisms for how vitamin D may help prevent or treat depression as outlined by Menon and colleagues in their paper titled, "Vitamin D and Depression: A Critical Appraisal of the Evidence and Future Directions".[24] Menon and colleagues report:

1. "An increased region-specific expression of vitamin D receptors in brain areas (such as prefrontal and cingulate cortices) known to play a key role in mood regulation[25]"
2. "The modulatory role proposed for vitamin D in the association between depression and inflammation (through a possible immune-modulatory mechanism)[26,27]"
3. "The neuroprotective properties of vitamin D (by virtue of its anti-inflammatory effects)[28,29]"

Regardless of the mechanism, there is ample evidence suggesting an association between vitamin D deficiency and depression.[24] However, more research is needed to determine the direction of causality and the exact mechanism. Spending 10 minutes outdoors in daylight before applying sunscreen provides 80% of your daily vitamin D. Thereafter, it's best to wear sunscreen for the rest of the day.

Dietary sources of vitamin D include egg yolks, mushrooms, oysters, salmon, herring, sardines, and shrimp.[12] A vitamin D supplement may also be used to raise vitamin D levels.

Iron

As discussed in a 2014 study by Kim and Wessling-Resnick, iron plays a role in the myelination of brain neurons as well as monoamine metabolism. "Glutamate and gamma-aminobutyric acid homeostasis is modified by changes in brain iron status. Such changes produce not only deficits in memory/learning capacity and motor skills, but also emotional and psychological problems".[30] Additionally, clinical studies have shown that low iron levels have been linked to depression.[12,31]

Iron-rich foods include "shellfish, lean red meats and organ meats (in moderation), legumes, pumpkin seeds, broccoli, and dark chocolate (though any sweet should be eaten in moderation)".[12]

Magnesium

Magnesium also plays a key role in facilitating proper brain function, and a large number of studies have implicated magnesium deficiency as a potential risk factor for depression.[12] The first report on the efficacy of magnesium treatment for depression was published in 1921, and the authors reported success in a remarkable 220 out of 250 cases.[32] In 2006, Eby and Eby published case studies reporting that patients experienced "rapid recovery (less than 7 days) from major depression using 125–300 mg of magnesium (as glycinate and taurinate) with each meal and at bedtime".[33]

To increase magnesium intake, patients can consume more "avocados, nuts and seeds, legumes, whole grains, and some omega-3-rich fish (such as salmon and mackerel)".[12]

Zinc

Zinc is another mineral that appears to reduce depression risk, putatively mediated by a reduction in brain inflammation.[34] A 2018 review reported a "positive association between zinc deficiency and the risk of depression and an inverse association between zinc supplementation and depressive symptoms".[35] Additionally, a 2013 meta-analysis of seventeen studies reported that depressed subjects had lower blood zinc concentrations than control subjects.[12,36] Zinc-rich foods include "seafood (especially cooked oysters), lean beef, and poultry".[12] Smaller amounts of zinc are also available from "beans, nuts, and whole grains".[12]

Omega-3s

Omega-3 fatty acids are critical to our mental health; they are a key component of cell membranes and are a precursor for "the hormones that regulate blood clotting, contraction and relaxation of artery walls, and inflammation".[12] Omega-3s also decrease inflammatory markers and help buffer our neurons against the harmful effects of inflammation.[12] There is some debate as to whether omega-3s meaningfully decrease depression risk, but the majority of studies support the affirmative. For example, a meta-analysis of thirteen randomized controlled trials conducted in 2016 reported a "beneficial effect" of omega-3s for patients with major depressive disorder, especially those patients who had a higher intake of EPA and/or were taking antidepressants.[12,37] EPA (eicosapentaenoic acid) and DHA (docosahexaenoic acid) are the two most important omega-3 fatty acids in the context of mood disorders, though a third type (alpha-linolenic acid, or ALA) also confers general health benefits.[12]

Importantly, the human body cannot produce omega-3s on its own, so they must be obtained from the diet (hence, omega-3s are considered "essential" fatty acids). Dietary sources of omega-3s include fatty fish (such as salmon, mackerel, anchovies, sardines, and herring), leafy green vegetables, walnuts, chia seeds, and flax seeds.[12] Plant sources of omega-3s primarily provide ALA, while animal sources (such as fatty fish) are rich sources of EPA and DHA. It is also critical to consider a patient's consumption of omega-6 fatty acids relative to that of omega-3 fatty acids. The ideal omega-6 to omega-3 ratio is approximately 4:1, though the average Western diet yields a ratio of about 15:1.[12,38] Notably, studies have shown that individuals who consume high-omega-6 foods have a four-fold higher risk of depression than those who regularly consume high-omega-3 foods, suggesting that decreasing omega-6 consumption and increasing omega-3 consumption may help prevent or reduce depressive symptoms.[12] Foods rich in omega-6 fatty acids include grain-fed red meat, full-fat cheese, palm oil, and corn oil.[12]

Prebiotics and Probiotics

Prebiotics and probiotics are often conflated for one another. They serve different purposes though both are supportive of overall gut health. Prebiotics are types of fiber that benefit gut bacteria by offering nutrients they can digest, but humans cannot. Prebiotics confer a number of health benefits, such as reducing the number of unhealthy gut microbes, decreasing endotoxin levels, lowering inflammatory markers, improving blood sugar and insulin concentrations, lowering total cholesterol, increasing satiety, and enhancing absorption of calcium and magnesium in the gut.[39]

Probiotics, on the other hand, are live bacterial species that can break down prebiotics, generating important metabolites called short-chain fatty acids (SCFAs). SCFAs help reduce inflammation in the gut, promote the growth of healthy cells, and hinder the growth of cancerous cells.[12] Probiotics have also been shown in multiple studies to ameliorate depressive symptoms. A 2010 study that randomly assigned 55 healthy subjects to either a placebo or a daily probiotic found that those in the probiotic group reported less depression and had lower levels of urinary cortisol after 30 days, "indicating that their brains were less stressed *and* less depressed".[12,40] One mechanism proposed for this observed improvement in depressive symptoms is that some species of gut bacteria are able to influence neurotransmitter levels in the brain. By modifying the levels of neurotransmitters like serotonin and GABA, these beneficial gut bacteria may expedite recovery from depression and other mental illnesses.[12,41]

Prebiotics are found in fiber-rich foods like whole grains, legumes, vegetables, fruits, and nuts and seeds, while probiotics are found in fermented foods like yogurt (with active cultures), kimchi, sauerkraut, miso, tempeh, kefir, and kombucha. Dietary sources of probiotics are preferable to probiotic supplements, which have been rapidly growing in popularity in recent years. One reason for this is that food sources also confer secondary health benefits that may not be found in supplements (e.g., the minerals and vitamins that come along with a whole food). Prioritizing probiotic food sources also increases your microbiome's exposure to a diversity of new bacteria, whereas a probiotic supplement will only provide one limited subset of bacterial species. Lastly, patients may struggle to take a supplement consistently, and when they stop taking a probiotic, the benefits to the gut also stop. The same is true for if the patients stop eating probiotic foods.

● THE ROLE OF NUTRITION IN THE PATHOPHYSIOLOGY OF ANXIETY

Tryptophan

The amino acid tryptophan is a precursor to serotonin, and supplementation with purified tryptophan has been shown to increase brain serotonin levels.[42] This finding has prompted research into the potential efficacy of tryptophan as an anxiolytic substance. A 2021 systematic review of 11 randomized controlled trials found that tryptophan supplementation "represses negative feelings and enhances positive feelings",[43] suggesting that it may help reduce anxiety.

Dietary Fiber

Though it may not be readily apparent, adequate dietary fiber intake is critical to mental health and well-being. When one considers the profound connection between the gut and the brain (which has only recently come into the forefront of scientific research), however, this comes as less of a surprise. Dietary fiber is especially important in preventing and/or reducing anxiety symptoms. This connection is partly mediated by gut bacteria and the gut-brain axis, as beneficial gut bacteria break down dietary fiber into SCFAs, smaller sugar molecules, and other metabolites that confer a number of health benefits to the human host.[12] Specifically, the breakdown of dietary fiber into these smaller sugar molecules promotes the growth of the beneficial gut bacterial species *Bifidobacterium* and *Lactobacillus*. These bacteria then activate brain and nerve signaling pathways that can reduce anxiety.[12,44]

Another mediating factor between dietary fiber (or the lack thereof) and anxiety is inflammation. Dietary fiber decreases inflammation throughout the body and brain, and substantial evidence suggests that patients with anxiety have high levels of systemic inflammation.[12,45] This inflammation can impact brain areas (such as the amygdala) that play a key role in anxiety disorders.

A 2018 review by Taylor and Holscher provides further evidence for the potential anxiolytic properties of dietary fiber. They found that "diets rich in dietary fiber and omega-3-polyunsaturated fatty acids may be linked to reduced risk of developing symptoms of depression, anxiety, and stress".[46] This brings us to our next key nutrient for combating anxiety: omega-3 fatty acids.

Omega-3s

Omega-3 fatty acids also appear to help prevent and combat anxiety, primarily via neurochemical and anti-inflammatory mechanisms.[47] Support for the anti-inflammatory mechanism comes from a 2011 randomized controlled trial which found that, in a population of 68 medical students, students assigned to the omega-3 supplementation group had lower levels of inflammation and anxiety compared to controls after twelve weeks.[48] Additionally, a 2018 meta-analysis of 19 clinical trials found that omega-3 supplementation was positively associated with decreased anxiety symptoms.[49]

Similar to depression treatment and prevention, the omega-3 fatty acid EPA appears to be particularly important for combating anxiety. Another 2018 study reported that higher levels of EPA consumption were associated with lower levels of anxiety.[50] This same study also found that a high omega-6 to omega-3 fatty acid ratio correlated with increased levels of anxiety; yet another parallel to the pathophysiology of depression.

Aged, Fermented, and Cultured Foods

Aged and fermented foods (such as kimchi, sauerkraut, yogurt with live cultures, and kombucha) may also have anxiolytic properties. Similar to probiotics, these foods are an excellent source of live bacterial species that can improve gut health and reduce anxiety.[13,51] The mechanism behind this effect is not yet clear, but the following three hypotheses have been suggested: "chemical by-products of intestinal bacteria and bioactive peptides may protect the nervous system; the changing gut bacteria might suppress the stress response through the HPA-axis; and neurotransmitters and 'brain tissue builders' such as brain-derived neurotrophic factor, gamma-aminobutyric acid, and serotonin may be increased".[12] Other examples of aged, fermented, and cultured foods include tempeh, miso, kefir, apple cider vinegar, and fermented vegetables.

Vitamin D and Other Vitamins

Vitamin D is a neurosteroid, which means it can cross the blood-brain barrier and diffusing into brain cells.[12,52] While inside the brain, vitamin D reduces inflammation and mediates "the release of nerve growth factor, which is essential for the survival of hippocampal and cortical neurons".[12] Abnormalities in the cortex, the hippocampus, and the amygdala (which is intricately connected to the hippocampus[53] are all implicated in anxiety disorders, so it has been suggested that vitamin D's anti-inflammatory and neurotrophic properties may be able to reduce anxious symptoms.

A 2019 randomized clinical trial assessed whether consuming a vitamin D capsule biweekly for 16 weeks could decrease anxiety in women with type 2 diabetes and vitamin D deficiency. By the end of the trial, the participants in the vitamin D group were significantly less anxious than those receiving the placebo.[12,54]

Vitamin D deficiency has become increasingly common in recent years as more people lead indoor lifestyles.[55] Approximately 80% of our vitamin D comes from skin exposure to direct sunlight, and, unfortunately, sunlight passing through windows does not count, since glass absorbs ultraviolet B radiation.[12] Consuming vitamin D-rich foods can help combat deficiency, but increased sun exposure and/or supplementation may be necessary to reach adequate levels. Vitamin D–rich foods include egg yolks, fortified milk, salmon, oysters, mushrooms, shrimp, and cod-liver oil.

Other Vitamins

The B vitamins (specifically, B1 and B6) and the antioxidant vitamins A, C, and E have also been shown to be helpful in reducing symptoms of anxiety. A 2008 study showed that up to 250 mg of vitamin B1 (thiamine) can be effective for decreasing anxiety, and a 2017 systematic review demonstrated that vitamin B6 (pyridoxine) may alleviate anxiety symptoms in older women and women with premenstrual stress.[56,57] In 2012, researchers found that levels of vitamins A, C, and E were all low in patients with generalized anxiety disorder.[58] They later reported a reduction of symptoms in these patients after 6 weeks of supplementation. Perhaps the most practical way to increase levels of all these key vitamins is to take an over-the-counter multivitamin. Two studies conducted in the year 2000 showed reductions in stress and/or anxiety levels after about 1 month of multivitamin supplementation, with one of the studies having a sample size of approximately 300 subjects.[59,60] In 2013, a meta-analysis further substantiated these findings.[61]

Magnesium

Magnesium deficiency has been associated with higher anxiety levels in humans, suggesting that supplementation may help ameliorate symptoms.[12] Support for this hypothesis comes from myriad studies, including a 2017 systematic review by Boyle and colleagues that reported magnesium supplementation may be especially helpful for those with a high vulnerability to anxiety.[62] One mechanism proposed for this beneficial effect is the magnesium-induced reduction of adrenocorticotropic hormone secretion in the brain, resulting in a dampened stress response.[63] The majority of studies supporting magnesium as an anxiolytic utilized a 6- to 12-week administration period, though more research is needed to determine the minimum effective intervention duration.[62] Dietary sources of magnesium include avocados, nuts, fatty fish, spinach, edamame, and legumes.

● AUTHOR'S CASE EXAMPLE

Anjali was a 28-year-old single domiciled consultant at Boston Consulting Group when she first came to see me. "Dr Naidoo I need Zoloft" were the first words out of her mouth. Her PCP had referred her for new onset anxiety. After taking a detailed medical history I discovered that she was highly successful at work and had been promoted 6 months prior. What changed in her lifestyle were the following:

- Traveling most days of the week by air
- No longer sipped on water throughout her workday
- Eating on the go, in airports and out of mini bar when she arrived late at the hotel
- No healthy packed lunches for work
- Less time walking her dog and spending time outdoors
- Wine every night at work dinners and networking

While these may not seem major changes, they were major for her microbiome and her mental well-being. Her consumption of processed and ultra-processed foods increased; she was consuming more alcohol, and this impacted her sleep; sleep was restless due to jet lag and alcohol impacting her sleep architecture; she had no time for yoga or Zumba classes, which she found relaxing; her stress level had increased. We talked about the gut microbiome and dysbiosis, an imbalance that may signal inflammation. She was very interested and was functioning well enough to avoid taking medication. Instead, I put her on a trial of nutrition and lifestyle measures.

I helped her implement the following:

1. She carried a sustained water bottle with a built-in filter so she hydrated herself wherever she was.
2. She packed small bags of healthy snacks like raw natural nuts and seeds along with some with small packets of nut butter for the airplane.
3. She ate fresh salads without the dressing at airports and asked for a healthy protein side and a piece of lemon for dressing.
4. She drank a maximum ⅓ to 1 glass of wine at any work event and then switched to a sparkling water with fruit in a wine glass so she would not feel out of place.
5. She stopped at a supermarket whenever she arrived somewhere and bought berries, chopped vegetables, hummus, and water for her mini fridge.
6. She restarted a mindful meditation to help lower her stress.

Over the first month with consistency, she noticed a drop in her level of anxiety, and by 3 months of continuing this plan she no longer felt anxiety. While her life had changed, she was now coping better and following a similar healthier lifestyle like she had been prior to her promotion.

Common Questions on Food, Fatigue and Fogginess:
What foods can help with feeling fatigued?

Most Americans consume the standard American diet or SAD diet, also called the Western diet, heavy in ultra-processed junk foods and fast foods. These foods lack true nutrition and are laden with added sugars, high fructose corn syrup, vegetable oils, preservatives, colorants, dyes, food stabilizers, and thickening agents. Worse, they may be fortified with single vitamins that might make them seem initially nutritious, but in reality they are giving us just one tiny component of a much larger picture of true nutrition. By consuming this type of diet, the body and brain are not receiving the types of nutrients from healthy whole foods to provide energy.

Some examples of foods to help with fatigue are:

Pumpkin seeds are a rich source of magnesium and zinc, key minerals in the production of mood and focus-boosting neurotransmitters. They also contain protein which helps to fuel the body.

Onions are an allium food and are a rich source of prebiotic fiber which feeds the gut microbes. They also contain polyphenols, vitamin C, and potassium, to help boost focus and energy.

Lentils are another incredible, high-fiber, nutrient-dense source of plant protein. They're rich in folate and iron, which have been shown to improve mood symptoms, while easy to digest proteins promote satiety, balanced energy, and muscular growth.

What foods can help with feeling foggy?

Vegetables and fruits such as celery, parsley, broccoli, onion leaves, carrots, peppers, cabbages, apple skins, and chrysanthemum flowers are luteolin-rich, meaning they are rich in an antioxidant compound, which research has shown may possess potent anti-cancer effects as well as fighting fatigue and providing energy.

SUMMARY

What we eat has an influence on our brain. Our meals can help us to prevent depression and anxiety. In fact, in some cases, our meals can work as medicine for these conditions. Medications for depression and anxiety are excellent tools for psychiatrists and primary care physicians to use when patients meet the diagnostic criteria for these conditions. In these cases, nutritional interventions, and a change in eating patterns, such as adopting a Mediterranean-style diet, can also have powerful effects on mood and anxiety levels. Screening for nutritional deficiencies can help identify patients who will most benefit from interventions focused on food.

THREE TAKE-HOME POINTS

1. **Encourage a Mediterranean eating pattern[64] with an emphasis on whole foods, omega-3s, and probiotics.**

In this chapter, we discussed the Mediterranean diet, but it is recommended that healthcare providers encourage patients to follow a Mediterranean eating pattern (MEP). The word "diet" can sound restrictive, while "eating pattern" may convey more flexibility and adaptability to the patient's preferences. A Mediterranean eating pattern entails the following:[64]

- A plant-rich diet focused on vegetables, fruits, whole grains, nuts, and seeds
- Minimally processed, consisting of locally grown and seasonal foods
- Limited amounts of added sugars, candy, sodas, and high fructose corn syrup
- Consumption of high-quality fats, e.g., avocado, olive oil
- Low-to-moderate intake of dairy, primarily consisting of yogurt and cheese
- Wild* seafood, when possible; grass-fed red meat; and pastured eggs (*these can be more costly so encouraging whole foods vs. processed is key e.g., regular beef or seafood is still better than deli meats, which are processed)
- Low-to-moderate consumption of wine with meals
- Herbs and spices used in lower the amount of salt needed to add flavor

Notice that the MEP prioritizes whole foods over refined, ultra-processed foods. Additionally, the moderate intake of seafood is consistent with our discussion of omega-3 fatty acids in the context of mental health. The MEP also includes yogurt, which can be a great source of probiotics (if the yogurt contains live, active cultures). If someone does not eat dairy, as many people are lactose intolerant, the plant-based yogurts may also contain live active cultures. However, suggesting a plain yogurt vs. fruited (which will have added sugars) is a better option. I would also encourage the incorporation of fermented foods such as kimchi, sauerkraut, kombucha, tempeh, or miso to increase the microbiome's exposure to a greater diversity of bacterial species.

2. **Screen for nutritional deficiencies**

As we have discussed, patients with nutritional deficiencies may present with symptoms of depression and/or anxiety. Rather than immediately prescribing a medication, it is worthwhile to screen for nutritional deficiencies in case there is a simpler, more cost-effective solution to try first (e.g., supplementation and/or dietary changes). With all the potential side effects that come along with psychiatric medications, a more holistic, nutritional approach may save the patient from unnecessary stress or adverse health consequences.

Nutritional interventions are clearly not a magic bullet. Nutritional deficiencies are not the only cause of these illnesses, and more traditional approaches (such as psychotherapy and/or medication) may be necessary.

3. **Make realistic, practical, and sustainable recommendations for behavior change—encourage small steps, not dramatic, sudden changes. "It's a marathon not a sprint mindset"**

As you may have experienced, lifestyle changes can be very difficult to implement and sustain. Rather than asking a patient to overhaul their entire diet in a matter of days, start by suggesting small, simple changes they can make to their regular eating habits. For example, if a patient currently has three creams and two sugars in their morning coffee, work with them to gradually decrease those amounts or help them identify a healthier alternative (such as unsweetened almond or oat milk). Once they succeed in that, identify another healthy change you can work on together. These small wins can eventually add up to a significantly improved diet and health status.

In clinical practice, it is ideal if you can tailor your dietary recommendations to a patient's food preferences and/or culture; doing so may make the changes easier to implement and adhere to long term. If rice dishes are regularly consumed in a patient's household, you could advise them to swap out white rice for brown rice, which has a lower glycemic index and more nutrients. If another patient often has wheat pasta or spaghetti, you could recommend they switch to a more blood sugar-friendly alternative like noodles made from zucchini ("zoodles") or spaghetti squash.

CASE STUDY ANSWERS

1.
- The first step would be to help her move away from fast food to whole food options instead. Suggest she select a green salad at the cafeteria along with a piece of healthy protein (chicken/salmon or tofu).

- Instead of a frozen meal, can she learn a simple recipe for a roast chicken with three sides of vegetables (which provide fiber and phytonutrients) or a stir fry tofu and vegetable dish?

- Can she learn to make a two-ingredient chia pudding to encourage an easy breakfast she can make ahead. Rich in both fiber and protein this is a great source of nutrients to start her day?

2. C; The Mediterranean diet has been studied with patients who have depression, and there is some evidence from observational cohort studies that this eating pattern helps reduce the risk of depression. Evidence for the potential efficacy of the Mediterranean diet in reducing depression risk comes from two large observational cohort studies: one following 10,094 participants for

a median of 4.4 years[6] and the other following 3,502 participants for a median of 7.2 years.[7] Both studies reported an inverse association between consumption of a "Mediterranean-type diet" and the incidence of depression. Notably, the former study found that the more closely a participant adhered to a "Mediterranean-type diet, the greater the reduction in depression risk.[6] There is not a "Depression Diet." The FODMAP diet is used in relation to Inflammatory Bowel conditions. The SAD diet is the Standard American Diet. A 2014 systematic review by Rahe and colleagues reported that "Western dietary patterns may be associated with higher odds of depression".[8] The Western diet is often also called the Standard American Diet (SAD).

3. True; Dietary fiber is especially important in preventing and/or reducing anxiety symptoms. This connection is partly mediated by gut bacteria and the gut-brain axis, as beneficial gut bacteria break down dietary fiber into SCFAs, smaller sugar molecules, and other metabolites that confer a number of health benefits to the human host.[12]

REFERENCES

1. American Psychiatric Association. *Diagnostic and Statistical Manual of Mental Disorders*, 5th ed. American Psychiatric Association; 2013. doi:10.1176/appi.books.9780890425596.

2. Martínez-González MA, Sánchez-Villegas A. Food patterns and the prevention of depression. *Proc Nutr Soc.* 2016;75(2):139-146.

3. Davis C, Bryan J, Hodgson J, Murphy K. Definition of the Mediterranean diet; a literature review. *Nutrients.* 2015;7(11):9139-9153.

4. Sánchez-Villegas A, Martínez-González MA, Estruch R, et al. Mediterranean dietary pattern and depression: the PREDIMED randomized trial. *BMC Med.* 2013;11(1):208.

5. Krauss RM, Eckel RH, Howard B, et al. AHA dietary guidelines: revision 2000: a statement for healthcare professionals from the Nutrition Committee of the American Heart Association. *Circulation.* 2000;102(18):2284-2299.

6. Sánchez-Villegas A, Delgado-Rodríguez M, Alonso A, et al. Association of the Mediterranean dietary pattern with the incidence of depression: The Seguimiento Universidad de Navarra/ University of Navarra Follow-up (SUN) Cohort. *Arch Gen Psychiatry.* 2009;66(10):1090-1098.

7. Skarupski KA, Tangney CC, Li H, Evans DA, Morris MC. Mediterranean diet and depressive symptoms among older adults over time. *J Nutr Health Aging.* 2013;17(5):441-445.

8. Rahe C, Unrath M, Berger K. Dietary patterns and the risk of depression in adults: a systematic review of observational studies. *Eur J Nutr.* 2014;53(4):997-1013.

9. Aucoin M, LaChance L, Naidoo U, et al. Diet and anxiety: a scoping review. *Nutrients.* 2021;13(12):4418.

10. Jacka FN, Pasco JA, Mykletun A, et al. Association of Western and traditional diets with depression and anxiety in women. *Am J Psychiatry.* 2010;167(3):305-311.

11. Schotte CKW, Van Den Bossche B, De Doncker D, Claes S, Cosyns P. A biopsychosocial model as a guide for psychoeducation and treatment of depression. *Depress Anxiety.* 2006;23(5):312-324.

12. Naidoo U. *This Is Your Brain on Food: An Indispensable Guide to the Surprising Foods That Fight Depression, Anxiety, PTSD, OCD, ADHD, and More*, 1st ed. Little, Brown Spark; 2020.

13. Gradin VB, Pomi A. The role of hippocampal atrophy in depression: a neurocomputational approach. *J Biol Phys.* 2008;34(1-2):107-120.

14. Albert PR, Benkelfat C, Descarries L. The neurobiology of depression—revisiting the serotonin hypothesis. I. Cellular and molecular mechanisms. *Phil Trans R Soc B.* 2012;367(1601):2378-2381.

15. Scott JM. Folate and vitamin B_{12}. *Proc Nutr Soc.* 1999;58(2):441-448.

16. Alpert JE, Fava M. Nutrition and depression: the role of folate. *Nutr Rev.* 1997;55(5):145-149.

17. Calderón-Ospina CA, Nava-Mesa MO. B Vitamins in the nervous system: current knowledge of the biochemical modes of action and synergies of thiamine, pyridoxine, and cobalamin. *CNS Neurosci Ther.* 2020;26(1):5-13.

18. Moncrieff J, Cooper RE, Stockmann T, Amendola S, Hengartner MP, Horowitz MA. The serotonin theory of depression: a systematic umbrella review of the evidence. *Mol Psychiatry.* 2023;28(8):3243-3256.

19. Olson CR, Mello CV. Significance of vitamin A to brain function, behavior and learning. *Mol Nutr Food Res*. 2010;54(4):489-495.

20. Misner DL, Jacobs S, Shimizu Y, et al. Vitamin A deprivation results in reversible loss of hippocampal long-term synaptic plasticity. *Proc Natl Acad Sci USA*. 2001;98(20):11714-11719.

21. Bremner JD, McCaffery P. The neurobiology of retinoic acid in affective disorders. *Prog Neuropsychopharmacol Biol Psychiatry*. 2008;32(2):315-331.

22. Pullar J, Carr A, Bozonet S, Vissers M. High vitamin C status is associated with elevated mood in male tertiary students. *Antioxidants (Basel)*. 2018;7(7):91.

23. Gariballa S. Poor Vitamin C status is associated with increased depression symptoms following acute illness in older people. *Int J Vitam Nutr Res*. 2014;84(1-2):12-17.

24. Menon V, Kar SK, Suthar N, Nebhinani N. Vitamin D and depression: a critical appraisal of the evidence and future directions. *Indian J Psychol Med*. 2020;42(1):11-21.

25. Prüfer K, Veenstra TD, Jirikowski GF, Kumar R. Distribution of 1,25-dihydroxyvitamin D3 receptor immunoreactivity in the rat brain and spinal cord. *J Chem Neuroanat*. 1999;16(2):135-145.

26. Mora JR, Iwata M, von Andrian UH. Vitamin effects on the immune system: vitamins A and D take centre stage. *Nat Rev Immunol*. 2008;8(9):685-698.

27. Van Etten E, Stoffels K, Gysemans C, Mathieu C, Overbergh L. Regulation of vitamin D homeostasis: implications for the immune system. *Nutr Rev*. 2008;66(s2):S125-S134.

28. Buell JS, Dawson-Hughes B. Vitamin D and neurocognitive dysfunction: preventing "D"ecline? *Mol Aspects Med*. 2008;29(6):415-422.

29. Song C, Wang H. Cytokines mediated inflammation and decreased neurogenesis in animal models of depression. *Prog Neuropsychopharmacol Biol Psychiatry*. 2011;35(3):760-768.

30. Kim J, Wessling-Resnick M. Iron and mechanisms of emotional behavior. *J Nutr Biochem*. 2014;25(11):1101-1107.

31. Hidese S, Saito K, Asano S, Kunugi H. Association between iron-deficiency anemia and depression: a web-based Japanese investigation. *Psychiatry Clin Neurosci*. 2018;72(7):513-521.

32. Eby GA, Eby KL, Murk H. Magnesium and major depression. In: Vink R, Nechifor M, eds. *Magnesium in The Central Nervous System*. University of Adelaide Press; 2011. Accessed October 24, 2022. Available at: http://www.ncbi.nlm.nih.gov/books/NBK507265/.

33. Eby GA, Eby KL. Rapid recovery from major depression using magnesium treatment. *Med Hypotheses*. 2006;67(2):362-370.

34. Szewczyk B, Kubera M, Nowak G. The role of zinc in neurodegenerative inflammatory pathways in depression. *Prog Neuropsychopharmacol Biol Psychiatry*. 2011;35(3):693-701.

35. Wang J, Um P, Dickerman B, Liu J. Zinc, magnesium, selenium and depression: a review of the evidence, potential mechanisms and implications. *Nutrients*. 2018;10(5):584.

36. Swardfager W, Herrmann N, Mazereeuw G, Goldberger K, Harimoto T, Lanctôt KL. Zinc in depression: a meta-analysis. *Biol Psychiatry*. 2013;74(12):872-878.

37. Mocking RJT, Harmsen I, Assies J, Koeter MWJ, Ruhé HG, Schene AH. Meta-analysis and meta-regression of omega-3 polyunsaturated fatty acid supplementation for major depressive disorder. *Transl Psychiatry*. 2016;6(3):e756-e756.

38. Simopoulos AP. The importance of the ratio of omega-6/omega-3 essential fatty acids. *Biomed Pharmacother*. 2002;56(8):365-379.

39. Valdes AM, Walter J, Segal E, Spector TD. Role of the gut microbiota in nutrition and health. *BMJ*. Published online June 13, 2018:k2179. doi:10.1136/bmj.k2179.

40. Messaoudi M, Lalonde R, Violle N, et al. Assessment of psychotropic-like properties of a probiotic formulation (*Lactobacillus helveticus* R0052 and *Bifidobacterium longum* R0175) in rats and human subjects. *Br J Nutr*. 2011;105(5):755-764.

41. Clapp M, Aurora N, Herrera L, Bhatia M, Wilen E, Wakefield S. Gut Microbiota's effect on mental health: the gut-brain axis. *Clin Pract*. 2017;7(4):987.

42. Young SN. How to increase serotonin in the human brain without drugs. *J Psychiatry Neurosci*. 2007;32(6):394-399.

43. Kikuchi AM, Tanabe A, Iwahori Y. A systematic review of the effect of L-tryptophan supplementation on mood and emotional functioning. *J Diet Suppl*. 2021;18(3):316-333.

44. Foster JA, McVey Neufeld KA. Gut–brain axis: how the microbiome influences anxiety and depression. *Trends Neurosci*. 2013;36(5):305-312.

45. Salim S, Chugh G, Asghar M. Inflammation in anxiety. In: *Advances in Protein Chemistry and Structural Biology*, Vol 88. Elsevier; 2012:1-25.

46. Taylor AM, Holscher HD. A review of dietary and microbial connections to depression, anxiety, and stress. *Nutr Neurosci*. 2020;23(3):237-250.

47. Su KP, Matsuoka Y, Pae CU. Omega-3 polyunsaturated fatty acids in prevention of mood and anxiety disorders. *Clin Psychopharmacol Neurosci*. 2015;13(2):129-137.

48. Kiecolt-Glaser JK, Belury MA, Andridge R, Malarkey WB, Glaser R. Omega-3 supplementation lowers inflammation and anxiety in medical students: a randomized controlled trial. *Brain Behav Immun*. 2011;25(8):1725-1734.

49. Su KP, Tseng PT, Lin PY, et al. Association of use of omega-3 polyunsaturated fatty acids with changes in severity of anxiety symptoms: a systematic review and meta-analysis. *JAMA Netw Open*. 2018;1(5):e182327.

50. Natacci L, Marchioni DM, Goulart AC, et al. Omega 3 consumption and anxiety disorders: a cross-sectional analysis of the Brazilian longitudinal study of adult health (ELSA-Brasil). *Nutrients*. 2018;10(6):663.

51. Selhub EM, Logan AC, Bested AC. Fermented foods, microbiota, and mental health: ancient practice meets nutritional psychiatry. *J Physiol Anthropol*. 2014;33(1):2.

52. Anjum I, Jaffery SS, Fayyaz M, Samoo Z, Anjum S. The role of vitamin D in brain health: a mini literature review. *Cureus*. 2018;10(7):e2960.

53. Shin LM, Liberzon I. The neurocircuitry of fear, stress, and anxiety disorders. *Neuropsychopharmacol*. 2010;35(1):169-191.

54. Fazelian S, Amani R, Paknahad Z, Kheiri S, Khajehali L. Effect of vitamin D supplement on mood status and inflammation in vitamin D deficient type 2 diabetic women with anxiety: a randomized clinical trial. *Int J Prev Med*. 2019;10:17.

55. Naeem Z. Vitamin d deficiency—an ignored epidemic. *Int J Health Sci (Qassim)*. 2010;4(1):V-VI.

56. Cornish S, Mehl-Madrona L. The role of vitamins and minerals in psychiatry. *Integr Med Insights*. 2008;3:33-42.

57. McCabe D, Lisy K, Lockwood C, Colbeck M. The impact of essential fatty acid, B vitamins, vitamin C, magnesium and zinc supplementation on stress levels in women: a systematic review. *JBI Database Syst Rev Implement Rep*. 2017;15(2):402-453

58. Gautam M, Agrawal M, Gautam M, Sharma P, Gautam A, Gautam S. Role of antioxidants in generalised anxiety disorder and depression. *Indian J Psychiatry*. 2012;54(3):244-247.

59. Carroll D, Ring C, Suter M, Willemsen G. The effects of an oral multivitamin combination with calcium, magnesium, and zinc on psychological well-being in healthy young male volunteers: a double-blind placebo-controlled trial. *Psychopharmacology*. 2000;150(2):220-225.

60. Schlebusch L, Bosch BA, Polglase G, Kleinschmidt I, Pillay BJ, Cassimjee MH. A double-blind, placebo-controlled, double-centre study of the effects of an oral multivitamin-mineral combination on stress. *S Afr Med J*. 2000;90(12):1216-1223.

61. Long SJ, Benton D. Effects of vitamin and mineral supplementation on stress, mild psychiatric symptoms, and mood in nonclinical samples: a meta-analysis. *Psychosom Med*. 2013;75(2):144-153.

62. Boyle N, Lawton C, Dye L. The effects of magnesium supplementation on subjective anxiety and stress—a systematic review. *Nutrients*. 2017;9(5):429.

63. Murck H, Steiger A. Mg 2+ reduces ACTH secretion and enhances spindle power without changing delta power during sleep in men - possible therapeutic implications. *Psychopharmacology*. 1998;137(3):247-252.

64. Boucher JL. Mediterranean eating pattern. *Diabetes Spectr*. 2017; 30(2):72-76.

Disordered Eating

Amanda Raffoul, PHD / S. Bryn Austin, ScD

Chapter Outline

CASE STUDY

A 23-year-old woman presents to you, her primary care provider, with concerns about her menstrual cycle becoming irregular over the past 6 months. She also reports experiencing acute dizziness and trouble sleeping. Since her last visit 2 years ago, she has lost 25 lbs. and her body mass index (BMI) has shifted from the "overweight" to the "normal" range. This patient has no significant medical history but has reported anxiety and depression during her adolescent years.

When you inquire about any changes to her daily routine in the past 6 months since her menstrual cycle has become irregular, she reports that she has started to "eat healthier" and began a new exercise routine, to which she credits her weight loss. The new diet that she is on includes only vegetables and specific types of proteins into a rigid structure and has explicit rules for foods that she avoids (e.g., cutting out any food/drinks with added sugars, avoiding all types of breads and pastas). She reports spending a lot of time thinking about her new diet and exercise routine, which she said helped her cope with the stress of trying to find a new job since she became unemployed 6 months ago. However, she does not believe that her new habits are related to the symptoms that she has developed, and instead blames general stress and anxiety.

1. What questions or screening tools could you ask or deliver to this patient that could assess the possibility of disordered eating?

2. What behaviors and preoccupations may indicate that patients who report eating "healthier" are engaging in harmful disordered eating?

3. Describe how the symptoms (i.e., amenorrhea, dizziness, weight loss) and life circumstances (e.g., unemployment, anxiety) that this patient is experiencing may be related to her new dietary habits and behaviors.

4. What nutritional complications related to the patient's weight loss and amenorrhea do you suspect? What management could you consider?

5. If the screening procedure you used suggests that the patient might be at risk for an eating disorder, how would you initiate a conversation with her?

DISORDERED EATING AND EATING DISORDERS

Eating disorders are psychiatric illnesses characterized by significant impairment to physical and psychosocial health and a disruption of eating- and weight-related behavior. They include a range of symptoms, outlined in the Diagnostic and Statistical Manual of Mental Disorders 5th Edition (DSM-5), that significantly impact daily life and result in negative physical, mental, and social consequences.[1] Eating disorders include anorexia nervosa (AN), avoidant/restrictive food intake disorder (ARFID), binge eating disorder (BED), bulimia nervosa (BN), and other specified feeding or eating disorder (OSFED), summarized in Table 25-1.[1,2] *Disordered eating* is a term used to capture eating- and weight-related behaviors that are harmful, serious, and may also impact an individual's daily life and overall well-being, but do not meet the diagnostic criteria for one of the eating disorders summarized in Table 25-1. Although all individuals with an eating disorder engage in disordered eating, not all forms of disordered eating meet diagnostic criteria for an eating disorder. Disordered eating may include thoughts and attitudes (e.g., poor body image, preoccupation with weight and appearance, fear of gaining weight) as well as behaviors (e.g., self-induced vomiting, abusing laxatives and diuretics, severe caloric restriction, binge eating), further described in the following sections. Subclinical ARFID symptoms may include avoidance of eating due to fear of choking or vomiting, poor appetite, and/or lack of interest, as well as eating a very narrow range of foods.[3]

Nine percent of the U.S. population will have an eating disorder in their lifetime.[4] The estimated lifetime prevalence for each eating disorder across the general population is 0.3–2.8% for AN, 0.3–2.3% for BED, 0.1–1.5% for BN, and 0.9–10.1% for OSFED;[5] however, these percentages are likely a gross underestimation of the prevalence of eating disorders. Eating disorders are underdiagnosed because of pervasive myths among the general population and medical practitioners about what an eating disorder "looks like" (e.g., that only thin individuals can have AN when in fact people of all weights can have atypical AN; Table 25-1),[6] the stigma surrounding eating disorders,[7] as well as gaps in medical education and training.[8] As a result, people with symptoms may not disclose symptoms to clinicians because of shame, may not have access to trained healthcare professionals who could provide a diagnosis, and/or may encounter health professionals who are not trained or knowledgeable about eating disorders.

Disordered eating, including vomiting to lose weight; using dangerous diet pills, laxatives, and diuretics; severe caloric restriction; and excessive exercise, affects a much larger segment of the population than those meeting full DSM-5 diagnostic criteria.

Eating disorders and disordered eating are prevalent across gender, sexual orientation, body weight, age, income status, race, ethnicity, and intersections of these identities,[9] but some socio-demographic groups may be at higher risk. Cisgender girls and women are more likely to have an eating disorder or engage in most types of disordered eating compared to

TABLE 25-1 • Summary of eating disorders diagnostic characteristics	
Eating disorder	**Diagnostic criteria**
Anorexia nervosa (AN)	• Restriction of energy intake leading to significant weight loss • Intense fear of gaining weight or "becoming fat" • Severely worried about body weight and shape, and has low self-esteem and/or concern about their low body weight
Avoidant/restrictive food intake disorder (ARFID)	• An eating or feeding disturbance that leads to failing to meet appropriate nutritional needs • May present with significant weight loss or falling off a growth curve and nutritional deficiencies • Eating or feeding disturbances are not explained by a lack of available food or another eating disorder
Binge eating disorder (BED)	• Recurring episodes of binge eating, characterized by eating a large amount of food and a lack of control during the episode • Binge eating episodes are characterized by eating rapidly, feeling uncomfortably full, eating when not hungry, eating alone because of embarrassment, and feeling disgust and/or guilt afterward • Binge eating occurs at least once a week for 3 months • Binge eating is *not* associated with the regular use of compensatory behaviors
Bulimia nervosa (BN)	• Recurring episodes of binge eating, characterized by eating a large amount of food and a lack of control during the episode • Recurring compensatory behaviors (e.g., self-induced vomiting; misuse of laxatives, diuretics, or other medications; fasting or excessive exercise) to prevent weight gain • Binge eating and compensatory behaviors occur at least once a week for 3 months • Self-evaluation is influenced by body shape and weight
Other specified feeding or eating disorder (OSFED)	• Individuals experience significant distress due to symptoms that are similar to AN, BN, BED, and ARFID, but do not meet the full criteria for a diagnosis (e.g., frequency of binge eating and compensatory behaviors occurs less than once a week for 3 months) • Includes atypical anorexia nervosa, or the presentation of all symptoms corresponding to AN with significant weight loss and without low body weight

cisgender boys and men.[5] Gender-diverse people, including transgender girls and women, transgender boys and men, and nonbinary people, have an elevated risk of disordered eating.[10] Higher risk of disordered eating has also been observed among LGBTQ+ populations when compared to heterosexual people.[10,11]

Some subpopulations may have elevated or similar risk of disordered eating but are less likely to receive a diagnosis and subsequently appropriate treatment for their condition. For example, from childhood through adolescence and adulthood, higher-weight individuals have elevated risk of disordered eating compared to lower-weight individuals, although they are less likely to receive diagnoses for AN, ARFID, and BN.[7,12] The same pattern is observed among individuals from marginalized racial and ethnic groups in the United States, including Black/African Americans, Latinx people, and South Asian people, who are more likely to face barriers to diagnosis and treatment than white Americans.[13] Finally, individuals from low-income backgrounds have similar rates of disordered eating compared to wealthier individuals, but also encounter difficulty in seeking diagnosis and treatment.[14]

EPIDEMIOLOGY AND HEALTH CONSEQUENCES

An array of risk factors may increase an individual's risk of disordered eating, ranging from the individual to broader sociocultural norms. Biological risk factors may include early-onset puberty (particularly for cisgender girls), altered neurobiology (e.g., chemical imbalances, altered reward modulation and inhibitory control), and genetic inheritability,[15] all of which have been studied more extensively in AN than in other eating disorders.[14] Biological and genetic contributors interact with environmental factors to increase an individual's risk for developing an eating disorder. Risk can be exacerbated among individuals who participate in activities that expose the body and/or impose weight standards for participation (e.g., dance, wrestling, fashion modeling).[16] Other behaviors, such as high levels of media consumption, especially social media, and the use of photo-editing mobile applications for modifying images of oneself are associated with a greater likelihood of disordered eating as well.[17] Finally, certain individual-level psychological factors may interact with the environment to affect a person's risk of developing an eating disorder, including body dissatisfaction and preoccupation with weight, perfectionism, negative affect, and thin-ideal internalization.[18] Certain experiences may also interact with individual risk factors to increase the risk of disordered eating, including experiencing abuse, weight discrimination, racist discrimination, bullying, and teasing.[19] Increasingly, research is highlighting how experiencing individual and household food insecurity and financial precarity may exacerbate disordered eating risk among youth and adults.[20]

Finally, an overall culture that emphasizes the value of thinness and appearance is a foundational contributor to disordered eating risk among populations. Appearance-based body ideals are present in all forms of media and messaging that we receive from childhood throughout our lives and emphasize a core message that being thin and attractive is associated with health and success. Messaging about appearance and body ideals affect all genders, but girls and women are particularly targeted. These cultural norms contribute to *weight stigma*, a set of negative stereotypes about people with higher weights (see also Chapter 17, "Overweight and Obesity"). Weight stigma contributes to weight-related harassment, violence, and weight discrimination, but may also help to explain the negative health consequences that some people with higher weights may experience, including an increased risk of disordered eating.[7] For example, studies have found that higher-weight individuals delay seeking medical care because they fear that their doctors will shame them for their weight, and as a result, they have a greater risk of missing screening and early diagnoses such as cervical cancer.[21] Further, higher-weight individuals face greater stress and discrimination than lower-weight people, and elevated cortisol and greater allostatic loads may contribute to worse health outcomes.[22]

Eating disorders have among the highest case fatality rates for any mental health condition,[23] leading to the deaths of approximately one person every 52 minutes in the United States.[4] Each type of eating disorder can present debilitating physical health consequences, including oral and dental (e.g., oral lacerations, dental erosion), cardiorespiratory (e.g., heart palpitations, dyspnea), gastrointestinal (e.g., hematemesis, constipation), endocrine (e.g., amenorrhea, infertility), and dermatologic (e.g., lanugo hair, Russell's sign).[24] Further, eating disorders are highly comorbid with other psychiatric illnesses, including substance use and mood disorders, and are associated with a lower quality of life.[25] Even when not meeting DSM-5 diagnostic criteria, disordered eating can also have a significant impact on individuals' daily functioning and lead to lasting health comorbidities and even death.

IMPACTS OF DISORDERED EATING ON NUTRITION AND PHYSIOLOGY

Disordered eating behaviors can result in inadequate nutritional intake, which may affect an individual's physiology and overall well-being. Each type of behavior and eating disorder influences diet quality and physiological changes (e.g., metabolism, hunger and satiety cues) in unique ways, and presents challenges for nutrition therapy and treatment. It is highly recommended that nutrition therapy for eating disorders be conducted by a nutrition professional trained in this specialty (see *Screening and Referral for Disordered Eating* below). Across disorders, restrictive behaviors often lead to a lack of key micro and macronutrients and can result in a state of malnutrition, including electrocardiographic abnormalities, anemia, and electrolyte imbalances.[6] Compensatory behaviors, including vomiting, excessive exercise, and laxative or diuretic use, can also present significant reductions in key micronutrients (e.g., potassium, chloride), as well as contribute to heightened pancreative enzymes that increase risk of pancreatitis.[24] Foods consumed during binge eating episodes are often high in calories and low in nutritional value,[26] which can lend to a decrease in overall diet quality among individuals with BN and BED. Across all eating disorders, rapid weight loss and/or weight cycling may present complications for metabolic processes, including the risk of metabolic adaptation and weight gain that can further exacerbate weight-related concerns in patients.[27] Even among people who do not have a diagnosable eating disorder, engagement in disordered eating behaviors over short-term and extended periods of time can also have impacts on nutrition and physiology.

● DISORDERED EATING BEHAVIORS

Disordered eating behaviors that are restrictive may include rigid food rules (e.g., not being "allowed" to consume foods high in sugar, fat, or salt), unreasonable food rituals (e.g., being able to eat only at certain times of the day), and/or an overall limit on caloric intake generally for the purpose of changing one's weight or shape. Individuals may report that their restriction of foods or liquids is part of a new diet for "health" purposes, and individually many of these dietary choices (e.g., reducing foods high in sugars) may be appropriate in moderation and lead to healthier status. However, health professionals should inquire the degree to which the patient is engaging in these behaviors (i.e., their level of flexibility in breaking their restrictive pattern) and if it coincides with the onset of other concerning signs and symptoms (see Table 25-2).[14,24]

Compensatory behaviors are often carried out by individuals after a binge eating episode (i.e., "compensate" for the calories consumed), and include purging behaviors (i.e., laxative or diuretic use, self-induced vomiting) and nonpurging behaviors (i.e., severe caloric restriction, excessive exercise). Compensatory behaviors may immediately follow a binge eating episode or be conducted after a more extended, but still brief, period of time (e.g., the next day). Even among individuals who do not have a diagnosed eating disorder, engagement in compensatory behaviors (such as laxative use) may be acutely dangerous in the near term and trigger and exacerbate eating disorder risk years later.[28,29]

Binge eating episodes are characterized by eating a large amount of food within a short period of time and feeling out of control over one's own eating during the episode. During a binge eating episode, an individual may eat very rapidly; feel uncomfortably full (i.e., to the point of feeling ill); eat in the absence of hunger; eat alone because of embarrassment and hide evidence of the binge eating episode; and feel disgust, guilt, and/or shame after the episode is over.

Individuals with eating disorders and disordered eating are at elevated risk of using dietary supplements and other diet-related products such as diet pills, muscle-building supplements, and cleanse and detox products (i.e., products to "cleanse" internal organs for the purpose of weight loss), and these products also present health risk more broadly (see also Chapter 7, "Herbs and Dietary Supplements"). In the United States and globally, these products face little government oversight. In the context of weak regulation, unscrupulous companies make deceptive claims about the efficacy and safety of their products, which have been found to contain toxic ingredients that can result in serious health consequences including adverse cardiovascular events, liver injury, and death.[30] In young women, the use of over-the-counter diet pills has been prospectively linked with four to six times elevated risk of diagnosis with an eating disorder within just a few years,[29,31] thus making detection of their use an important target for screening and early intervention.

● SCREENING AND REFERRAL FOR DISORDERED EATING

Given the severity of eating disorders, the early identification of disordered eating is a significant factor in improving treatment outcomes.[32] Unfortunately, many health professionals and primary care providers do not have adequate training in eating disorder screening and lack knowledge of referral resources.[33,34] Even brief training modules have been shown to increase primary care providers' knowledge of eating disorder symptoms and referral practices,[35] and may improve patient prognosis. Table 25-2 summarizes notable presenting signs and symptoms of eating disorders from the Academy for Eating Disorders Medical Care Standards[24] that health professionals should be aware of when interacting with patients of all ages, genders, body sizes, and races/ethnicities. In particular, health professionals may choose to screen for disordered eating if individuals present significant changes or fluctuations in weight, drastic and sudden changes in eating behaviors, body image or self-esteem disturbances, as well as inappropriate use of the diet-related products summarized in the previous section.

Screening

Several brief screening tools have been developed for health professionals to conduct among patients in their practice; see Table 25-3 for an overview of screening tools. The most widely used tool, SCOFF, is a five-item validated short tool to assess eating disorder risk among nonclinical populations of adults.[36] SCOFF, first developed in the United Kingdom, includes the following questions: **S** – Do you make yourself sick (vomit) because you feel uncomfortably full? **C** – Do you worry you have lost control over how much you eat? **O** – Have you recently lost more than one stone (6.35 kg or 14 lbs.) in a 3-month period? **F** – Do you believe yourself to be fat when others say you are too thin? **F** – Would you say food dominates your life? A score of 2 or higher may be indicative of disordered eating and warrant patient referral.

Other brief screening items may also be used to screen for specific disorders of behaviors. For example, the Eating Disorders in Youth Questionnaire (EDY-Q) is a 14-item measure that can be used to screen for disordered eating in children and adolescents, and is specifically used to assess for ARFID.[37] Screening tools for other psychiatric conditions, such as the Patient Health Questionnaire 9 (PHQ-9) which is typically

TABLE 25-2 • Presenting signs and symptoms of eating disorders

Category	Symptoms
General	• Marked weight loss, gain, fluctuations or unexplained change in growth curve or body mass index (BMI) percentiles in a child or adolescent who is still growing and developing • Cold intolerance • Weakness • Fatigue or lethargy • Presyncope (dizziness) • Syncope (fainting) • Hot flashes, sweating episodes
Oral and dental	• Oral trauma/lacerations • Perimyolysis (dental erosion on posterior tooth surfaces) and dental caries (cavities) • Parotid (salivary) gland enlargement
Cardiorespiratory	• Chest pain • Heart palpitations • Orthostatic tachycardia/ hypotension (low blood pressure) • Dyspnea (shortness of breath) • Edema (swelling)
Gastrointestinal	• Epigastric discomfort • Abdominal bloating • Early satiety (fullness) • Gastroesophageal reflux (heartburn) • Hematemesis (blood in vomit) • Hemorrhoids and rectal prolapse • Constipation
Endocrine	• Amenorrhea or oligomenorrhea (absent or irregular menses) • Low sex drive • Stress fractures • Low bone mineral density • Infertility
Neuropsychiatric	• Depressive/Anxious/Obsessive/Compulsive symptoms and behaviors • Memory loss • Poor concentration • Insomnia • Self-harm • Suicidal thoughts, plans or attempts • Seizures
Dermatologic	• Lanugo hair (fine hair growth on the body and face) • Hair loss • Carotenoderma (yellowish discoloration of skin) • Russell's sign (calluses or scars on the back of the hand from self-induced vomiting) • Poor wound healing • Dry brittle hair and nails
Metabolic and electrolytes imbalances detectable	• Low sodium (may indicate laxative use) • Low potassium (self-induced vomiting, laxative use, diuretic use) • Low chloride (self-induced vomiting, laxative use) • Elevated blood bicarbonate (self-induced vomiting), decreased blood bicarbonate (laxative use) • Elevated blood urea nitrogen (dehydration) • Elevated creatinine (dehydration, renal dysfunction), or low creatinine (poor muscle mass) • Slightly low calcium (poor nutrition) • Low phosphate (poor nutrition) • Low magnesium (poor nutrition, laxative use) • Elevated total protein/albumin in early malnutrition, low total protein/albumin in later malnutrition

Adapted from the Academy for Eating Disorders Medical Care Standards Committee. *Eating Disorders: A Guide to Medical Care. Critical Points for Early Recognition & Medical Risk Management in the Care of Individuals with Eating Disorders.* 4th ed. 2021.

TABLE 25-3 • Select brief screening tools for eating disorders that can be used by health professionals	
Tool name	Questions
SCOFF	Responses include "yes" and "no." 1. Do you make yourself sick (vomit) because you feel uncomfortably full? 2. Do you worry you have lost control over how much you eat? 3. Have you recently lost more than one stone (6.35 kg or 14 lbs.) in a 3-month period? 4. Do you believe yourself to be fat when others say you are too thin? 5. Would you say food dominates your life?
Eating Disorders in Youth Questionnaire (EDY-Q)	Responses range from "never true" to "always true." 1. If I was allowed to, I would not eat. 2. Food/eating does not interest me. 3. I do not eat when I'm sad, worried, or anxious. 4. Other people think that I weigh too little. 5. I would like to weigh more. 6. I feel fat, even if other people do not agree with me. 7. As long as I do not look too fat or weigh too much, everything else does not matter. 8. I am a picky eater. 9. I do not like to try new food. 10. I am afraid of choking or vomiting while eating. 11. I am afraid of swallowing food. 12. I do not like to try food with a specific smell, taste, appearance, or a certain consistency (e.g., crispy or soft). 13. I like to eat things that are not meant for eating (e.g., sand). 14. I regurgitate food that I have already swallowed.

used to screen for depression, also include items relevant to eating patterns that may introduce conversations about disordered eating with patients. Even brief questions about weight or shape concerns (e.g., "Do you have any worries about your body weight?" "Have you tried to make any changes to your body weight since your last visit?") may lead to discussions about patients' engagement in disordered eating. Health professionals should be especially alert to how discussions about body weight, nutrition, and physical activity are received by patients, especially those who are most vulnerable to disordered eating. Overall, the Academy for Eating Disorders Medical Care Standards[24] is a valuable resource containing information on symptoms and screening for non-specialist health professionals.

Referral

Eating disorders are complex conditions that require extensive, multidisciplinary treatment by trained specialists. Fortunately, openly available resources for referral are easily accessible to health professionals in the United States. The Alliance for Eating Disorders Awareness' Treatment Center & Practitioner Directory is a user-friendly way to find providers according to a number of criteria. Using this free tool, health professionals can search by insurance accepted, gender, treatment modality, language, and special populations (e.g., specialists training to treat athletes and/or LGBTQ patients).

THREE TAKE-HOME POINTS

1. Eating disorders and disordered eating are serious conditions that pose significant risk to physical and mental health, as well as nutritional intake and diet quality.

2. Eating disorders and disordered eating can affect individuals from a range of identities and backgrounds, although some population subgroups may be at an elevated risk of certain behaviors.

3. Health professionals should screen for disordered eating-related attitudes (e.g., concerns about body shape/weight) and behaviors (e.g., restriction, binge eating, laxative misuse) when discussing food or diet, exercise, or body weight with patients. Health professionals should also look for signs and symptoms of disordered eating that impair physiologic or social functions.

CASE STUDY ANSWERS

1. Consider administering a validated screening measure, such as SCOFF, to assess the patient's risk of an eating disorder. If she endorses at least two items on SCOFF, she would be a candidate for referral to treatment services. You may also consider asking general questions about body and weight concerns and the use of diet pills, as well as the rigidity of her new diet and exercise plans. Given her previous history of anxiety and depression, and her overall stress related to job loss, the administration of the PHQ-9 may also assist in assessing her overall mental health.

2. Rigid rules surrounding food types may be a warning sign that a patient is engaging in disordered eating rather than trying to improve their overall diet quality and health. Combined with rapid weight change, drastic overhauls to one's diet that are linked to "health" may still be indicative of disordered eating for the purpose of changing one's appearance. Regardless of whether an individual is making diet/behavior changes for health or for appearance, they may be at risk for an eating disorder. Many dietary behaviors individually may be healthier choices (e.g., reducing food with added sugars); however, red flags should be raised when the behaviors are implemented with high rigidity and lead to nutritional deficiencies or signs/symptoms of concerns (Table 25-2).

3. The patient's physical symptoms are likely a result of her caloric deficit, and further questioning about the types and quantity of foods she consumes will provide clarity into whether macro- and micronutrient needs are being met. The stress of her job loss may contribute to her risk of disordered eating, as individuals may cope with such behaviors in times of distress.

4. When malnutrition leads to irregular periods or amenorrhea, physicians should be concerned about decreased estrogen production, which is vital for the patient's bone mineral density. Although weight-bearing exercise is helpful, you should evaluate the extent of the patient's exercise, too much exercise would end up hurting her bones and increasing her risk for stress fractures. You may also consider calcium and vitamin D supplementation to support bone health in these cases. Further, even if the patient is eating protein, oftentimes the proteins are leaner (i.e., containing less iron) and you may elect to check her iron levels. Anemia is the most common hematologic abnormality for people with eating disorders because of changes to the bone marrow caused by malnutrition. This resolves with improved weight and diet, so although iron supplementation is not necessarily required, it may help.

5. Always begin with an open-ended question such as: "How has your new diet and exercise regimen affected your life?" Sometimes, like in this case, patients are not ready to change their disordered behaviors, but most do acknowledge the difficulty they experience in upholding rigid thoughts and behaviors. Open-ended questions help you and the patient to understand the effect an eating disorder has on their quality of life. Additional questions that help may include: "What happens if you can't exercise when you want?" or "What happens if you're invited to a friend's house for pizza?" If a patient answers with clearly rigid thoughts or behaviors such as, "I get really anxious if I can't exercise and I will exercise twice as hard the next day" or "I just won't go to my friend's house," you can explore this more to help them understand that these functional impairments and changes to her quality of life are associated with disordered eating thoughts. Other times, patients need to hear the negative effects on their physical health, so focusing on the impact of malnutrition on her periods, fertility, and bone health may help.

Acknowledgments: The authors would like to acknowledge Jessica Lin, MD (Cincinnati Children's Hospital) for her support in drafting responses to the Case Study questions.

REFERENCES

1. American Psychiatric Association. Feeding and eating disorders. *Diagnostic and Statistical Manual of Mental Disorders*, 5th ed. American Psychiatric Publishing; 2013:329-354.

2. Walsh BT, Hagan KE, Lockwood C. A systematic review comparing atypical anorexia nervosa and anorexia nervosa. *Int J Eat Disord.* 2023;56(4):798-820.

3. Zickgraf HF, Murray HB, Kratz HE, Franklin ME. Characteristics of outpatients diagnosed with the selective/neophobic presentation of avoidant/restrictive food intake disorder. *Int J Eat Disord.* 2019;52(4):367-377.

4. Streatfeild J, Hickson J, Austin SB, et al. Social and economic cost of eating disorders in the United States: evidence to inform policy action. *Int J Eat Disord.* 2021;54(5):851-868.

5. Galmiche M, Déchelotte P, Lambert G, Tavolacci MP. Prevalence of eating disorders over the 2000–2018 period: a systematic literature review. *Am J Clin Nutr.* 2019;109(5):1402-1413.

6. Hornberger LL, Lane MA. Identification and management of eating disorders in children and adolescents. *Pediatrics.* 2021;147(1):e2020040279-e.

7. Puhl R, Suh Y. Stigma and eating and weight disorders. *Curr Psychiatry Rep*. 2015;17(3):552.

8. Kalindjian N, Hirot F, Stona A-C, Huas C, Godart N. Early detection of eating disorders: a scoping review. *Eat Weight Disord*. 2022;27(1):21-68.

9. Burke NL, Schaefer LM, Hazzard VM, Rodgers RF. Where identities converge: the importance of intersectionality in eating disorders research. *Int J Eat Disord*. 2020;53(10):1605-1609.

10. Nagata JM, Ganson KT, Austin SB. Emerging trends in eating disorders among sexual and gender minorities. *Curr Opin Psychiatry*. 2020;33:562-567.

11. Calzo JP, Blashill AJ, Brown TA, Argenal RL. Eating disorders and disordered weight and shape control behaviors in sexual minority populations. *Curr Psychiatry Rep*. 2017;19(8):49.

12. Nagata JM, Garber AK, Tabler JL, Murray SB, Bibbins-Domingo K. Prevalence and correlates of disordered eating behaviors among young adults with overweight or obesity. *J Gen Intern Med*. 2018;33(8):1337-1343.

13. Sonneville KR, Lipson SK. Disparities in eating disorder diagnosis and treatment according to weight status, race/ethnicity, socioeconomic background, and sex among college students. *Int J Eat Disord*. 2018;51(6):518-526.

14. Schaumberg K, Welch E, Breithaupt L, et al. The science behind the Academy for Eating Disorders' Nine Truths About Eating Disorders. *Eur Eat Disord Rev*. 2017;25(6):432-450.

15. Yilmaz Z, Hardaway JA, Bulik CM. Genetics and epigenetics of eating disorders. *Adv Genomics Genet*. 2015;5:131-150.

16. Mitchison D, Hay PJ. The epidemiology of eating disorders: genetic, environmental, and societal factors. *Clin Epidemiol*. 2014;6:89-97.

17. Marks RJ, De Foe A, Collett J. The pursuit of wellness: social media, body image and eating disorders. *Child Youth Serv Rev*. 2020;119:105659.

18. Stice E, Gau JM, Rohde P, Shaw H. Risk factors that predict future onset of each DSM-5 eating disorder: predictive specificity in high-risk adolescent females. *J Abnorm Psychol*. 2017;126(1):38-51.

19. Lie SØ, Rø Ø, Bang L. Is bullying and teasing associated with eating disorders? A systematic review and meta-analysis. *Int J Eat Disord*. 2019;52(5):497-514.

20. Hazzard VM, Loth KA, Hooper L, Becker CB. Food insecurity and eating disorders: a review of emerging evidence. *Curr Psychiatry Rep*. 2020;22(12):74.

21. Puhl RM, Heuer CA. Obesity stigma: important considerations for public health. *Am J Public Health*. 2010;100(6):1019-1028.

22. Vadiveloo M, Mattei J. Perceived weight discrimination and 10-year risk of allostatic load among US adults. *Ann Behav Med*. 2017;51(1):94-104.

23. Arcelus J, Mitchell AJ, Wales J, Nielsen S. Mortality rates in patients with anorexia nervosa and other eating disorders: a meta-analysis of 36 studies. *Arch Gen Psychiatry*. 2011;68(7):724-731.

24. Academy for Eating Disorders Medical Care Standards Committee. *Eating Disorders: A Guide to Medical Care. Critical Points for Early Recognition & Medical Risk Management in the Care of Individuals with Eating Disorders*. Academy for Eating Disorders; 2016.

25. van Hoeken D, Hoek HW. Review of the burden of eating disorders: mortality, disability, costs, quality of life, and family burden. *Curr Opin Psychiatry*. 2020;33(6):521-527.

26. Chao AM, Wadden TA, Walsh OA, et al. Perceptions of a large amount of food based on binge-eating disorder diagnosis. *Int J Eat Disord*. 2019;52(7):801-808.

27. Lowe MR, Piers AD, Benson L. Weight suppression in eating disorders: a research and conceptual update. *Curr Psychiatry Rep*. 2018;20(10):80.

28. Schaumberg K, Anderson LM, Reilly E, Anderson DA. Patterns of compensatory behaviors and disordered eating in college students. *J Am Coll Health*. 2014;62(8):526-533.

29. Levinson JA, Sarda V, Sonneville K, Calzo JP, Ambwani S, Bryn Austin S. Diet pill and laxative use for weight control and subsequent incident eating disorder in US young women: 2001-2016. *Am J Public Health*. 2020;110(1):109-111.

30. Austin SB, Yu K, Tran A, Mayer B. Research-to-policy translation for prevention of disordered weight and shape control behaviors: a case example targeting dietary supplements sold for weight loss and muscle building. *Eat Behav*. 2017;25:9-14.

31. Hazzard VM, Simone M, Austin SB, Larson N, Neumark-Sztainer D. Diet pill and laxative use for weight control predicts first-time receipt of an eating disorder diagnosis within the next 5 years among female adolescents and young adults. *Int J Eat Disord*. 2021;54(7):1289-1294.

32. Cadwallader JS, Godart N, Chastang J, Falissard B, Huas C. Detecting eating disorder patients in a general practice setting: a systematic review of heterogeneous data on clinical outcomes and care trajectories. *Eat Weight Disord*. 2016;21(3):365-381.

33. Banas DA, Redfern R, Wanjiku S, Lazebnik R, Rome ES. Eating disorder training and attitudes among primary care residents. *Clin Pediatr*. 2013;52(4):355-361.

34. Lebow J, Narr C, Mattke A, et al. Engaging primary care providers in managing pediatric eating disorders: a mixed methods study. *J Eat Disord*. 2021;9(1):1-8.

35. Raffoul A, Vitagliano JA, Sarda V, et al. Evaluation of a one-hour asynchronous video training for eating disorder screening and referral in U.S. Pediatric Primary Care: a pilot study. *Int J Eat Disord*. 2022;55(9):1245-1251.

36. Hill LS, Reid F, Morgan JF, Lacey JH. SCOFF, the development of an eating disorder screening questionnaire. *Int J Eat Disord*. 2010;43(4):344-351.

37. Kurz S, van Dyck Z, Dremmel D, Munsch S, Hilbert A. Early-onset restrictive eating disturbances in primary school boys and girls. *Eur Child Adolesc Psychiatry*. 2015;24(7):779-785.

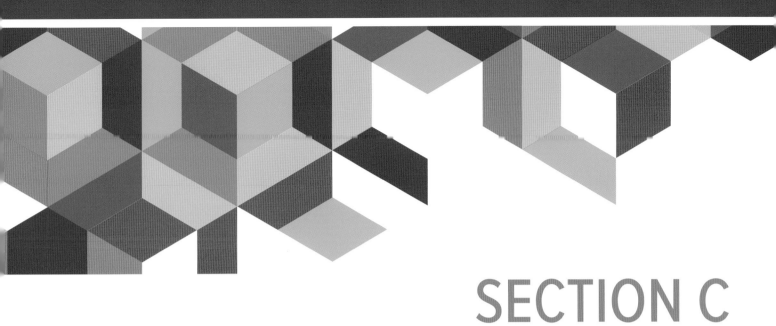

SECTION C

Counseling and Coaching for Behavior Change

chapter 26

Introduction to Behavior Change

Beth Frates, MD, FACLM, DipABLM

Chapter Outline

CASE STUDY

Anna is a 45-year-old Caucasian woman whose chief complaint is back pain. She has a history of type 2 diabetes. Anna recently gained weight after quitting smoking, and now has a BMI of 31, a waist circumference of 38 inches and a waist-to-hip ratio of greater than 1. "Quitting smoking made me gain weight and get this back pain again," she asserts.

For the past 15 years, Anna has worked as a cashier at a fast-food chain. She loves her work and loves the food there. Anna openly admits, "Vegetables taste terrible, and I've never liked them." She states the only two vegetables she eats are "French Fries and ketchup," and she refuses to try any others. Because she has no time for shopping, does not know how to cook, and does not have the time to spend following recipes,

she eats out a lot. Anna is a single parent and works long hours. After work, she goes directly home to take care of her three children. As an employee benefit, she is often able to bring an entire family meal home.

In the past, losing weight helped to cure her back pain. She tells you that gaining weight makes the back pain worse. Anna feels strongly that the way for her to lose weight is to smoke again.

1. In what stage of change is the patient with regards to eating vegetables?
   A. Precontemplative
   B. Contemplative
   C. Preparation
   D. Action

(Continued)

CASE STUDY *(Continued)*

2. When discussing weight with the patient, what counseling strategies can be useful?
   A. Motivational interviewing
   B. Tell and sell approach
   C. Anticipation interviewing
   D. Reaction recreation approach

3. Working with this patient on healthy eating patterns will include factoring in her home environment, her workplace, as well as her own attitudes and preferences about food. One behavior change theory that covers all these different areas is the
   A. Rational-Irrational Thought Theory
   B. Workplace Wellness Strategies First
   C. Socioecological Model of Change
   D. Healthy Options First Model

4. There are certain ways of being during an interview with a patient that help to empower the patient to adopt and sustain change. They can be summed up by a mnemonic.
   A. COACH—Curious, Open, Appreciative, Compassionate and Honest
   B. REAL—Rational, Enthusiastic, Accurate and Lively
   C. SMART—Specific, Measurable, Action-Oriented, Realistic and Time Sensitive
   D. EXPERT—Examine, X-Ray, Problem Solve, Explain, Repeat, Tell and Sell

5. What are two to three open-ended questions that you could ask this patient to open up a conversation and counseling session about nutrition?

6. What are two to three phrases that could create resistance in this patient and close off the conversation?

INTRODUCTION

Behavior change science has been an area of interest for healthcare professionals who specialize in nutrition, exercise, and lifestyle medicine for decades. Health and wellness coaching is defined as "A patient-centered approach wherein patients at least partially determine their goals, use self-discovery or active learning processes together with content education to work toward their goals, and self-monitor behaviors to increase accountability, all within the context of an interpersonal relationship with a coach. The coach is a healthcare professional trained in behavior change theory, motivational strategies, and communication techniques, which are used to assist patients to develop intrinsic motivation and obtain skills to create sustainable change for improved health and well-being".[1] Coaching patients on lifestyle keeps patients engaged, inspired, curious, and hopeful about their future. Board certification for health coaches is available through the National Board of Health and Wellness Coaches. All physicians and healthcare professionals can apply principles of coaching and motivational interviewing to support healthy behaviors during their patient encounters without being board certified. One does not need to be certified to use the COACH Approach™ which is covered in detail in this chapter. Some physicians choose to hire a health coach to partner with them in their practice. Health and wellness coaches can serve as part of the multidisciplinary team that works with patients to make lifestyle changes including adopting and sustaining healthy eating patterns.

In the early 2000s, health and wellness coaching became more and more popular. Some physicians were getting trained and certified in this field in the late 2000s. Several randomized controlled trials demonstrating the use of health and wellness coaching revealed a statistically significant improvement over usual care for a variety of conditions including elevated cholesterol, diabetes, and other chronic conditions. See Table 26-1 for details.

Wolever and colleagues reviewed 284 health and wellness coaching studies to better understand the operationalization of coaching and found that health and wellness coaching was described as patient centered in 86% in the studies, involved self-discovery and active learning in 63%, provided education

TABLE 26-1 • Landmark studies in health coaching from the early 2000s		
Study author and date	Number of subjects	Primary outcomes
Vale et al. 2003[2]	792 patients with cardiac disease	Serum cholesterol reduced 21 mg/dL vs. 7 mg/dL (p < .0001)
Whittemore et al. 2004[3]	53 women with diabetes	Better diet self-management, less diabetes related distress, higher satisfaction with care
Wolever et al. 2010[4]	56 patients with Type 2 diabetics	Significant reduction in hemoglobin A1C among subjects with baseline > 7%
Fischer et al. 2009[5]	191 children with asthma (parents and children coached)	Decreased re-hospitalization rate compared to controls 35.6% vs. 59.1% (p < .01)
Oliver et al. 2001[6]	67 patients with cancer pain	Improved pain severity compared to controls (p = .014)

in 91%, encouraged accountability in 86%, and involved a consistent ongoing relationship in 78% of the studies.[1]

When reviewing the original landmark randomized controlled trials (RCTs), it is clear that there were some commonalities within the health and wellness coaching interventions: they all had a one-on-one relationship with the coach, the counseling used negotiation and collaboration skills, there was goal setting in each description of coaching, and the coaches used accountability as a strategy to keep patients on track. It is also apparent that more research is needed with larger numbers of subjects, follow up times longer than 6 months, and a consistent explanation of the coaching process including how the coaches were trained as well as what theories and techniques they used. Some of these limitations have been addressed with more recent research such as a better description of coaching and the coaches, but long-term follow-up and large-scale studies are still needed.

Over the past two decades, the research on coaching grew to the point that reviews of the RCTs could be completed. There are several systematic reviews in different populations including patients with cardiovascular disease, COPD, cancer, multiple chronic conditions, aging workers, and patients in rehabilitation settings as well as in preventative care settings. Table 26-2 lists systematic reviews with the important findings. Still, more research needs to be completed to better understand the dose of coaching, meaning length and frequency of sessions, as well as the total duration of the coaching engagement. Further research needs to address and discover what types of people respond to coaching, and if people with certain conditions benefit more from coaching than others.

Students and healthcare professionals embarking on coaching for lifestyle and nutrition topics can use the 5-Step Cycle of Collaboration as a road map.[15] The 5-Step Cycle of Collaboration involves empathy, motivation, confidence, goal setting, and accountability. This cycle reflects the behavioral theories and techniques that define health and wellness coaching and will be reviewed in detail in this chapter. The cycle will provide a step-by-step approach to a nutrition counseling session, whether it is for 10 minutes or a half an hour.

TABLE 26-2 • Systematic review of randomized controlled trials in health coaching and conclusions		
Study author and date	Number of participants	Conclusions about health coaching
An & Song 2020[7]	15 randomized trials of adults with cardiovascular risk	Significant effect on physical activity, dietary behaviors, management of stress, health responsibility
Stara et al. 2020[8]	Two randomized controlled trial (RCT) with digital health coaching programs for aging workers	Improved well-being based on physical criteria cardiovascular activity, body mass index, eating practices by motivating older workers to engage in healthy diet, physical activity, and less tobacco use.
Obro et al. 2021[9]	Review of nine studies (including randomized controlled trials and other interventions) on chronic disease with mobile health and health coaching.	Patients prefer physical interactions compared to interactions on mobile devices.
Singh et al. 2020[10]	12 peer-reviewed journal articles using pharmacist as coaches	Analysis noted improved clinical (such as hemoglobin A1C, blood pressure) and nonclinical outcomes (such as confidence in managing condition, attitude about medication, satisfaction with consultation) by pharmacist coaches when managing patients with chronic conditions including diabetes, depression, hypertension, and those with a number of chronic conditions.
Long et al. 2019[11]	Meta analysis with 10 RCT's on COPD	Improved QOL (p = .02), reduced COPD hospital admissions (p = .0001), but no reduction in all cause hospital admission (p = .20)
Dejonghe et al. 2017[12]	14 RCTs in preventative (7 studies) and rehab settings (7 studies)	Improved outcomes with statistically significant differences in long term outcomes in 3 out of 7 studies in each group. For the preventative group, there was improvement in knowledge level (work hazards and proper technique in manual handling operations), objective measures of sickness, and multiple risk behavior scores. For the rehab setting group, there was improvement in hemoglobin A1C, depression severity, and change in BMI.
Barakat et al. 2018[13]	12 studies including 1,038 cancer survivors (6 RCTs and 6 pre and post studies)	67% of included studies reported statistically significant outcomes that support quality of life, acceptance and spirituality, 75% decreased fatigue and pain, 67% increased physical activity, and 33% improved the social deprivation index.
Kivelä et al. 2014[14]	13 studies on health coaching for adult patients with chronic conditions (11 RCTs, 2 quasi-experimental design)	Statistically significant results for better weight management, increased physical activity and improved physical and mental health status.

● BEHAVIOR CHANGE THEORIES

Transtheoretical Model of Change

The transtheoretical model of change helps physicians and healthcare professionals to meet patients where they are in their journeys of change. Change is a process. For many people, it takes time. By understanding which stage of change a patient is in, the healthcare professional can use time in the clinical encounter to support the patient with strategies appropriate for that specific stage of change. There are five stages of change: *precontemplation, contemplation, preparation, action, and maintenance*. See Table 26-3, which lists the different stages of change and the common sentiments expressed in each stage. A patient in precontemplation needs different interventions, and they need to be asked different questions than a patient in preparation in order to make progress in their behavior change journey. Dr. James Prochaska and colleagues discuss this in detail in the book *Change for Good*.[16]

Precontemplation In precontemplation, patients are not ready or willing to change their behaviors. In this stage of change, healthcare professionals can waste time and effort for both the patients and themselves by telling these patients they need to change and laying out specific plans as to how they can achieve the change. Usually, patients in this stage are not even listening to these words. They often do not believe there is a problem with their eating, exercising, or smoking. Many people in this stage are in denial.

One of the strategies that can work in the precontemplation stage is dramatic relief. Dramatic relief invites the patient to watch a video, listen to a case presentation, or read about a person who had a similar situation to theirs. The case usually details how the patients overcame an obstacle and eventually enjoyed success. Often patients in precontemplation can see success for themselves after hearing about someone else. This could help them move from precontemplation to contemplation. Asking questions, listening to the answers, and expressing empathy may be the most important actions the healthcare professional can take with someone in precontemplation. Asking the patient how their behavior impacts others in their life like children, pets, roommates, or partners is another strategy that can encourage the person to see things from a different point of view. Policies such as banning fast foods from hospitals as was done with smoking years ago is another strategy that helps people in precontemplation.

Contemplation In contemplation, the patient is considering change and its pros and cons. They often acknowledge their problem or issue and voice a desire to behave differently. At the same time, they share all the obstacles in the way and list the various reasons why they cannot change. There is ambivalence in this stage. One strategy that can help with patients in contemplation is to write down a list of pros and cons. It is important that the healthcare professional does not make the list for the patient. Envisioning is another exercise healthcare professionals can utilize with patients in this stage. Envisioning involves asking patients what life would be like if they did make the healthy changes they are considering. Inviting patients to set forth a vision of themselves in 5, 10, or 20 years often helps them see the value of making the change so they can reach this vision of themselves. Asking about motivators is also helpful in this stage.

Preparation In preparation, the patient has acknowledged there is a problem and the problem is important enough to the patient to address it. The pros of making the healthy behavior change outweigh the cons. In this stage, patients are often ready to make the change, but they lack a solid plan. In some cases, they may have an obstacle in the way such as they have bought fresh produce in the past and not used it in time before it perished. Thus, they feel they are wasting money every time they buy fresh produce, and they actively avoid this scenario. In this preparation stage, the healthcare professional can help by asking, "What needs to be in place for you to start eating more produce and less processed meats?" Crafting a concrete plan that is achievable will help the patient move from preparation to action. Helping the patient set specific goals that are achievable like SMART (Specific, Measurable, Action-Oriented, Realistic, and Time Sensitive) goals, as discussed below, can help patients in preparation move forward to action.

Action Patients in action are already practicing the healthy habit. They have been doing so for 6 months or less. They are practicing new strategies and are actively engaged in healthy lifestyle behaviors. People in action often need encouragement to continue. Questions to ask include "What is going well? What have you learned? What changes have you noticed in yourself since starting the new healthy behavior?" Having a monitoring strategy in place can also help people in action. Suggesting a food log or keeping a record of the number of vegetables consumed in the day can help people stay engaged in the new healthy habit. There are many wearable devices that can track several behaviors. Lab values like low density lipoprotein cholesterol (LDL), hemoglobin A1C, and others may also help depending on the condition the patient is managing. Congratulating the patient is also important in this stage.

Maintenance If a patient has been practicing a healthy behavior for more than 6 months, then they are in maintenance. People in maintenance cannot be ignored. Asking them what keeps them motivated can help them stay engaged. Asking about what they foresee as future barriers or obstacles for maintaining the healthy behavior will empower them to brainstorm possible solutions prior to the barriers manifesting. This will

TABLE 26-3 • The transtheoretical model of change and common sentiments expressed	
Stage	**Common sentiments expressed**
Precontemplation	"I can't." "I won't." "There's no way!"
Contemplation	"I may." "I might." "It is possible." "Maybe."
Preparation	"I will." "I want to." "I plan to start soon."
Action	"I am." "I am engaged." "I am doing this now."
Maintenance	"I have been." "I am still doing this."

work to keep them on track. For example, if they are going on vacation, figuring out a plan for meals in advance by looking at menus online may help people to stick to their healthy eating pattern when they are away from home. Inviting the person to act as a mentor for someone who is just starting to adopt the healthy behavior can also help in this maintenance stage. Ask if they are thinking of trying something new to keep things fresh and add variety (Table 26-4).

Lapses It is important to remember that people can have slips or lapses, meaning that they may move from action to contemplation. This is a common occurrence for people on a behavior change journey. If there is a stressful event, someone might change their routine and that could impair their ability to consistently follow through with healthy behaviors. When this happens, it is important to support the person and help them reach their goals when they are ready and able to get back on track. It is important to emphasize that a lapse is common and the goal is to get back on track as soon as possible and avoid reverting back to the old behavior or old routine.

Self-Efficacy Theory

Self-efficacy is the belief that a person can accomplish a task or complete an action successfully.[17] Building up a person's self-efficacy helps them to adopt and sustain healthy behavior patterns and practices. Self-efficacy is influenced by a history of personal accomplishments as well as experiences watching others succeed or fail. In addition, people's physiologic states, whether they are sleep deprived, ill, hurt, hungry, feeling fatigued, suffering pain, or experiencing high levels of stress in their own lives, may impair their level of self-efficacy. Understanding the patient's circumstances and addressing areas that can be improved will allow the person to learn, grow and work toward goals. Setting appropriate goals that are easily achieved by the patient will help to increase their feeling of self-efficacy.

Self-Determination Theory

For motivation to last, there needs to be three key components according to the self-determination theory: autonomy, relatedness (or connection), and competence.[18] Working to help patients feel that they are responsible for their own behaviors and that they have choices is important for healthy behaviors to be maintained over time. Presenting a variety of solutions to barriers is key. This way the patient has autonomy to choose the best option for them. People want to feel they have some control. They do not respond when they feel controlled or when they feel they do not have a choice. Patients also need to feel a connection, also described as a sense of relatedness, to stay motivated. The healthcare professional can create that connection for the patient or a loved one may provide this connection. Helping the patient connect to others on a similar journey may also be useful. Group visits, as discussed in Chapter 30, may help. Feeling competence often takes practice. This is another reason why setting small, specific goals that the patient can achieve is important. It builds a feeling of success, accomplishment, pride, and proficiency. Success breeds success. Healthcare professionals can support patients looking to make behavior change by giving them choices of actions or goals they can pursue so that they have autonomy, routinely checking in on the patient's plans and progress to keep a strong connection and helping to co-create SMART goals to increase a sense of competency.

TABLE 26-4 • Stages, interventions for the specific stage, questions to ask people in specific stages of change		
Stages	**Interventions**	**Questions**
Precontemplation	Dramatic Relief	Want to hear about someone just like you who made a successful change?
	Suggest books or movies	Are you interested in watching a movie about how lifestyle behaviors impact health?
	Think about others	How is this behavior having an impact on loved ones, colleagues, friends?
	Express empathy	I am here for you when you are interested in addressing this.
Contemplation	List Pros and Cons	What are the pros of change? What are the Cons of change?
	Identify motivators	What is your motivation for changing?
Preparation	Create a plan	What needs to be in place for you to take action?
	Identify obstacles	What is holding you back?
	Set a SMART goal	What would be a possible SMART goal for you?
Action	Congratulate	Great job with these changes! What are you most proud about?
	Check in on monitoring.	What are you using to monitor or track your progress?
	Identify positive changes	What biometrics or labs have changed? What changes have you noticed?
Maintenance	Investigate	What is something new you may want to try?
	Identify future obstacles	What obstacles might be coming your way?
	Connect with motivators	What keeps you motivated?
	Ask about mentoring others	Would you consider helping someone who is starting on their behavior change journey?

Goal Setting Theory

Goals help motivate people. This has been utilized in the business world for decades using Edwin Locke's Goal Setting Theory from the 1960s.[19,20] The goal setting theory states that when people have a goal to work toward, they are more apt to focus and spend time and energy on the project so that they can meet the goal and be successful. Without goals, people can become aimless and simply reactive. Originally this SMART goal approach was intended for people in the workplace. Locke defined SMART goals as specific, measurable, achievable, relevant, and time bound. Oftentimes, business managers are making the goals for employees. Thus, they must make sure it is relevant. The health goal SMART mnemonic is specific, measurable, action oriented, realistic, and time sensitive. With health goals, the patient is setting them which will ensure they are relevant. For this reason, the mnemonic is altered slightly. Table 26-5 lists the SMART Goal mnemonic for use with behavior change and lifestyle medicine topics such as nutrition.

Social Ecological Model of Change

The social ecological model of change demonstrates that a person has three spheres of influence all around them, including relationship, community, and societal. It is important to counsel the patient one-on-one or in a group, but the healthcare professional must remember that the individual is connected to relationships such as family and friends. For the community level, patients have neighborhoods and possibly work environments as well as local norms and cultural norms. Considering societal impacts, there are laws and policies at the city, state, and country levels too.

Each person has attitudes, knowledge, skills, and beliefs. Working one-on-one with a patient to enhance these areas of personal growth and influence is important. Also essential is taking into consideration the person's interpersonal life, including their home environment and work environment. For healthy eating, a healthcare professional can ask, "What is in your cabinets right now? What is in your refrigerator? What food is available at work? What grocery stores and restaurants are around you?" Another area of influence is the organizational level or the environment and ethos in which the patient lives. What type of environment is in the neighborhood? What are the patterns and practices of neighbors, friends, family?

TABLE 26-5 • SMART goals for lifestyle medicine	
S = Specific	
M = Measurable	
A = Action Oriented	
R = Realistic	
T = Time-sensitive	

Are fresh fruits and vegetables available? Are there community gardens? Also, the influence of community including culture and traditions around food plays a role in shaping patterns and practices. Beyond that, public policy with city and state laws influence an individual. Is there a ban on trans-fats? What are the requirements for food labels? There are national guidelines and laws that impact behaviors and need to be taken into consideration. When a healthcare professional counsels a patient on healthy eating, that healthcare professional needs to know a lot about the individual as well as the individual's surroundings. Figure 26-1 is a graphic describing the socioecological model of change.

● BEHAVIOR CHANGE COUNSELING STRATEGIES

Motivational Interviewing

Motivational interviewing (MI) is a specific type of counseling that was created to help people work through ambivalence to change with compassion and guidance while encouraging self-direction and enhancing motivation to change.[21–24] With MI, the healthcare professional works to elicit change talk. Change talk happens when the patient discusses their own reasons for change. The patients are telling the healthcare professionals why they want to change. Usually, the healthcare professionals are busy telling the patients why they should change and giving them every reason to adopt healthy eating. However, this "tell and sell" strategy is not going to work in all situations. For example, when a patient is in contemplation or precontemplation, motivational interviewing will be helpful to empower the patient to think about change and convince themselves that change would be a good idea. With MI, the patient does the convincing of themselves by talking about

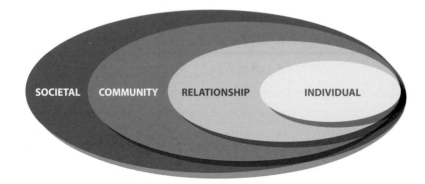

FIGURE 26-1 • Socioecological model of change.
(Used with permission from Frates B, Bonnet JP, Joseph R, Peterson JA. *Lifestyle Medicine Handbook: An Introduction to the Power of Healthy Habits.* 2nd ed. Monterey, CA: Healthy Learning; 2021:Chapter 3, page 100.)

the benefits of changing. The opposite of change talk is sustain talk. Often when a healthcare professional starts listing all the reasons a patient should change, the patient answers with sustain talk and explains all the reasons why they cannot change and reasons they must sustain their current unhealthy behavior. This "sustain" talk can build resistance to change.

The way to elicit change talk is to ask open-ended questions, share affirmations, use reflections, and state summaries. The mnemonic for this is OARS,[21,22] which is listed in Table 26-6.

Open-Ended Questions The O in OARS is for open-ended questions. In health care, healthcare professionals are often in a rush to obtain all the necessary information, especially in an acute crisis. In this case, closed-ended questions are essential. Review of systems is a good example of a battery of closed-ended questions. With MI, the goal is to avoid closed-ended questions and strive for open-ended questions which invite the patient to think and talk. When the patient talks, the healthcare professional listens. With MI, the patient talks more than the healthcare professional.

Affirmations Appreciating any change talk is critical and this allows for affirmations. This is the A for affirmations in OARS. If the patient mentions that they had thought about eating vegetables weeks ago, the healthcare professional might pick up on that and inquire, "I heard you say you were thinking of eating vegetables weeks ago. What made you think like that?" This way no amount of change talk is left uncovered and unappreciated with MI. The healthcare professional affirms and highlights any steps in a healthy direction.

Reflections R stands for Reflections. Reflections allow the patient to hear their own words. The patient may say, "I am really busy, but I know I would feel better and more energized if I made the time to cook food at home." The healthcare professional could share a simple reflection by saying, "You are really busy, but you know you would feel better and more energized if you made the time to cook food at home." Or the healthcare professional could change the statement and reflect, "It sounds like you know if you made the time, you would be able to cook a few delicious homemade meals and that would help you to feel healthier and more energized." An amplified reflection would be, "You know you need to start cooking at home to feel better, but there is absolutely no way that you can make the time. It's impossible." In this case, the patient may react to the amplification with change talk. "I didn't say, 'Impossible.' I could take 15 minutes to prepare a nice salad for myself. It's not that much time." The patient is giving reasons why it is not that difficult to make a homemade salad. This will have a much different effect than if the healthcare professional said, "Come on!

It only takes less than 15 minutes to prepare a salad. Are you telling me you can't even make a salad?" That is not an example of MI. That is actually MI-inconsistent behavior.

Summaries Lastly, the S in OARS stands for summaries. Summaries give the healthcare professional a chance to show the patient that they have been mindfully paying attention to the whole conversation and they can repeat back the essential parts of the conversations. The healthcare professional would include the patient's own change talk in the summary, if there was change talk. Motivational interviewing takes time and patience.

Appreciative Inquiry

Appreciative inquiry (AI) is a useful way of interviewing patients who are looking to change their way of eating. This form of interviewing was originally used with businesses[25,26] and has been used in healthcare settings with success.[27] With appreciative inquiry, the healthcare professional focuses on the positive core. There is likely something going well in a person's life. The healthcare professional can ask open-ended questions to discover the things that are going well and the patient's strengths. Everyone has strengths, and there are usually one or two things that are going well in a person's life. The AI model has a 5D cycle, which includes define, discover, dream, design, and deliver. Figure 26-2 shows this 5D cycle.

Define In the define stage, the healthcare professional asks what the focus of the consultation is. This defines the problem.

Discover Then, the healthcare professional discovers what is working well and what is the best of what is. This is the positive core that they will build on in the process of the interview.

Dream After the discovery phase, the healthcare professional and patient dream what might be and what life could be like. They envision.

Design Then, they get concrete with what they will build on in the process of the interview. This is a co-construction phrase. This involves the SMART goals, possibly 3-month goals or even 6-month goals, too.

Deliver Lastly, the healthcare professional and patient continue the innovation process with delivery. The co-constructed plan will work or will likely require reworking and alteration. After the patient has time to have the design play out with destiny, they get back together to review progress. This brings them back to the define and discover phases. Throughout the 5D cycle there is an emphasis on the positive core, what's working well and how to build on it.

The COACH Approach Way of Being

It is important to understand the way of being that is recommended when using these behavior change theories and techniques. This way of being is encapsulated in the COACH Approach™.[28] It allows for negotiation and collaboration while

TABLE 26-6 • OARS Mnemonic for motivational interviewing
O = Open-ended Questions
A = Affirmations
R = Reflections
S = Summaries

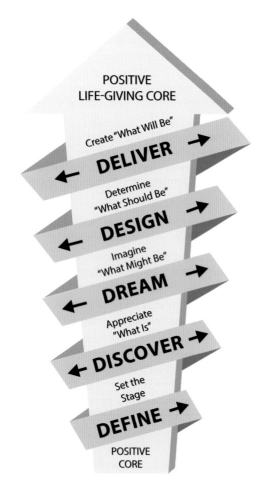

FIGURE 26-2 • Appreciative inquiry 5Ds.
(Used with permission from Frates B, Bonnet JP, Joseph R, Peterson JA. *Lifestyle Medicine Handbook: An Introduction to the Power of Healthy Habits*. 2nd ed. Monterey, CA: Healthy Learning; 2021, Chapter 3, page 98.)

counseling patients on eating patterns. This gives a sense of autonomy to the patient which is a critical component for their commitment to the change process.[15] The key ingredients to empower people to change are summed up in the COACH Approach™ mnemonic which includes curiosity, openness, appreciation, compassion, and honesty (Table 26-7).

When counseling people on changing eating practices, healthcare professionals will be more successful in the long term and enjoy the process more if they adopt a COACH Approach™. This approach is used with patients who have

TABLE 26-7 • The COACH approach™ mnemonic
C = Curiosity
O = Openness
A = Appreciation
C = Compassion
H = Honesty

Used with permission from Frates B, Bonnet JP, Joseph R, Peterson JA. *Lifestyle Medicine Handbook: An Introduction to the Power of Healthy Habits*. 2nd ed. Monterey, CA: Healthy Learning; 2021.

chronic conditions like cardiovascular disease, diabetes, hypertension, obesity, and stroke.

Curiosity With the COACH Approach™ , the healthcare professional is first and foremost *curious* about the patient. What stage of change is the person in? What is important to the patient? What motivates the patient? What does the patient cherish? What are the patient's strengths? When has the patient been successful in the past? Getting to know the patient is key. One cannot learn without listening. As with motivational interviewing, asking open-ended questions will encourage the patient to talk and share vital information with the healthcare professional.

Openness Being *open* and nonjudgmental is essential to the COACH Approach™. Each person is unique. They have wisdom and experience to share. They are the experts in their own lives, their desires, their dreams, their failures, their successes, their obstacles, and their own solutions. By honoring each patient and remaining open-minded, ready to learn, the healthcare professional is in a valuable position to help the patient feel understood and appreciated, not judged, shamed, or blamed. Shame, blame, and guilt will build distance between the patient and healthcare professional. To build a therapeutic alliance, the healthcare professional needs to create a safe space for the patient. For a patient to open up and be vulnerable, healthcare professionals must be fully present with the intention to fully understand and respect the human being in front of them.

Appreciation *Appreciating* any movement forward by the patient will encourage continued effort. What we appreciate, appreciates. Just as in motivational interviewing where affirmations are an integral part of the process, with the COACH Approach™, appreciating any step forward in the direction of change will help the patient gain hope and pride. Pride is a type of positive emotion that can help patients to gain motivation. Using appreciative inquiry, healthcare professionals can appreciate the positive core, create opportunities for pride and positivity, and then build on that with every patient encounter.

Compassion Compassion is defined as "sympathetic consciousness of others' distress together with a desire to alleviate it."[29] *Compassion* is only possible when a healthcare professional is mindfully present in the moment. To be mindful, one cannot have a full mind–a mind full of to-do lists, projects, research protocols, manuscripts, clinic concerns, or family matters. This means that healthcare professionals need to put away all distractions including their phones, worries, and paperwork so that they can be fully present for the patient in front of them. This presence is a gift on multiple levels.

Creating a space filled with compassion is a key part of genuinely connecting with the patient who is trying to make behavior change. Many people have tried to change multiple times in the past. They tried to eat healthy, but the fast food was so easy and cheap. They tried multiple diets in the past but feel they failed. Helping the patient feel safe and accepted for the person they are right now is critical in behavior change counseling. Listening to the patient and working to understand them helps create an atmosphere of compassion. Patients do not want to be judged. They have felt judged many times by others. They will do better when they feel loved and understood. Everyone longs to be understood. This can take time. However, even in a 10-minute intervention, a healthcare professional can share compassion by looking the patient in the eye and listening. Repeating what the patient said as in the reflections from motivational interviewing helps with demonstrating compassion. A little dose of compassion can go a long way and could help to open the door for future conversations at the next clinic visit. Being compassionate may be the only action a healthcare professional can accomplish in one visit with a person in precontemplation. Compassion creates connection. In addition, this compassion may serve to open the patient's mind to a consultation with a nutrition specialist or health and wellness coach who can spend an hour with the patient.

Honesty Everyone has heard that *honesty* is the best policy. It is certainly true with behavior change counseling. For students, this means if the patient asks a question and you do not know the answer, then it is important to respond with "That is a great question. I do not know the answer to that question right now. But, I can find out. Thank you for bringing this to my attention. We can both learn from this." In fact, attendings and seasoned faculty members also need to use this approach when they do not know the answer to a question. Sometimes it feels like a physician is supposed to know everything, but this is a fallacy. Healthcare professionals including physicians cannot know everything. There will be times when healthcare professionals forget facts or their knowledge is tested. That is OK. It is best to be honest and say, "I know I knew that once, but I seem to be forgetting it right now. Let me get back to you."

Honesty is also important when patients ask, "Is eating fast food *really* that bad?" or "My blood sugars are only up a little bit and my mom had diabetes for years. She lived to be 85. So, I don't think I really need to worry too much." These are times when the patient is seeking reassurance for staying the same. Healthcare professionals do need to share the facts and the threats that unhealthy eating can cause to the body. This can be done in an honest, sincere, and compassionate way.

● FIVE STEP CYCLE FOR COLLABORATION

What do you do when you are one-on-one with a patient? You may not recall all the specifics of the behavior change theories and models or the motivational interviewing strategies covered in this chapter, but you can keep the 5 Step Cycle in mind. Print out a copy of it and put it in your pocket or notes page on your phone so you can easily review it when the time comes to counsel a patient on nutrition. Collaboration and negotiation are the key.[30]

The 5 Step Cycle for Collaboration is depicted in Figure 26-3.[15] It has been successfully adopted by hundreds of physicians and students alike. Some students find it helpful to try to coach

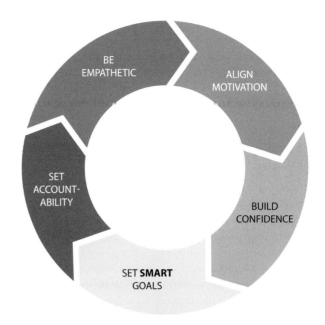

FIGURE 26-3 • 5-Step cycle for collaboration. (Used with permission from: Frates B, Bonnet JP, Joseph R, Peterson JA. *Lifestyle Medicine Handbook: An Introduction to the Power of Healthy Habits.* 2nd ed. Monterey, CA: Healthy Learning; 2021: Chapter 3, page 101.)

friends and family on nutrition prior to coming face to face with a patient in the hospital or clinic. This type of counseling takes time and practice to master.

Express Empathy

The first step in the five-step cycle is to express empathy. Merriam Webster Dictionary defines empathy as the capacity to understand, be aware of, be sensitive to, and vicariously experience the feelings, thoughts, and experience of another.[31] With one-on-one counseling, we start with the most important principle and action. Everyone wants to feel understood and appreciated. In several theories and behavior change techniques reviewed in this chapter already, the concept of compassion and empathy has been covered. This is where a healthcare professional starts and ends the visit centered on lifestyle modification such as nutrition counseling. Information is power. Empathy is powerful too. And, when sharing information is combined with empathy, it can penetrate even deeper.

Feeling empathy is one thing, and expressing it is another. Looking a patient in the eyes, being at eye level with them, and focusing on them and their words will demonstrate empathy. It is important to think about how the room is set up for the interview. The healthcare professional should not be looking at a computer with their back to the patient, which is unfortunately how some offices and clinics are set up.

Paying attention not just to the patient's words and language but also to their body language will allow the healthcare professional to better understand the patient's situation and how they are feeling about it. Stating simple reflections will help patients to feel the empathy from a healthcare professional.

Summaries also show empathy. One cannot summarize a 30-minute clinic visit unless he or she is listening carefully and mindfully. This type of care, concern, attention, and empathy helps patients feel safe to fully share their story.

Align Motivation

The second step in the cycle is to align motivation, which means to help patients connect with a powerful motivator that is important to them and relevant to their health goals. With patients in precontemplation or contemplation, motivational interviewing will be one of the most effective ways to make progress. Evoking change talk from the patient and asking questions that allow for the patient to explore their own motivators to change their eating patterns is the critical component of this second step in the five-step cycle.

Figuring out what is most important to the patient right now and how changing their nutritional patterns could align with their priorities helps patients feel motivated to move forward. Questions one may ask in this step include "Why is your nutrition important to you right now? What is the most important thing in your world right now and how is your nutrition connected to that? If you were to eat more healthy meals, how would that serve you? In what ways would altering your eating patterns help you achieve the goals that you have?"

Build Confidence

Once the healthcare professional has assisted the patient in aligning their motivation, then it is time to build confidence and bring in the self-efficacy theory discussed at the start of the chapter. The third step in the five-step cycle is to highlight the patient's strengths. People need to believe that they can be successful with the task at hand. If the healthcare professional can ask questions that draw out the patient's strengths, then the patient can start to envision success with adopting healthy eating practices.

Reviewing a time when the patient was successful with change in the past will help them to gain confidence by replaying that event and to identify strengths that can help them achieve their goals at this time in their lives. Asking patients to list their strengths is sometimes uncomfortable but asking them to share a time when they set a goal and met that goal will help draw out their strengths organically. The healthcare professional can listen carefully and then list strengths that the patient used in their story. At times, the healthcare professional needs to list some examples of strengths like determination, creativity, organization, sociability, grit, dedication, friendliness, compassion, perseverance, positivity, optimism, resilience, collaboration, negotiation, generosity, kindness, curiosity, dedication, loyalty, forgiveness, flexibility, love, or others. There are countless examples of possible strengths. Talking about people's strengths builds their confidence level.

Set Smart Goals

The fourth step is setting SMART goals. As discussed in the behavior change theory section, Locke's goal setting theory from the 1960s is still valuable to this day. When a patient makes a goal and commits to it out loud with a healthcare professional or another person, then they are more apt to work toward that goal. For nutrition goals, it is not SMART to set the goal, "I will eat better." This is a good goal in theory, but what does it mean? It is vague and general. There is nothing to measure. There is no action assigned to it. There are no time constraints. It is not possible to judge if this goal is realistic. So, the first step here is to get specific. What will the patient do differently this week compared to last week? This gives it a time frame. For example, a SMART goal might be, "I will eat three servings of vegetables on Monday, Wednesday, and Friday at dinner time." This is specific, measurable, action oriented, and time sensitive. One will only know if it is realistic if one asks. The healthcare professional could ask, "How confident are you that you can achieve this goal on a scale of 1–10 and 10 is the highest confidence?" If the patient provides a number lower than a 7, then this is not a realistic goal. It would be a valuable exercise to adjust the goal so that the patient feels more confident. A follow-up question could be "How can you change the goal so that you feel more confident?" The patient might answer, "I will eat two servings of vegetables on Monday and Friday at dinner time." This is an example of SMART Goal Setting.

Set Accountability

The last step in the five-step cycle is setting accountability. If a healthcare professional and patient co-create a goal for the patient and never follow up, the chances of the patient taking the goal seriously are very low. If the healthcare professional makes time to check in on the goal, this will keep the patient accountable for that goal. This could happen at a follow-up visit. This could also happen via email, text, or a healthcare app. There are many ways to help patients stay accountable. The most important action for a healthcare professional to do is make note of the SMART goal and have a plan to ask about it.

Sometimes setting accountability for the patient day to day is helpful. This could be accomplished by identifying an accountability buddy or friend who will help the patient keep track of behaviors. This could also be done with a supportive community or family members. Even an online community or Facebook group could help with accountability.

Some people want to keep themselves accountable by measuring and tracking their own progress. Working with the patient to determine an appropriate way to measure progress will be useful. This could be pen and paper logging and tracking; for example, the number of vegetables consumed each day. It could be a food log for a week or longer. It could be the use of an online tracker like My Fitness Pal or others. There are many wearable devices or applications that can be used to help keep patients on track.

This 5-Step Cycle of Collaboration begins and ends with empathy. No matter what happens in the time between the last clinic visit and the current one, the healthcare professional starts the cycle off with empathy. The patients may not have eaten the vegetables they had planned to eat, but maybe they started a garden in their backyard, and nothing has grown yet. Exploring their progress with empathy will set the stage for continued progress toward healthy eating patterns.

SUMMARY

Behavior change is part of nutrition counseling and the "food as medicine" movement. Giving people healthy food is a good start, but teaching people how to shop for healthy options, find healthy options, prepare healthy options, and fully savor the healthy meals is also part of the power of food. People need autonomy, connection, and competence as the self-determination theory explains. There is no one size fits all with nutrition counseling. The patient's individual experiences, stage of change, beliefs, social situation, neighborhood, economic situation, and education level all play a part in one's ability to adopt and sustain healthy eating patterns. The whole person needs to be heard and understood for progress to be made. Using a COACH Approach™ with curiosity, openness, appreciation, compassion, and honesty will help to set the tone for a productive and collaborative clinic visit.

TAKE-HOME POINTS

1. Meeting the patient where they are and collaborating with them to find healthy steps forward toward a healthier eating pattern is key.
2. The patient will benefit from information and empathy delivered together.
3. Individualizing the counseling session on nutrition to match the patients' stage of change; building their self-efficacy; providing them with autonomy, connection, and competence; setting SMART goals; and taking into account the social situation surrounding the patient are all essential elements.
4. Entering the consultation or clinic visit with a COACH Approach™ filled with curiosity, openness, appreciation, compassion, and honesty will set the stage for a deep connection that allows forward progress with adopting and sustaining healthy lifestyles.
5. The 5-Step Cycle for Collaboration includes expressing empathy, aligning motivation, building confidence, setting SMART goals, and setting accountability.

CASE STUDY ANSWERS

1. A
2. A
3. C
4. A
5.
   - What is one thing you could do differently with your meals that might help you to reach your goal of losing weight?
   - What kinds of preparation and seasoning have you tried with vegetables?
   - What would need to happen in order for you to start eating a new type of vegetable?
   - How do you feel about fruits?
   - What is your favorite meal to cook at home?
   - What is your favorite meal to eat?
6.
   - Smoking is awful and so is fast food. You should know that!
   - If you start smoking again, your children will start smoking.
   - You really must eat vegetables because they have so many vitamins, nutrients, and healthy fiber.
   - Stop eating fast food now.
   - You are killing your children by feeding them this junk fast food.
   - You are ignoring your duties as a parent! You are supposed to protect your children, not put them in harm's way by feeding them this heart attack food.
   - Do you want to die early? You will, if you keep eating this way.
   - Do you want your kids to be very sick adults? They will, if they keep eating this awful fast food.

REFERENCES

1. Wolever RQ, Simmons LA, Sforzo GA, et al. A systematic review of the literature on health and wellness coaching: defining a key behavioral intervention in healthcare. *Global Adv Health Med.* 2013;2(4):38-57.

2. Vale MJ, Jelinek MV, Best JD, et al. Coaching patients on achieving cardiovascular health (COACH): a multicenter randomized trial in patients with coronary heart disease. *Arch Intern Med.* 2003;163(22):2775-2783.

3. Whittemore R, Melkus GD, Sullivan A, Grey M. A nurse-coaching intervention for women with type 2 diabetes. *Diabetes Educ.* 2004; 30(5):795-804.

4. Wolever RQ, Dreusicke M, Fikkan J, et al. Integrative health coaching for patients with type 2 diabetes: a randomized clinical trial. *Diabetes Educ.* 2010;36(4):629-639.

5. Fisher EB, Strunk RC, Highstein GR, et al. A randomized controlled evaluation of the effect of community health workers on hospitalization for asthma: the asthma coach [published correction appears in *Arch Pediatr Adolesc Med.* 2009 May;163(5):493]. *Arch Pediatr Adolesc Med.* 2009;163(3):225-232.

6. Oliver JW, Kravitz RL, Kaplan SH, Meyers FJ. Individualized patient education and coaching to improve pain control among cancer outpatients. *J Clin Oncol.* 2001;19(8):2206-2212.

7. An S, Song R. Effects of health coaching on behavioral modification among adults with cardiovascular risk factors: systematic review and meta-analysis. *Patient Educ Couns.* 2020;103(10):2029-2038.

8. Stara V, Santini S, Kropf J, D'Amen B. Digital health coaching programs among older employees in transition to retirement: systematic literature review [published correction appears in *J Med Internet Res.* 2020 Dec 14;22(12):e25065]. *J Med Internet Res.* 2020;22(9):e17809.

9. Obro LF, Heiselberg K, Krogh PG, et al. Combining mHealth and health-coaching for improving self-management in chronic care. A scoping review [published correction appears in *Patient Educ Couns.* 2021 Oct;104(10):2601]. *Patient Educ Couns.* 2021;104(4):680-688.

10. Singh H, Kennedy GA, Stupans I. Does the modality used in health coaching matter? A systematic review of health coaching outcomes. *Patient Prefer Adherence.* 2020;14:1477-1492.

11. Long H, Howells K, Peters S, Blakemore A. Does health coaching improve health-related quality of life and reduce hospital admissions in people with chronic obstructive pulmonary disease? A systematic review and meta-analysis. *Br J Health Psychol.* 2019;24(3):515-546.

12. Dejonghe LAL, Becker J, Froboese I, Schaller A. Long-term effectiveness of health coaching in rehabilitation and prevention: a systematic review. *Patient Educ Couns.* 2017;100(9):1643-1653.

13. Barakat S, Boehmer K, Abdelrahim M, et al. Does health coaching grow capacity in cancer survivors? A systematic review. *Popul Health Manag.* 2018;21(1):63-81.

14. Kivelä K, Elo S, Kyngäs H, Kääriäinen M. The effects of health coaching on adult patients with chronic diseases: a systematic review. *Patient Educ Couns.* 2014;97(2):147-157.

15. Frates EP, Moore MA, Lopez CN, McMahon GT. Coaching for behavior change in physiatry. *Am J Phys Med Rehabil.* 2011;90(12):1074-1082.

16. Prochaska JO, Norcross JC, DiClemente CC. *Changing for Good: The Revolutionary Program That Explains the Six Stages of Change and Teaches You How to Free Yourself from Bad Habits.* Quill; 2007.

17. Bandura A. *Self-efficacy: The Exercise of Control.* W H Freeman/Times Books/Henry Holt & Co.; 1997.

18. Deci EL, Ryan R. *Intrinsic Motivation and Self-determination in Human Behavior.* Plenum; 1985.

19. Locke EA, Latham GP. *A Theory of Goal Setting and Task Performance.* Prentice-Hall; 1990.

20. Locke EA. Toward a theory of task motivation and incentives. *Organ Behav Hum Perform.* 1968;3(2):157-189.

21. Miller WR, Rollnick S. *Motivational Interviewing: Preparing People for Change.* Guilford Press; 2002.

22. Miller WR, Rollnick S. *Motivational Interviewing: Helping People Change.* Guilford Publications Inc.; 2022.

23. Frost H, Campbell P, Maxwell M, et al. Effectiveness of motivational interviewing on adult behaviour change in health and social care settings: a systematic review of reviews. *PLoS One.* 2018 Oct 18;13(10):e0204890.

24. Bischof G, Bischof A, Rumpf HJ. Motivational interviewing: an evidence-based approach for use in medical practice. *Dtsch Arztebl Int.* 2021 Feb 19;118(7):109-115.

25. Cooperrider DL, Whitney D, Stavros JM. *Appreciative Inquiry Handbook: The First in a Series of AI Workbooks for Leaders of Change.* Lakeshore Communications; 2003.

26. Cooperrider DL, Whitney DK, Stavros JM. *Essentials of Appreciative Inquiry.* Crown Custom Publishing; 2008.

27. Merriel A, Wilson A, Decker E, et al. Systematic review and narrative synthesis of the impact of appreciative inquiry in healthcare. *BMJ Open Qual.* 2022 Jun;11(2):e001911.

28. Frates B, Bonnet J, Joseph R, Peterson J. *Lifestyle Medicine Handbook: An Introduction to the Power of Healthy Habits.* Healthy Learning; 2020, Chapter 2.

29. Merriam-Webster. Definition of compassion. Merriam-Webster.com. Published 2009 accessed July 8, 2023. Available at: https://www.merriam-webster.com/dictionary/compassion.

30. Frates EP, Bonnet J. Collaboration and negotiation: the key to therapeutic lifestyle change. *Am J Lifestyle Med.* 2016 Jul 8;10(5):302-312.

31. Merriam Webster. Empathy. Merriam-webster.com. Published 2008. Available at: https://www.merriam-webster.com/dictionary/empathy.

chapter 27

Sustaining Change – Challenging Cases

Kathy McManus, MS, RD, LDN

Chapter Outline

I. Case Study
II. Case 1 Issue: Lapse, relapse, collapse
III. Case 2 Issue: Rolling with resistance
IV. Case 3 Issue: All or nothing thinking and the power of self-talk

V. Case 4 Issue: Food insecurity
VI. Case 5 Issue: Managing patient's expectations
VII. Case 6 Issue: Sustaining behavioral changes and maintenance of lost weight
VIII. Answers to Case Introduction

CASE STUDY

MN is a 65-year-old cis female (pronouns she, her, hers) retired office manager. Her daughter was divorced 2 years ago and has 3 children, a son who is 16 and in his junior year, a daughter who is 14 and a freshman in high school and a son 11 years old in 6th grade. MN moved in with her daughter and children to help with caring for her grandchildren. Her daughter works two jobs to support the family. She has a full-time position (7:00AM–3:30PM) as a transport attendant at a large city hospital and then has a part-time job as a cashier at a convenience store from (4:00PM–8:00PM). MN takes the children to school including some later days when the oldest son has baseball practice. Prior to her moving in with her daughter, MN prepared her meals at home and would walk with her neighbor four to five times a week. Currently, she makes herself and the children a quick breakfast in the morning, often a sugar-sweetened cereal and toast. For dinner, she will either do a drive through at a fast-food restaurant or make macaroni and cheese or other pasta dish with red sauce. MN feels as though she does not have the energy or the desire to make herself meals and eats whatever she makes for her grandchildren. The children do not like vegetables, so she rarely prepares them. MN gained 30 pounds over the past 2 years and currently weighs 230 pounds. Ht: 5′8″ with a BMI 35 kg/m². Her PCP retired and she is seeing you for the first time. Her main compliant today is knee pain. She has been thinking that she needs to lose weight and get "healthy" but knows it will be difficult with her current life.

1. **What stage of change is MN currently in?**
   A. Precontemplation
   B. Contemplation
   C. Preparation

2. **In the past she was told to "eat less and move more." Is that consistent with principles of motivational interviewing?**
   A. Yes
   B. No
   If you answered "No" – What are two open-ended questions to ask that would be more in line with motivational interviewing?

3. **If MN said "I am really stuck with my need to care for my grandchildren and don't think losing weight for me is even doable."**
   What are two questions you could ask to help MN at this time?

● INTRODUCTION

This chapter discusses cases that providers may experience while caring for patients who are trying to improve their health. The cases focus on specific issues related to diet and nutrition and offer ideas and approaches that can support their change process. The cases are purposely more detailed in background since in modifying behavior it is critical to understand the patient's "story". Beyond the objective information of anthropometric data, lab values, medications, and co-morbidities, we want to try to better understand the context of where our patients exist, which can include but is not limited to their family, workspace, daily habits, living situation, and the cultural and religious parts of their lives. We used weight-related issues in the chapter, given that it is a common challenging medical condition for which the core management involved dietary changes (even when pharmacologic and/or surgical approaches are part of the treatment plan). However, the principles of MI and the "challenges" in behavior changes can be applied in any patient-provider interactions (i.e., not restricted to weight management). It is important to note that although weight reduction may be the primary goal for patients, improving the quality of food can lead to better health outcomes even in the absence of weight changes. Patients who work towards a more plant-based whole-food eating pattern that includes fruits, vegetables, whole grains, healthy fats, beans, legumes, and nuts in place of diets that contain more animal-based products, sweets, and solid fats can improve their health even if they do not lose weight. This quality diet pattern as seen in the Diet Approaches to Stop Hypertension (DASH) diet and the Mediterranean diet has been shown to reduce cardiovascular risk factors, CVD disease, and the development of type 2 diabetes (See Chapter 18, "Diabetes Mellitus," Chapter 19, "Stroke and Hypertension," and Chapter 20, "Cardiovascular Disease").

Motivational interviewing (MI) was introduced in Chapter 26, "Introduction to Behavior Change." It has been used as a technique in the treatment of addictive disorders and there is a growing body of evidence for consultation in weight and lifestyle management.[1] It is an evidenced-based style of healthy behavior change consultation to support increased effectiveness of clinician patient communication. MI involves a directive person-centered approach designed to explore ambivalence and activate motivation for change. One of the key components of MI is that it acknowledges that clients have every right to make no change.

Motivational interviewing is a guiding communication style that invites people to consider their own situation and find their own solutions to situations that they identify as problematic that are preventing change. It is a collaborative approach where the expertise of the practitioner plays a part, but it is the patient's journey as they decide where to go and how to get there.

These cases explore some of the places where patients get "stuck" in their change process and offer ideas to support and guide them through the process. There is a difference between adopting a behavioral change and sustaining that change. The core principle of implementing healthy behavior change is making the healthy choice the "easy" choice (or the choice that becomes the "natural" option). Putting this principle into practice requires the removal of barriers that patients face when trying to live a healthy lifestyle.

Supporting patients' awareness about their current behavior patterns, helping them become aware of the skills they already have, and respecting any initial resistance is critical to conducting a positive conversation.

As you review this chapter, there are a few take-home messages.

Help patients:

- Prepare for a long-term, sustainable healthy lifestyle.
- Identify specific behaviors that contribute to unhealthy lifestyle and specific behaviors that can support them during their change (tracking foods or activity, accessibility to healthy foods, less processed foods, etc.).
- Roll with resistance to guide and support. Let the patient know you believe in them; a lapse does not mean a collapse.
- Help patients to set realistic expectations around goals and how they define "success."
- Long-term weight loss or any change in unhealthy behavior is doable with ongoing attention and support.

● CASE 1 ISSUE: LAPSE, RELAPSE, COLLAPSE

RG is a 30-year-old gay male (pronouns he, him, his) engineer who has a long history of a BMI in the overweight category. His waist-to-hip circumference is 1.0. He grew up in a family of three sisters and a single mom. As a young boy, he was often bullied at school and had difficulty making friends. He discovered that food made him happy and would oftentimes come home from school and eat large amounts of food in front of the television. His mother worked two jobs and would bring home fast food for the family to eat. After college, RG joined a large development firm, but rarely socialized with his colleagues. He would typically go out for lunch to a fast-food restaurant, buy a double cheeseburger with fries and a milkshake, and sit alone at his desk to eat. He never ate vegetables growing up and dislikes the taste of most of them. Because of his body size, he did not date much until his late 20s. At a work seminar by the HR department, he heard about a weight loss program that was subsidized by his company and he decided to join it. Another motivator for him was that his sister was getting married and he was in the wedding party. He went on a strict diet given to him by the weight loss program that included one egg with whole wheat toast and ½ cup berries for breakfast, a salad with chicken for lunch, and a small portion of fish with green beans and a small baked potato for dinner. He started to work out with a trainer at his company's gym 3 days a week and purchased a stationary bike to work out the remaining days. After 4 months, he lost 30 pounds.

Introduction

Too often, when patients experience a minor slip or misstep in their food or physical activity guidelines, they view it as total failure and feel they have lost control. However, these slips can serve as learning experiences.

Defining Terms

- Lapse – a small mistake or slip. It is one unplanned eating behavior.
- Relapse – happens when there is more than one lapse – two or three strung together over a few days
- Collapse – a total loss of self-management skills, disregard of weight fluctuations or an unwillingness to re-institute self-monitoring tools.

The challenge for patients is to break the cycle – to prevent slips from occurring and to respond in a constructive way when they do. Recognizing that changing behaviors does not follow a straight path. Flexible thinking is the first step in developing a tolerance for failure.

Situation

At his sister's wedding, RG ate more than he had planned at both the rehearsal dinner and wedding. His guilt was high, and he blew off his weight management strategies for the rest of the weekend, along with canceling his appointment with his trainer. Instead, he stopped at the grocery store on the way home and picked up an extra-large pizza along with bags of snacks.

Analysis

RG's tolerance for failure is low. He is exhibiting black-and-white thinking, seeing the highs and lows as total successes or failures. Such totality is difficult to overcome. Being overwhelmed with a mistake makes it difficult for the patient to confront the mistake and problem solve.

What happened? RG went to his sister's wedding without a plan. When he indulged, he felt guilty, but instead of letting it go and learning from past experiences of how to plan for occasions in life, he kept his guilt level high.

RG put himself in a high-risk situation by stopping at the grocery store without planning for a healthy dinner at home. He exposed himself to a multitude of choices, feeling overwhelmed by food that was not within his food guidelines.

How to help the patient respond. Help him use strategies to gain control:

- Building tolerance for failure means being flexible and willing to view lapses as valuable feedback and learning experiences. Helping patients identify and examine their lapse: Where were you? What was your lapse? What did you do? What can you do next time?
- Support patients in identifying their high-risk situations. Are they challenged when they are in social situations, at home alone, stressed at work? Help them develop a plan or alternative activity to combat the risk.
- Help patients recognize that lapses are normal. No one eats "perfectly" all the time. It is the response to the lapse that counts. A lapse does not have to lead to a relapse.

Summary

1. Patients who feel guilty over a slip or mistake can soon repeat the lapse, which becomes relapse and risk of collapse.
2. Changing a behavior is a journey, not a destination. Patients who continue to work at skill building and developing alternative plans for high-risk situations can see success over time.

● CASE 2 ISSUE: ROLLING WITH RESISTANCE

PT is a 62-year-old married cis male (pronouns he, his, him) who works as a bus driver. He has two children in college. PT played high school and college football. Back then, he was encouraged to eat "a lot" to increase his muscle mass. During the off season, he never changed his eating habits and would enter the next season 10–15 pounds heavier. PT and his wife have a busy social life, going out with friends most weekends. He grew up in the Mid-west and his family's diet was mostly meat and potatoes. He has always enjoyed beer and on weekends usually consumes six to seven beers a night. During the week, he has coffee with sugar and cream in the morning, a steak and cheese sub for lunch, and a large bowl of spaghetti and meatballs for dinner with three pieces of garlic bread. After dinner, he usually has a large bowl of ice cream with fudge sauce. PT has a strong family history of cardiovascular disease, hypertension, and hyperlipidemia. His father passed away from an MI at age 60 and his uncle recently underwent cardiac surgery.

- Anthropometrics: Ht.: 6′; Wt.: 250 pounds; BMI: 33.5 kg/m^2
- Labs: Chol: 270 mg/dL; HDL: 34 mg/dL; LDL: 135 mg/dL; Trig: 300 mg/dL BP: 145/95
- Medications: Lipitor, Lisinopril

Introduction

Resistance is what happens when the clinician or someone else other than the patient pushes for change and the patient is not ready for that change. It arises as a normal, expected product of the interaction. When resistance emerges, there are good reasons the patient is not ready to change. Oftentimes, the reasons may not be clear to the clinician or the patient.

Situation

PT is 10 minutes late to his scheduled appointment with you. He reports "I tried to do what you told me last time, but it didn't work." Your response, "Why didn't it work? I gave you the list of foods to stay away from. It is important that you make these change to lower your blood pressure and cholesterol." PT responds, "I can't do this. You don't understand the pressure I am under, and you expect me to change my diet on top of everything else?"

Analysis

The patient is showing signs of resistance in his reply. It is both issue-related (diet) and relation-related (provider). There is discord in the interaction with the clinician. Patient is thinking: "You don't understand me, you are not hearing me, you can't help me."

In reviewing the Transtheoretical Model of Change[2] introduced in Chapter 26, "Introduction to Behavior Change," the issue may be that the patient is in precontemplation and not ready or willing to change their behavior. They are not even contemplating it. If this is so, telling patients they need to change and making a plan for them is wasted time. The provider should consider other strategies to help move them from precontemplation to contemplation. This will not lead to change in the short term, but it is an essential step towards future behavior change. If on the other hand some "change talk" is evident that suggests the patient has moved into a contemplation or preparation stage but is exhibiting some resistance some responses can help. Change talk refers to the patient's statements about their desires or reasons for making a change. Some examples of change talk are:

- "I just need to find the time to exercise."
- "I am concerned about my breathing when I walk up the stairs. I know I need to stop smoking."

How to Respond to Resistance

What Doesn't Work" Trying to persuade the patient about the importance of the problem or the benefits of changing the behavior. This can result in more talk from the provider and less listening. The patient does not feel heard.

Trying to make things right. The clinician wants to fix the patient's behavior, and argues or pushes back. This usually results in the patient continuing to talk about reasons not to change.

What Can Work Express empathy; this assures the patient he is being heard and shows the patient you recognize the barriers he faces. The way information is relayed is essential. It needs to be in a compassionate tone that is non-judgmental, open, honest and considerate of the person and their issues. Use the COACH Approach introduced in Chapter 26.

Reflective listening; build rapport and emphasize personal choice and control. Patients are influenced by their own experience, knowledge, and goals as well as their environment. Listen to their stories with presence; acknowledge their situations without interruption; and reflect back what they say in a supportive, curious, respectful manner.

Support self-efficacy; promote belief in patient's ability to do the behavior needed. Self-efficacy is influenced by past experiences, both negative and positive. Help them identify areas that they have been successful. As an example, maybe they have given up smoking or received a promotion at work. Setting small goals that are easily achievable can be a first step (see SMART goals in Chapter 26) to building self-efficacy.

Develop discrepancy; reflect back in a nonconfrontational way how their views fit in with goals that they have expressed.

Ask a key transition question: "What are you thinking about doing or not doing? What is the next step, if any? Where do we go from here?" "How would you like things to turn out?"

Next Visit

Clinician (issue-related resistance): Begin the session with reflection and empathy: "You don't like this idea. . ., You seem to feel hopeless about . . . On the one hand you want . . .on the other hand you don't think you can."

Clinician (provider-related resistance): Begin the session with acknowledging that you misstepped." I've gotten us off track here. It's up to you. You're the one in charge."

Summary

1. Explore positive and negative consequence of change or continuing current behavior. Acknowledge and accept the patient's decisions and choices, even if the choice is not to change.
2. Clinicians have medical knowledge, but the patient is the "expert" with their own behaviors and what works for them once/if they are deciding to change.
3. Help patients identify "WHY" they want to change.
4. Listen more and talk less.

● CASE 3 ISSUE: ALL OR NOTHING THINKING AND THE POWER OF SELF-TALK

MG is a 32-year-old single woman (pronouns she/her/hers) who lives alone and works as a teacher. Growing up, MG's mother was always on a diet. She would oftentimes tell MG that she shouldn't eat a particular food because it will make her fat. MG started restricting food on her own at age 10 and would weigh herself two to three times a day. If she gained a pound, she would not eat dinner. This pattern continued through college and her 20s. She has been on every diet from Atkins to the Zone. The diets have produced temporary weight loss of between 15–20 pounds, but once she "goes off" the diet, she gains all the weight back. She is on Facebook throughout the day and constantly compares herself to others, always in search of the next new diet. For breakfast she has a protein bar, lunch is a green salad with tuna or chicken with dressing on the side, dinner is take-out Chinese, and her snack at night starts with a small bowl of corn chips, but she oftentimes will go back to the kitchen and finish the bag of corn chips, adding some melted cheese. On weekends she has two to three cocktails.

She is currently at her highest weight and for the first time is asking her provider for help.

Ht.: 5′3″; Wt.: 170 pounds; BMI 30 kg/m²

Introduction

Many patients see the world in all-or-nothing terms. Having a few pieces of candy means you must eat the whole bag. Similarly, if you do not have time to exercise for your usual 60 minutes, you don't exercise at all.

Situation

MG visits her grandmother and vows not to touch any of her homemade desserts. Her grandmother's reaction: "What do you mean you are on a diet; you look fine," "I made these just for you." MG has two cookies and then decides to eat four more before the end of the visit.

Self-Talk

After leaving her grandmother's home, MG starts, "What the heck? I already blew my diet so I might as well stop on the way home and pick up a burger, fries, and milkshake. I just don't have any will power. I will never lose this weight."

Analysis

The underlying belief is that "I must be perfect." MG allowed herself no middle ground or flexibility. Having the cookies may have added some calories to her day, but an insignificant number in the total week. However, the *reaction* to the extra calories was the problem. She was feeling guilty and frustrated about slipping and ended up eating additional calories on fast food.

Blaming thoughts -→ feeling guilty -→feeling defeated and like a failure → more eating

The clinician can begin the session with the question: Would you share your recent experience with me regarding the visit to their grandmother's or the struggle with snacking at night?

Constructive Self-Talk

MG can assess the reality of what is the "cost." "The six cookies are about 400 extra calories for my day. I can make up for these calories by exercising longer and watching my calories closely tomorrow. It is not a major contribution when I look at my entire week. And it's not just about the calories. It's about the quality of the food, too. Maybe I can figure out some foods that are healthy and that I really like to eat. So, the next time I feel a craving for something hyperpalatable, high in fat, salt, and sugar, I have some options."

Developing Skills of Constructive Self-Talk

Patients can practice understanding and describing their internal dialogue. Self-talk is a powerful force. Oftentimes by saying the same messages repeatedly, the mind comes to believe they are true. Statements become self-fulfilling prophecies. For example, the more often you tell yourself that you are unable to go to a restaurant and not have dessert, the more likely you'll give in to temptation every time you go out to eat. Instead, if you tell yourself, you have a solid plan to eat at a restaurant and then enjoy fruit for dessert or know if they don't have fruit at the restaurant, you will have some at home when you return. You can also enjoy a cup of herbal tea while others eat dessert.

Helping the patient practice developing the skill of positive self-talk by writing down rather than just thinking about these three elements can be useful:

- Problem situation: briefly describe the event leading to the destructive self-talk
- Destructive self-talk: write the automatic thoughts that accompany the event
- Constructive self-talk: write a constructive response to the automatic thoughts

Example

- Situation: MG has been on numerous diets over the past 10 years.
- Negative self-talk: "I've tried many diets to lose weight, but I just can't keep it off. It is too hard."
- Positive self-talk: "My past does not dictate my future. This is a new start, and I can learn over time how to make it work. If I break my goals into small, manageable steps I will not be overwhelmed. Many people learn to manage their weight despite past failures."

Summary

1. Patients can learn to look at the slips or lapses (see Case 1) as learning opportunities instead of failures. The reaction to the eating episode is more important than the episode itself. Most people will not gain weight from one lapse.
2. Certain events or mood states can trigger destructive self-talk. The key to turning putdowns and negative self-talk into positives is to identify the negative thought as soon as you think it, challenge it, and turn it into a positive.

● CASE 4 ISSUE: FOOD INSECURITY

CF is a 65-year-old single African American cis male (pronouns he, him, his) who lives in subsidized housing. He is divorced and unemployed. CF has two children who live on the West Coast, and he has not been in touch with them in more than 10 years. He goes to his church every Sunday and enjoys singing in the choir. He receives Social Security, but it does not keep up with inflation and often times he runs out of money before the end of the month. CF has hypertension, type 2 diabetes, gout, sleep apnea, and a history of alcohol abuse. He reports that he gave up drinking last year. He is not on any medication because he can't afford it. This is his first visit to a healthcare provider in 2 years. He reports he has not eaten since yesterday. He says he has lost weight over the past year, but not sure how much. He describes breakfast as coffee with a slice of toast and margarine, lunch a donut with orange soda, and dinner at the senior center or a bologna sandwich with potato chips.

Introduction

Many years of research have shown that hypertension and diabetes affect racial and ethnic minorities and low-income adult populations in the United States disproportionately resulting in higher risk of diabetes, rates of diabetes complications, and mortality.[3,4] With a healthcare shift toward greater emphasis on population-based health and value-based care, social determinants of health (SDOH) have become a critical intervention to achieve health equity.[5–8]

Underlying social and economic conditions of communities that affect health include affordable housing, stable employment, reliable transportation, the food environment, and safety. The food environment, which encompasses food insecurity, food access, food availability, and food affordability, are essential issues for supporting patients to improve their diet.

Action Plan

- Have an open discussion with CF, starting with assessment of his food situation: Incorporate a quick screening tool such as the Validated 2-item screening tool:

    1. Within the past 12 months, I worried whether my food would run out before I got money to buy more.
    2. Within the past 12 months, the food I bought just didn't last and I didn't have money to buy more.

    The item-item screen (HFSS-2) derived from the U.S. Department of Agriculture Household Food Security Scale (HFSS-18) was validated in an adult general medicine ambulatory population. An affirmative response to either of the two items has a sensitivity of 98% and specificity of 91%. Food insecurity was associated with increased odds of coronary heart disease and diabetes.[9]

- Identify team members that can help in addressing some of these complex issues. This may include social workers, dietitians, resource specialists, continuing care nurses, and psychologists, to name a few. This is reviewed in Chapter 28, "A Multidisciplinary Approach for Nutrition Counseling."
- Connect the patient with community resources to support a healthy lifestyle such as community healthcare workers, peer supporters, and lay leaders to assist in the delivery of services.
- Food assistance comes in various forms. Some people need monthly assistance and others need temporary support with an occasional meal or bag of groceries. Below are a few examples of national and state programs:
- National: FNS Nutrition Programs

The USDA Food and Nutrition Service has a website that includes programs to end hunger and obesity through the administration of 16 federal nutrition program. Examples of some of these programs include Child Nutrition Programs, Food Distribution Programs, and the Supplemental Nutrition Assistance Program (SNAP).

Summary

1. Many patients will not be able to begin to modify their risk factors if their basic needs are not addressed first.
2. Helping patients connect with hospital and clinic support along with additional community resources can be the most important "prescription" the clinician offers.

● CASE 5 ISSUE: MANAGING PATIENT'S EXPECTATIONS

KD is a 54-year-old nurse who is a cis female (pronouns she, her, hers) and lives with her partner and two teenage daughters. During her first pregnancy, she gained 50 pounds and delivered at 200 pounds. Although she tried to lose weight after her daughter was born, she was not successful. She became pregnant 18 months later and gained 40 pounds with her second daughter. For the past 14 years, she has been busy raising her family and working full time.

KD lives an active life. She works the early shift so that she can be home in the afternoon to take her girls to dance class along with basketball practice and games on the weekends. She goes to the grocery store on Sundays to buy food for the week. Money is limited so she tries to buy in bulk and items that are on sale. During the week, she has coffee and a pastry for breakfast, lunch is a roast beef sandwich or take-out fried chicken with French fries. After work, she is shuttling her girls to practice and has a candy bar and another cup of coffee. Dinner is chicken thighs with rice and peas. She does strength training on Sundays at the gym for 60 minutes. Currently her weight is 275 pounds, Ht: 5′8″ BMI: 42 kg/m². Waist circumference is 88 cm (34.6 inches)

Introduction

Despite much professional consensus that modest weight loss of 5% to 10% is a success and can result in reduction of comorbid conditions associated with obesity, some patients often want weight losses to be two to three times greater than this. This discrepancy between the patient's desired outcome and actual weight loss can result in unrealistic and negative assessment of the treatment. A study conducted in a university weight loss clinic in individuals with obesity concluded that the amount of weight loss produced by the best behavioral and pharmacologic treatments was viewed as "disappointing".[10] Patients with the highest pretreatment weights were likely to have the most unrealistic expectations for success.

Situation

KD presents in clinic today and wants to lose weight. She tells you her goal is to weigh 150 pounds, back to her weight when she was in her 20s, prior to her first pregnancy. KD believes she is very motivated at this time and tells you that she wants a plan that will help her lose at least 2–3 pounds per week.

The Conversation

The next few words from the clinician can make or break the relationship with the patient. Utilizing motivational interviewing skills is critical at this beginning juncture. One of the first goals is to build rapport with KD through empathetic listening. Meeting patients where they are and understanding their current motivators and expectations is key. Having an open discussion about why the patient wants to lose weight at this time can start to build trust. Identify connections with open-ended questions:

- What matters to you? Why does it matter to you?
- Avoid the "I" and "Y" words to start a sentence: "I think . . . ." "You should. . . ."

Aim at not focusing on a number on the scale, but rather the big picture of what and why losing weight matters to them. How will they feel if they start eating healthy foods? How will they feel if they start exercising? How do they see themselves in 5 or 10 years? What would it take to change eating practices and patterns?

Summary

Help patients set realistic goals that are focused on behavior that is sustainable. Let them make the decision about where to start and how they would like to measure their goal. One way to help patients develop goals is to help them using the SMART goal checklist. Below are some questions patients can ask themselves to determine if their goal is SMART.

- **Specific** – What behavior are you specifically focusing on? What specific steps will you take to accomplish this goal? When do you plan on starting this?
- **Measurable** – What do you plan on tracking and how will you accomplish this? How often and how much will you do?
- **Action oriented** – What behavior are you changing? Is it food or activity related or is it related to feelings or emotional behavior?
- **Realistic** – Can you realistically complete this goal? Try to set smaller goals that can lead to a bigger goal.
- **Time-sensitive** – Can you reach this goal within your time frame? Is this a behavior change you are committed to or a temporary goal?

Example of KD's SMART Goal: For the next 2 weeks, I will bring my lunch to work on Tuesdays and Thursdays. I will pack my lunch the night before and leave a note on the refrigerator as a reminder. I will track my progress using a phone app and will start May 5th and reassess May 19th.

1. Communicate that you recognize what a challenging and frustrating task weight control presents but that you will stay with them through their journey.
2. Making small, incremental change lays the foundation for larger, long-term success.
3. Obesity is a chronic disease that requires lifelong care.

● CASE 6 ISSUE: SUSTAINING BEHAVIORAL CHANGES AND MAINTENANCE OF LOST WEIGHT

SS is a 52-year-old cis female (pronouns she, her, hers) who has lost and gained weight since she was 18 years old. Her two brothers and sister have significant excess weight. She grew up in a family where food was the center of every occasion. On Sundays, the entire extended family would get together for large feasts with plenty of food and drink. Cooking would start in the early morning and continue until all 20 relatives sat down for the meal in the late afternoon. SS has many fond memories of these weekly dinners and misses these times with family. She is single and works as an administrative assistant at a small private company. She gets together with her siblings about twice a month, oftentimes at a new restaurant in the city. Three years ago, her mother died from a heart attack after living with type 2 diabetes for 20 years. A few months later, SS started on a (another) weight loss diet. She began walking and is now walking 10 miles a week, about 2 miles each day. When she started her plan, she weighed herself at least one/week. Since starting to regain weight, she has not been on the scale. A typical day includes breakfast of cereal with skim milk and fruit, lunch of half a turkey sandwich and vegetable soup, snack of ½ cup yogurt, and dinner of broiled chicken with broccoli and a sweet potato. After dinner, she watches TV. About 6 months ago, she started going back to snacking in the evening. She starts with grapes and one cheese stick, but then will have crackers and peanut butter, ½ pint of ice cream, and a bowl of pretzels. After 18 months on her diet, SS had lost 60 pounds. At her last visit, she weighed 180 pounds. Today, she comes for her annual physical, having regained 25 pounds.

Weight History: January 2020: 109 kg; BMI: 44 kg/m^2; June 2021: 81.8 kg; BMI: 33 kg/m^2; June 2022: 93.2 kg; BMI: 37.5 kg/m^2

Initial Discussion

SS: "I just can't seem to do it anymore. I can't stop eating after dinner. I crave sweets all the time. I don't see the point of trying anymore."

Clinician: "I know it is not easy, but you just need to work harder and take control." Hoping to motivate her, the clinician reminds her of how bad she will feel if she continues to regain her lost weight and that she may need to go back on her blood pressure medication. The clinician offers her a GLP-1 receptor agonist, but she declines, feeling that it would mean "she failed."

Conclusions from Research Studies

A study examining attitudes and behavior of people with obesity showed that sustained weight loss success was seen in people who had a personal motivation to lose weight, were willing to talk to a diabetes educator about their weight and had their weight loss attempts recognized by their healthcare provider.[11] A systematic review of weight loss registries in five countries revealed the following eating strategies supported weight loss maintenance: having healthy food available at home, regular breakfast intake, increasing vegetable consumption, decreasing sugary and fatty foods, and limiting certain foods.[12]

Results from the National Weight Control Registry Study showed that weight regain was fastest in the early years of follow-up, with decreasing rates after the first 5 years. Key behaviors for success were leisure time physical activity, dietary restraint, and frequent weighing.[13]

In the case of SS, she has continued with some of her healthy behaviors that are consistent with the ability to sustain long-term weight loss, including having a personal motivation to lose weight (mother's death from complications of diabetes), willing to talk to her provider about weight issues, eating breakfast, consuming vegetables, regular leisure time activity, and having healthy foods at home. The continued connection to her healthcare provider is critical at this time. Using some of the strategies in the COACH Approach™ from the "Introduction to Behavior Change," Chapter 26, can serve as a helpful tool.

Curiosity: What is motivating the patient now? Is she still concerned about her own health?

Openness: With recent regain of some weight it is crucial for the provider to be nonjudgmental and help the patient feel understood and not shamed or blamed.

Appreciation: Appreciating any movement forward by the patient will encourage continued effort. Reminding and praising the patient for what they have accomplished; losing 35 pounds not focusing on the 25 pounds that were regained. Reviewing the behaviors that they have continued to do to support a healthy lifestyle.

Compassion: Listening to the patient and working to understand them can create an atmosphere of compassion. Helping them feel accepted, even when they feel frustrated and dejected by their recent resumption of old behaviors.

Honesty: It is important to share information in a compassionate way. After the patient said, "I don't see the point of trying anymore," it is an indication that they are seeking reassurance for staying the same. Sharing the facts regarding complications from diabetes is important, but communicating them in an empathetic way that allows for the patient to see you are on their side and will continue to be with them through their journey.

Recommendations for Long-Term Weight Maintenance[14]

Long-Term Commitment

- The obesity treatment guidelines recommend weight loss interventions should include a long-term comprehensive weight loss maintenance program that continues for **at least 1 year.** Consider referral to a registered dietitian, an obesity medicine specialist, a comprehensive weight management clinic, a community weight management group such as the Diabetes Prevention Program for prediabetes (covered by CMS), or a commercial program such as Weight Watchers.

Strengthen Satisfaction with Outcomes

- People tend to focus on what they have not achieved, rather than what they have accomplished. Call attention to the patient's progress.
- Acknowledge the significant weight that the patient has kept off. Put into context the health benefits (improved lipids, BP, a1C, etc.).

Relapse Prevention Training

- Help patients anticipate and manage high risk situations. When a lapse occurs, help them get back on track.

- Weighing daily is an important strategy to support weight maintenance. Identify with patient a threshold that signals re-engaging with team (i.e., weight gain of 5 pounds)
- Problem solving to identify challenges; evaluate options.

Appeal to Patient's Deeper Motivations

- External, superficial rewards are unlikely to support long-term weight management.
- Longer-term sustained motivation is more likely when patients take ownership of their behavior changes and engage in them because they are meaningful and enjoyable.
- Helping patients shift their locus of motivation from weight loss alone to intrinsically meaningful areas such as health can improve long-term outcomes.

Alternative Discussion

PCP: "I understand your frustration. I know how challenging this is. You have worked so hard, and you think you have nothing to show for it" SS: "That's right. Why bother?"

PCP: "From what I see, you are doing really well. You have lost 35 lbs. and kept it off for more than a year. That is 15% of your baseline weight. Studies show that under the best of circumstances average weight loss is 5–10% of starting body weight. You are doing better than most. Studies also show that losing 7% of body weight lowers the risk of diabetes by 60%. Remember, you have also been able to stay off your blood pressure medications. Weight goes up and down, and our bodies fight back against weight loss, so this is never easy. Some regain and relapse is inevitable." Then, pause to let patient think or speak. Conclude with a statement like, "Let's plan out some next steps and we'll meet again in a few weeks and see if we need to consider additional strategies." Would you be willing to consider any of these ideas?

1. Tracking your food intake for a week using an app such as My Fitness Pal or Lose It. Another option is to jot the information down on paper including time, portion, and food eaten.
2. Using your phone or another wearable device to count your steps each day.

Then, ask the patient if they have other ideas for strategies to try. Ultimately, the patient will decide the next step that is best for them at this time.

SUMMARY

Help patients with the following:
- Prepare for long-term healthy, sustainable lifestyle.
- Identify specific behaviors that contribute to unhealthy lifestyle and specific behaviors that can support them during their change (tracking, accessibility to healthy foods).

- Set realistic expectations around goals, timeline, how they define "success."
- Build flexibility. When things do not go according to plan, what is plan B?
- Long-term behavior change is doable with ongoing attention and support.

ANSWERS TO CASE INTRODUCTION

1. Contemplation—MN is aware that a problem exists and is considering change. One strategy in this stage is to have the patient write a list of pros and cons to making a change. Have the patient envision what life would be like if she did make the change.

2. No; Sample open-ended questions:
   - If you did decide to change, what would need to be in place for you to change?

   - It appears in the past you had some success with healthy eating. Tell me how you were feeling during that time.

3. Sample open-ended questions if feeling some resistance:
   - You certainly do have much on your plate currently. If you did decide to take a step- what might be one thing you would want to start with?
   - Where would you like to go from here?

REFERENCES

1. Rollnick S, Miller WR. What is motivational interviewing? *Behav Cogn Psychother.* 1995;23:325-334.

2. Prochaska JO, DiClemente CC. Transtheoretical therapy: towards a more integrative model of change. *Psychotherapy Theory Res Pract.* 1982;19:276-288.

3. Aggarwal R, Chiu N, Wadhera AE, et al. Racial/ethnic disparities in hypertension prevalence, awareness, treatment and control in the United States, 2013 to 2018. *Hypertension.* 2021;78:1719-1726.

4. Golden SH, Brown A, Cauley JA, et al. Health disparities in endocrine disorders: biological, clinical, and nonclinical factors—an Endocrine Society scientific statement. *J Clin Endocrinol Metab.* 2012;97:E1579-E1639.

5. Hill-Briggs F, Adler NE, Berkowitz SA, et al. Social determinants of health and diabetes: a scientific review. *Diabetes Care.* 2021;44(1):258-279.

6. Centers for Medicare & Medicaid Services, Office of Minority Health the CMS Equity Plan for Improving Quality in Medicare, September 2015.

7. U.S. Department of Health and Human Services, Office of the Secretary, Office of the Assistant Secretary for Planning and Evaluation, and Office of Minority Health. *HHS Action Plan to Reduce Racial and Ethnic Health Disparities: Implementation Progress Report 2011-2014,* Washington, DC, Office of the Assistant Secretary for Planning and Evaluation; 2015.

8. Chin MH. Creating the business case for achieving health equity. *J Gen Intern Med.* 2016;31:792-796.

9. Harrison C, Goldstein JN, Gbadebo A, et al. Validation of a 2-item food insecurity screen among adult general medicine outpatients. *Popul Health Manag.* 2021;24:4.

10. Foster GD, Wadden TA, Phelan S, et al. Obese patients' perceptions of treatment outcomes and the factors that influence them. *Arch Intern Med.* 2001;161(17):2133-2139.

11. Dhurandhar NV, Kyle T, Stevenin B, et al. Predictors of weight loss outcomes in obesity care; results of the national ACTION study. *BMC Public Health.* 2019;19:1422.

12. Paixao C, Dias CM, Jorge R, et al. Successful weight loss maintenance: a systematic review of weight control registries. *Obes Rev.* 2020;21(5):e13003.

13. Thomas JG, Bond DS, Phelan S, et al. Weight-loss maintenance for 10 years in the national weight control registry. *Am J Prev Med.* 2014;46(1):17-23.

14. Greaves C, Poltawski L, Garside R, et al. Understanding the challenge of weight loss maintenance: a systematic review and synthesis of qualitative research on weight loss maintenance. *Health Psychol Rev.* 2017;11(2):145-163.

A Multidisciplinary Approach for Nutrition Counseling

Jamieson D. Johnson, MSS, CLMC, CITC, CPWC, CEP / Ashley C. Draviam, MS, RD, LDN, CSO / Loren N. Winters, MSN, ANP-BC, OCN, DipABLM / Amy Comander, MD, DipABLM

Chapter Outline

"The degree to which I can create relationships, which facilitate the growth of others as separate persons, is a measure of the growth I have achieved in myself."

CARL ROGERS

CASE STUDY

WB is a 56-year-old, cis male, pronouns (he, him, his), with a diagnosis of stage IVB anaplastic thyroid cancer who initially presented to his PCP with acute headaches and dizziness. He underwent a total thyroidectomy and left neck dissection, followed by 7 weeks of radiation and chemotherapy (carboplatin and paclitaxel). WB's medical history includes obesity (class II), non-insulin-dependent diabetes mellitus, and developmental delay. His medications include metformin, atorvastatin, lisinopril, Synthroid, and diazepam. He has no known food or drug allergies.

WB lives alone in a boarding house and has minimal social support. He has family that lives nearby, but they are only involved in his medical care when necessary. He takes The Ride, a free, small-vehicle public transport for people with a disability. He is unemployed;

(Continued)

however, he used to work bagging groceries at his local grocery store and plans to resume this after his oncology treatment is complete. WB is sedentary at baseline.

WB has poor dietary habits at baseline. His boarding house room has only a microwave and mini refrigerator with a freezer; therefore, he is not able to cook meals. He eats mostly frozen meals or take-out from local sub shops and restaurants. His diet lacks variety and is high in processed foods and saturated fats, and low in plant-based foods such as fruits and vegetables. At the initiation of treatment, he reports normal appetite and no changes to his diet. He denies any difficulty eating or swallowing. He reports no use of alcohol or other substances.

1. Match each of the following multidisciplinary team members with their most likely role/responsibility in WB's case.
   A. Nurse
   B. Registered Dietitian
   C. Speech Language Pathologist
   D. Social Worker
   E. Physician
      a. Assess patient's current understanding of treatment plan, provide education regarding medications, treatment schedule and side effects.
      b. Assess patient's swallowing ability and identify deficits, provide treatment recommendations to referring provider (MD/APP).
      c. Oversee medical management, refer to specialists and apply specialist recommendations to treatment plan.
      d. Assess patient's current dietary habits, nutrition status, and nutrition needs, and provide nutrition treatment plan.

      e. Assess patient's basic needs in home environment, including access to food and the ability to prepare meals.

2. To identify potential areas for behavior change, you must first listen to the patient. Which statement identifies a potential area for change?
   A. The patient tells you, their expectations.
   B. The patient complains about a problem.
   C. The patient judges your ability to help.
   D. The patient reveals self-sabotaging thoughts.

3. What might be the first nutrition-related issue the multidisciplinary team addresses for patient WB?
   A. Whether he needs a feeding tube.
   B. Care for his diabetes.
   C. The healthfulness of his current diet.
   D. How will he access food or necessary supplements during treatment.

4. Patient WB described in this chapter has the diagnosis of an aggressive Stage IVB anaplastic thyroid carcinoma. He has required aggressive treatment which compromised his nutrition status. A multidisciplinary team is integral for the care of patients like WB for the following reasons:
   A. To provide optimal support for the patient's nutrition needs during his active treatment and recovery.
   B. To ensure that WB has appropriate resources, including insurance coverage, for his needs during treatment.
   C. To enhance WB's ability to complete his treatment, manage side effects, and optimize quality of life.
   D. All the above.

IMPORTANCE OF AND STRATEGIES FOR CREATING A MULTIDISCIPLINARY TEAM

We are slowly becoming a society of people incapable of managing our own health and well-being, incapable of living with a personal vision for being healthy, happy, and able to vigorously thrive and prosper. A multidisciplinary team approach to nutrition care is an opportunity to encourage a framework within the healthcare system that creates superior, sustainable solutions for serving and empowering patients.

Empowering patients to adopt and sustain healthy eating patterns takes a team approach. The physician is often the leader of the team. Other members of the team, caring for a patient with a nutrition concern, may include a nutrition specialist such as a registered dietitian, a speech pathologist depending on the diagnosis, and a health coach. Nurses, nurse

practitioners, physician assistants, social workers, mental healthcare providers, as well as caregivers and family members of the patient are part of the patient's healthcare team. This is a multidisciplinary team, and each member brings their own expertise, scope of practice. Communication and collaboration are key to the effectiveness of any team. Lifestyle medicine, as reviewed in Chapter 31, incorporates all members of the team, and patients working to adopt and sustain healthy lifestyles, including healthy eating patterns. This also may include seeking lifestyle medicine specialists to help them reach their goals.

As evidenced by the *American Journal of Lifestyle Medicine, Case Series in Lifestyle Medicine: A Team Approach to Behavior Changes,* "the combined efforts of a multidisciplinary lifestyle medicine team provided *important, collaborative* support to help patients adopt and maintain change."[1] The main question asked was, "Would patients who have, or are at greater risk for chronic diseases, benefit from the support of a multidisciplinary, lifestyle medicine team in making healthier lifestyle choices?"[1] It was evidenced that, "patients were able to *significantly improve* their lifestyles and their lab values with the three-month intervention of a lifestyle medicine team including a physician trained in lifestyle medicine, a certified health and wellness coach, a licensed nutritionist specialist, a physical therapist and a licensed mental health professional".[1] It was also noted, "a nutrition specialist, physical therapist, and mental health professional add to the lifestyle medicine team's *power* by addressing the needs of each patient in these areas".[1]

A multidisciplinary team helps a patient develop a *willingness* to take steps in discovering how to manage their myriad health challenges. Working on lifestyle modification such as healthy eating patterns requires paying attention to the whole person. "It is about encouraging an *open mindset* for the possibility of creating a more physically fit body, more loving heart and peaceful mind," as described in *PAVING the Path to Wellness Workbook: The Guide to Thriving with a Healthy Body, Peaceful Mind, and Joyful Heart* co-authored by three lifestyle medicine specialists.[2] It's not just about how much people eat or what they eat. It's also about how easy it is to obtain fresh produce, how confident people are with their cooking skills, whether there is enough money to buy food for the month, how people feel about what you eat, how people feel when they eat, and how their body feels after they eat. And, sleep, exercise, stress, social connections, and substance use can impact what people eat, as described in Chapter 31. This is another reason why a multidisciplinary team is helpful for empowering people to adopt and sustain change.

The multidisciplinary team approach supports an important premise that a patient feels understood and appreciated, being able to accept his condition in the present moment. This essential acceptance encourages a patient to be more open and willing to do his best work to improve and solve his health challenges. Growing a patient's capacity is the foundation and focus of a multidisciplinary team. By asking the question: "What are the things that you value that will contribute to your vision of improved health, happiness, and success?' The patient then can open the door of opportunity to influence and inspire the direction for his own healing and health".[2]

The words and language a multidisciplinary team uses to *communicate* are vital and have a *direct impact* on the patient's sustained performance and success. A multidisciplinary team creates an opportunity for sustainable success when the team appreciates a patient's efforts, not for what the multidisciplinary team values, but for what the *patient's vision and values* are.[3]

In addition, when the multidisciplinary team *appreciates* their **own** team members, this simple empowering act clearly *communicates* to team members that their *work is getting noticed* and they are *on the right track*, aligned with the *mission* of the team. Without judgment or criticism, a safe, *trusting* environment begins to flourish. It is important that each team member is *genuinely acknowledged* and *valued* for their individual expertise. This way, the multidisciplinary team becomes more connected, cohesive, collaborative, and confident in sharing their opinions more openly. This validating communication, in turn, fuels an increase of natural effort among team members. A new sensitivity to the patient's needs flourishes, and each team member becomes empowered too.

The multidisciplinary team is built on individual team members' strengths and expertise. The respect for and appreciation of each team member opens opportunities for each person to build self-confidence, grow their capacity to learn new skills and talents within their realm of expertise, all the while supporting their patients.

Not only are multidisciplinary teams an asset to a patient's health and well-being, but the positive benefit to a *team member's* experience, health and well-being is also enhanced. Successful multidisciplinary teams generate win-win situations encouraging everyone to become better versions of themselves. See Table 28-1 for strategies for creating a successful multidisciplinary team. Multidisciplinary teams are slowly helping society discover the need for patients to become better managers of their own health, capable of living with an enhanced vision of being healthy, happy, and able to vigorously thrive and prosper.

The first step for creating a multidisciplinary team is to *bring together a team of health care providers with the common mission of serving each other and the patients*. What is the *mission/ vision of the multidisciplinary team*? What will success look like? When a patient's needs are identified, each member of the team will provide unique resources that support the patient within a team member's field of expertise, and scope of practice. Any member of the multidisciplinary team, regardless of job or title, has the *capacity to lead* a team. This opportunity not only accelerates each team member's growth, but also supports a patient's capacity to take their first step towards better health and well-being.

Creating a positive learning community is a key characteristic of a multidisciplinary team. Members learn and grow together while respecting and empowering each other. When a multidisciplinary team member has input into what *they* want to learn, this input inspires each team member to learn and grow on their own, thus creating stronger self-esteem and a more robust autonomous spirit. It is important to respect and encourage a team member's need for learning and growth.

● IMPORTANCE AND ROLE OF EACH MULTIDISCIPLINARY TEAM MEMBER FOR THE CASE STUDY

Each member of the multidisciplinary team had an important individual as well as collective role in WB's care throughout his oncology treatment and recovery. The physician, a medical oncologist, established WB's medical treatment plan and made necessary adjustments as needed based on side effects and nutrition impact symptoms. The nurse practitioner worked with the physician and team members to implement the treatment plan and provided medical management as well as co-management of complex care issues including those requiring urgent care, hospitalization, and home services. The speech language pathologist evaluated WB for dysphagia with a modified barium swallow study and provided him with recommendations for safe swallowing techniques and for a safe diet during

TABLE 28-1 • Strategies for creating a multidisciplinary team		
1. The Team's Mission: Virtuous Cycle, Holistic Care	Reinforce the need for a holistic approach; provide patients with healthcare services, education, through empowerment; create a virtuous cycle	Benefit = positive impact
2. Clarify the Role of Each Team Member	A team leader identifies the expertise and talent that is needed from each team member; noted will be strengths of the team member, their value to the team and why their input matters	Benefits = builds trust in team member's talents, capabilities, and judgments
3. Identify Each Team Member's Strengths and Capabilities	Acknowledge the positive, professional influence a team member has and how their strengths connect to the success of the team's work	Benefits = talents, strengths, and learning edges are identified
4. Express Appreciation	Verbally highlight, during a team meeting, the benefit of each team member's work, the benefit to the patient and for themselves	Benefits = affirmation and acknowledgment of team member's value
5. Grow an Open mindset	Opportunities for engaging dialogues; using active listening: affirm, acknowledge, and appreciate team members when they share ideas and contribute to meetings, with patients or team members	Benefits = builds confidence to grow and learn; mistakes are a means to growth
6. Utilize the COACH Approach TM	Encourage team members to be open to the possibilities for success by understanding and utilizing the coach approach vs. the expert approach	Benefits = empowers, educates, and engages a patient for taking his next step to improve his health, his vision
7. Build Relationships	Make time to ask empowering open-ended questions of team members and patients, showing you are genuinely interested in listening and learning about their aspirations and interests	Benefits = builds character, empowers choices, makes connections
8. Inspire Learning and Growth	Be able to engage, involve and empower patients to co-discover a willingness to learn, foster a positive learning environment where team members co-create choices of what the patient wants to learn to improve their health and wellbeing	Benefits = deeper satisfaction, increased positive healthcare experience autonomous spirit emerges

treatment and recovery. The social worker provided emotional support to WB throughout treatment, communicated with WB's family, helped WB get access to food through a food pantry, and assisted with transportation resources. The nurse practitioner referred WB to visiting nursing services for assistance with medication management and close symptom monitoring. Following completion of treatment, the multidisciplinary team followed up closely with WB and continued to coordinate necessary care and provide ongoing education in his recovery.

In the care of patient WB, the RD provided nutrition counseling to optimize nutrition and to manage side effects during treatment, including odynophagia, dysgeusia, xerostomia, and constipation, and to help control blood sugars. The RD recommended liquid nutrition supplements and got these covered by insurance. The RD assessed the patient's need for enteral or parenteral nutrition, and with the collaboration of the team determined it was not necessary. She followed up during the recovery period to help WB resume intake of solid foods. At the end of treatment, the RD also provided WB with education on survivorship nutrition to reduce risk of recurrence, manage his diabetes and fatigue, and optimize long-term health.

Interprofessional collaboration has been associated with patient-centered measures of success. The patient's care is influenced by how well the members of the multidisciplinary care team perform within their own scope of practice as well as understand and value what the other team members contribute to the team. Leadership and importance of team member's

roles are dynamic and shift throughout the course of the patient's journey through the healthcare system. Different team members contribute within their scope of practice and may take the lead in providing expertise depending on the phase of a patient's care or the current challenge. Table 28-2 describes the roles and scope of practice of the multidisciplinary team members highlighted in this case study.

Continuing education is required for all healthcare providers to remain current in their fields as well as to maintain their certification and licenses. Continued education provides many opportunities to expand knowledge of nutrition, to improve effectiveness of interdisciplinary care, and to expand professional development.

Education and Credentials of Each Team Member

The multidisciplinary healthcare team, collectively, provides the patient with a broad and deep span of knowledge, skills, and experience. Each team member has completed educational programs and competencies (e.g., exams, skills, supervised clinical hours) for their role, as described in Table 28-3. This training is required to maintain licenses and certifications with continuing education, and team members can choose to access additional education, anytime, to expand and enrich knowledge and skills. Each team member brings a thorough understanding of their unique field of knowledge and skillset, while also recognizing the potential of knowledge deficits.

TABLE 28-2 • Scope of practice and roles of multidisciplinary team members for this case	
Physician	Manages and treats medical conditions and provides continuous care across hospital, clinic, and community settings. Nutrition: assess for nutrition needs, provide medical management for nutrition related problems or side effects, make referrals to other care providers, and provide nutrition education to patient and family. Can bill for medical nutrition therapy when the diagnosis code is applicable. Can bill for nutrition counseling for certain diagnoses as well as preventative counseling.
Advanced practice provider (APP – NP or PA)	Manages and treats medical conditions in collaboration with supervising physician and provides continuous care across multiple settings, often the "lead communicator" in the multidisciplinary team. Nutrition: assess for nutrition needs, provide medical management for nutrition related problems or side effects, make referrals to other care providers, and provide nutrition education to patient and family. Cannot bill for medical nutrition therapy. Can bill for nutrition counseling for certain diagnosis as well as preventative counseling.
Nurse	Provides direct patient care, case management, triage and/or care coordination. Nutrition: can provide nutrition education as it pertains to the patient's diagnosis but cannot provide or bill for medical nutrition therapy.
Registered Dietitian (RD)	Provides medical nutrition therapy to manage acute or chronic medical conditions, reduce risk of other chronic disease, and/or manage side effects of treatment. Can bill for medical nutrition therapy when services are ordered by the MD/APP.
Speech language pathologist (SLP)	Treats communication and swallowing problems when services are ordered by the MD/APP.
Social worker (SW)	Helps patients meet basic and complex needs, provides direct services or therapy, links to community resources. Referred by MD/APP.
Mental healthcare provider	Treats psychological problems and behavioral dysfunctions related to physical or mental health. Referred by primary team to specialist care.
Health coach	Assists clients in co-creating health changes to promote improvement in health and well-being. Cannot provide or bill for medical nutrition therapy or counseling.
Community resources	Aid/help obtain access to basic needs such as social support, transportation, food access, health education
Family and/or caregivers	Serve as advocates and care coordinators, provide help with personal care, transportation, and household chores, provide social and emotional support.

Nutrition Curriculum Deficit

Despite the clear evidenced connection between diet and disease, current medical and nursing school curricula contain very limited nutrition focused course hours. Most medical and nursing programs do not require nutrition courses for students.[4–6] Deficits in nutrition education leave future medical providers unprepared to care for their patients optimally and confidently.[7] Currently, there is a wide range of medical and nursing curriculums. Within disciplinary and interdisciplinary continuing education offerings, there is a call to action to teach non-RD providers how to include nutrition education in patient care, how and when to involve the RD, and how to work effectively within an interdisciplinary team to improve patient outcomes. At this time, each individual clinician must take proactive steps to augment their knowledge base about the use of nutrition interventions for health care. Interdisciplinary Resources for Nutrition related CME can be found on a variety of these medical organization's websites including but not limited to:

- American College of Lifestyle Medicine (ACLM) Continuing Education Store

- Harvard T.H. Chan School of Public Health Continuing Nutrition Education
- Mayo Clinic School of Continuing Professional Development

More medical schools and some nursing schools are starting to embrace a field of medicine known as "lifestyle medicine". The American College of Lifestyle Medicine (ACLM), defines lifestyle medicine as a medical specialty that uses therapeutic lifestyle interventions as a primary modality to treat, reverse and prevent chronic conditions including CVD, type 2 diabetes, and obesity. Through the ACLM, physicians and allied health professionals receive training, CMEs, and an option to complete certification and apply evidence-based lifestyle changes to treat and/or reverse medical conditions. Nutrition counseling, emphasizing a whole food, predominantly plant-based eating pattern, is one of the six pillars of lifestyle medicine. The other five pillars are physical activity, restorative sleep, stress management, avoidance of risky behaviors and positive social connections and are discussed in Chapter 31. The ACLM also provides many opportunities for healthcare providers to share research, join special interest groups, attend conferences, and form collaborative communities.

TABLE 28-3 · Education and credentials of each team member

Team member	Undergraduate	Nutrition course hours	Graduate	Postgraduate	Board exam	Credentials
Physician	4-year bachelor's degree	Not required, approximately 25–30 hours	Medical school	Residency, fellowship in specialty	USMLE, specialty exams, state license	MD
Nurse Practitioner	4-year bachelor's degree in nursing or other	Included in assessment and pathophysiology courses	Degree in advanced practice nursing subspecialty	Optional PhD in nursing or Doctor of Nursing practice (DNP)	National board certification, specialty exams, state license	Adult: ANP Pediatric: CPNP Women's health: WHNP Psychiatric: PMHNP Family: FNP
Physician Assistant	4-year bachelor's degree and prerequisite courses in behavioral and basic sciences	Modeled after medical school education, varies by program	Required, 3 years of classroom and clinical instruction		National board exam, state license	PA-C
Nurse	Associate degree or 4-year bachelor's degree in nursing	Included as part of nursing assessment course	Optional master's in nursing (MSN)	PhD in nursing, Doctor of Nursing practice (DNP), or Doctor of Nursing Science (DNS)	NCLEX, specialty certifications	RN
Registered Dietician	4-year bachelor's degree, complete an accredited, supervised practice program	Coursework approved by the Academy of Nutrition and Dietetics Accreditation Council for Education in Nutrition and Dietetics (ACEND)	Required as of 2024	Optional PhD for RDs interested in nutrition related research (not required for clinical practice)	National exam, specialty practice training and exams (such as diabetes, oncology)	RD
Speech Language Pathologist	4-year bachelor's degree in related field (communication sciences and disorders)	Some included in assessment of dysphagia, swallowing disorders coursework	Master of science in SLP	Clinical fellowship required	Praxis Examination in Speech-Language Pathology, state license	MS, CCC-SLP or MA, CCC-SLP
Social Worker	4-year bachelor's degree in social work (specialties include child and family services, mental health, geriatrics, hospice, school)	Coursework includes content on interdisciplinary collaboration with RDs	Many states require (MSW)		National board exam: ASWB Exam	LICSW

Choosing Teams for Hospital, Primary Care Clinic, and Community Settings

Choosing the team that will provide care is a critical initial step in putting together a patient centered and effective treatment care plan. In the hospital setting, the team will be comprised of healthcare staff tasked to address issues of high acuity and to prepare the patient for discharge to home or post-hospital care. RDs are assigned to patient units in the hospital and should be consulted early in the patient's care when nutrition needs are first identified or anticipated. Early access to RDs helps to prevent or slow nutrition deficits caused by the patient's state of health and/or treatment.

In the primary care setting, the clinic team members such as the physician or APP may be affiliated with a hospital, but largely provide care in the community. Some, but not all primary care clinics have an RD on staff, therefore some nutrition education is offered by MD/APPs or RNs. Primary care providers that don't have an RD on staff can provide referrals to RDs as well as to community-based nutrition programs.

Community-based nutrition programs serve patients in their community and are typically grant-funded at a national or state level, and often rely on volunteers. Community-based nutrition programs provide services such as nutrition education, how to get access to affordable and accessible food, or help accessing emergency food supplies.[8]

For patients who may need and could benefit from ongoing support in co-creating and achieving health and wellness goals, including improving diet and healthy eating habits, certified health and wellness coaches provide an important component to the multidisciplinary healthcare team. Certified health and wellness coaches can provide both group and individual coaching sessions with clients and work collaboratively within the healthcare practice or system. While health coaches do not diagnose, or treat illnesses, they can help inspire and teach patients how to co-create goals with action steps. These goals are authentic and achievable based on what is most important to the *patient* and utilizing what resources they have available. There is a virtuous cycle that is depicted in Figure 28-1 which encourages health and wellness coaches to use positivity and optimism to build confidence and a belief in one's self like the self-efficacy reviewed in Chapter 26. Coaches respect self-determination and encourage persistence, which leads to learning and increased effectiveness. This then leads to achievements and success which feeds into optimism and positivity.

Multidisciplinary healthcare teams will vary in size and expertise needed from each team member. Teams are created to address the *patient's* needs and are based upon what resources are available in the healthcare setting. Knowledge and skills as well as competence and confidence in nutrition and coaching among multidisciplinary team members will increase the opportunity for success, improving dietary behaviors of individuals and populations.

While the registered dietitian is the expert on nutrition and nutrition counseling, other team members can obtain further education to expand their knowledge, skills, and

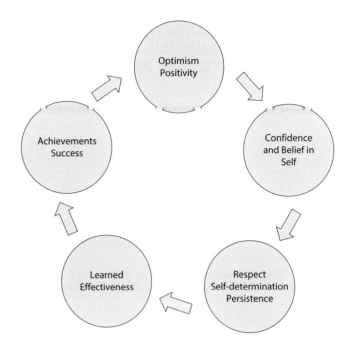

FIGURE 28-1 • A virtuous circle

confidence, to counsel patients about nutrition within their scope of practice. These nutrition education and certification opportunities have become available through the ACLM and other medical organizations such as to improve a team member's effectiveness and competency in nutrition counseling and education.

The Benefits of Varied Backgrounds, Experience, and Expertise

For a patient with a diagnosis of malnutrition, no single provider can adequately assess, treat, provide ongoing care and support particularly once the patient leaves the acute care setting. The unique strengths of each team member are what fosters collaboration and innovation when coming up with patient care strategies and solving health problems. Without differing perspectives, backgrounds, and experience, health problems could remain uncovered and thus negatively impact patient outcomes. The acquisition of clinical competencies in nutrition as well as using a multidisciplinary approach to care for patients is essential for all healthcare providers. In this way, patients will be able to receive optimal nutrition care.

Insurance Coverage for Nutrition Counseling

In the inpatient setting, nutrition counseling and medical nutrition therapy (MNT) are covered by insurance under the included services of inpatient care. In the ambulatory setting, insurance coverage for nutrition services can vary widely, depending on type of insurance, the reason for referral or diagnosis, location (state), and the type of nutrition care needed. Patients are often required to check with their health insurance company regarding coverage for nutrition services before appointments can be scheduled.

THE ROLE OF CONSISTENT MESSAGING AND OPEN COMMUNICATION AMONG TEAM MEMBERS AND PATIENTS

Communication among members of the multidisciplinary team was essential throughout WB's oncology treatment and recovery. Weekly Head and Neck team rounds allowed providers to communicate their concerns and recommend ways to support this complicated patient. Frequent emails or messages in the electronic medical record also allowed for ongoing communication and updates. In one instance, there was a debate about whether WB would need an enteral feeding tube to maintain his nutrition status throughout treatment, given the many nutrition-related side effects of his treatment regimen

(including odynophagia, dysphagia, dysgeusia, anorexia, nausea/vomiting, constipation, and general increased protein and calorie needs related to the hypermetabolic demands of chemotherapy and radiation). The open channels of communication allowed all providers to give input and stay apprised of information that would inform a decision to place a feeding tube (e.g., everyone knew about his oral intake, medication regimen, and treatment side effects that would impact his nutrition status). As such, all team members were able to provide competent, consistent messaging and recommendations to the patient as one unified voice, as described in Table 28-4.

Despite the barriers, WB was able to complete treatment without a feeding tube, due in large part to the other supports the team was able to implement such as: giving him a weekly

TABLE 28-4 • Challenges and barriers: How to create a learning environment of excellence	
Challenges and barriers	**How to improve**
Not having a mindset of excellence	Develop a *willingness* to improve = *optimism*
No respect for self or team members (e.g., it doesn't matter if I'm late)	*Take responsibility for words, thoughts, and behaviors.* (show up to meetings on time)= being on time shows respect for self and others
No awareness of your strengths or teammates strengths	Recognize your strengths that are valued—(a learned behavior that can be improved; having a willingness to reflect). *True strengths are illuminated by gaining mastery through action.*
No awareness of uncomfortable feelings = an opportunity to ID a learning edge or weakness	Open to *constructive feedback to learn and grow* = builds confidence and competence
Not capable to engage with teammates	Recognize and lead with your signature strengths = increases *power and competence* to live more fully
Not willing to create space and time to ask yourself—about being on a multidisciplinary team—what energizes you?	Share stories that empower and inspire teammates. Share your truth.
Not feeling secure because there is a fear of being judged	After listening, affirm, acknowledge, appreciate what you heard someone say; we each need acceptance and validation of self-worth
Not recognizing what makes you a unique member of the multidisciplinary team	Look inside yourself and ID your signature strengths (What creates *infectious enthusiasm* from your heart?)
No energy or life in your team	Bring your infectious energy to weekly meetings, team members, relationships; this will help you shine, build ally's or deepen connections
Violent communication is used: unkind words, actions are used, mostly complaints	Breathe, keep your cool, *listen for the unmet need and what the person cares about* in a complaint you hear; extend kindness affirm, acknowledge & appreciate what you see and hear
Negative thinking or self-talk (fear, self-doubt challenges you) limits beliefs and habits (hostile work environment)	Reframe a situation (take a new perspective); using different language empowers, energizes, uplifts; well-being shifts to feeling more positive and capable
No routine	Create a routine for yourself, setting you up for success
Feelings of stress and anxiety exist about performance & winning; trying to force outcomes	Ask yourself, what progress have I made with a team member or patient? Are you learning/embracing a curious mindset?
No celebrations of wins at work	How are you showing up to work with your best efforts? Recognize the rewarding and things you do and pleasure you get from being on the team.
Diminishing others, NOT making others good	Notice what is right about your teammates; empower/support the people you work with; compliment others and affirm, acknowledge, and appreciate
Feeling threatened, anger, insecure, jealous, competitive	Notice a teammate's success, powerfulness increases; notice and observe behaviors; what is the unmet need? What does the teammate care about?
Demands are made through criticism of self or others	Be able to ID the difference between a demand and request

supply of oral nutrition supplements, setting him up with home meal delivery, providing medical nutrition therapy to adjust his diet and maximize calorie and protein intake, making changes to his medication regimen for symptom management, and monitoring the safety of his swallowing. Because WB was able to maintain oral intake and adequate nutrition throughout treatment, his recovery was quicker, and he was able to resume a normal solid oral diet within six weeks of completing treatment.

Members of the team continued following up with WB in person and through patient messages and phone calls during his recovery from treatment. This included and was not limited to communicating his progress and changes, his oral intake, or medications, and collaborating on strategies to help him recover and improve his overall nutrition and health status moving forward into the survivorship period.

Forms of Communication Among Team Members

Multidisciplinary teams may use a variety of forms of communication to plan and coordinate care for patients with nutrition needs. It is essential that any form of written communication that includes patient identifiers to be handled in a HIPPA-compliant manner. While there are still a handful of hospitals that utilize a paper medical record, most U.S. hospitals utilize an (EMR) electronic medical record.[9] Within the EMR, team members can communicate within the patient's chart allowing for information to be better organized, shared and referenced among team members. Because messages can be tracked when sent within the patient's chart, EMR offers an advantage over email which excludes anyone not included in the message and is trackable only to those included. Email is also not as secure as EMR. A better use for email may include circulating pertinent article references or updated treatment guidelines, coordinating team meetings, or sending calendar invites for offerings such as educational and/or team building opportunities.

Team meetings are essential to optimal care coordination and can be challenging to implement as seen in Table 28-5. For patients admitted to hospital, standardized multidisciplinary rounds have been associated with positive patient-centered outcome measures.[10] While multidisciplinary team meetings/rounds in hospitals are most often done in person, team meetings/rounds done in person, team meetings in the ambulatory care setting, especially if involving community-based team members, may out of necessity take place by phone or more recently via video conference. Whether in person or via phone/video, each team member in the meeting is encouraged and has an opportunity to share their assessment of the patient, share their expertise and perspective towards the diagnosis and treatment plan. They each can pose clarifying questions to other team members to increase understandings, ensure clear communication and together, further fine tune and coordinate the patient's care.

Family meetings bring together the members of a patient's family and the multidisciplinary team. Family meetings allow for the team to assess the family's understanding of the patient's diagnosis, prognosis, and treatment options. The family may also express concerns about their loved one's care, and their ability to provide for care needs at home. Team preparation and coordination ahead of the family meeting is essential to maximize cohesion and efficacy of the team. Some key components of team practices that are likely to optimize diverse team members' skills in a family meeting are knowledge of the meeting goals, one's own role and skills, other team member's role and skills, of the family members' roles as well as team attitudes (positive morale, mutual trust, and a mutual commitment to understanding the goals and plan for the patient.[11] Family meetings also are an opportunity for the team to assess what support and resources are needed at home to support positive outcomes.

Finally, it is important for team members to document in the patient's medical record, the multidisciplinary team's

TABLE 28-5 • Making others good—a compass for guiding a multidisciplinary team[a]		
Making others bad	**Making others good**	**Strategies for using non-violent communication**
Judge, criticize, target = protect myself	Collaborate openly, engage, affirm	Listen mindfully, *affirm* what someone is saying
Undermining others, assuming bad intentions	Use a caring, and kind attitude	*Acknowledge* other's feelings and what you *observe*
Gossiping	Use direct and honest communication	*Affirm* positive qualities and *strengths* of the other person
Writing others off	Honor a person's opinion	*Affirm* something positive about the other person in your mind
Being right all the time	Become curious, create a learning situation	Ask *open-ended* questions
Avoiding conflict, being vague, not engaging	Use clear, direct, concise language	*Acknowledge* what someone is saying, *validate* their feelings
Not listening	Appreciate what you have learned	*Appreciate* and *validate* something you hear
Hearing a complaint, taking offense	Hearing the unmet need and what the person cares about	*Affirm* what the person cares about

[a]*"We change best when we are strongest and most positive, not when we feel the weakest, most negative, or helpless."* David Cooperrider.

collaborative assessment, care plan with specific roles and responsibilities, and planned follow-up. Generously sharing the limelight and being mindful to give credit to all who contribute to the success of the team, empowers team members and the organization.[12]

As a team, it is about enlarging our vision, bringing answers together that are the consensus of the multidisciplinary team, while helping patients and team members lead healthier lives. Genuinely listening with a willingness to be open to creating a new way of interacting can produce astounding results.[13] We can inspire and encourage each other on our multidisciplinary team to make a difference in all the lives we touch.

THE NEW PERSPECTIVE LOOKING AHEAD: THE VALUE AND IMPACT OF A MULTIDISCIPLINARY TEAM APPROACH

"In making decisions and moving forward in medicine, business and life, it's better to make the decision that everyone can agree on rather than the one a single person might think is best, even when that person is the leader."

DR. CATO LAURENCIN

Multidisciplinary care for patients with complicated medical diagnoses has been increasingly implemented across healthcare settings throughout the world.[14,15] As illustrated in the case of WB, comprehensive care of this patient required collaborative decision making and involvement of clinical experience from numerous specialties. The multidisciplinary team approach was essential to ensure appropriate attention was given to his nutrition needs during his active treatment, and during the recovery phase. The involvement of a multidisciplinary team, involving this patient's physician, advanced practice provider, nurse, registered dietitian, social worker, speech language pathologist, and family, ensured that WB was able to tolerate his intensive chemotherapy and radiation therapy regimen, and then recover from treatment. Table 28-6 reviews key strategies that influence the daily work of a multidisciplinary team.

The implementation of an effective, multidisciplinary team approach to address nutrition needs of patients like WB is a challenge, requiring time, effort, and dedicated financial resources. However, as this case illustrates, a multidisciplinary approach to nutrition care allows for coordination of complex care and provides continuity during treatment. It is important to ensure the best possible clinical outcome for patients like WB. According to researchers like Dr. Laurencin, there are always new questions, many involving how we can achieve better outcomes for our patients.[16] Future research in this area of complex care of patients will further illuminate the benefits of multidisciplinary nutrition care. Benefits of a multidisciplinary team approach include improvement in assessment and management of a patient's nutrition-related needs, improvement in sustainable patient outcomes and improvement in patient satisfaction and quality of life. Table 28-7 provides a new perspective on pillars of a dynamic multidisciplinary team as reviewed in this chapter.

TABLE 28-6 • Key strategies that influence the daily work of a multidisciplinary team

1. Acknowledge, affirm, and validate team members:
   -notice and make a positive observation of their work, communication, or interactions with team members
   -highlight a difference they are making with a patient;
   -share what you value about them being part of the team
2. Embody, capture, and elucidate moments of a connected spirit, happiness that inspires joy, notice something that amazes you; acknowledge, affirm, and appreciate a team member's work
3. Celebrate professional or personal growth: -acknowledge the positive changes and influences you see
4. Express gratitude that is heartfelt: -write a thank you note or e-mail that highlights the positive contributions of a team member
5. Encourage opportunities for engaging dialogues: -listen deeper; acknowledge, affirm, and appreciate when team members share thoughts and ideas
6. Invite collaboration -encourage team members to share their skills, passions and talents with the team, department, or community; -provide opportunities for team members to share ideas at weekly staff meetings, -mentor a new team member; -support another multidisciplinary team in their area of strength
7. Build relationships create time to ask empowering questions showing team members you are interested in learning about their aspirations and interests
8. Inspire learning and growth engage and involve team members to discover a willingness to learn on their own; -foster a positive learning environment by empowering team members to share their focus and input into what they want to learn

---

TABLE 28-7 • Pillars of a dynamic multidisciplinary team[a]

A new perspective
Trust
Empathy
Mindful listening
Authentic leadership presence
Recognized purpose, meaning and passion
Generosity, open collaboration and engagement
Acknowledgment of appreciation and gratitude
Inspiration for learning and growth
Open mindset
Resilience

[a]*"Connection is the energy that exists between people when they feel seen, heard and valued; when they can give and receive without judgment; and when they derive sustenance and strength from the relationship."* Brown

SUMMARY

The goal of a multidisciplinary team approach for nutrition care of complex patients is to ensure that patients receive appropriate assessment and management of nutrition-related needs, so the team can then collaborate and formulate a management approach that will ultimately improve patient outcomes, as well as patient satisfaction and quality of life. While the multidisciplinary team approach requires additional time and resources in a healthcare setting, the care provided in this case, for a patient with a complex cancer diagnosis, was optimized.

A multidisciplinary approach is key for supporting patients' willingness to learn how to create sustainable, healthier lives and relationships, regardless of social or economic status. Such models can be implemented in a wide array of healthcare settings to address a patient's nutrition issues, while ultimately improving patient outcomes, satisfaction, and quality of life.

TAKE-HOME POINTS: MERITS OF A MULTIDISCIPLINARY APPROACH FOR NUTRITION COUNSELING

1. Promotes a framework within the healthcare system:
   - capable of creating superior, sustainable, solutions, to optimize nutrition.
   - allowing for coordination and continuity of complex care involving, but not being limited to using a primary care provider and registered dietician.
   - *honoring patient-centered care* to manage acute or chronic health needs during all phases of care.
2. Supports the important premise of using *validating communication*, among the multidisciplinary team members, the patient, and caregivers, from which a patient's vision and values are acknowledged, understood, and appreciated.
3. Recognizes and appreciates each team member's unique expertise, strengths, and skill sets aligned with the multidisciplinary team mission, fostering collaboration and innovation.
4. Encourages a positive, supportive learning community among team members, especially supporting additional education and training in nutrition: learning and growing together while respecting and empowering one's autonomous spirit.

CASE STUDY ANSWERS

1. **Match each of the following multidisciplinary team members with their most likely role/responsibility in patient's care:**
   A. **Nurse: (a)** Assesses patient's current understanding of patient's treatment plan, provides education regarding medications, closing schedule and side effects.
   B. **Registered Dietitian: (d)** Assesses patient's current dietary habits, nutrition status and needs, and provide a nutrition treatment plan.
   C. **Speech Language Pathologist: (b)** Assesses patient's swallowing ability and identify deficits, provide treatment recommendations to referring provider (MD/APP)
   D. **Social Worker: (e)** Assesses patient's basic needs in home environment, including access to food and the ability to prepare meals.
   E. **Physician: (c)** Oversees medical management, refers to specialists, and applies specialist recommendations to treatment plan.

2. **To identify potential areas for behavior change, you must first listen to the patient or multidisciplinary team member. Which statement identifies a potential area for change?**
   B. The patient or multidisciplinary team member complains about a problem.

When a multidisciplinary team member hears a compliant being expressed (by a patient), this moment is a valuable opening for learning and uncovering what the patient's need is that hasn't been met. This way of listening supports the patient and affirms that the patient or (anyone) is heard. Perceptions, assumptions, and false stories can be identified and cleared up. The result is improved collaboration and more open communication.

3. **What might be the first nutrition-related issue the team addresses for the patient?**
   D. How he will access food or necessary supplements during treatment

4. **Patient WB described in this chapter has the diagnosis of an aggressive Stage IVB anaplastic thyroid carcinoma, and he has required aggressive treatment which has compromised his nutrition status. A multidisciplinary team is integral for the care of patients like WB for the following reasons:**
   D. All the above

This case illustrates that for patients with complicated medical diagnoses, such as patient WB, a multidisciplinary team approach for nutrition counseling ensures that patients receive appropriate assessment and management of nutrition needs, access to key resources, and coordinated care that will improve a patient's outcome, satisfaction, and quality of life.

REFERENCES

1. Kent K, Johnson JD, Simeon K, Frates EP. Case series in lifestyle medicine. *Am J Lifestyle Med.* 2016;10(6):388-397.

2. Frates B, Tollefson M, Comander A. *Paving the Path to Wellness Workbook: A Guide to Thriving with a Healthy Body, Peaceful Mind, and Joyful Heart.* Healthy Learning; 2022.

3. Bark L. *The Wisdom of the Whole: Coaching for Joy, Health, and Success.* Create Space Press; 2011.

4. Adams L. Status of nutrition education in medical schools. *Am J Clin Nutr.* 2006;83(4):941S-944S.

5. DiMaria-Ghalili RA, Mirtallo JM, Tobin BW, Hark L, Van Horn L, Palmer CA. Challenges and opportunities for nutrition education and training in the health care professions: intraprofessional and interprofessional call to action. *Am J Clin Nutr.* 2014 May;99(5 Suppl):1184S-93S.

6. Laing BB, Crowley J. Is undergraduate nursing education sufficient for patient's nutrition care in today's pandemics? Assessing the nutrition knowledge of nursing students: An integrative review. *Nurse Educ Pract.* 2021;54:103137.

7. Crowley J, Ball L, Hiddink GJ. Nutrition in medical education: a systematic review. *Lancet Planet Health.* 2019;3(9):e379-e389.

8. United States Department of Agriculture, Nutrition programs, National Institute of Food and Agriculture, https://www.nifa.usda.gov/grants/programs/nutrition-programs, accessed December 12, 2023.

9. Parasrampuria, S., Henry, J. Hospitals' use of electronic health records data, 2015-2017. The Office of the National Coordinator for Health Information Technology. ONC Data Brief. 2019 April No. 46. https://digirepo.nlm.nih.gov/master/borndig/9918332987406676/9918332987406676.pdf

10. Lau C, Dhamoon AS. The impact of a multidisciplinary care coordination protocol on patient-centered outcomes at an academic medical center. *J Clin Pathways.* Published online 2017. https://www.hmpgloballearningnetwork.com/site/jcp/article/impact-multidisciplinary-care-coordination-protocol-patient-centered-outcomes-academic.

11. Walter JK, Arnold RM, Curley MAQ, Feudtner C. Teamwork when conducting family meetings: concepts, terminology, and the importance of team-team practices. *J Pain Symptom Manage.* 2019;58(2):336-343.

12. Goleman D, Langer E, David S, Congleton C; Harvard Business Review. *Mindfulness.* Harvard Business School; 2017:86.

13. Hughes S. *Making Others Good: The Crucial Tool for Transforming Dysfunction in Your Organization.* Learning as Leadership Press; 1970:36.

14. Taylor C, Munro AJ, Glynne-Jones R, et al. Multidisciplinary team working in cancer: what is the evidence? *BMJ.* 2010;340(Mar 23 2):c951-c951.

15. Pillay B, Wootten AC, Crowe H, et al. The impact of multidisciplinary team meetings on patient assessment, management, and outcomes in oncology settings: a systematic review of the literature. *Cancer Treat Rev.* 2016;42(42):56-72.

16. Laurencin CT. *Success Is What You Leave Behind: Fostering Leadership and Innovation.* Elsevier Academic Press; 2022.

chapter 29

Culinary Medicine

Michelle Hauser, MD, MS, MPA, FACP, FACLM / Shirly (Shalu) Ramchandani, MD / David Eisenberg, MD

Chapter Outline

CASE STUDY

Maria is a 40-year-old, married, cis female (pronouns she, her, hers) psychologist, who presents for an annual exam as a new patient. She is a mother to two girls, ages 2 and 4 years old. She has a history of infertility requiring IVF and anxiety well controlled with a selective serotonin reuptake inhibitor. She has gained 40 pounds since having her children.

Maria is concerned about her weight gain given her family history of diabetes. She has tried various commercial diet plans and has aimed to increase her level of physical activity; however, her work is mostly sedentary. She has always regained the weight she lost plus a few extra pounds after stopping the previous diets. Sheepishly, Maria admits that a barrier to losing weight has been stress eating, particularly highly processed, carbohydrate-rich foods. When preparing meals at home, she often relies on pasta-based dishes due to their ease and acceptance by her children. As a family,
they consume few vegetables. Maria is interested in losing weight and asks for advice.

Brief 24-hour dietary recall:
Breakfast: bagel with cream cheese, coffee with cream and sugar
Lunch: large bowl of pasta with cream sauce, cranberry juice
Dinner: chicken breast with white rice, water
Snacks: chocolate chip cookie, thick slice of banana bread, 2 cupcakes
Other drinks: water and diet soda
Vital signs and labs: Weight: 186 lbs; Height 5'6"; Body Mass Index (BMI) 30 kg/m², Fasting glucose: 98 mg/dL, Blood Pressure (BP): 138/86 mm Hg

1. You decide to gather more information from the patient to formulate a treatment plan. Which of the following questions or statements is the *least* helpful?

(Continued)

CASE STUDY   *(Continued)*

A. Why do you want to work on weight loss right now?

B. You could do more cardio to burn calories.

C. Is there anything about your current dietary pattern that you think should change to help you meet your weight loss goals?

2. Shifting toward a predominantly whole food, plant-based diet means one would eat only plant-based products and could not consume any packaged processed foods. True or False?

3. Maria acknowledges that her diet is low in vegetables and understands that eating more vegetables would support improved health in a variety of ways. However, she cites a few barriers to eating more vegetables. Which of the following is *not* a commonly cited barrier to eating more vegetables?

A. "Produce is expensive."

B. "Vegetables aren't satisfying."

C. "Vegetables are simple and easy to prepare."

D. "Vegetables are bland and tasteless."

INTRODUCTION TO CULINARY MEDICINE

History, Definitions, and Importance of Culinary Medicine

Culinary medicine (CM) is a relatively new field that evolved from centuries old ideas, namely using food to prevent and treat disease while recognizing the enjoyment that delicious food instills in our lives. It gained the moniker, culinary medicine, only in recent years. Other related terms include culinary nutrition and "food as medicine." While there is no single, globally recognized definition of CM, leaders in the field touch largely on the same points in their definitions. Culinary medicine was first described by physician-chef John La Puma as an "evidence-based field in medicine that blends the art of food and cooking with the science of medicine".[1] Physician-chef Michelle Hauser defines CM as, "an evidence-based field that brings together nutrition and culinary knowledge and skills to assist patients in maintaining health and preventing and treating disease by choosing high-quality, healthy food in conjunction with appropriate medical care".[2,3]

The field of CM arose to fill a void between the limited way nutrition is taught in most health professional training programs and the need to gain knowledge and skills to effectively partner with patients to help change their dietary habits to achieve their health goals and improve longevity, wellness, and performance. It incorporates important skills needed for effective patient counseling, including how to take a dietary history, assess food access, glean information on cultural aspects of diet and incorporate these into any recommendations, engage in motivational interviewing around making healthy dietary changes, and counsel on how to prepare and otherwise acquire and eat foods that are healthy, delicious, and meet the time, budget, and skills available to a given patient.

Nutrition education represents a critical missed opportunity in medical education in the United States and in many countries around the world. In the United States, only 25% of medical schools have a dedicated nutrition course[4] and most schools fall short of recommended hours of nutrition education.[3,5] This is despite diet being the single most important risk factor for morbidity and mortality in the United States[6] and is associated with 11 million deaths around the world annually.[7] With the overwhelming preponderance of obesity[8] and cardiovascular disease,[9] there has never been a more important time to equip healthcare professionals with the tools needed to best address diet-related diseases. In May 2022, House Resolution 1118 passed, recognizing "the mounting personal and financial burden of diet-related disease in the United States" and called on "medical schools, graduate medical education programs, and other health professional training programs to provide meaningful physician and health professional education on nutrition and diet".[10]

Home Cooking Skills Are Waning

Home cooking improves health outcomes and has also been associated with lower BMI and lower risk of developing obesity and type 2 diabetes.[11] However, the U.S. population has moved away from food preparation at home. Between the 1960s and 2000s, overall calorie consumption increased and so did the proportion of calories eaten outside the home. Low-income households went from eating 95% to only 72% of calories at home. Middle-income households dropped from eating 92% to 69% of calories at home, and high-income households now eat only 65% of calories at home, down from 88%.[12] These trends in home cooking in U.S. households are due in part to a lack of cooking skills and food preparation knowledge.[13] It can no longer be assumed that people were taught by their parents to cook, nor that they or someone they live with has confidence in preparing a home-cooked meal from scratch. Culinary medicine emphasizes the importance of all family members participating in household food activities.

Culinary Medicine—Beyond Dietary Counseling

Culinary medicine is an appealing way to approach dietary behavior change, not only because it includes effective counseling strategies, but also because it focuses on practical food preparation and acquisition skills. It could reasonably be argued that ignoring the cultural importance of food and innate human cravings for certain flavors and textures are key reasons that dietary counseling alone often fails to change behavior. For example, most people have learned at some point that vegetables are good for them. However, only 1 in 10 eat the recommended number of servings each day.[14,15] Common barriers to increasing vegetable intake (and making other healthy dietary changes) include cost, lack of knowledge and skills to select and prepare healthful foods, time, and (inaccurate) socialization that foods can be healthy or delicious but not both. A strength of CM is that it is a particularly effective method of addressing these key barriers to dietary behavior change by teaching that healthy food can be tasty, fast, and inexpensive if you know how to cook and meal plan. When incorporating CM into teaching or counseling, it can be very effective to focus on deliciousness and craveability first to capture interest and then highlight health aspects of what is being covered—a stealth health approach.[16] When considering cost, screening for food insecurity and food access issues are important. (See Chapter 4, "Food Insecurity.") Additionally, sharing tips on eating healthy on a budget can be helpful as well as dispelling myths that healthful foods are always more expensive than less nutritious options. Among the healthy food patterns recommended in the 2015–2020 Dietary Guidelines for Americans (DGA),[17] the least expensive was the one richest in vegetables and other whole plant foods—the healthy vegetarian dietary pattern.[18] In this analysis, legumes, whole grains, nuts, seeds, and soy were found to be more economical per calorie than dairy, meat, poultry, eggs, and seafood.[18] This pattern is also recommended in the 2020–2025 DGA.

Key Components of Culinary Medicine and Practice Settings

Key components of CM include practical nutrition education, cooking skills, behavior change and related motivational interviewing, counseling, or coaching (see Chapter 26, "Introduction to Behavior Change"). Using a CM approach to dietary behavior change, one aims to engage patients in shared solution development, decision making, knowledge acquisition, and skill building. This can be done in a variety of settings including teaching kitchens, traditional (1:1) clinic appointments, shared medical appointments (SMAs)/group visits (see Chapter 30, "Nutrition Counseling with Group Visits") and community and other educational settings.

Clinical cases are presented in this chapter, and they focus on the practical details of patient counseling and using CM to improve dietary quality. This section of the chapter explores screening for food insecurity, investigates motivators and barriers to healthful dietary behaviors, uses motivational interviewing (MI) to assist in dietary behavior change, and adds CM to clinical encounters.

Incorporating CM into the Traditional Office Visit Format

When a patient comes to the clinic for a routine 1:1 visit, assessing their stage of change for improving their eating patterns, using motivational interviewing strategies, and collaborating with the patient in a COACH Approach ™ (see Chapter 26, "Introduction to Behavior Change") will help the clinician to connect with the patient and develop a rapport for continued conversations at subsequent visits. The COACH Approach ™ invites the clinician to use curiosity, openness, appreciation, compassion, and honesty while collaborating and negotiating with the patient rather than simply telling the patient what to do and how to do it.

CM Resources

Many diets studied in scientific literature show improved health outcomes as one shifts away from a Western diet and towards a diet that is based on less processed plant foods.[19] It can be helpful to share this concept in a visual format. One example is in Figure 29-1. Many patients have an "all-or-nothing" concept of dieting. They think of dietary changes as something to throw themselves into wholeheartedly for a while, but often return to a more familiar diet when enthusiasm wanes if sustainable dietary practices are not implemented. Making sure to explicitly discuss sustainability of dietary practices is important when counseling on behavior changes. Taking steps at one's own pace along a dietary spectrum from a highly processed diet to a diet rich in whole foods is often less daunting and more sustainable than a rapid diet overhaul.

Adopting a predominantly whole food, plant-based diet (WFPB) can be achieved through a variety of eating patterns, including an entirely WFPB, Healthy Mediterranean, Dietary Approaches to Stop Hypertension (DASH), low-fat vegan, and numerous other plant-predominant diet recommendations and guidelines.[19] While adopting a predominantly WFPB diet, it is important to emphasize the intake of minimally processed foods such as vegetables, fruits, whole grains, beans, nuts, and seeds. Focusing on what to add or focus on (i.e., positive framing) can be more helpful and informative than focusing on what to cut out of the diet (i.e., negative framing).

● CASE EXAMPLES OF CULINARY MEDICINE COUNSELING

Case 1

Foluke, a 42-year-old African American (pronouns he, him, his) with a history of hypertension (HTN), prediabetes, and dyslipidemia presents to his PCP for his annual physical exam. His BP is 138/90 mm Hg, waist circumference is 40 inches, and labs are notable for fasting glucose of 106 mg/dL, glycosylated hemoglobin (HbA1c) 5.8%, triglycerides 350 mg/dL, and high-density lipoprotein (HDL) cholesterol 35 mg/dL. He has a family history of type 2 diabetes (T2D) and coronary artery disease (CAD). He is interested in learning more about dietary changes that can help prevent diabetes, improve his health, and reduce his reliance on medications. He currently takes two anti-hypertensive medications and has been told he may need to start a new medication for his hypertriglyceridemia.

A dietary assessment is obtained from Foluke using a brief, 24-hour dietary recall. He describes eating in a typical Western dietary pattern, high in ultra-processed foods and low in whole, plant foods. He frequently eats fast food, including subs and pizza, but feels he is doing well eating one serving of vegetables each day.

DIETARY SPECTRUM

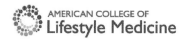

AMERICAN COLLEGE OF
Lifestyle Medicine

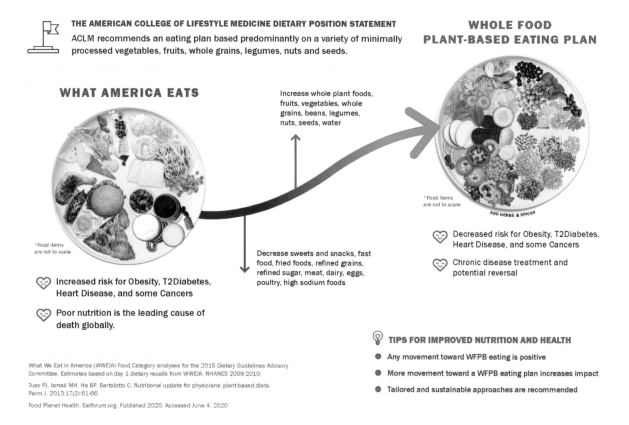

THE AMERICAN COLLEGE OF LIFESTYLE MEDICINE DIETARY POSITION STATEMENT
ACLM recommends an eating plan based predominantly on a variety of minimally
processed vegetables, fruits, whole grains, legumes, nuts and seeds.

**WHOLE FOOD
PLANT-BASED EATING PLAN**

WHAT AMERICA EATS

Increase whole plant foods,
fruits, vegetables, whole
grains, beans, legumes,
nuts, seeds, water

*Food items
are not to scale

ADD HERBS & SPICES

Decrease sweets and snacks, fast
food, fried foods, refined grains,
refined sugar, meat, dairy, eggs,
poultry, high sodium foods

*Food items
are not to scale

Increased risk for Obesity, T2Diabetes,
Heart Disease, and some Cancers

Poor nutrition is the leading cause of
death globally.

Decreased risk for Obesity, T2Diabetes,
Heart Disease, and some Cancers

Chronic disease treatment and
potential reversal

TIPS FOR IMPROVED NUTRITION AND HEALTH

● Any movement toward WFPB eating is positive

● More movement toward a WFPB eating plan increases impact

● Tailored and sustainable approaches are recommended

What We Eat in America (WWEIA) Food Category analyses for the 2015 Dietary Guidelines Advisory
Committee. Estimates based on day 1 dietary recalls from WWEIA, NHANES 2009 2010.

Tuso PJ, Ismail MH, Ha BP, Bartolotto C. Nutritional update for physicians: plant-based diets.
Perm J. 2013;17(2):61-66.

Food Planet Health. Eatforum.org. Published 2020. Accessed June 4. 2020

FIGURE 29-1 • The ACLM dietary position statement and the spectrum of dietary patterns from a standard American diet to a
predominantly whole food, plant-based dietary pattern.
(**Source:** Reproduced with permission from Tuso PJ, Ismail MH, Ha BP, Bartolotto C. Nutritional update for physicians: plant-based
diets. *American College of Lifestyle Medicine*. 2013;17(2):61-66. Courtesy of American College of Lifestyle Medicine.)

**Question: How might his PCP help him to increase his
vegetable intake?**

Foluke's presentation is consistent with metabolic syndrome.
Metabolic syndrome is classified as a group of conditions that
together increase risk of cardiovascular disease (CVD) and
related serious health problems. Criteria vary between organizations, but the most widely used, the National Cholesterol
Education Program ATP III guidelines, requires the presence of
three or more of the following criteria: abdominal obesity (waist
circumference ≥ 35 inches for women, ≥ 40 inches for men),
elevated fasting blood glucose (≥ 100 mg/dL), elevated BP
(≥ 130/85 mm Hg), elevated triglycerides (≥ 150 mg/dL), and/
or low HDL cholesterol (< 40 for men, < 50 for women).[20]

Foluke is at elevated risk of developing atherosclerotic CVD
and T2D. It is important for the PCP to confirm this and to
express that they're glad he is interested in making dietary
changes to improve his health. The PCP validates that diets
that move along the Dietary Spectrum from a highly processed
to a less processed diet rich in whole plant foods, along with
addressing other lifestyle factors, can reduce risk of developing these conditions and potentially improve his current risk

factors including HTN, dyslipidemia, elevated fasting glucose,
and abdominal obesity.

One can move along the Dietary Spectrum by making
changes aimed at following several evidence-based healthful
dietary patterns including the DASH, Healthy Mediterranean,
Whole Food Plant-based (WFPB), and others.[19] (See Chapter 6,
"Popular Diets" and Chapter 9, "Healthy and Sustainable Diets"
for more details about these diets and the evidence to support
them.) Foluke was referred to a group visit with the clinic's registered dietitian nutritionist (RDN) who reviewed these diets
and their potential health benefits. Once any knowledge gaps
about what a healthful diet consists of are addressed, then the
more challenging work begins—addressing barriers the patient
faces in making dietary behavior changes.

In a follow-up visit with his PCP, Foluke acknowledged the
need to increase his intake of plant foods for the treatment of
metabolic syndrome as well as prevention of T2D and other
CVD outcomes. When given a choice, he feels more satiated
with subs and pizza over salad. He also enjoys the flavor of
these foods and finds them convenient to pick up on his way
home from work. Additionally, he wonders about the cost of

eating more whole foods as he has heard that they are very expensive.

His PCP acknowledges these are barriers to making dietary changes that many patients face. Then, they explain the CM group visit models including Sharing Medical Appointments (SMAs) offered in the clinic on a regular basis. (See Chapter 30, "Nutrition Counseling with Group Visits" for more on this topic.) The PCP describes how they see a group of patients at once—either in person or by virtual visit—and cook together to show how to make eating a wide variety of foods in the recommended dietary patterns in ways that are delicious, quick, and affordable. The PCP explains that by joining in-person sessions using a pop-up teaching kitchen set up in a conference room in the clinic, they can taste the items prepared together as a group. Or, if joining by virtual visit, he would be provided with recipes and a grocery list ahead of time and could purchase the ingredients and cook along in his own kitchen or even join during a break from work to watch the session as a demonstration. Then, he could try preparing any items he finds intriguing on his own.

He is open to considering the CM group visit model in person or virtual option. He feels the virtual option will allow him to join without taking too much time off work. He admits little experience in the kitchen, having grown up with his grandmother doing the family's cooking. He doesn't feel confident or efficient in the kitchen and these have been major barriers to cooking.

Now that Foluke understands the risks associated with HTN, prediabetes, abdominal obesity, and dyslipidemia, and has learned how healthy diet and other lifestyle changes can improve, and in some cases reverse, these conditions, he is very motivated to learn ways to implement these changes in his life. He wants to enjoy the food he prepares at home more and learn some new cooking skills. His PCP congratulates him on taking the first steps to improve his health and looks forward to hearing how the CM group visits unfold. This case will be continued in Chapter 30, "Nutrition Counseling with Group Visits."

Case 2

Camilla is a 32-year-old (pronouns she, her, hers) from the Dominican Republic who presents to her PCP for an annual wellness visit. She is 30 weeks' pregnant and has been diagnosed with gestational diabetes mellitus (GDM). She acknowledges that she has gained a lot of weight. She worries her risk of developing T2D has increased and is looking for advice on how to best prevent developing T2D. She also has a 3-year-old whose eating habits she would like to improve to put them on a healthier trajectory.

Pregnancy is a relatively insulin-resistant state. However, when insulin resistance is too great, GDM can develop. This is sometimes due to excess weight gain in pregnancy. Gestational diabetes is associated with nine times the risk of developing T2D in the future. Lifestyle changes—such as improving dietary quality and increasing physical activity—are imperative to reducing the risk of developing T2D as well as other negative outcomes for mother and baby, such as preterm birth,[21] preeclampsia,[22] need for Cesarean section,[23] and long-term health risks of metabolic disease.[24]

The PCP completes a brief dietary assessment with Camilla. She tells her PCP that she primarily eats a traditional Dominican diet. She grew up eating white rice with every meal. Her dinner yesterday was no exception. Half her plate was filled with white rice and 1/3 of the plate with meat. Sometimes they eat vegetables as well, but not yesterday. She worries she will be hungry if she cuts back on her portion of rice. For other meals, she will have her son's leftovers. Yesterday, her lunch consisted of his leftover macaroni and cheese with hot dogs.

The PCP asks about outside meals, sugar-sweetened beverages (SSBs), and juices. Camilla reports that she works full time and often doesn't have time to cook. So, she orders in Dominican food two to three times a week. She drinks water with her meals, but her son has juice with at least two meals daily.

Question: How can the PCP effectively counsel Camilla to reduce her reliance on foods prepared outside the home and increase the number of meals prepared at home?

People who cook at home more often have higher-quality diets, consume fewer calories (including overall calories and calories from carbohydrates, fat, and sugar), consume fewer calories away from home, eat less fast food, spend less money on food, and have less weight gain over time than those who dine out and eat prepared foods on a regular basis.[25] Sharing the Healthy Eating Plate from the Nutrition Source website by the Harvard TH Chan School of Public Health is a useful guide for creating healthy, balanced meals (Figure 29-2).

Camilla learned that ½ of her plate should be produce, aiming to incorporate different colors and variety whenever possible. When discussing the whole grains section, the PCP highlights the benefits of whole grains over refined grains, including increased satiety, reduced impact on blood sugar, and higher fiber content. Her PCP discusses that both changes—increasing produce and switching to whole grains from processed grains—increase fiber in the diet which can improve satiety, cholesterol levels, foster a healthy microbiome, keep bowel movements regular, reduce risk of metabolic disease, and help maintain a healthy weight, among many other benefits. They discuss specifically how this can improve insulin sensitivity and glucose tolerance[26]—key concerns in the setting of her diagnosis of GDM. A balanced plate also includes a healthy source of protein. There is often a misconception that one must eat animal products to meet protein requirements. The PCP and Camilla discuss beans—staples in the Dominican diet—are versatile and healthy protein sources that also have some of the benefits of vegetables. Incorporating more beans and reducing meat portions would be a great way to increase fiber in her diet in a familiar way. Of the available protein options, her PCP explains that the plant-based (e.g., beans and nuts) and lean protein (e.g., poultry, fish, and seafood) options are best for health and that reducing red and processed meat (e.g., bacon and sausage) can have additional health benefits. Regularly eating even small amounts of red meat and processed red meat is associated with increased risk of heart disease, stroke, CVD and overall morbidity, whereas replacing these with beans, soy foods, nuts, fish, and poultry reduces these risks.[27-29]

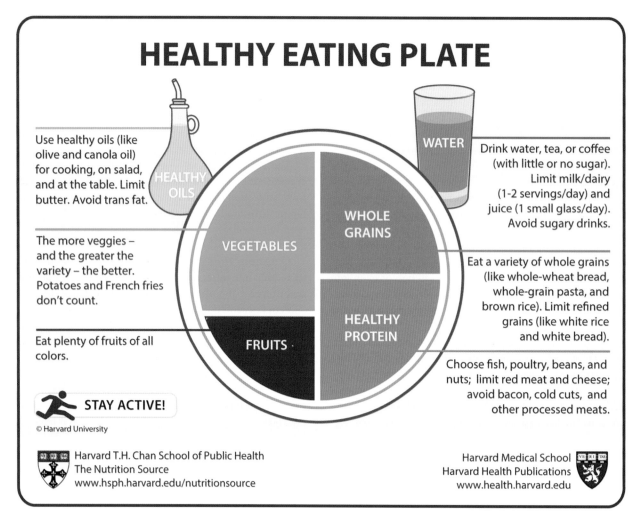

FIGURE 29-2 · Harvard healthy plate
(**Source:** https://www.hsph.harvard.edu/nutritionsource/wp-content/uploads/sites/30/2012/09/HEPJan2015.jpg.)

She has also heard that high protein diets may be good for reducing diabetes risk and wonders if adding more plant foods to her diet will be bad for her. The PCP reassures her that plant-predominant diets are associated with decreased risk of developing T2D across all age and sex categories.[30] In addition to higher red and processed meat consumption being associated with an increased risk of diabetes, those that increased consumption above their usual level (e.g., to follow a high-protein diet, for example, had a 50% increased risk over the following 4 years of developing diabetes.[31]

Finally, her PCP advises against the excessive use of oils, which are high in calorie density. Foods high in calorie density are those with a relatively high number of calories in a relatively small volume, whereas foods low in calorie density are those with a relatively low number of calories in a relatively large volume of food. Calorie density typically negatively correlates with water and fiber content, whereas fat content is positively correlated with calorie density. [Refer to Culinary Medicine Curriculum E-Book (2) for Table on Categories of foods that are low, moderate, and high in calorie density.] Reducing the quantity of high calorie density items and increasing the amount of low and moderate calorie density foods helps one to

feel satiated with fewer calories. This means avoiding pan- or deep-frying foods and instead using oils liquid at room temperature, which are more heart-healthy than solid fats, and using just what is needed to cook food using healthier cooking methods such as steaming, sauteing, simmering, braising, roasting, or baking.

This is a lot of information for one day, but Camilla agrees that these changes are important. She is not sure how well she will do trying to work more cooking into her schedule but would like to try what she's learned. Her PCP agrees on a plan for her to try working to shift her plate to be more like the portions and foods on the Healthy Eating Plate and offers her a follow-up appointment in 1 month.

One month later, at Camilla's follow-up visit with her PCP, she reports being pleased with her progress. She has started cooking one to two times per week following the Healthy Eating Plate proportions. She found the ideas she got from community cooking classes (recommended by her PCP) especially helpful. On the days she cooks, she reports less evening snacking and more energy. Her weight is not going up as quickly as during prior weeks but is still increasing faster than her obstetrician recommends. She still struggles to find time to cook at home, but is motivated to do it. Additionally, the main dietary change she is struggling with is replacing white rice with a whole-grain option like brown rice or quinoa.

On subsequent visits, Camilla reports being pleased with improving her cooking skills and is motivated to try brown rice. Her PCP shares with her that some patients find it an acquired taste which can be facilitated by mixing brown and white rice in varying proportions, increasing the proportion of brown rice over time, until they are able to enjoy 100% brown rice. For optimal flavor, she recommends making separate batches of brown and white and mixing after cooking. However, for ease in the kitchen, they can be cooked together, but the brown rice takes longer to cook and should be used to judge when the dish is appropriately cooked. Batch cooking whole grains, portioning, and freezing is a cost-effective and time-saving strategy to keep nearly instant whole grains on hand for busy weeknight meals.

Camilla also started to include her toddler in food preparation tasks. Encouraging children with age-appropriate kitchen tasks from meal planning to preparation has been shown to encourage lifelong healthy eating habits. Children are more likely to try foods they help prepare. Try to incorporate fun in the process (e.g., arranging a variety of vegetables on a platter and allowing the child to use these items to decorate their meal). We also know that home cooking has benefits beyond improving nutrition quality and reducing cost. It helps families connect with one another. Parental dietary behaviors are among the most important factors in establishing or changing children's eating habits.[32]

Finally, the PCP discusses with Camilla the importance of limiting or avoiding SSBs and juices. They explain that SSBs are associated with increased risk of weight gain and childhood obesity.[33] Additionally, these processed, high-sugar drinks lead to sharp increases, followed by crashes, in blood sugar which promotes cravings for high-carbohydrate foods and drinks and increases appetite. The PCP circles back to the Healthy Eating Plate, recommending that calories come primarily from whole and minimally processed foods. Water should be the primary beverage but recommended amounts of dairy or plant-based milks (varies by age and gender, avoid those with added sugars) to meet calcium needs can also be included. Camilla is also interested in CM group visits and will join them after her baby is born. Her story will continue in Chapter 30, "Nutrition Counseling with Group Visits."

Case 3

A healthy, 19-year-old (pronouns he, him, his) Caucasian student (Damian) with a family history of CAD comes into his PCPs office for an annual exam. He reports a desire to optimize his performance in academics and athletics and prevent CAD and other chronic diseases. He is single and does not cook, citing barriers of time and the expense of healthy foods. He has mostly been eating frozen meals and fast food, with a preference for burritos, burgers, and fries.

As part of his annual visit, he is screened for food insecurity with the Hunger Vital Sign.[34] Food insecurity is highly prevalent in the United States and elsewhere. See Chapter 4, "Food Insecurity," for more details on the validated screening questionnaire.

Question: How can the clinician help this patient to reduce their reliance on prepared and fast food and increase home cooking to improve dietary quality?

Damian's PCP explores his current lifestyle, culinary knowledge and skills, and addresses the positive food insecurity screen. The PCP provides the following resources: contact information to the local food bank system (which can help sign patients up for applicable government resources, such as SNAP, WIC, etc.), the web address to the Feeding America where one can enter their zip code and find nearby free food resources, a prescription to a local food pharmacy that provides a free, biweekly food box containing vegetables, fruits, whole grain items, and lean proteins, and a Healthy Eating on a Budget handout (see Table 29-1) filled with tips to save money when food shopping or eating out. Additionally, the PCP contacted the local food bank, who delivers print materials for their medical office (including business cards with food resource information, prescription pads for food resources, and flyers about free food options).

On further discussion with Damian, his PCP learns that he would like to improve his diet and would consider cooking at home if healthy foods were available and quick to prepare. His PCP inquires about whether Damian has any prior experience with meal preparation. Damian recalls cooking a vegetable curry recipe he found online. However, he is reluctant to cook this again because the long, expensive list of ingredients is filled with spices he won't use again. In addition, the recipe required multiple steps which he found too time consuming for the preparation of a single meal.

The PCP recommends saving time by stocking his kitchen with some basic, healthy staples needed frequently in the meal preparation, which will also aid the efficiency and cost of home cooking. They discuss whole grains and legumes being some of the least expensive foods, despite being rich in fiber, protein, vitamins, and minerals. Finally, the PCP reviews how to "bulk up" prepared items with more healthful ingredients (e.g., adding fresh or frozen vegetables) to improve the overall quality of a meal with very little added time. In terms of Damian's current health status and future risk factors for CAD, his BP is borderline. His PCP discusses that his current diet high in fast and prepared foods is very high in sodium and may be increasing his BP. Preparing more meals at home; incorporating more herbs, spices, and other salt-free ingredients to flavor food in lieu of salt and other high-sodium condiments; and increasing produce intake could help decrease his blood pressure to the normal range and help prevent the development of HTN, a key contributor to heart disease.

Damian's PCP explains that he does not have to follow recipes exactly nor purchase multiple spices he may not use again. His PCP also shares a handout about meal ideas for plant-based eating on a budget. Many suggestions for eating healthy and shopping on a budget are shared in Table 29-1. The PCP reviews resources with Damian and he is surprised to learn that a serving of potato chickpea curry could cost him less than $2.00. In addition to supporting his health goals, this is far less expensive than his go-to freezer meals and fast food.

TABLE 29-1 • Shopping for healthy food on a budget

Tips for shopping healthy on a budget:

- Buy in bulk if you're able to. If you won't go through the food in time, try to find others to split the food and cost with.
- Don't buy prepared foods.
- Find the time and learn the skills needed to cook. The more you cook, the healthier you'll eat and the less money you'll spend.
- Don't pay for beverages. Water is the healthiest drink and most tap water is safe and free.
- If you do purchase beverages, stick with coffee and tea that you make at home. These healthy options are naturally sugar-free and nearly calorie-free.
- Meat is expensive—eating less can save you $$ and improve your health. Opt for plant-based proteins more often.
- Dairy can be very expensive—stick with 2 servings per day (or other calcium-rich, non-dairy alternatives).
- Look for sales and in-season items to find deals on produce.
- Go to farmer's markets and get "seconds". These are items that either need to be used quickly to prevent spoiling or that have an imperfect appearance, but still taste good.
- If using CalFresh/SNAP, you can double your dollars at the main market stand at many farmer's markets.
- Food banks in some areas offer locations and services with healthy food options (see details at end of handout).
- Look for grocery stores in your area that carry produce that has limited shelf-life remaining to find steep discounts.
- Avoid canned fruit—it's often more expensive than fresh or frozen by weight and packed in juice or sugary syrup that adds empty calories. If you do buy it, get packed in juice; avoid those with syrups.
- Avoid empty calories like white bread, cakes, cookies, other items that are highly-processed and filled with white flour and added sugars because these are unhealthy, lead to food cravings, and have limited nutritional value beyond extra calories.
- Use oils instead of butter when cooking.
- Avoid food waste-Know what fresh items you have and make a plan to use or freeze them.
- Use water instead of stock in recipes or make your own stock from vegetables scraps and/or bones.

What to buy:

• Grains/Starches: • Brown Rice • Quinoa • Old-fashioned Oatmeal • Steel-cut oats • Polenta • Any other whole grains that you buy to cook yourself • Whole wheat couscous • Sprouted grain bread (keep frozen) • Whole wheat pitas	• 100% whole wheat bread • Corn tortillas (keep in fridge) • Frozen whole-wheat pizza dough (or make your own!) • Whole wheat (or other whole grain) pasta • Whole grain flours for baking • Other baking dry good ingredients like baking powder, soda, sugar, etc.

Proteins:

• Dried beans • Dried lentils • Canned beans • Eggs • Nuts & seeds (store in freezer to prevent spoiling if not using within a few weeks) • Frozen edamame • Tofu	• Tempeh • Canned fish • Bulk sales on chicken, turkey, or meat (freeze what you can't use right away) • Frozen cooked shrimp (smaller sized shrimp are cheaper) • Frozen fish fillets (look for sales or bulk)

Fruit:

• Frozen fruit (avoid those in syrup) • Apples • Pears • Oranges and other citrus fruit • Lemons/Limes • Bananas (peel and freeze if they start to brown—these are great for smoothies, baking, and frozen desserts)	• Watermelon and other melons • Kiwi • Grapes • Pineapple • Dried fruit (avoid those with added sugar) • Anything on sale or in-season

TABLE 29-1 • Shopping for healthy food on a budget (*Continued*)

Veggies:

• Carrots • Cucumbers • Zucchini • Summer squash • Sweet potatoes • White or yellow potatoes • Beets or other root veggies • Cabbage • Winter squash • Frozen corn • Frozen peas	• Frozen spinach • Fresh baby spinach—can often get a large package inexpensively • Romaine or leaf lettuce (when stored properly, lasts much longer than spring mix) • Canned tomatoes (Whole, diced, crushed—look for low- or no-sodium added) • Canned or jarred tomato sauce • Anything on sale and in-season • Many other veggies spoil quickly or don't taste great when cooked from frozen. Buy just what you need each week and include at least one fresh veggie with every meal, if possible

Dairy/Dairy alternatives:

• Greek yogurt, unsweetened
• Low-fat, 1%, or 2% milk (avoid flavored or sweetened varieties)
• Soy or non-dairy milk, unsweetened (soy has the most protein and is most similar to dairy milk in nutrients)
• Parmesan or another hard cheese for flavoring—a little goes a long way
• Unsalted butter or butter alternative (avoid those with "hydrogenated" ingredients), limited quantities
• Block of real cheese (shred your own if needed, avoid processed styles like American), limited quantities

More seasonings/flavoring items/condiments:

• Canola oil • Olive oil • Toasted sesame oil • Dijon mustard or other mustards • Salsa • Nut butters • Tahini • Honey • Flaxseed (ground) or chia seed (whole)	• Low-sodium soy sauce or tamari • Pure vanilla extract • Vinegars (Red wine, apple cider, rice wine, white wine, etc.) • Nutritional yeast (for vegans/vegetarians) • Coconut milk (avoid low-fat, get full-fat and use less to reduce calories and maintain taste) • Chili paste or sauce (e.g., Sriracha, chili garlic sauce, etc.) to spice up your food

Sweets:

• Dark chocolate (at least 70%)

Some Super Basic herbs and spices (see World Flavors—Herbs & Spices for an expanded list):

• Bay leaves • Cayenne pepper, ground • Chili powder • Cinnamon, ground • Coriander, ground • Crushed red pepper • Cumin, ground or whole seeds • Curry powder	• Ginger, ground • Italian seasoning • Nutmeg, whole or ground • Oregano • Paprika • Rosemary • Thyme • Get whatever you like!

Second Harvest Food Bank offers free, healthy food to anyone who needs it and is referred from a medical clinic. Call, text, or email Second Harvest Food Bank at the numbers/addresses below and tell them your doctor referred you.

• Call (Weekdays 8am to 5pm) 1-800-984-3663
• Text "HEALTH" to 1-408-455-5181
• Email: food@shfb.org
• Learn more online: SHFB.org/getfood

Source: Michelle Hauser owns the copyright.

Counseling patients on adopting healthier diets requires not only an understanding of culture, nutrition, and cooking skills but also of how economic barriers contribute to the underconsumption of healthy foods. A key step when working with patients is to acknowledge cost as a barrier to healthy eating and discuss individual concerns and limitations with patients when introducing steps toward a healthier eating pattern which is rich in whole plant foods. Discussing the process of dietary behavior change as moving along a spectrum toward a healthier diet is particularly useful in working with those of limited means and other barriers because it acknowledges the varying levels of difficulty that people face in making dietary changes, encourages changes of any size, and acknowledges any step toward healthier lifestyle as positive and beneficial.[2] In addressing social determinants of health, such as food insecurity, it is important to recognize the large impact that unmet needs have on health outcomes. Make sure to identify resources to address common unmet needs. Have educational materials and contact information on hand (in multiple languages, if needed) to provide to patients during counseling. More information on Damian and his journey will be shared in Chapter 30, "Nutrition Counseling with Group Visits."

PART 3: TEACHING KITCHENS—THE GOLD STANDARD OF CULINARY MEDICINE EDUCATION: HISTORY, CONCEPTUAL ORIGINS, AND CORE EDUCATIONAL COMPONENTS

Teaching kitchens (TKs) are where CM shines. The conceptual origins of modern-day TKs relate to fundamental teachings from traditional Chinese medical texts. Specifically, in the traditional Chinese medical classic, *The Yellow Emperor's Classic of Internal Medicine*,[35] there are two core tenants. These are that prevention is always superior to intervention and the way we eat, move, and think impacts our health and determines our recuperative capacity.

Modern-day TKs have evolved as a reflection and reinterpretation of these long-standing principles. Teaching kitchens typically include (a) nutrition education based on the latest science; (b) hands-on culinary instruction to teach trainees (health professionals and patients) the culinary skills to prepare healthy, delicious, easy-to-make, affordable, sustainable recipes and meals; and (c) strategies to encourage sustained behavior change, informed by motivational interviewing and health coaching.[36] Additionally, many teaching kitchens also incorporate lessons on other lifestyle topics (e.g., such as the importance of physical activity).

History and Examples of Culinary Medicine and Teaching Kitchens in All Levels of Medical Education (and beyond)

Examples of CM can increasingly be found at all levels of health professional education. These courses or sessions are often aimed both at helping the clinician improve their own diet and learning to help patients improve theirs. The first elective course incorporating both nutrition and cooking in a U.S. medical school was taught in 2003 by physician-chef John La Puma and colleagues at the State University of New York-Upstate campus. The first continuing medical education conference (Healthy Kitchens, Healthy Lives [HKHL]) focused on CM was held in 2007, spearheaded by David Eisenberg, one of the authors and then–associate professor of medicine at Harvard Medical School, in collaboration with the Culinary Institute of America in St. Helena, California. In 2014, physician-chef Rani Polak developed the Culinary Health Education Fundamentals (CHEF) Coaching program for clinicians to use in telemedicine to improve nutrition by combining culinary training and health coaching principles. The first permanent TK established in a medical school was at the Goldring Center for Culinary Medicine (GCCM) at Tulane University School of Medicine in 2012, led by physician-chef Timothy Harlan. The GCCM curriculum has been licensed to over 30 medical schools across the United States.[37] In 2018, Dr. Harlan and his team developed the first Culinary Medicine Specialist Certification for clinicians interested in a designation that, "identifies clinicians who have a unique foundation for incorporating healthy eating into patients' diets".[38] In 2019, physician-chef Michelle Hauser, clinical associate professor at Stanford University School of Medicine, along with the American College of Lifestyle Medicine, published the first open-source CM curriculum (CMC).[2] This CMC is based on the popular elective course for medical and physician assistant students at Stanford. A key goal of publishing the CMC was to reduce barriers for those interested in starting CM courses by making the information needed to do so freely available to everyone. To date, the CMC has been downloaded by thousands of health professionals in over 100 countries.

Given the continued growth in diet-related disease and the limited nutrition education historically offered in health professional training programs, the demand for and availability of CM courses is rapidly expanding. Health professionals in a variety of fields who are trained in CM offer courses in clinical, university, community, and workplace settings. These courses are diverse in their organization, duration, format, type of instructor(s), location, and dietary strategy employed. Many teaching the sessions modify content or curricula from sources mentioned above to best meet the needs of their learners. All manner of pop-up, mixed-use, and stand-alone TKs are used for the sessions. For items needed to create a pop-up TK, refer to Table 29-2.

The Teaching Kitchen Collaborative (TKC) was established in 2014 as an offshoot of the HKHL conference. It is an invitational collaborative which currently includes dozens of institutional members with TKs across the United States, Canada, Italy, Germany, and Japan. Members include hospitals, medical schools, healthcare delivery systems, grade schools, colleges, universities, corporations, YMCAs, Veterans Affairs hospitals, public libraries, and botanical gardens. Key goals of the TKC are to develop TK best practices and create a research network to evaluate the impact of TK-related programs across various

TABLE 29-2 • Example portable pop-up teaching kitchen equipment list (from hauser cmc, appendix 2)

The following example works for 12 participants working in 6 groups, plus an instructor demo station.
- Make sure as many items as possible are NSF-rated and dishwasher safe.
- Must wash items in commercial dishwasher or 3-compartment sink per Serve-Safe Sanitation protocol

Checklist of items (most items can be stored in the tubs listed):
- Folding cart that can hold at least 2–3 storage bins
- Bungee cords long enough to connect to cart and wrap all the way around the storage bins to secure them to the cart for safe transport
- 12- to 18-gallon storage bins (4–6)
- Bus tubs for dirty dishes (2–4)
- Broom, dustpan, mop/Swiffer WetJet or Wet + Dry
- Paper towels
- Disinfectant wipes
- Hand sanitizer (2–3 bottles)
- Gloves, medium and large sizes (non-latex)
- Mini first aid kit: gloves, Band-Aids, finger cots, cleansing wipes, burn cream, hair ties for anyone with long hair)
- Paper salad plates or 5–8 oz disposable cups for tasting-sized servings
- 10-in disposable plates and disposable bowls if having meal-sized servings
- Disposable cups for meals (or ask participants to bring their own water bottles)
- Containers or heavy-duty Ziplock bags for leftovers to take away
- Plastic wrap
- Parchment paper
- Aluminum foil
- Utensils for tasting (spoons, forks, butter knives, as needed)
- Tasting spoons (to use while cooking)
- Garbage bags
- Induction burners—7 for hot items if everyone cooks, or just 1 if only demonstrating hot items
- Can opener
- Assorted mixing bowls (0.75, 1.5, 3, 5, 8 qt sizes are useful but not all are needed for each kit; aim for 1 larger and 1 smaller mixing bowl per kit)
- 12″ × 18″ cutting boards (7)
- Non-slip mats for cutting boards (7)
- 8″ chef's knives (7)
- 8″ knife blade guards (7)
- 3-1/2″ or 4″ paring knives (7)
- 4″ knife blade guards (7)
- 10–12″ high heat silicone spatulas (7)
- 11–13″ basting spoons (7)
- 11–13″ slotted basting spoons (7)
- 10–12″ stainless-steel piano whisks/whips (7)
- 12″ stainless-steel tongs (7)
- Ladles (2-3)
- 11–14″ high-heat nylon turner (or stainless steel with temperature safe handle) (7)
- 4-piece measuring cup set (1-cup, ½ cup, 1/3 cup, ¼ cup) (7)
- 4-piece measuring spoon set (1 tbsp, 1 tsp, ½ tsp, ¼ tsp) (7)
- 9″ heavy-duty stainless steel, 4-sided box grater (2–3)
- Bowl/bench scrapers (7)
- Vegetable peelers, Y-style or swivel (stainless-steel blades) (7)
- ~8″ Fine mesh strainers (2–3)
- 2- or 3-quart saucepans with lids (must work with induction burners) (7)
- 10–12″ sauté pans (7)
- 6- or 8-quart stockpots with lids (generally only for pasta) (2)
- Salad spinner (1–2)
- Food processor
- Blender
- Aprons (1/participant, generally 14 for 12 students + 2 instructors)
- Kitchen towels (14, 2 per station including instructor station)

(Continued)

TABLE 29-2 • Example portable pop-up teaching kitchen equipment list (from hauser cmc, appendix 2) *(Continued)*
Optional, Nice to have items
• Oven
• Sheet pans
• Parchment paper (for sheet pans/baking)
• Wine opener, optional (if needing to open corked items)
• Steel (for knives)
• Knife sharpener (for upkeep of knives, allows use of inexpensive knives)
• Electric grill/griddle–can be used in the roasting class to teach how to grill in lieu of roasting if no ovens are available in the kitchen/teaching space you plan to use.

Reproduced with permission from Hauser ME. *Culinary Medicine Curriculum.* St. Louis, MO: American College of Lifestyle Medicine; 2019.

settings and populations. Additionally, since many TKC members are involved with the education of medical students and practicing health professionals, the TKC has embarked on efforts to co-create educational materials and resources for medical students, residents, fellows, and practicing clinicians. The article, "Perspective: Teaching Kitchens: Conceptual Origins, Applications and Potential for Impact within Food Is Medicine," describes how TK can be used as educational classrooms and translational research labs.[39]

Culinary Medicine and Teaching Kitchen Research

In PubMed, a search for "cooking" AND "health," filtered by clinical trials and randomized controlled clinical trials on humans in English returned 527 related studies [date of search August 14, 2022], the vast majority of which are from the past decade. These studies covered the entire life span from pregnancy and breastfed infants to older adults, included pop-up and permanent TKs, demonstration, and hands-on sessions; virtual, in person, and hybrid instruction; as well as other forms of teaching cooking skills alongside nutrition and behavior change. The studies looked at an array of common health outcomes, quality of life, behaviors, and more. As more evidence emerges in the field, it is likely that aspects of CM will become more differentiated and firmly defined.

There have been several clinical studies[40–42] evaluating the impact of teaching kitchens. One involved the impact of a TK curriculum on employees (n = 39) of a self-insured educational institution.[40] Another involved patients (n = 72) with increased CVD risk[41]; a third involved patients with CVD (n = 429).[42] These studies documented improvements in weight, BP, lipids, and/or glycemic control in response to educational interventions which mirror the core concepts of TKs and include nutrition education, culinary instruction, mindfulness, and behavior change strategies along with other behavioral lifestyle interventions. In addition, there have been studies that reported a positive association of hands-on culinary instruction in combination with nutrition education on the knowledge and dietary pattern counseling competency of medical students[43,44] and medical trainees,[44] as well as the beneficial effects a medical school-based TK program had on cardiometabolic biomarkers in patients with T2D[45] and diet quality.[46]

Variations in the Design of Teaching Kitchens and the Future of Culinary Medicine

Recent publications have summarized the spectrum of existing TK designs, including those that offer culinary demonstrations only; those offering both demonstrations and hands-on culinary instruction; those involving built-in kitchens, portable (i.e., "pop-up") facilities; those offering instruction in-person only; those providing virtual, interactive training only; and TKs capable of providing both in-person and virtual, interactive classes.[2,36] The TKC also offers descriptions of different styles of teaching kitchens along with example photos on their website.

One method proposed to expand teaching kitchens in healthcare settings has been to incorporate them into new or existing cafeterias (aka, production kitchens with adjacent dining areas).[2,36] This method, also called a *mixed-use space*, addresses some common barriers to installing teaching kitchens, including space constraints, various associated costs, and staffing. This is because the production kitchen and dining areas can be used as a cafeteria when most lucrative for point-of-sale purchases. Teaching occurs during times the kitchen is not in use or when there is excess capacity. This allows the space and equipment to be maximized for two purposes, with less down time than either a cafeteria or teaching kitchen alone. Also, TKs tend to cost more, with less influx of money than a cafeteria or other dining establishment. Therefore, this is an especially good option when in high cost-of-living areas where space is at a premium and having a stand-alone TK may be cost prohibitive.

In this way, future TKs based in cafeterias (e.g., of hospitals, universities, office buildings, etc.) could be used to train medical and other health professional students, medical staff, residents, fellows, patients (some of whom may agree to participate in controlled clinical trials), employees of the hospital, as well as community-based populations. Moreover, a TK in a hospital cafeteria could also showcase healthy, delicious, affordable foods. These delicious, healthy foods could also be made available as part of the hospital's inpatient, on-demand, dining program. This is in stark contrast to many hospitals that have fast-food restaurants and serve food items associated with many of the diseases they are treating.

SUMMARY

Culinary medicine (CM) is a new field that builds on centuries-old principles of preparing, sharing, and enjoying nutritious and delicious meals. A goal of CM is to help patients prevent and treat chronic conditions in their own kitchens in a way that is practical and joyful. Clinicians can use their clinic visits to explore barriers to cooking and empower patients to adopt home cooking practices. Culinary medicine in 1:1 traditional clinic visits includes taking a dietary history, assessing food access, gleaning information on cultural aspects of diet, engaging in motivational interviewing around making healthy dietary changes, and counseling on how to prepare and otherwise acquire and eat foods that are healthy, delicious, and meet the time, budget, and skills available to an individual patient. With CM, clinicians can be instrumental in teaching patients that healthy food can be tasty, fast, and inexpensive once they feel confident about meal planning and cooking. Teaching kitchens are places to successfully engage in CM with patients, especially in groups. They have a long history and are growing in popularity. There is a wide array of options for teaching kitchens including built-in kitchens, portable or pop-up facilities, and virtual teaching kitchens. The spaces used for cooking, experimenting, teaching, learning, and creating appetizing meals provide opportunities to make the process of preparing food delightful and inspiring. The more clinicians can encourage and empower patients to cook nutritious and delicious meals for themselves and their families, the healthier they will be.

TAKE-HOME POINTS

1. Culinary medicine is an effective method to address key barriers to dietary behavior change by teaching that healthy food can be tasty, fast, and inexpensive if you know how to cook and meal plan.

2. In using a CM approach to dietary behavior change, one aims to engage patients in shared solution development, decision making, knowledge acquisition, and skill building. This can be done in a variety of settings, including teaching kitchens, traditional (1:1) clinic appointments or group visits (covered in Chapter 30, "Nutrition Counseling with Group Visits"), and community and other educational settings.

3. Counseling patients on adopting healthier diets requires not only an understanding of culture, nutrition, and cooking skills, but also an understanding of how economic barriers contribute to the underconsumption of healthy foods.

4. Teaching kitchens typically teach (a) nutrition based on the latest science; (b) hands-on culinary instruction to teach trainees culinary skills needed to prepare healthy, delicious, easy-to-make, affordable, sustainable recipes and meals; and (c) strategies to encourage sustained behavior change, informed by motivational interviewing and health coaching.

CASE STUDY ANSWERS

1. **B**; Key components of CM include practical nutrition education, cooking skills, behavior change and related motivational interviewing, counseling, and coaching. Using a CM approach to dietary behavior change, one aims to engage patients to identify barriers and facilitators of behavior change and engage in shared solution development, decision making, knowledge acquisition, and skill building. Answer b offers advice without first gathering information, which is not in keeping with the CM approach.

2. **"False."** This statement is incorrect because one does not need to eliminate all processed foods when shifting toward a predominantly whole food, plant-based (WFPB) diet. Many patients engage in "all-or-nothing" dieting. When engaging in dietary behavior change counseling or coaching, it's important to emphasize the sustainability of dietary practices.

3. **C**; While there are affordable ways to acquire produce and ways to prepare it that are delicious and filling, this information is not always well known. The calorie density of nonstarchy vegetables is much lower than other foods; if preparing a plate of nonstarchy vegetables without the addition of items with more calories (such as starchy vegetables, whole grains, nuts, or seeds), the low number of calories consumed can leave one hungry again soon after eating. This is not due to vegetables being unsatisfying, but rather eating an inappropriately low-calorie dish for the situation. On the other hand, when a meal is appropriately put together, vegetables ADD TO satiety by adding fiber to a meal.

REFERENCES

1. La Puma J. What is culinary medicine and what does it do? *Popul Health Manag.* 2016;19:1-3.

2. Hauser ME. *Culinary Medicine Curriculum.* St. Louis, MO: American College of Lifestyle Medicine; 2019. www.lifestyle-medicine.org/culinary-medicine.

3. Hauser ME. Culinary medicine basics and applications in medical education in the U.S. In: Black MM, Delichatsios HK, Story MT, eds. *Nutrition Education: Strategies for Improving Nutrition and Healthy Eating in Individuals and Communities. Nestlé Nutr Inst Workshop Ser.* 2019;92:161-170. doi:10.1159/000499559.

4. National Research Council Committee on Nutrition in Medical Education. *Nutrition Education in U.S. Medical Schools.* National Academy Press; 1985.

5. Adams KM, Kohlmeier M, Zeisel SH. Nutrition education in U.S. medical schools: latest update of a national survey. *Acad Med.* 2010;85:1537-1542.

6. US Burden of Disease Collaborators; Mokdad AH, Ballestros K, et al. The state of US health, 1990-2016: burden of diseases, injuries, and risk factors among US States. *JAMA.* 2018;319:1444-1472.

7. Afshin A, Sur PJ, Fay KA, et al. Health effects of dietary risks in 195 countries, 1990–2017: a systematic analysis for the Global Burden of Disease Study 2017. *Lancet.* 2019;393(10184):1958-1972.

8. Flegal KM, Kruszon-Moran D, Carroll MD, Fryar CD, Ogden CL. Trends in obesity among adults in the United States, 2005 to 2014. *JAMA.* 2016;315(21):2284-2291.

9. Heron M. Deaths: leading causes for 2014. *Natl Vital Stat Rep.* 2016;65(5):1-96.

10. H.Res.1118 - 117th Congress (2021-2022): Expressing the sense of the House of Representatives that the United States recognizes the mounting personal and financial burden of diet-related disease in the United States and calls on medical schools, graduate medical education programs, and other health professional training programs to provide meaningful physician and health professional education on nutrition and diet. HR 1118, 117th Cong, (2022). Available at: https://www.congress.gov/bill/117th-congress/house-resolution/1118.

11. Zong G, Eisenberg DM, Hu FB, Sun Q. Consumption of meals prepared at home and risk of type 2 diabetes: an analysis of two prospective cohort studies. *PLoS Med.* 2016;13(7):e1002052.

12. Smith LP, Ng SW, Popkin BM. Trends in US home food preparation and consumption: analysis of national nutrition surveys and time use studies from 1965–1966 to 2007–2008. *Nutr J.* 2013;12. doi:10.1186/1475-2891-12-45.

13. Soliah LAL, Walter JM, Jones SA. Benefits and barriers to healthful eating: what are the consequences of decreased food preparation ability? *Am J Lifestyle Med.* 2012;6(2):152-158.

14. Lee-Kwan SH, Moore LV, Blanck HM, Harris DM, Galuska D. Disparities in state-specific adult fruit and vegetable consumption—United States, 2015. *MMWR Morb Mortal Wkly Rep.* 2017;66(45):1241-1247.

15. Kim SA, Moore LV, Galuska D, et al. Vital signs: fruit and vegetable intake among children—United States, 2003-2010. *MMWR Morb Mortal Wkly Rep.* 2014;63(31):671-676.

16. Gardner CD, Hauser ME. Food revolution. *Am J Lifestyle Med.* 2017;11(5):387-396.

17. U.S. Department of Health and Human Services and U.S. Department of Agriculture. 2015–2020 Dietary Guidelines for Americans. 8th Edition. December 2015. Available at: http://health.gov/dietaryguidelines/2015/guidelines/.

18. Fulgoni V 3rd, Drewnowski A. An economic gap between the recommended healthy food patterns and existing diets of minority groups in the US national health and nutrition examination survey 2013-14. *Front Nutr.* 2019;6:37.

19. Hauser ME, McMacken M, Lim A, Shetty P. Nutrition—an evidence-based, practical approach to chronic disease prevention and treatment. *J Fam Pract.* 2022;71(Suppl 1 Lifestyle):S5-S16.

20. Alberti KG, Eckel RH, Grundy SM, et al. Harmonizing the metabolic syndrome: a joint interim statement of the International Diabetes Federation Task Force on Epidemiology and Prevention; National Heart, Lung, and Blood Institute; American Heart Association; World Heart Federation; International Atherosclerosis Society; and International Association for the Study of Obesity. *Circulation.* 2009;120(16):1640-1645.

21. Zhu Y, Hedderson MM, Brown SD, et al. Healthy preconception and early-pregnancy lifestyle and risk of preterm birth: a prospective cohort study. *Am J Clin Nutr.* 2021;114(2):813-821.

22. Allen R, Rogozinska E, Sivarajasingam P, Khan KS, Thangaratinam S. Effect of diet- and lifestyle-based metabolic risk-modifying interventions on preeclampsia: a meta-analysis. *Acta Obstet Gynecol Scand.* 2014;93(10):973-985.

23. International Weight Management in Pregnancy (i-WIP) Collaborative Group. Effect of diet- and physical activity-based interventions in pregnancy on gestational weight gain and pregnancy outcomes: meta-analysis of individual participant data from randomised trials [published correction appears in BMJ. 2017 Aug 23;358:j3991]. *BMJ.* 2017;358:j3119.

24. Mourtakos SP, Tambalis KD, Panagiotakos DB, et al. Maternal lifestyle characteristics during pregnancy, and the risk of obesity in the offspring: a study of 5,125 children. *BMC Pregnancy Childbirth.* 2015;15:66.

25. Wolfson JA, Bleich SN. Is cooking at home associated with better diet quality or weight-loss intention? *Public Health Nutr.* 2015;18(8):1397-1406.

26. Alejandro EU, Mamerto TP, Chung G, et al. Gestational diabetes mellitus: a harbinger of the vicious cycle of diabetes. *Int J Mol Sci.* 2020;21(14):5003.

27. Bernstein AM, Sun Q, Hu FB, Stampfer MJ, Manson JE, Willett WC. Major dietary protein sources and risk of coronary heart disease in women. *Circulation.* 2010;122(9):876-883.

28. Pan A, Sun Q, Bernstein AM, et al. Red meat consumption and mortality: results from 2 prospective cohort studies. *Arch Intern Med.* 2012;172(7):555-563.

29. Bernstein AM, Pan A, Rexrode KM, et al. Dietary protein sources and the risk of stroke in men and women. *Stroke.* 2012;43(3):637-644.

30. McMacken M, Shah S. A plant-based diet for the prevention and treatment of type 2 diabetes. *J Geriatr Cardiol.* 2017;14(5):342-354.

31. Pan A, Sun Q, Bernstein AM, Manson JE, Willett WC, Hu FB. Changes in red meat consumption and subsequent risk of type 2 diabetes mellitus: three cohorts of US men and women. *JAMA Intern Med.* 2013;173(14):1328-1335.

32. Mahmood L, Flores-Barrantes P, Moreno LA, Manios Y, Gonzalez-Gil EM. The influence of parental dietary behaviors and practices on children's eating babits. *Nutrients.* 2021;13(4):1138.

33. Keller A, Bucher Della Torre S. Sugar-sweetened beverages and obesity among children and adolescents: a review of systematic literature reviews. *Child Obes.* 2015;11(4):338-346.

34. Hager ER, Quigg AM, Black MM, et al. Development and validity of a 2-item screen to identify families at risk for food insecurity. *Pediatrics*. 2010;126(1):e26-e32.

35. Barnes LL, Veith I. *The Yellow Emperor's Classic of Internal Medicine*. University of California Press; 2015.

36. Eisenberg DM, Imamura BEnvD A. Teaching kitchens in the learning and work environments: the future is now. *Glob Adv Health Med*. 2020;9:2164956120962442.

37. Durkin M. Setting a course for food as medicine. *ACP Internist*. June 1, 2018. Accessed July 24, 2023. Available at: https://acpinternist.org/archives/2018/06/setting-a-course-for-food-as-medicine.htm.

38. The Certified Culinary Medicine Specialist Program. CulinaryMedicine.org. April 14, 2023. Available at: https://culinary-medicine.org/certified-culinary-medicine-specialist-program/.

39. Eisenberg DM, Pacheco LS, McClure AC, McWhorter JW, Janisch K, Massa J. Perspective: teaching kitchens: conceptual origins, applications and potential for impact within food is medicine research. *Nutrients*. 2023;15(13):2859.

40. Eisenberg DM, Righter AC, Matthews B, Zhang W, Willett WC, Massa J. Feasibility pilot study of a teaching kitchen and self-care curriculum in a workplace setting. *Am J Lifestyle Med*. 2019;13(3):319-330.

41. Dasgupta K, Hajna S, Joseph L, Da Costa D, Christopoulos S, Gougeon R. Effects of meal preparation training on body weight, glycemia, and blood pressure: results of a phase 2 trial in type 2 diabetes. *Int J Behav Nutr Phys Act*. 2012;9:125.

42. Ricanati EH, Golubić M, Yang D, Saager L, Mascha EJ, Roizen MF. Mitigating preventable chronic disease: progress report of the Cleveland Clinic's Lifestyle 180 program. *Nutr Metab (Lond)*. 2011;8:83.

43. Leong B, Ren D, Monlezun D, Ly D, Sarris L, Harlan TS. Teaching third- and fourth-year medical students how to cook: an innovative approach to training students in lifestyle modification for chronic disease management. *Medical Science Educator*. 2014;24(1):43.

44. Monlezun DJ, Urday P, Baranwal P, et al. Cooking up better doctors as teachers globally: a novel integrated nutrition and cooking class curriculum for pediatric residents to boost their competencies and attitudes in patient counseling. *J Med Person*. 2014;13(2):125-128.

45. Razavi AC, Monlezun DJ, Sapin A, et al. Multisite culinary medicine curriculum is associated with cardioprotective dietary patterns and lifestyle medicine competencies among medical trainees [published correction appears in *Am J Lifestyle Med*. 2020 Mar 11;14(2):234]. *Am J Lifestyle Med*. 2020;14(2):225-233.

46. Stauber Z, Razavi AC, Sarris L, Harlan TS, Monlezun DJ. Multisite medical student-led community Culinary Medicine classes improve patients' diets: machine learning-augmented propensity score-adjusted fixed effects cohort analysis of 1381 subjects. *Am J Lifestyle Med*. 2019;16(2):214-220.

Nutrition Counseling with Group Visits

Shirly (Shalu) Ramchandani, MD / Helen Delichatsios, MD, SM, DipABLM / Beth Frates, MD, FACLM, DipABLM / Michelle Hauser, MD, MS, MPA, FACP, FACLM

Chapter Outline

CASE STUDY

Andrea is a 48-year-old female who presents for an annual visit. She reports a significant amount of weight gain during the COVID-19 pandemic and wants to control her weight. She worries about her health since multiple family members have diabetes. She has joined structured weight loss programs in the past. She acknowledges the importance of preparing home-cooked meals but cites lack of confidence and time as barriers and admits to not always making healthy choices. She has multiple life stressors including work projects, a recent divorce, and a move which have interrupted her routine. A brief, 24-hour diet recall includes a fast-food bacon, egg, and cheese breakfast sandwich; fries and a hamburger for lunch; and a frozen meal for dinner. She gained 40 pounds in the last 2 years and currently weighs 218 pounds (Body Mass Index [BMI] = 38 kg/m²). Her waist circumference is 38 inches. Her blood pressure is 142/88 mm Hg and glycosylated hemoglobin (HbA1c) is 5.7%. She wants to lose weight to prevent starting antihypertensive medication and developing diabetes, and to improve her stamina during physical activities. Her level of motivation to change her eating habits is 7/10, but reports low confidence at 5/10.

Her primary care provider (PCP) encourages her to attend nutrition and culinary focused group visits in person or virtually, called shared medical appointments (SMAs), along with a group of other patients who have similar health concerns and are working to eat healthy foods.

For the questions below, choose the best answer.

1. Group visits, called shared medical appointments, are conducted in person or virtually and may help this patient because_____. Select all that apply.
   A. She can learn to make healthy meals by watching cooking demonstrations or she can cook along in her kitchen.
   B. She will gain a better understanding of healthy ingredients and improve her confidence and culinary skills.
   C. She will get helpful tips from other patients, such as where she can find the cheapest produce.
   D. She will benefit from the support of other patients with similar health concerns.

(Continued)

2. To treat her elevated blood pressure (BP), her PCP reviews with her the Dietary Approaches to Stop Hypertension (DASH) diet recommendation to limit her sodium intake to less than 2,300 mg per day and increase produce intake. To follow DASH diet recommendations to improve her BP, she should do all of the following EXCEPT:
   A. Increase intake of apples, oranges, and bananas.
   B. Cook more at home and eat out less.
   C. Use spices and herbs to flavor her food in lieu of salt.
   D. Decrease intake of spinach, tomatoes, and eggplant.

3. Which of the following is NOT an outcome expected from shared medical appointments?
   A. Gaining knowledge and skills related to disease prevention and management
   B. Becoming a health coach through the process
   C. Enjoying camaraderie around making healthy lifestyle changes
   D. Increasing confidence about taking action toward positive healthy changes

WHAT ARE GROUP VISITS?

Traditionally in medicine, the interaction between patients and healthcare professionals has been one-on-one. Healthcare professionals have often observed that they repeatedly provide brief counseling to patients on lifestyle changes but don't regularly see significant improvements. Patients with and at risk for chronic diseases such as heart disease, diabetes, and cancer often need more time, education, and different approaches than brief one-on-one visits can provide.

Group visits are a helpful option for patients with chronic conditions. All group visits have an element of group support and education, but they also allow time for group participation and coaching for behavior change. Group visits have different names. Two common names are shared medical appointments (SMAs) and group medical visits (GMVs). If these group visits are conducted virtually, they are called virtual group visits or (VGVs). Other names for group visits in medicine are drop-in group medical appointments (DIGMAs), lifestyle medicine group interventions, and culinary medicine group visits. Culinary medicine group visits could also be SMAs, if they include the required medical appointment documentation.

The group visits that include a specific one-on-one medical appointment time represent a type of healthcare delivery model pioneered by Edward Noffsinger in the early 1990s.[1] SMAs and DIGMAs specifically combine a medical visit with patient education and management of chronic medical conditions in a group setting. The one-on-one time may be within the group or in a separate room with the clinician while the rest of the group is working on behavior change with a health coach or other behavior change specialist. When virtual, the clinician and patient may hold the medical visit component in a breakout room. These types of medical group visits can be in person or virtual and be paid for by insurance when the proper coding and billing are used.

During all group visits, one or more group facilitators meet with a small group of patients (often 8–12) simultaneously for 60–120 minutes to manage their conditions. Using a team-based approach, group visits focus on patient-centered care, allowing for patient empowerment, confidence building, goal setting, and accountability for successful health behavior adoption.[2] This team approach often includes the members of the multidisciplinary team which are reviewed in detail in Chapter 28.

Early group visit models were successfully used in pediatric well-child visits and prenatal care.[3] Subsequently, they became popular among various medical specialties for the care of patients with numerous chronic conditions, especially with patients who have type 2 diabetes.[4] During group visits, the clinician can reach multiple patients at the same time to provide medical care and education as well as enable peer support.[5] More recently, fueled by loneliness as a result of the COVID-19 pandemic[6] and social distancing protocols, conducting group visits virtually using two-way, audio-video conferencing software has become popular. As mentioned earlier, these virtual group visits are sometimes referred to as VGVs. An important benefit of VGVs is that they expand access to group visits to those who might not be able to join in person. In addition, they reduce barriers to attending since they don't require the costs and time of transportation or parking to attend. More research is needed to further support the clinical effectiveness of group visits, the financial viability in the long run, and improved access for people who are the most vulnerable.[7]

In a group setting, the availability of more time for the clinician to listen and interact with patients makes the medical experience less intimidating for patients and more rewarding for all.[2,5,8,9] Many patients find significant added value in the facilitated interaction with their peers through sharing struggles and successes. Patients can also develop a strong connection with their clinician because patients observe their expertise and empathy in dealing with many patients, thus resulting in improved patient and physician satisfaction.

To maintain privacy, patients sign a confidentiality agreement before starting any type of group visit. It is critical that patients feel they are sharing their experiences in a safe environment. Patients only divulge what they feel comfortable sharing, and often patients relay quite sensitive and personal information. Fellow patients respect this and know not to share personal information beyond the group, as they have signed a confidentiality agreement. Patients overwhelmingly give positive feedback for the group visit experience.[8–10] Additional benefits of group visits include reduced healthcare costs due to improved access for reduced emergency room visits and specialty care visits.[11] Lastly, as was highlighted during the COVID-19 pandemic, social isolation is a significant stressor.[6] The group visit model enables the creation of social connections and a reduction in patient isolation. The types of group visits and their benefits have been described and published broadly, especially over the past two decades.[8,9]

In our experience in leading group visits for patients with chronic diseases, we find that this interactive, supportive environment with extended facetime is beneficial for patients to improve their self-care. The format of group visits provides an opportunity to review evidence-based guidelines for the six pillars of lifestyle medicine. These pillars include nutrition, physical activity, stress management, restorative sleep, social connections, and avoiding risky substances, as discussed in Chapter 31. Given the commonality of various chronic disease etiologies, it is possible to see patients with numerous conditions in the same visit. It is helpful to review healthy habits and tips on adopting these behaviors as well as to discuss their barriers and facilitators to change. Behavior change techniques, theories, and approaches used in group visits include motivational interviewing, appreciative inquiry, the transtheoretical model of change, the social-ecological model of change, positive psychology, goal setting theory, accountability, and tracking. These have been reviewed in depth in Chapter 26, "Introduction to Behavior Change."

Research suggests that asking for feedback from the patients helps to tailor the program and improve it.[12]

GROUP VISIT LOGISTICS

When deciding to implement group visits, initial considerations include the topic(s) of your group visits or series of visits, which disease entities patients who attend will have, whether patients will attend a specific session(s) or a full series of sessions, the timing and interval of the group visits, whether to hold the visits in person or virtually, and a recruitment strategy, among other considerations. A common practice is to hold weekly meetings for 6–12 weeks. Members of the team that make group visits run successfully generally include a clinician facilitator and medical assistant. For SMAs, billing as a medical appointment using standard evaluation and management codes, the clinician facilitator is usually a medical doctor, doctor of osteopathy, nurse practitioner, or physician assistant. The medical assistant can take vital signs and address other clinical processes, such as questionnaires, with patients. Other team members may be included such as a registered nurse, registered dietitian, physical therapist, or health coach. These team members are described in detail in Chapter 28, "A Multidisciplinary Approach for Nutrition Counseling." Additionally, scheduling is done differently than one-on-one visits, and the clinician needs to work closely with those scheduling visits to ensure they are done correctly.

Each group visit session includes time for the clinician facilitator to conduct a brief follow-up with each patient to have one-on-one time (usually a clinician speaking directly to an individual patient while others in the group observe) for assessment and billing purposes. The group visits include more time for education, coaching for behavior change, and group discussions which may be led by the clinician facilitator or other member of the multidisciplinary team. Again, SMAs are reimbursed at standard evaluation and management billing levels (like one-on-one visits with a clinician) and require related elements of documentation. Other types of group visits may be paid for out of pocket, through a research fund, through a philanthropic fund, or are provided as part of a package in a concierge-type practice. This chapter is focused on culinary medicine (CM) group visits where different topics are addressed including cooking skills, food shopping, dietary behavior change to manage chronic diseases, and risk factors for these diseases. For more details about the logistics of group medical visits, please refer to the excellent resources in the references.[13–15]

THE ART OF RUNNING GROUP VISITS

The rationale for group visits is that a unique process occurs when people come together in a group. In our experience, we have seen many benefits of group visits including people feeling inspired by seeing others who are coping well. In addition, the group dynamics lead patients and clinicians to develop more equitable relationships.

The clinician facilitator typically determines what is covered during the educational portion of a group visit. When focusing on nutrition and culinary topics (such as in CM group visits), the clinician facilitator, or another team member (such as a behavior health specialist or health coach) may spend time covering strategies to eat healthy meals that are both delicious and nutritious and to set goals for the week around meal planning.

Part of the art of running group visits is knowing when to use the COACH Approach™ (as discussed in Chapter 26) to empower patients to change.[2] With the COACH Approach™ the goal is collaboration and negotiation with the patient with the clinician emphasizing *curiosity, openness, appreciation, compassion, and honesty,* which helps tap into the patient's own motivation for change. The clinician using the COACH Approach™ uses open-ended questions in accordance with motivational interviewing (as discussed in Chapter 26), listens more than they talk, and they work toward understanding the whole person. During the medical check in and the education parts of the visit, the EXPERT Approach is used. At these times, the clinician may use closed-ended questions, collect data, talk more than they listen, and at times work to have the patient understand the medical plan. For the behavior change and group discussion, the COACH Approach™ is required. Asking inspiring questions and supporting any steps in the direction of healthy change is important. The COACH Approach™ is used during the facilitated discussions and aims to help those attending identify barriers and solutions around them. The clinician facilitator can encourage group members to share or brainstorm strategies to address barriers that have been brought up in the group. For example, one patient may suggest buying pre-cut vegetables to another patient who may not be able to chop vegetables due to time limitation or dexterity issues. Patients enjoy learning from each other and feel a sense of connection as they share experiences and face similar challenges. Clinician facilitators set the stage for these peer-to-peer interactions by creating a room, virtual or in person, that is free of judgment, shame, blame, and guilt.

It takes experience and practice to master smooth facilitation of group visits. It helps to observe one or more sessions that colleagues are already running. Included in the resources are training programs for those who wish to learn more.[13–15]

HEALTH OUTCOMES WITH GROUP VISITS

There is a growing body of medical literature that demonstrates positive health outcomes associated with group visits. Most of the available research is observational with an increasing number of randomized trials. These studies demonstrate improvement in various chronic conditions and risk factors such as pre diabetes,[16] diabetes,[17] and hypertension.[18] For example, a retrospective cohort study compared patients with prediabetes attending SMAs to usual care and demonstrated a statistically significant improvement in weight loss in the SMA group (2.88 kg vs. 1.29 kg, P = 0.003), reduction in HbA1c (−0.87% vs. +0.87%, P = 0.001) and systolic blood pressure (−4.35 mm Hg vs. +0.52 mm Hg, P = 0.044).[16]

In a small retrospective study, researchers evaluated the effectiveness of a comprehensive lifestyle medicine intervention on chronic disease risk factors and quality of life in breast cancer survivors. More than three-quarters of the 21 breast cancer survivors who attended five or more of the seven group visits had statistically significant reductions in their body weight, and positive changes in psychosocial variables of perceived stress, depression, patient activation, and quality of life trended, but did not reach statistical significance.[19] In addition to health outcomes, patients have reported improved health behaviors, better medication adherence, increased self-efficacy, and improved quality of life.[2]

Examples of five randomized controlled trials (RCTs) on health outcomes using group visits are described in Table 30-1. More RCTs are needed to assess the effectiveness of group visits in reducing overall costs and improving health outcomes long term beyond 6 months postintervention. Further research is also needed to evaluate the most effective model for group visits and to assess how best to implement them in clinical practice.

BEYOND THE GROUP

In addition to group visits, patients also typically attend one-on-one visits with their PCP, other specialists, and allied health professionals on their medical team. When addressing dietary behavior change, visits with registered dietitians and health coaches may be helpful. Group visits work in concert with one-on-one visits.

TABLE 30-1 • Examples of randomized controlled trials with group visits		
Study	**Number of participants**	**Primary outcomes**
Gardiner et al. (2022)[20]	159 low- income racially diverse adults with nonspecific chronic pain and depressive symptoms.	Integrative Medical Group Visits (IM combines mindfulness techniques, evidence based integrative medicine vs. 1:1 Primary Care Physician visit. IMGV group had fewer emergency department visits (RR 0.32, 95% CI: 0.12, 0.83) compared to controls. At 21 weeks, the IMGV group reported reduction in pain medication use (Odds Ratio: 0.42, CI: 0.18–0.98) compared to controls.
Bisno et al. (2022)[21]	53 patients with T1DM	Participants were randomized to Colorado Young Adults with Type 1 Diabetes (CoYoT1) Clinic TeleHealth (TH)+Virtual Group Visit (VGV) or individual Telehealth (TH)-only. Participants in TH+VGV reported relative reductions in Physician (ES = -2.87, P = .02) and Regimen-related distress compared to those in TH-only (ES = -0.35, P = .01). Participants in TH+ VGV reported improved self-management of T1D-related problem solving (ES = 0.47, P = .051) and communication with care providers (ES = 0.39, P = 0.07).
Sönmez et al. (2023)[22]	1,000 patients with glaucoma	SMA compared to one-on-one visits for four successive visits. Patients who participated in SMAs showed higher satisfaction (p = 0.0002) and higher knowledge (p= 0.002). Patients who participated in SMAs exhibited higher medication compliance rates (p = 0.013).
Woodard et al. (2022)[23]	280 participants with type 2 diabetes	Effectiveness of Empowering Patients in Chronic Care (EPICC) with 6 group sessions based on collaborative goal-setting followed up with a 1:1 visit after each group vs. usual care with added educational component EUC). Participants in group visit EPICC had significant post intervention improvements in HbA1c levels (P = .003) and Diabetes Distress Scale (DDS) (P = .003) compared with EUC. 6-month follow-up demonstrated continued improvement with DDS but not HbA1c levels.
Heisler et al. (2021)[24]	1537 adults with type 2 diabetes and elevated HbA1c	SMA participants achieved clinically and statistically significant greater reductions in HbA1c compared with those in the control group which was continuation of usual care between baseline and 6 months (HbA1c reductions 0.35% points greater than the control group with p = .001), but differences between groups were no longer statistically significant at 12 months.

● CULINARY MEDICINE GROUP VISITS

Culinary medicine (CM) group visits offer a unique opportunity to review nutrition science, teach culinary skills, introduce healthy ingredients, and share time-saving as well as cost-saving strategies with patients in a medical appointment that can be covered by insurance using standard billing practices.

Culinary medicine is covered in detail in Chapter 29 and is a growing area of interest for healthcare professionals and patients alike. There are clinics across the country that have developed these nutrition-focused group visits including teaching kitchens (see Chapter 29 for more information on teaching kitchens) to increase access to practical nutrition education and aid in facilitating dietary behavior change.[10,13] For clinical practices with limited space, CM group visits can be done virtually using a telehealth model. All that is needed is a willing clinician facilitator with appropriate nutrition knowledge and adequate cooking skills (or clinician facilitator along with another facilitator with nutrition and cooking skills), interested patients, a conference room, and a few basic and inexpensive pieces of equipment (such as a cutting board, knife, mixing spoons, measuring cups and spoons, and bowls). Food costs are limited—cooking demonstrations of simple dishes allowing everyone to taste the food can be completed for as little as $12-$20 per class.[10]

For telehealth CM group visits, several items are needed, including a laptop, good internet connection, good lighting, Bluetooth headphones/microphone that reduce background noise, a virtual meeting platform, and a space to set up a laptop in view of a cooking space. To allow patients to cook along, it is best to send them an email prior to the session that includes recipes, shopping and equipment lists, as well as instructions for basic preparation steps to be done ahead of time. Conducting CM group sessions can also be done in the community or other educational settings; these would not be SMAs and therefore would not include the medical appointment aspects such as taking vital signs, clinical documentation, or other clinical processes.

The trend in less frequent home cooking in U.S. households is due in part to a lack of confidence, cooking skills, and food preparation knowledge.[25] Using CM group visits fills this educational gap by focusing on practical dietary behavior changes, pertinent education about food, and basic cooking skills needed to move toward a healthier diet. The nutrition focus of the sessions are on the lessons covered throughout this text and described in more detail in Chapter 29, namely increasing intake of unprocessed and minimally processed healthful ingredients such as vegetables, fruits, whole grains, beans, nuts, and seeds. One of the main goals of the CM group visits is to empower patients to enjoy home cooking. Additionally, the CM group visits can address overcoming potential limitations related to time availability, financial resources, and cultural considerations. The act of demonstrating how simple, healthy, and delicious dishes can be prepared is fodder for patients to prepare these meals at home for themselves and their families.

● CULINARY SKILLS DELIVERED IN GROUP VISITS

The emphasis of CM group visits is on practical culinary skills that can be incorporated into group visits held either in person or virtually. Any topic falling under the purview of CM can be covered using a group visit format. If participants in CM group visits are new to cooking, basics such as food safety, including storing of foods, safe use of knives, securing hair and loose clothing, preventing burns, and proper cleanup are important. Strategies for meal prepping are often reviewed which help improve self-efficacy and confidence to get patients started on their culinary journeys. Time management skills can help patients. These can include (1) *mise-en-place*, a French term referring to organizing, collecting ingredients and tools, and doing basic food preparation before starting to cook, (2) batch cooking, and (3) repurposing which refers to the use of one ingredient in different recipes like chopping onions for three dishes at once or preparing a salad dressing that can later be used as a marinade or dip.[26] Batch cooking can be done easily for some long-cooked ingredients such as whole grains and legumes. In this way, leftovers of these staples can be repurposed for a different dish. Repurposing also limits time needed to wash and rewash dishes. Batch cooking full meals that lend themselves well to freezing, eating cold, or reheating also reduces the number of times meals need preparation. Cooking one-pot meals is another time-saving strategy.

CM group visits can help patients prepare healthy meals by teaching how to incorporate more vegetables and plant-based proteins, use less salt, reduce intake of saturated fat, and minimize the added sugars. Often, patients report not enjoying eating certain foods, such as raw, steamed, or canned vegetables. Thus, teaching them how to prepare these foods in other ways they might find delicious is key.

During CM group visits, healthy cooking techniques such as steaming, poaching, boiling, roasting, and sautéing are covered. Avoiding methods that involve blackening or browning for animal proteins can greatly decrease production of advanced glycosylation end products (AGEs) in these foods. Dietary AGEs were shown to be correlated with metabolic syndrome, T2DM, and its comorbidities.[27] CM group visits can increase uptake of healthy cooking behaviors by allowing patients a space to practice skills and taste dishes which can improve confidence in the kitchen, create buy-in around healthful foods being delicious, and reduce concerns about spending money on new foods that may not seem tasty to the patient due to lack of experience with that particular ingredient.

CM group visits can be designed to address individual barriers to healthy eating that patients may encounter. Common barriers include lack of time, lack of skills, the cost of healthy food, and perception that healthy food cannot be tasty. Patients sometimes also report being overwhelmed by the multitude of recipes online, multi-step directions, and the process of shopping for ingredients. The task of making multiple healthy meals daily is not practical for many people, often resulting in the increased frequency of take-out meals. Since these are common barriers, the group visits sessions are planned out so that they cover all these concerns. CM group visits also focus on the deliciousness of foods used in the sessions to "hook" the learner and then cover health benefits of items included. There is no dearth of people watching mouthwatering foods prepared on TV cooking shows; focusing on deliciousness is essential to keep patients engaged.

CASES IN CULINARY MEDICINE GROUP VISITS

The following patients are described in detail in Chapter 29, "Culinary Medicine," and will be participating in the CM group visit series discussed here. There are often 8–12 patients in these visits. For this example, we will share details for only the three patients who were introduced in Chapter 29. The patients include Foluke who is a 42-year-old African American male with metabolic syndrome. He is interested in learning about dietary changes to prevent diabetes, improve his health, and reduce his reliance on medications to treat chronic, lifestyle-related conditions. Previously, Foluke was eating a lot of subs and pizzas as they were tasty, convenient, and cheap. He has little cooking experience and is therefore uncomfortable in the kitchen.

Camilla is a 32-year-old female from the Dominican Republic who has a newborn and a 3-year-old son. During her pregnancy, she gained weight and was diagnosed with gestational diabetes mellitus (GDM). She wants advice on incorporating healthier meal options for the family. Her PCP recommended she go to community cooking classes which she has enjoyed. Camilla wants to continue to learn about healthy cooking techniques and time-saving strategies. She wants to continue to enjoy common Dominican dishes without compromising their flavors.

Damian is a healthy, 19-year-old, Caucasian student with a family history of coronary artery disease (CAD) who wants to maximize his performance in academics and athletics and also prevent CAD and other chronic diseases. He was told by his PCP that his BP is borderline. He wants to avoid getting hypertension like his father. Damian wishes to stock his home with staple items that have a long shelf life that will enable him to make quick, low-cost dishes. Damian had expressed concerns about the cost of buying multiple spices and herbs for different recipes. He also admits to fatigue and difficulty focusing on his studying around 3 pm each afternoon.

In this CM group visit, patients are learning to make a quinoa and black bean bowl with tofu bites, kale, tomatoes, onions, and a chipotle dressing. During the preparation of the meal, the clinician facilitator first describes how the flavors of the ingredients and cooking techniques complement each other to produce a fresh, hearty, tasty dish. Then, they discuss the health benefits of the ingredients, including highlighting how high-fiber foods like beans can help reduce cholesterol levels. This material resonates with Foluke who has metabolic syndrome, and Damian who is looking to lower his risk for heart disease. Foluke jumps in and asks about how many calories they will be consuming. Camilla quickly chimes in that her PCP has emphasized considering the quality of the food

over the calories in the food. The clinician facilitator then leads a discussion among the group about shifting overall eating patterns to those that are plant-predominant and rich in whole foods, rather than simply counting calories. This is an excellent strategy for addressing conditions like metabolic syndrome, diabetes, high blood pressure and heart disease, all of which are on the minds of the patients in the group. They also emphasize that there are many ways of achieving this goal that can include using ingredients from many different cultural food backgrounds.

While preparing the kale, the clinician reviews the use of the Harvard Healthy Eating Plate as a useful guide for structuring balanced meals with more vegetables; whole grains like quinoa; and healthy, high-protein foods such as tofu, legumes, nuts, and seeds. Camilla explains that she printed out a copy of the Healthy Eating Plate from the Harvard TH Chan School of Public Health's Nutrition Source website and has used it ever since her PCP recommended it to her. She says it helps her and her 3-year-old son create balanced meals. Damian voices concern about the cost of fresh ingredients like the ones they are using today. The clinician facilitator takes this opportunity to discuss how legumes and beans are actually inexpensive and healthy sources of protein which can save him money and lower his risk of heart disease at the same time. Camilla adds that her PCP told her lowering intake of red and processed meats helps lower the risk of heart disease and diabetes. The other patients seem surprised to hear about this connection. Camilla feels happy she could share something valuable with the group.

Foluke says, "Healthy food tastes so bland," and Damian quickly agrees. Camilla shares her experience using herbs and spices when she is able to prepare her mother's Dominican recipes. Foluke is interested in Camilla's spices as he is looking to lower his use of salt so that he can lower his blood pressure and avoid the diagnosis of hypertension. Camilla shares some of her favorite spices including malagueta, also known as allspice, clavo (cloves), and nuez moscada (nutmeg). She tells the others what foods taste good with what spices. Both Foluke and Damian are extremely attentive while Camilla speaks.

Foluke then shares with Damian that many of his dietary patterns and lifestyle behaviors started around Damian's age, especially after Foluke graduated from college and started working full time. Foluke then takes the opportunity to congratulate Damian on intervening early in his life and making positive lifestyle changes at his young age. It is clear that Foluke's words impact Damian as he thanks Foluke and smiles with a sense of pride that everyone can see. Camilla quickly adds that she is working on teaching her 3-year-old son healthy eating, and she smiles, too.

Foluke then shares that he was recently advised to increase his consumption of complex carbohydrates from whole grains, vegetables, fruits, and legumes, and minimize refined grains and added sugars in order to help control his metabolic syndrome. The clinician facilitator discusses quinoa and brown rice as options for improving carbohydrate quality. Camilla shares that she has been shifting from white rice to brown rice recently by making meals that are half white rice and half brown rice.

The clinician facilitator reviews several beneficial effects of lower glycemic index and higher fiber diets including lowering of postprandial glucose and insulin responses, improvements in lipid profile, and, possibly, reduced insulin resistance.[28] Foluke was also advised that increasing fiber intake would increase his satiety compared with highly processed, caloric dense, fast-food meals. Camilla shares that she feels the brown rice keeps her full longer than the white rice. Foluke expresses an interest in using brown rice and learning how to incorporate more fiber to reduce his cholesterol.

At this point, the clinician facilitator asks if the group wants to hear about the guidelines for fiber consumption. They are all eager to learn, and the facilitator reports, "The United States Department of Agriculture (USDA) recommended daily amount of fiber is 25 grams for women and 38 grams for men. On average, American adults eat 10–15 grams of fiber per day." The facilitator states that incorporating more whole grains like brown rice and quinoa, legumes, vegetables, fruits, and nuts will help them meet their daily requirements for fiber and also control blood sugars.

During this CM group visit, quinoa is cooked in a batch and divided into 1-cup portions to freeze and store for multiple meals later on. This allows for significant cost savings. Damian especially enjoys the toothsome texture of the quinoa and crispness of the tofu. He learns he can also roast a variety of vegetables to create that savory flavor and texture (crisp on the outside, tender on the inside) that he really enjoyed in this dish. Learning a new cooking technique (roasting) now gives him endless meal options that allow utilization of the cost-saving and meal prepping techniques that were reviewed in the session.

These three patients learned that they can combine cooked and raw vegetables with a protein and use a whole-grain base to create balanced meals that are satiating and delicious at minimal cost. Camilla says, "It's great to save money, but I really need to focus on saving time too." Camilla presents like many other working parents, having difficulty finding time to prepare home-cooked meals and feeling compelled to eat prepared foods, which are expensive and increase the chances of eating foods high in sodium, added sugars, and saturated fats. The clinician facilitator reviews ways to organize the pantry and use time management skills like *mise-en-place*, repurposing, batch-cooking, and using leftovers to minimize food waste.

Camilla is also trying to incorporate more plant-based proteins into her diet. Batch cooking dried beans is a great recommendation for her, as soaking can be done while she's working and cooking can be done largely hands' off while she's attending to other things when at home with her family. During the CM group visit, the clinician facilitator asks if the other patients eat beans. Damian admits he is learning about the benefits of beans, and he has enjoyed beans at local fast-food places where he picks up burritos to go. Then, the clinician facilitator asks if the group wants to hear about some interesting facts about beans. They all agree. So, the facilitator shares that dried beans are the least expensive, protein-rich food that one can prepare without constant, direct supervision. Examples of largely hands' off methods of preparing beans include simmering over low heat on the stove or using an instant pot or pressure cooker. The clinician facilitator also shares that portioning, freezing, and reheating works well for beans and bean-based dishes. Damian states he saw beans at the local food pantry and plans to pick some up next time he is there.

This first CM group visit is successful in that all participants enjoyed the food that was prepared. They each learned something specific for their individual circumstances, and they were able to enjoy the act of preparing and eating the meal together as well as the joy of creating new social connections.

Because they all enjoyed the session, they elected to join follow-up CM group visits. In the follow-up sessions, the clinician facilitator starts by reviewing how to set up a pantry with staple ingredients. This allows one to prepare balanced meals entirely from these staples or with the addition of a limited number of fresh ingredients. The following are some examples of items that can be used to stock a pantry, freezer, and refrigerator.

- Dry ingredients: quinoa and other whole grains, bulgur, whole-wheat couscous, cornmeal, lentils (brown, green, red, or black), beans, nuts, seeds (e.g., pepitas, sunflower, sesame, hemp, flax), dried spices and herbs, tahini paste (and other nut and seed butters), whole-grain flours, whole-grain or bean/lentil-based noodles, shelf-stable soy milk or dairy milk, dried fruits, low-sodium condiments, canned ingredients, vinegars, oils, low-sodium tomato sauce, and canned beans and lentils.
- Frozen ingredients: vegetables, fruits, cooked beans and whole grains, plant-based proteins, fish and seafood, chicken and turkey, chopped garlic and ginger, and some herbs or herb pastes (like pesto).
- Refrigerated ingredients (that don't spoil quickly): plant milks, yogurt, hard cheeses, eggs, cabbages, potatoes, sweet potatoes, winter squashes, onions, garlic, carrots and other root vegetables, citrus fruits and apples, and tortillas.

During a follow-up CM group visit, Damian and the others learn that spices have a wide range of health benefits, such as antioxidant and anti-inflammatory properties and can be used in place of salt to enhance flavor. Then, the clinician facilitator demonstrates preparing a dish with a variety of herbs and spices as key flavoring ingredients. The patients then taste the dish.

Some of the patients in the earlier session elected to join the follow-up session virtually. While they lamented not being able to interact, cook, and taste the dishes with the others in person, joining from their home kitchen allowed the facilitator to review which spices in the patient's pantries may be substituted for those they're less familiar with or those they wouldn't be likely to use in other recipes. Sharing information like this with patients opens their culinary world and can make recipes more appealing by encouraging them to try new spices and reassuring them that they can swap out spices for ones they know they enjoy.

See Table 30-2 for examples of some herbs and spices common to different world cuisines. For a more extensive list with

TABLE 30-2 • Common herbs and spices of world cuisines				
Indian	**Italian**	**Mexican**	**Spanish**	**North african**
Cardamom	Basil	Cayenne	Cayenne	Cilantro
Cinnamon	Bayleaf	Chipotle	Leaf	Cumin Seeds
Cumin	Oregano	Cilantro	Oregano	Mint
Coriander	Rosemary	Cloves	Paprika	Red Pepper
Curry	Sage	Cinnamon	Rosemary	Saffron
Turmeric	Thyme	Coriander	Saffron	Turmeric
Saffron		Cumin	Parsley	Cinnamon
		Chiles		

more details on running CM group visits and educational sessions, refer to the Culinary Medicine Curriculum e-book.[29]

All three patients benefited from attending the CM group visit and learned numerous strategies to prepare tasty, inexpensive, balanced meals taking into account their taste preferences and health goals.

After attending a series of six CM group visits addressing a number of culinary medicine topics, the group gathers to share their progress. Foluke is happy to report that he learned to create delicious meals filled with whole, plant foods. He successfully lost another 12 pounds, which resulted in improvement of his BP, HbA1c, and lipid profile.

Camilla is now routinely following the Harvard Healthy Eating Plate recommendations and is creating healthy bowls with a rainbow of colors with her child, who now eats a wider variety of produce. She has successfully lost half her pregnancy weight postpartum and has a goal to lose it all in the next year.

Damian is excited to report on the money he has saved as he is now making four home-cooked meals per week and eating leftovers for several other meals. He has learned to be flexible with the ingredients he uses in cooking and prides himself on finding ways to use an item he prepares in multiple ways, in different meals throughout the week, to save money and time as well as reduce food waste. He finds his stamina throughout the day has improved. He doesn't have an afternoon crash in energy levels and has been able to focus more while studying.

These cases illustrate common clinical scenarios and the significant improvements that can be made in short- and long-term health and well-being when clinicians learn to incorporate culinary medicine into their clinical practices.

SUMMARY

Group visits enable more time for education and provide a supportive, collaborative environment, facilitating behavior change, and increasing self-efficacy. Some of the outcomes of these visits include reduced BP, BMI, cholesterol, and blood glucose levels. By joining a group visit, patients will enjoy the camaraderie of others while giving and receiving social support.

Healthcare delivery models are constantly evolving. Group visits, whether in person or virtual, offer an opportunity to reach many patients at once and more frequently than typical one-on-one visits. With group visits, especially CM group visits, all the information in the chapters of this nutrition text can be shared and discussed with patients more efficiently, leading to improved health outcomes. Facilitating group visits with patients is a skill worth practicing both for improving patient care and also improving clinician's personal health and reducing burnout.

TAKE-HOME POINTS

1. Group visits enable more time for education and provide a supportive environment, facilitating behavior change around the six pillars of lifestyle medicine: nutrition, physical activity, stress management, social connectedness, reducing risky substance use, and restorative sleep.

2. There is evidence in the medical literature that shared medical appointments improve health outcomes and reduce cost for chronic disease management.

3. Culinary medicine shared medical appointments provide an opportunity to focus on practical dietary behavior changes, food knowledge, and cooking skills needed to move toward a healthier diet.

CASE STUDY ANSWERS

1. A, B, D, C; Culinary medicine group visits focus on practical dietary behavior changes, food knowledge, and cooking skills needed to move toward a healthier diet. All of these are true.

2. D; By making their own meals patients have control over the ingredients which is especially helpful in reducing her intake of sodium. The use of spices and herbs is helpful in adding flavor without adding excess sodium. Processed foods and restaurant foods generally contain more sodium, added sugars, and saturated fat and are generally more expensive than home-cooked meals. Patients need to add more fruits and vegetables including spinach, tomatoes, eggplants, apples, oranges, bananas, and others.

3. B; All of the choices are expected outcomes from shared medical appointments except becoming a health coach. Health coach strategies will be utilized and demonstrated during group visits. Patients may end up asking open-ended questions of each other, praising each other's attempts at healthy eating, and working to strategize around obstacles in each other's way which are all part of the COACH Approach™. But, there are training programs and certification in health coaching that are recommended for anyone who is seeking a career in health and wellness coaching.

REFERENCES

1. Noffsinger EB. 'Today's three major group visit models', The ABCs of Group Visits. 2012:23–111.

2. Frates EP, Morris EC, Sannidhi D, Dysinger WS. The art and science of group visits in lifestyle medicine. *Am J Lifestyle Med.* 2017;11(5):408-413.

3. Rising S. Centering pregnancy an interdisciplinary model of empowerment. *J Nurse-Midwifery.* 1998;43(1):46-54.

4. Trento M, Passera P, Bajardi M, et al. Lifestyle intervention by group care prevents deterioration of type II diabetes: a 4-year randomized controlled clinical trial. *Diabetologia.* 2002;45(9):1231-1239.

5. Ramdas K, Darzi A. Adopting innovations in care delivery—the case of shared medical appointments. *N Engl J Med.* 2017;376(12):1105-1107.

6. Hwang T-J, Rabheru K, Peisah C, Reichman W, Ikeda M. Loneliness and social isolation during the COVID-19 pandemic. *Inter Psychogeriatr.* 2020;32(10):1217-1220.

7. Mirsky JB, Thorndike AN. Virtual group visits: hope for improving chronic disease management in primary care during and after the COVID-19 pandemic. *Am J Health Promot.* 2021;35(7):904-907.

8. Noffsinger, EB. 'Introduction to group visits', Running Group Visits in Your Practice. 2009:3–19.

9. Lacagnina S, Tips J, Pauly K, Cara K, Karlsen M. Lifestyle Medicine shared medical appointments. *Am J Lifestyle Med.* 2020;15(1):23-27.

10. Delichatsios HK, Hauser ME, Burgess JD, Eisenberg DM. Shared medical appointments: a portal for nutrition and culinary education in primary care—a pilot feasibility project. *Glob Adv Health Med.* 2015;4(6):22-26.

11. Wagner, E.H. et al. 'Chronic care clinics for diabetes in primary care: a system-wide randomized trial. Diabetes Care', *Diabetes Care,* 2001b;24(4):695-700.

12. Lacagnina, S. et al. 'Lifestyle Medicine Shared Medical appointments'. *Am J Lifestyle Med.* 2020;15(1):23-27.

13. Kakareka R, Stone TA, Plsek P, Imamura A, Hwang E. Fresh and savory: Integrating teaching kitchens with shared medical appointments. *J Altern Complement Med.* 2019;25(7):709-718.

14. Virtual group consultations—the British Society of Lifestyle Medicine. *Brit Soc Lifestyle Med.* June 23, 2023. Accessed July 24, 2023. Available at: https://bslm.org.uk/vgc.

15. Medical group visits, online course on building a successful program. UMass Chan Medical School. September 26, 2022. Accessed July 2023. Available at: https://www.umassmed.edu/cipc/continuing-education/MGVTraining/.

16. Papadakis A, Pfoh ER, Hu B, Liu X, Rothberg MB, Misra-Hebert AD. Shared medical appointments and prediabetes: the power of the group. *Ann Fam Med.* 2021;19(3):258-261.

17. Guirguis AB, Lugovich J, Jay J, et al. Improving diabetes control using shared medical appointments. *Am J Med.* 2013;126(12):1043-1044.

18. Mirsky JB, Bui TX, Grady CB, Pagliaro JA, Bhatt A. Hypertension control and medication titration associated with lifestyle medicine virtual group visits and home blood pressure monitoring. *Am J Lifestyle Med.* Published online 2022:155982762211080. doi:10.1177/15598276221108060.

19. Schneeberger D, Golubíc M, Moore HCF, et al. Lifestyle medicine-focused shared medical appointments to improve risk factors for chronic diseases and quality of life in breast cancer survivors. *J Altern Component Med.* 2019;25(1):40-47.

20. Gardiner P, Luo M, D'Amico S, et al. Effectiveness of integrative medicine group visits in chronic pain and depressive symptoms: a randomized controlled trial. *PLoS One.* 2019;14(12):e0225540.

21. Bisno DI, Reid MW, Fogel JL, Pyatak EA, Majidi S, Raymond JK. Virtual group appointments reduce distress and improve care management in young adults with type 1 diabetes. *J Diabetes Sci Technol.* 2022;16(6):1419-1427.

22. Sönmez N, Srinivasan K, Venkatesh R, Buell RW, Ramdas K. Evidence from the first shared medical appointments (SMAS) randomized controlled trial in India: SMAS increase the satisfaction, knowledge, and medication compliance of patients with glaucoma. *PLOS Global Public Health.* 2023;3(7):e0001648.

23. Woodard L, Amspoker AB, Hundt NE, et al. Comparison of collaborative goal setting with enhanced education for managing diabetes-associated distress and hemoglobin A1c levels: a randomized clinical trial. *JAMA Netw Open.* 2022;5(5):e229975.

24. Heisler M, Burgess J, Cass J, et al. Evaluating the effectiveness of diabetes shared medical appointments (SMAs) as implemented in five veterans affairs health systems: a multi-site cluster randomized pragmatic trial. *J Gen Intern Med.* 2021;36(6): 1648-1655.

25. Soliah LA, Walter JM, Jones SA. Benefits and barriers to healthful eating. *Am J Lifestyle Med.* 2012;6(2):152-158.

26. Clinicians Chef Coaching. Institute of Lifestyle Medicine. Accessed July 24, 2023. Available at: https://www.instituteoflifestylemedicine.org/?page_id=890%E2%80%AF.

27. Jiang T, Zhang Y, Dai F, Liu C, Hu H, Zhang Q. Advanced glycation end products and diabetes and other metabolic indicators. *Diabetol Metab Syndr.* 2022 Jul 25;14(1):104.

28. Riccardi G, Rivellese AA, Giacco R. Role of glycemic index and glycemic load in the healthy state, in prediabetes, and in diabetes. *Am J Clin Nutr.* 2008;87(1):269S-274S.

29. Hauser ME. *Culinary Medicine Curriculum.* St. Louis, MO: American College of Lifestyle Medicine; 2019. Available at: www.lifestylemedicine.org/culinary-medicine.

The Six Pillars of Lifestyle Medicine and Nutrition

Beth Frates, MD, FACLM, DipABLM / Coral Rudie, MS, RD, LDN, CNSC

Chapter Outline

CASE STUDY

Magdalena, a 28-year-old woman (pronouns she, her, hers), is a second-year medical school student. Of late, she has stopped exercising, eats mainly packaged or fast food, and has been staying up late to study and keep up with her Step 1 review. Prior to medical school, Magdalena was an avid runner who would regularly go on 5-mile runs. She stopped running this year, due to time constraints and the mindset that anything less than 5 miles is not worth doing. Cooking was never her thing, and she does not have a real kitchen in her current dorm room. Often, Magdalena finds herself feeling extremely hungry and exhausted by the end of the day, especially on days when she skips lunch. On these nights, she finds herself munching on whatever is in her cupboard. Being on a student budget, she looks for lower-priced food and sale items from the grocery store. Many of these are more processed foods such as cookies, cakes, and potato chips. Her days are long with classes and studying. In addition, she has been too tired to connect with her friends. Her exhaustion is likely related to her sleep disruption, as she finds herself waking up at night worrying about memorizing the

roots and cords of the brachial plexus. Since medical school, her dentist told her she was grinding her teeth, which is a sign of her stress level. Now, she wears a mouth guard at night. She has been averaging about 4–5 hours of sleep per night for several weeks.

1. **How could Magdalena's lack of sleep be connected to her eating pattern?**
   With sleep insufficiency:
   A. Serum ghrelin increases and leptin decreases
   B. Insulin resistance decreases
   C. Intake of hyperpalatable foods decreases
   D. Insulin sensitivity increases

2. **How could exercise help Magdalena with her nutrition in this case?**
   A. Serum Lac Phe and Irisin have been shown to increase with exercise
   B. Dopamine levels in the brain decrease with exercise
   C. Platelet adhesion increases with exercise
   D. Serotonin levels in the brain decrease with exercise

(Continued)

CASE STUDY *(Continued)*

3. How does stress play a role in Magdalena's eating patterns?
   A. Disrupting her sleep and altering levels of cortisol, ghrelin, and leptin
   B. Disrupting her social connections and lowering cortisol
   C. Increasing Growth Related Brain Factor (GRBF)
   D. Decreasing Growth Related Brain Factor (GRBF)

4. Exercise could help Magdalena in many ways, including
   A. Decreasing Brain Derived Neurotophic Factor (BDNF), which can lead to increased neurogenesis

   B. Increasing norepinephrine in the brain, which can increase attention and focus
   C. Decreasing serotonin in the brain, which can decrease symptoms of depression
   D. Decreasing the size of the hippocampus with time

5. List two to three practical ways that Magdalena could change her eating patterns.

6. Explain how increasing her social connections could help Magdalena with her eating pattern.

INTRODUCTION

Food and healthy eating patterns play a critical role in health as well as in the prevention and treatment of several chronic diseases including diabetes, heart disease, obesity, metabolic syndrome, stroke, and hypertension. There are many factors that influence what we eat. Social determinants of health including a person's education access and quality, economic stability, neighborhood and built environment, social and community context, and healthcare access and quality can all have direct effects on diet and lifestyle patterns. Factors such as unsafe neighborhoods and food deserts may make people more susceptible to unhealthy eating patterns. Lifestyle behaviors can also impact the food people consume. For example, exercise routines, sleep habits, stress management, social connections, and substance use can all play a role in how people nourish their bodies. Thus, to help patients adopt and sustain healthy eating patterns, a person's whole lifestyle needs to be assessed and often recalibrated to improve health and well-being.

According to the American College of Lifestyle Medicine, "Lifestyle medicine is a medical specialty that uses therapeutic lifestyle interventions as a primary modality to treat chronic conditions including, but not limited to, cardiovascular diseases, type 2 diabetes, and obesity. Lifestyle medicine certified clinicians are trained to apply evidence-based, whole-person, prescriptive lifestyle change to treat and, when used intensively, often reverse such conditions. Applying the six pillars of lifestyle medicine—a whole-food, plant-predominant eating pattern, physical activity, restorative sleep, stress management, avoidance of risky substances and positive social connections—also provides effective prevention for these conditions".[1] The American College of Lifestyle Medicine's Pillar puzzle is a graphic showing the six pillars that can be shared with healthcare professionals and patients (Figure 31-1).

These six pillars are all interrelated, and to enjoy optimal health, it is important to address each one. Evidence-based guidelines and recommendations exist for these pillars and can be used as practical targets. It is best to meet patients at their stage of change for each individual pillar, since they may be in different stages of behavior change for different pillars. The five

stages of change from the Transtheoretical Model of Change can be used to assess an individual's readiness for change and are described in the "Introduction to Behavior Change" (Chapter 26).

For many pillars, some is better than none, as with minutes of exercise, hours of sleep, minutes of mind-body practices, number of vegetables consumed, and number of connections with friends or loved ones. For risky substance use, usually none is better than some. For example, the recommendations are clear for cigarette smoking: quit. However, there is a J-shaped curve with alcohol, in that moderate intake may be beneficial for some health outcomes, but excessive use is associated with higher risk of mortality and morbidity.[2] Each lifestyle medicine pillar will be discussed in detail in this chapter.

PILLAR #1: NUTRITION BASICS

> Practice Guidelines: *Enjoy a delicious and nutritious whole food, plant predominant eating pattern with a focus on including vegetables, fruits, whole grains, legumes, nuts and seeds. Avoid processed foods, saturated fats, trans fats, sweets, added sodium, and sugar-sweetened beverages.*

A whole-food plant-based (also called *WFPB*, plant forward, plant slant, or plant predominant) eating pattern is recommended by many major medical organizations, including the American College of Lifestyle Medicine, American Heart Association, and the American Cancer Society. This pattern emphasizes consuming foods that are nutrient dense (i.e., naturally high in vitamins, minerals, antioxidants, phytonutrients, polyphenols, and flavonoids). Two examples of eating patterns that fall into this category include the Mediterranean-style diet and the DASH diet. Chapter 9, "Healthy and Sustainable Diets," and Chapter 6, "Popular Diets," provide specific information on different diets.

There are guidelines for people who choose to consume animal products. If people eat fish, the recommendations

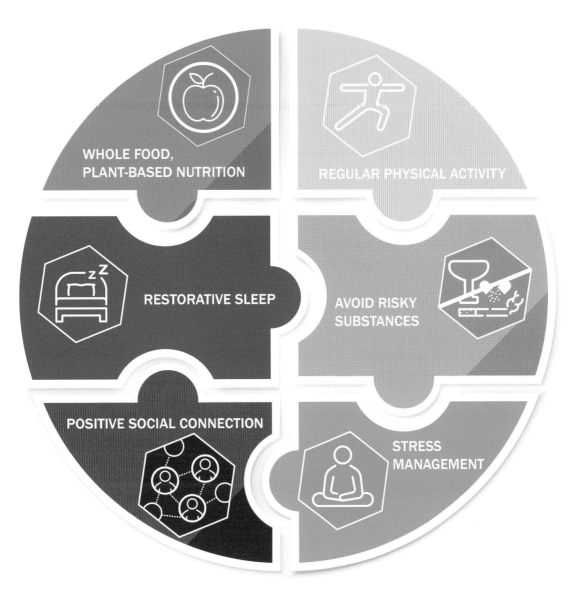

FIGURE 31-1 • American College of Lifestyle Medicine's six pillar puzzle graphic (Reproduced with permission from American College of Lifestyle Medicine; 2023.)

are to consume fish high in omega-3 fatty acids like salmon, tuna, mackerel, herring, and trout.[3] It is important to be careful about the level of mercury in fish, especially for women who are pregnant or breastfeeding and for children.[4] If people choose to eat meat, the recommendations are to select lean meats that are minimally processed.[3] For those opting to consume dairy, the recommendations are to select low fat or nonfat milk and milk products.[3] Nondairy milks that are plant based are also available. People who are not consuming animal products need to focus on getting B12 from nutritional yeast, fortified foods and or take a B12 supplement to ensure adequate intake of vitamin B12.

The four overarching principles in the U.S. Dietary Guidelines 2020–2025 are helpful general recommendations to share with all patients whether they choose to eat only plants or they choose to eat some animal products. They are:

1. to follow a healthy dietary pattern at every life stage,
2. to customize and enjoy nutrient-dense food and beverage choices to reflect personal preferences, cultural traditions, and budgetary considerations,
3. to focus on meeting food group needs with nutrient-dense foods and beverages, and
4. to stay within calorie limits and limit foods and beverages higher in added sugars, saturated fat, and sodium, and limit alcoholic beverages.[5]

Every bite someone takes can be a step closer to health or closer to disease. Most adults make food choices multiple times a day. "Knowledge is power," as Sir Francis Bacon said. Thus, sometimes sharing information, data, numbers, and recent research findings with patients and health care professionals, helps to empower them with inspiration to make a change. Other times knowledge is not powerful enough to instill lasting change. Individuals may need the COACH Approach™ as described in "Introduction to Behavior Change," Chapter 26. Whereas for some, their environment is the barrier that needs addressing. Patients may live in a food desert where there are limited options for fresh produce or a food swamp where the area is swamped with fast food restaurants. (Frozen fruits and vegetables may be a reasonable source of nutrition in some cases.) Eating on a budget is covered in Chapter 29, "Culinary Medicine," and Chapter 30, "Nutrition Counseling with Group Visits." Screening for food insecurity helps identify individuals who could benefit from social services and access to nutritious food. Chapter 4 covers food insecurity.

The socio-ecological model of change (introduced in Chapter 26, "Introduction to Behavior Change") reminds healthcare professionals to consider the person's family structure, work environment, neighborhood, cultural norms, city policies, and state laws that can influence the food choices and options available to the person. Eating healthy foods regularly is not an issue of willpower; it is complex and multifactorial.

A registered dietician (RD) is an expert on nutrition interventions and counseling (see Chapter 28 for more on the role of the RD). If a physician does not have the time, knowledge, or experience with nutrition counseling, then partnering with an RD is critical. An RD will help patients adopt meal plans that are tailored to their needs. Common referrals to an RD may include weight management for people with obesity or overweight (as discussed in Chapter 27, "Sustaining Change – Challenging Cases" with RD Kathy McMannus), chronic kidney disease, kidney stones, hypertension, gastroesophageal reflux disease, inflammatory bowel disease, celiac disease, small intestinal bacterial overgrowth (SIBO), food intolerance, food allergy, hyperlipidemia, diabetes, prediabetes, and pregnancy for weight management, gestational diabetes, or pregnancy induced hypertension. The Academy of Nutrition and Dietetics is a useful resource for learning more about nutrition experts and locating an RD in your area.

● PILLAR #2: PHYSICAL ACTIVITY AND NUTRITION

Practice Guidelines: *According to the World Health Organization and the U.S. Health and Human Services Department's Physical Activity for Adults, the recommendations are to engage in 2.5–5 hours of moderate intensity physical activity per week.*[6,7]

According to the sing test, moderate intensity means someone cannot sing but they can talk while exercising. If someone can sing, they are at low intensity. If someone cannot sing or talk, they are at vigorous intensity.

These two pillars are related by the relationship between energy expenditure (via physical activity) and energy consumption (via diet). The current focus of nutrition counseling, however, is not solely on the quantity of calories but rather their quality,

with high-quality calories coming from whole, unprocessed foods that are full of nutrients.

Another way these two pillars are connected is through the potential impact of exercise on cravings and appetite. In a small cross-over study, Ledochowski and colleagues examined the impact of a 15-minute walk versus 15 minutes of passive sitting on urges to consume sugary snacks in 47 subjects with BMI over 25 kg/m² and found that the walking intervention significantly reduced urges for sugary snacks.[8] Irisin is a myokine, a cytokine produced by muscle cells, that impacts many different organs including the brain, and serum levels of irisin increase with exercise. Irisin may have an impact on appetite regulation.[9] Another recently identified metabolite called n-lactoyl phenylalanine, or Lac Phe, may also play a role in decreasing food consumption and appetite after exercise. Blood levels of Lac Phe increase as the intensity of exercise increases, and this is associated with reduced food intake.[10]

Certain types of physical activity have been shown to have positive effects on stress levels, body image, and food consumption. For example, in a systematic review of five studies investigating the impact yoga has on stress, the researchers concluded that yoga may increase self-compassion (meaning treating yourself with compassion when you notice failures, mistakes, or short-comings), lower salivary cortisol, and lower the autonomic stress response by impacting the posterior hypothalamus leading to lower blood pressure.[11] A small trial of 45 adult women who met criteria for binge eating and had a BMI > 25 kg/m² examined the effects of a 12-week yoga program on binge eating. The women were either assigned to attend a weekly 1-hour yoga class (intervention) or waitlist (control). Women in the intervention group had a statistically significant reduction in self-reported binge eating as well as an increase in self-reported levels of physical activity.[12] What about the association of yoga and consumption of healthy foods? A mixed-methods study of 1,820 young adults demonstrated that those practicing yoga ate more fruits and vegetables and consumed less processed food as well as fewer sugar-sweetened beverages.[13] More research is needed to determine the strength of these associations.

Exercise in many different forms (including walking, running, swimming, and other aerobic activities) is known to have many important positive impacts on the body and brain. At the recommended doses, physical exercise helps reduce the risk of high blood pressure, stroke, heart disease, diabetes, breast cancer and colon cancer, and depression.[6,7] A study of 176 participants undergoing creative thinking tests while sitting or walking (outside or on a treadmill) revealed that any type of walking helped to increase creativity.[14] Exercise can increase several neurochemicals: norepinephrine which helps with focus and attention, dopamine which helps with motivation and reward, serotonin which helps with mood, endorphins which create a type of "runner's high," and brain derived neurotrophic factor (BDNF), which increases neurogenesis, the growth of new neurons.[15] In a randomized trial of 120 older adults, aerobic exercise was demonstrated to increase the size of the hippocampus, which was associated with improved spatial memory.[16]

The other part of the physical activity equation is physical inactivity. Sedentary behavior includes activities in which people sit, recline, or rest horizontally for long periods of time and is associated with lower lipoprotein lipase, higher triglycerides, lower HDL, and disruption of blood glucose control.[17,18] This indicates that movement or lack of movement impacts how food is managed by the body.

Many people sit for prolonged periods in the day due to their work, participating in online meetings, writing, doing paperwork, reading, or driving. Stopping prolonged periods of sitting is the solution to avoid the dangers of sedentary physiology, but when that is not possible, people can take short breaks from sitting. For instance, a study employing stable isotopes found that taking "activity snacks" of brief walks or body weight squats every 30 minutes improved measures of muscle protein synthesis compared to those who did not take these breaks.[19] It is recommended that people break up sitting with periods of standing and light activity each hour.[20] The American Diabetes Association recommends that people with prediabetes or diabetes break up sitting more frequently with "mini exercise bursts" every half an hour.[21] Ultimately, people need to sit less and move more for their health.

PILLAR #3: SLEEP AND NUTRITION

> **Practice Guidelines:** *According to the National Sleep Foundation, the recommendations are for adults to get 7–9 hours of sleep per night.*[22]

Getting a good night's sleep is key to a healthy body and peaceful mind. Sleep impacts almost every organ of the body, and sleep insufficiency is connected to many chronic conditions, including diabetes, heart disease, high blood pressure, stroke, and obesity.[23] For years, the American Heart Association advocated for controlling weight, blood pressure, blood sugars, blood lipids, increasing physical activity, healthy nutrition, and quitting smoking. They put together a prescription for health called, Life's Simple 7. In 2022, they changed Life's Simple 7 to Life's Simple 8 to include sleep as the eighth factor of cardiovascular health based on the available evidence.[23]

During sleep, the body consolidates memories which means it transforms temporary memories into more stable, long-term ones.[24] Evidence from animal and human studies shows that poor sleep is associated with Alzheimer's disease in a bidirectional manner.[25] Helping people experience restorative sleep may reduce their risk for this condition. There is more about Dementia in Chapter 23.

How are nutrition and sleep connected? When people eat, how much they eat and what they eat close to bedtime can impact their sleep patterns. For example, eating large meals right before bed can be associated with difficulty falling asleep due to symptoms of indigestion or acid reflux, especially with spicy foods or those high in fat. It is recommended that people should not eat large meals within three hours of bedtime.

There is a bidirectional relationship between food and sleep: eating patterns can hinder our sleep and poor sleep can hinder our eating patterns. Greer, Goldstein and Walker, demonstrated that people who were sleep-deprived were more likely to desire high-calorie food items.[26] Twenty-three healthy young adults were studied in a repeated-measures, counterbalanced cross-over design, which involved a regular night of sleep (8 hours) and a monitored night of total sleep deprivation. The different conditions were separated by at least 7 days. Functional MRI scans during food desirability choices revealed that sleep deprivation significantly decreased activity in appetitive evaluation regions of the brain in the frontal cortex and insular cortex. At the same time, it was noted there was a heightening of activity in the amygdala (involved with emotional processing). The researchers reported a significant increase in consumption of weight-gain promoting high-calorie foods when subjects were sleep deprived.[26] In a small cross-over inpatient study of 30 adults, the researchers found that when subjects slept 4 hours per night, they consumed close to 300 more calories compared to when they slept 7-9 hours per night.[27] These trials show association, and more research needs to be performed to identify the strength of the relationship.

Some eating patterns can enhance sleep duration and quality. A review of 17 articles concluded that a dietary pattern consistent with the Mediterranean diet, including "a healthy profile of fat, proteins, and carbohydrates and peculiar richness in polyphenols and vitamins, mainly provided by moderate to high intake of fruits, vegetables, nuts, olive oil, cereals, and fish" was associated with adequate sleep duration and improved sleep quality.[28] A cross-sectional study of 172 middle-aged adults in Naples, Italy, revealed that subjects considered good sleepers by the Pittsburgh Sleep Quality Index (PRQI) had lower BMIs, lower waist circumferences, and greater adherence to the Mediterranean diet as assessed by the PREDIMED questionnaire score than those subjects who were classified as poor sleepers by the PRQI.[29]

When considering sleep and managing blood glucose levels, there is evidence that lack of sleep can have a negative effect on glucose regulation and insulin sensitivity. Sleep impacts the beta cells of the pancreas that produce insulin, and thus regulate blood glucose. There are several different pathways linking sleep insufficiency, sleep fragmentation, obstructive sleep apnea, and hypoxemia to abnormal glucose metabolism and type 2 diabetes.[30] Epidemiologic studies of adults and children have demonstrated that sleep deprivation results in reduced glucose tolerance, reduced insulin sensitivity, increased insulin resistance, higher evening cortisol concentrations, higher ghrelin levels, lower leptin levels, and increased hunger and appetite.[31]

When discussing nutrition and sleep, the caffeine content of beverages is important to consider as it can impact sleep. As the body uses and breaks down adenosine triphosphate (ATP) for energy, adenosine accumulates in the brain, which increases sleepiness. Caffeine binds to the same receptor as adenosine, but it has the opposite effect, reducing sleepiness. One of the ways it does this is by sending signals to the pituitary gland, which then releases adrenocorticotropic hormone (ACTH). ACTH sends signals to the adrenal gland to release adrenaline, which increases alertness. Caffeine has a half-life of about 3–5 hours, but metabolism does vary. If someone drinks caffeinated coffee at 3 pm, half of it could be in their system at 8 pm. If someone drinks it at 7 pm, half of it could be in their system at 11 pm or midnight. The recommendation for caffeinated beverages is to drink them in the morning, before noon. Logging caffeine consumption can help when patients are having trouble with sleep.

● PILLAR #4: STRESS RESILIENCE AND NUTRITION

Practice Guidelines: *Try different stress management techniques. Engage in 10 to 20 minutes of meditation per day.*[32–35]

Stress management is a pillar of lifestyle medicine that is relevant for all individuals. Practicing stress resiliency, reduction, or management is recommended by many medical organizations and institutions such as the American Heart Association, the American College of Lifestyle Medicine, the American Psychological Association, Cleveland Clinic, Harvard Health, Nutrition Source by the Harvard TH Chan School of Public Health, and Mayo Clinic. A specific recommendation with respect to type of stress reduction technique or minutes of engagement has not been solidified or agreed upon. There are many different types to try. As with exercise and vegetables, some is better than none. The key is finding one or two stress reduction techniques, such as meditation, deep breathing, mindfulness, or yoga that resonates with the individual.

One stress management technique that is popular and has several research studies to support its use is meditation. *Meditation* is a broad term for spending time in a calm, quiet place, focusing on breathing, a word, or phrase. Meditation can include mindfulness meditation, prayer, transcendental meditation, mantra meditation, walking meditation, body scan, and other practices. One small randomized trial by Basso and colleagues included 42 adults ages 18–45, who were new to meditation and randomly assigned them to follow a guided meditation session 13 minutes daily (intervention) or to listen to a podcast for 13 minutes daily (control). After 8 weeks, compared to the control group, the daily meditation group experienced a decrease in negative mood state and enhanced attention, working memory, and recognition memory as well as decreased state anxiety scores.[32] Other studies of meditation in the military,[33] adults with cognitive decline,[34] and adults taking the GRE[35] all support a target time frame between 10–20 minutes. Most cite 12–13 minutes in order to reduce stress and have positive effects on the body and brain. Consistency is key. It takes 8–12 weeks of routine practice to achieve these results. More research is needed to continue to evaluate the dose of meditation and determine the strength of the association, but aiming for between 10–20 minutes is a solid recommendation.

Psychological stress is connected to many chronic conditions, as it can negatively alter metabolism. It is associated with higher cortisol levels, which may be partly responsible for the increased desire for hyperpalatable foods when stress levels are

high.[36] In a small observational study, there were 20 subjects ages 18–45 enrolled in a controlled, hospital based, 3-day study examining stress and cravings for highly palatable food. They defined highly palatable food as "those high in sugar, with sweet taste, highly processed foods high in saturated fats or high carbohydrates making up savory tastes and combinations of food groups prepared in ways that enhance taste and value or 'salience' of such foods to an individual."[36] The researchers found exposure to food cues and stress before a snack led to increased food cravings and was predictive of higher intake of highly palatable food items. Also, in this study, cortisol went up during the food cue exposure, and increased cortisol was associated with both higher highly palatable food cravings and higher highly palatable food intake.[36] Cortisol can also signal the body to alter its metabolism to store fat.[37]

High stress levels are associated with muscle tension, migraine headaches, glucose imbalances, inflammatory bowel disease, reproductive problems, and decreased immune function.[38] Chronic stress can negatively impact the brain. For example, animal and human research has demonstrated a negative impact of stress on the hippocampus, the area in the limbic system intimately involved with consolidating memories.[39] Additionally, stress can impact cardiovascular health. High levels of stress and cortisol can lead to high blood pressure and cardiovascular events.[40] Broken heart syndrome, also referred to as stress cardiomyopathy or Takotsubo cardiomyopathy, is thought to result from stressful situations creating extreme emotional responses.

If someone is eating healthy foods and continuing to experience high levels of stress, then this stress will still have a negative impact. Additionally, stress reduction is critical for adopting and sustaining healthy eating patterns. Making a habit of deep breathing before eating can help the body and brain move into parasympathetic drive prior to consuming food, which will help set the system up for rest and digestion. Mindful eating is a way to slow down and savor food. One exercise that helps people experience mindful eating is to slowly eat a raisin by taking the time to use all five senses to fully appreciate the one tiny raisin that is full of flavor. Slowing down to savor food has many advantages and has been demonstrated to reduce the risk of obesity.[41]

Slowly and mindfully eating can help reduce stress. Expressing gratitude for food and thanking all those that touch the food from the farm to table helps to put people into a calm state that can reset the body, take it out of the stress response of fight or flight and prepare it for consuming food during a time when the parasympathetic response predominates allowing for proper digestion. Feeling a sense of deep appreciation and connection can help lower stress, as the brain has difficulty holding both a grateful feeling and a stressful feeling at the same time.

What people eat may also have an impact on stress. One cross-sectional survey study examining depressive and stress symptoms in 3,706 university students in the United Kingdom reported that consuming "unhealthy" foods, such as cookies, sweets, snacks, and fast food, was significantly associated with perceived stress in female students and depressive symptoms in both male and female students.[42] The researchers also reported that there was an association between consuming 'healthy' foods like fresh fruits, salads, and cooked vegetables and reports of less perceived stress and lower depressive symptom scores for both male and female students.[42] There is more information about depression and food in Chapter 24.

Realizing the relationship between stress and food is the first step for healthcare professionals and patients. Assessing stress and addressing it is the next step. People may be stressed about when they are going to get their next meal. In this case, the nutrition counseling session will focus on locating local food pantries and working toward food security. Finding ways to adopt and sustain a healthy eating pattern on a budget may be one important way to help people reduce stress.

● PILLAR #5: SOCIAL CONNECTION AND NUTRITION

> **Practice Guidelines:** *Cultivate close supportive relationships with spouse/partner and relatives and connect with six to seven friends each week.*[43]

Social connections impact our health in many ways. The research on this lifestyle medicine pillar is ongoing, and there are no official recommendations or guidelines from major medical organizations about the specifics for social connection. However, there is a lot of data that demonstrates the power of social connection for health.[44,45]

The practice guideline presented here is based on a study published in Mayo Clinic Proceedings on social interactions. Becofsky and colleagues conducted a prospective mail-in survey study of 12,709 adults and followed them for 13 years or until death.[43] The subjects answered questions about social support from relatives, friends, and spouse/partner, and the number of friends and relatives they had contact with at least once per week. The results demonstrated that receiving social support from spouse/partner or from relatives provided the same benefit, with support from either group being associated with a nearly 20% lower risk of mortality. Social contact with six to seven friends on a weekly basis was associated with a 24% lower mortality risk compared to those who had social contact with one friend or less.[43]

As the authors state, "In order for these findings to inform behavioral care and intervention work, a conceptual shift must occur that awards improving social relations the same health behavior status as physical activity, diet and tobacco use, just as an active lifestyle and healthy diet lower mortality risk, so too does receiving support from loved ones and staying socially engaged".[43]

As described in Chapter 26 ("Introduction to Behavior Change"), the socio-ecological model of change factors in the individual's home environment, work environment, neighborhood, social norms, cultural influences, state laws, and country policies. A person's family, friends, and loved ones can have an impact on their lifestyle behaviors. Moreover, social connection is a pillar of lifestyle medicine because it has been documented that those people who have the least social connections are the ones with the highest risk of mortality as reported in a seminal study on this topic in 1979 by Berkman and Syme[46] in which they followed a random sample of 6,928 adults in Alameda County, California, over a 9-year period. For every age group from 30 to 69, those with the fewest social connections were the most likely to die.

A review of the literature in this area highlighted that a lack of social connection was associated with development and progression of heart disease, recurrent heart attack, high blood pressure, atherosclerosis, slower wound healing, cancer, and delayed cancer recovery.[47] Cultivating social connections and spending time with family and friends is good for health; this can happen around food at mealtimes.

Cooking and eating meals with the family can increase opportunities for social connection. Additionally, cooking at home is associated with healthier eating patterns, as reviewed in "Culinary Medicine," Chapter 29. When people eat alone, they may eat standing up, sitting in front of a television, or driving a car. Whereas when people eat as a family or with others, they sit down at a table, and this slows people down. Mealtime conversations can help to create bonds between people. It allows for sharing highlights and stressors from the day which can even help alleviate stress. Mealtimes can nourish people with food, interesting conversations, and the opportunity for deep connection, gratitude, and joy.

Our social connections can also influence our eating patterns. When friends, family members or colleagues order pizza, the smell alone can get people salivating. Eating pizza, fast food, and take-out from restaurants is often easy, tasty, and cheap. It is an all-too-common practice for lunch meetings at work or social gatherings with friends. Fast food seems to save money as well as time on preparation and clean up, but it has additional costs to the body and brain.

Another social factor to consider is that the person who shops for food and the person who cooks it have a great deal of power with regards to the eating pattern of the entire family. In addition, parents and grandparents lay the groundwork for early experiences with food. The country of origin and culture of the parents and grandparents often influence the cuisine of the family. Understanding a person's family is helpful when working with someone on their nutrition as these social connections have an important influence.

Friends, family, and loved ones are often excellent sources of support. When someone discusses their struggles and obstacles with friends and family, these social connections may be able to share helpful strategies around obstacles that they have tried for themselves. Additionally, when people set goals for themselves like eating more vegetables each day and they share those goals with friends, they often feel more compelled to follow through with the goals. Having an accountability buddy helps with behavior change, as noted in Chapter 26, "Introduction to Behavior Change." Group visits, as discussed in Chapter 30, help patients to create a social connection. Culinary medicine group visits allow for this social connection to develop in addition to learning cooking skills to bring home and share with family and friends.

● PILLAR #6: SUBSTANCE USE AND NUTRITION

Practice Guidelines:

1) *Quit smoking*

2) *If you don't drink, don't start. If you drink, limit Alcohol to one drink per day for women and one to two drinks per day for men according to the American Heart Association.*[48]

One drink is one 12-ounce regular beer; 5 ounces of wine; or 1.5 ounces of 80-proof spirits, such as bourbon, vodka, or gin.

There are no health benefits to smoking tobacco. Smoking is associated with high blood pressure, heart disease, chronic obstructive lung disease, emphysema, stroke, and several types of cancers. Some people report that smoking helps to relieve stress. Stress management with exercise, yoga, or deep breathing are healthier options. Others report that they feel smoking helps them to lose weight or keep their weight in control. Healthy options for weight management are reviewed in Chapter 17, "Overweight and Obesity." Quitting smoking is the best thing a smoker can do for their health. It may take time with multiple quit attempts, and there may be a period of cutting down, but ultimately the goal is zero cigarettes.

The situation with alcohol is different. In the 1980s, many cardiologists encouraged patients with coronary artery disease to drink a glass of red wine with dinner as the benefits of resveratrol and other components with antioxidant properties in alcohol were thought to be heart healthy.[49] The J curve for alcohol was described years ago and expresses the fact that a small dose of alcohol may have benefits, but more than that could be deleterious to the person's health.[2] Nowadays, the American Heart Association does not recommend people start drinking. They recommend that if people do drink, that they limit their drinking to one drink per day for a woman and two drinks for a man.[48]

When people consume alcohol, they are consuming non-nutrient (so-called "empty") calories. In fact, people with alcohol substance use disorder can experience nutrient deficiencies as they prioritize alcohol over food. Common nutritional deficiencies include thiamin (vitamin B1), vitamin B12, folic acid, and zinc.

Alcohol may affect the amount of food people consume. One small observational study demonstrated that when subjects consumed alcohol before a meal, they consumed about 30% more calories at that meal.[50] The authors suggested that alcohol might have a stimulatory effect on appetite.[50] With alcohol intake, there is a loss of inhibition due to the activation of gaba aminobutyric acid (GABA), an inhibitory neurotransmitter, which works in the same way that benzodiazepines like valium and lorazepam work to reduce anxiety.[51] With less inhibition, people are more likely to indulge in unhealthy food options that they would normally have the self-control to avoid.

Galanin, a neuropeptide in the central nervous system that is made in the hypothalamus, might be partially responsible for an increase in the intake of unhealthy foods when people are drinking alcohol. The hypothalamus helps connect the endocrine system and the nervous system as well as regulate activities of the autonomic nervous system. It helps control body temperature, sleep, hunger levels, thirst levels, satiety levels, sex drive, and mood. Galanin is associated with an increase in the desire for and often the consumption of fat and alcohol.[52] Interestingly, the more fat and alcohol people consume, the more galanin is expressed. This can create a vicious cycle of more alcohol and more fatty foods. Perhaps this is why people often gravitate to a rich dessert after consuming a few drinks with dinner.

Another way alcohol may impact nutrition is through dehydration because it also acts as a diuretic by blocking vasopressin, also known as antidiuretic hormone (ADH). Dehydration can lead to increased consumption of calories, as some people mistake the signal for thirst as a signal for hunger.[53] Thus, they eat more food when really their body requires more water.

Another pillar that alcohol relates to is sleep. People often drink before bed to help them fall asleep faster. This may reduce sleep latency, meaning the time it takes them to fall asleep is reduced. However, people tend to have disrupted, poor-quality sleep overall, after consumption of alcohol.[54,55] In fact, people often complain that they wake up in the middle of the night and cannot fall back asleep after drinking alcohol. They also report that they do not feel refreshed upon awakening. Acute alcohol intake is associated with reduced rapid eye movement (REM) sleep.[54,55] It is during REM sleep that the brain spends time processing emotions, consolidating memories, and dreaming. Sleep disturbances and the development of insomnia are common among people diagnosed with alcohol substance use disorder.[55]

Alcohol has been shown to have an impact on the microbiome, the distribution of adipose tissue in the body, liver health, and risk of cancer. Research in animals and humans reveals that alcohol may have a negative effect on the microbiome.[56] Alcohol has been associated with increased gastrointestinal tract inflammation and increased intestinal permeability, allowing endotoxins to enter the blood.[56] Of note, increased alcohol consumption is associated with increased abdominal adiposity[57] which is associated with an increased risk of heart disease, diabetes, and high blood pressure. Alcohol is known to cause liver disease, cirrhosis, and liver cancer, as well as other cancers. In fact, according to the National Toxicology Program of the U.S. Department of Health and Human Services, alcohol is considered a known human carcinogen. Research studies demonstrate that the more a person drinks throughout a lifetime, the higher the risk for cancer.[58] According to a recent article in the *Lancet Public Health*, "no safe amount of alcohol consumption for cancers and health can be established".[58] It is also important to remember that alcohol has addictive potential, as some people struggle with alcohol use or have alcohol substance use disorder. Assessing and addressing a patient's alcohol consumption is an integral part of nutrition counseling.

SUMMARY OF PRACTICE GUIDELINES

For a sustainable healthy nutrition plan, it is important to assess all six pillars of lifestyle medicine including nutrition, exercise, sleep, stress resilience, social connections, and alcohol use, as they are all interconnected. Encouraging someone to exercise may help them to control cravings and lower their appetite. Without assessing people's sleep, a healthcare professional may miss an opportunity to help balance important hormones and help a patient improve their eating pattern. Stress can lead to increased consumption of hyper-palatable foods. Social connections can help or hinder healthy eating patterns. Alcohol can lead to overeating, increased empty calorie consumption, poor sleep, weight gain, and even substance use disorder. When counseling patients on nutrition, addressing the six pillars of lifestyle medicine will help the patient to adopt and sustain healthy eating practices. The recommendations for all six pillars of lifestyle medicine as described in this chapter are summarized in Table 31-1.

TABLE 31-1 Summary of practice guidelines

Pillar	Practice guidelines
Nutrition	Enjoy a delicious and nutritious whole food, plant predominant eating pattern.
Physical Activity	Engage in 2.5–5 hours of moderate intensity physical activity[a] per week
Sleep	Get 7–9 hours of sleep per night
Stress Reduction	Try different stress management strategies. For meditation, do 10–20 minutes a day.
Social Connection	Cultivate close supportive relationships with spouse/partner and relatives and connect with six to seven friends each week
Substance Use	Quit Smoking If you don't drink, do not start. Limit alcohol to 1 drink[b] per day for women and 1–2 drinks per day for men

[a]According to the sing test, moderate intensity means someone cannot sing but they can talk while exercising. If someone can sing, they are at low intensity. If someone cannot sing or talk, they are at vigorous intensity.

[b]One drink is one 12-ounce regular beer; 5 ounces of wine; or 1.5 ounces of 80-proof spirits, such as bourbon, vodka, or gin.

THREE TAKE-HOME POINTS

1. Nutrition is connected to a person's environment, movement, sleep, stress levels, social connections, and alcohol use.
2. When counseling on nutrition, make sure to inquire about physical activity levels, sleep quantity and quality, stress levels and stress management techniques, social connections both quality and quantity, and substance use, especially alcohol.
3. Slowing down to savor one's food during mealtimes when sitting at a table with friends and family while sharing a conversation and creating connections is an important part of a healthy eating pattern.

CASE STUDY ANSWERS

1. **A;** Sleep insufficiency leads to an imbalance of the hormones ghrelin and leptin. Ghrelin is the hormone that increases hunger signals. Leptin is the hormone that keeps people satiated. With lack of sleep, ghrelin goes up and leptin goes down, setting people up for hunger. Insulin sensitivity decreases with sleep insufficiency. Insulin resistance increases. Desire for hyperpalatable foods increases with sleep insufficiency.

2. **A;** Since she is experiencing cravings, Lac Phe and Irisin may help. Both of these are associated with decreased appetite according to research studies.
   - Platelet adhesiveness decreases with exercise, which helps to prevent stroke.
   - Serotonin increases with routine exercise which helps with mood regulation. Dopamine increases with exercise.

(Continued)

CASE STUDY ANSWERS *(Continued)*

3. A; Stress is associated with increased cortisol levels. Stress often impacts sleep negatively. Sleep insufficiency is associated with increased cortisol. It's also associated with increased ghrelin and decreased leptin. This combination can lead to increased hunger which can influence eating patterns. Stress may disrupt social connections, and this could increase stress even more. Increased stress leads to increased cortisol levels. GRBF was a distractor.

4. B; Exercise increases brain-derived neurotrophic factor (BDNF). It also increases norepinephrine which can increase attention and focus, and it increases serotonin, which can help decrease symptoms of depression. Also, exercise has been shown to increase the volume of the hippocampus.

5.
   - Stock up on healthy options like carrots and celery with hummus or apple slices with a nut butter.
   - Stop buying cookies, cakes, sweets, and chips and buy walnuts or pumpkin seeds instead.
   - Consider asking a friend or classmate if they want to venture into cooking together on days off and batch cook healthy soups or other items that are easy to reheat.
   - Take healthy snacks to work such as an apple, pear, banana, or orange.
   - Get a small blender to make a green smoothie at home, which would help her with increasing her intake of fruits and vegetables.
   - Think about preparing a salad that's easy like greens, beans, carrots, and cucumber to start.

   Selecting a healthy and delicious salad dressing will help.
   - Work on her stress resilience strategies and try meditation or yoga.
   - Prioritize her sleep and work to get the recommended 7–9 hours.
   - Consider walking or running for shorter distances when she has time. Get rid of the all-or-none mindset and realize that if a 5-mile run is not possible, a 3-mile run or walk is still healthy and may even help with creativity.
   - Consider doing exercise classes in her dorm. There are free classes on the internet.
   - Connect with friends and share her worries. She could make a study schedule to help her feel more comfortable about the brachial plexus, which could lower her stress so that she could sleep better.

6. Our friends and family often influence our food choices. By talking with friends about her own struggles with eating, she may come up with some excellent strategies that other medical students are using. Making goals and sharing them with friends helps to keep people accountable. Also, talking to supportive friends reduces stress. Eating with other people helps to slow down the process of consuming food. She could invite a friend to mindfully eat a raisin with her and see how that feels and tastes. By sharing gratitudes together before the meal, Magdalena can set herself and her friends up for a calm meal with low stress and high positive emotion, allowing for the parasympathetic system to predominate for resting and digesting.

REFERENCES

1. Overview: American College of Lifestyle Medicine. Accessed July 14, 2023. Available at: https://lifestylemedicine.org/overview/.

2. de Gaetano G, Costanzo S. Alcohol and health. *J Am Coll Cardiol.* 2017;70(8):923-925.

3. American Heart Association. *The American Heart Association's Diet and Lifestyle Recommendations.* Published November 1, 2021. Accessed July 14, 2023. Available at: https://www.heart.org/en/healthy-living/healthy-eating/eat-smart/nutrition-basics/aha-diet-and-lifestyle-recommendations.

4. Center for Food Safety and Applied Nutrition. Advice About Eating Fish. U.S. Food and Drug Administration. Published 2019. Available at: https://www.fda.gov/food/consumers/advice-about-eating-fish.

5. Dietary Guidelines for Americans. Published 2022. Accessed July 28, 2023. Available at: https://health.gov/our-work/nutrition-physical-activity/dietary-guidelines.

6. World Health Organization. Physical activity. World Health Organization. Published 2022. Accessed July 14, 2023. Available at: https://www.who.int/news-room/fact-sheets/detail/physical-activity.

7. U.S. Department of Health and Human Services. *Physical Activity Guidelines for Americans* 2nd ed; 2018. Accessed July 14, 2023. Available at: https://health.gov/sites/default/files/2019-09/Physical_Activity_Guidelines_2nd_edition.pdf.

8. Ledochowski L, Ruedl G, Taylor AH, Kopp M. Acute effects of brisk walking on sugary snack cravings in overweight people, affect and responses to a manipulated stress situation and to a sugary snack cue: a crossover study. *PLoS One.* 2015;10(3):e0119278.

9. Arhire LI, Mihalache L, Covasa M. Irisin: a hope in understanding and managing obesity and metabolic syndrome. *Front Endocrinol.* 2019;10:524.

10. Li VL, He Y, Contrepois K, et al. An exercise-inducible metabolite that suppresses feeding and obesity. *Nature.* 2022;606(7915):785-790.

11. Riley KE, Park CL. How does yoga reduce stress? A systematic review of mechanisms of change and guide to future inquiry. *Health Psychol Rev.* 2015;9(3):379-396.

12. McIver S, O'Halloran P, McGartland M. Yoga as a treatment for binge eating disorder: a preliminary study. *Complement Ther Med.* 2009;17(4):196-202.

13. Watts AW, Rydell SA, Eisenberg ME, Laska MN, Neumark-Sztainer D. Yoga's potential for promoting healthy eating and physical activity behaviors among young adults: a mixed-methods study. *Int J Behav Nutr Phys Act.* 2018;15(1):42.

14. Oppezzo M, Schwartz DL. Give your ideas some legs: the positive effect of walking on creative thinking. *J Exp Psychol Mem Cogn: Learning, Memory, and Cognition.* 2014;40(4):1142-1152.

15. Lin TW, Kuo YM. Exercise benefits brain function: the monoamine connection. *Brain Sci.* 2013;3(4):39-53

16. Erickson KI, Voss MW, Prakash RS, et al. Exercise training increases size of hippocampus and improves memory. *Proc Natl Acad Sci U S A.* 2011;108(7):3017-3022.

17. Hamilton MT, Hamilton DG, Zderic TW. Role of low energy expenditure and sitting in obesity, metabolic syndrome, type 2 diabetes, and cardiovascular disease. *Diabetes.* 2007;56(11):2655-2667.

18. Crichton GE, Alkerwi A. Physical activity, sedentary behavior time and lipid levels in the observation of cardiovascular risk factors in Luxembourg study. *Lipids Health Dis.* 2015;14:87.

19. Moore DR, Williamson EE, Hodson N, et al. Walking or body weight squat "activity snacks" increase dietary amino acid utilization for myofibrillar protein synthesis during prolonged sitting. *J Appl Physiol.* 2022;133(3):777-785.

20. Is Sitting The New Smoking? by Hannah at The Heart Foundation Published August 10, 2019. Accessed December 11, 2023. Available at: https://theheartfoundation.org/2019/08/10/is-sitting-the-new-smoking/.

21. *Breaking Sitting Streaks.* ADA. diabetes.org. Accessed July 15, 2023.Available at: https://diabetes.org/healthy-living/fitness/break-sitting-streak#:~:text=The%20Standards%20of%20Medical%20Care.

22. *National Sleep Foundation Recommends New Sleep Times.* National Sleep Foundation; 2015. Accessed July 15, 2023. Available at: https://els-jbs-prod-cdn.jbs.elsevierhealth.com/pb/assets/raw/Health%20Advance/journals/sleh/NSF_press_release_on_new_sleep_durations_2-2-15.pdf.

23. Lloyd-Jones DM, Allen NB, Anderson CAM, et al. Life's essential 8: updating and enhancing the American Heart Association's construct of cardiovascular health: a presidential advisory from the American Heart Association. *Circulation.* 2022;146(5):e18-e43.

24. Klinzing JG, Niethard N, Born J. Mechanisms of systems memory consolidation during sleep. *Nat Neurosci.* 2019;22(10):1598-1610.

25. Wang C, Holtzman DM. Bidirectional relationship between sleep and Alzheimer's disease: role of amyloid, tau, and other factors. *Neuropsychopharmacology.* 2020;45(1):104-120.

26. Greer SM, Goldstein AN, Walker MP. The impact of sleep deprivation on food desire in the human brain. *Nat Commun.* 2013;4:2259.

27. St-Onge MP, Roberts AL, Chen J, et al. Short sleep duration increases energy intakes but does not change energy expenditure in normal-weight individuals. *Am J Clin Nutr.* 2011;94(2):410-416.

28. Scoditti E, Tumolo MR, Garbarino S. Mediterranean diet on sleep: a health alliance. *Nutrients.* 2022;14(14):2998.

29. Muscogiuri G, Barrea L, Aprano S, et al. Sleep quality in obesity: does adherence to the Mediterranean diet matter? *Nutrients.* 2020;12(5):1364.

30. Makarem N, Alcántara C, Williams N, Bello NA, Abdalla M. Effect of sleep disturbances on blood pressure. *Hypertension.* 2021;77(4):1036-1046.

31. Leproult R, Van Cauter E. Role of sleep and sleep loss in hormonal release and metabolism. *Endocr Dev.* 2010;17:11-21.

32. Basso JC, McHale A, Ende V, Oberlin DJ, Suzuki WA. Brief, daily meditation enhances attention, memory, mood, and emotional regulation in non-experienced meditators. *Behav Brain Res.* 2019;356(356):208-220.

33. Jha AP, Witkin JE, Morrison AB, Rostrup N, Stanley E. Short-form mindfulness training protects against working memory degradation over high-demand intervals. *J Cogn Enhanc.* 2017;1(2):154-171.

34. Innes KE, Selfe TK, Brundage K, et al. Effects of meditation and music-listening on blood biomarkers of cellular aging and Alzheimer's disease in adults with subjective cognitive decline: an exploratory randomized clinical trial. In: Ashford JW, ed. *J Alz Dis.* 2018;66(3):947-970.

35. Mrazek MD, Franklin MS, Phillips DT, Baird B, Schooler JW. Mindfulness training improves working memory capacity and GRE performance while reducing mind wandering. *Psycholog Sci.* 2013;24(5):776-781.

36. Sinha R, Gu P, Hart R, Guarnaccia JB. Food craving, cortisol and ghrelin responses in modeling highly palatable snack intake in the laboratory. *Physiol Behav.* 2019;208:112563.

37. Heckman W. *Stress, Cortisol and Abdominal Fat.* The American Institute of Stress. Accessed July 14, 2023. Available at: https://www.stress.org/stress-cortisol-and-abdominal-fat.

38. American Psychological Association. *Stress Effects on the Body.* American Psychological Association. Published March 8, 2023. Accessed July 28, 2023. Available at: https://www.apa.org/topics/stress/body.

39. Kim EJ, Pellman B, Kim JJ. Stress effects on the hippocampus: a critical review. *Learn Mem.* 2015;22(9):411-416.

40. Inoue K, Horwich T, Bhatnagar R, et al. Urinary stress hormones, hypertension, and cardiovascular events: the multi-ethnic study of atherosclerosis. *Hypertension.* 2021;78(5)1640-1647.

41. Hurst Y, Fukuda H. Effects of changes in eating speed on obesity in patients with diabetes: a secondary analysis of longitudinal health check-up data. *BMJ Open.* 2018;8(1):e019589.

42. El Ansari W, Adetunji H, Oskrochi R. Food and mental health: relationship between food and perceived stress and depressive symptoms among university students in the United Kingdom. *Cent Eur J Public Health.* 2014;22(2):90-97.

43. Becofsky KM, Shook RP, Sui X, Wilcox S, Lavie CJ, Blair SN. Influence of the source of social support and size of social network on all-cause mortality. *Mayo Clin Proc.* 2015;90(7):895-902.

44. *Do social ties affect our health?* NIH News in Health. Published February 27, 2017. Accessed July 18, 2023. Available at: https://newsinhealth.nih.gov/2017/02/do-social-ties-affect-our-health.

45. Don BP, Gordon AM, Berry Mendes W. The good, the bad, and the variable: examining stress and blood pressure responses to close relationships. *Soc Psychol Personal Sci.* Published online March 27, 2023:194855062311560. Available at: doi:https://doi.org/10.1177/19485506231156018.

46. Berkman LF, Syme SL. Social networks, host resistance, and mortality: a nine-year follow-up study of Alameda County residents. *Am J Epidemiol.* 1979;109(2):186-204.

47. Umberson D, Karas Montez J. Social relationships and health: a flashpoint for health policy. *J Health Soc Behav.* 2010;51(1):54-66.

48. American Heart Association. Alcohol and heart health. www.heart.org. Published 2014. Accessed July 28, 2023. Available at: https://www.heart.org/en/healthy-living/healthy-eating/eat-smart/nutrition-basics/alcohol-and-heart-health.

49. *Drinking red wine for heart health? Read this before you toast.* www.heart.org. Published May 24, 2019. Accessed July 27, 2023. Available at: https://www.heart.org/en/news/2019/05/24/drinking-red-wine-for-heart-health-read-this-before-you-toast#:~:text=Federal%20guidelines%20and%20the%20American.

50. Hetherington MM, Cameron F, Wallis DJ, Pirie LM. Stimulation of appetite by alcohol. *Physiol Behav.* 2001;74(3):283-289.

51. Davis M. The role of GABAA receptors in mediating the effects of alcohol in the central nervous system. *J Psychiatry Neurosci.* 2003;28(4):263-274.

52. Barson JR, Morganstern I, Leibowitz SF. Galanin and consummatory behavior: special relationship with dietary fat, alcohol and circulating lipids. *Exp Suppl.* 2010:87-111.

53. McKiernan F, Houchins JA, Mattes RD. Relationships between human thirst, hunger, drinking, and feeding. *Physiol Behav.* 2008;94(5):700-708.

54. Koob GF, Colrain IM. Alcohol use disorder and sleep disturbances: a feed-forward allostatic framework. *Neuropsychopharmacology.* 2019;45(1):141-165.

55. Colrain IM, Nicholas CL, Baker FC. Alcohol and the sleeping brain. *Handb Clin Neurol.* 2014;125:415-431.

56. Phillip E, Green S, Voigt R, Forsyth C, Keshavarzian A. The gastrointestinal microbiome: alcohol effects on the composition of intestinal microbiota. *Alcohol Res.* 2015;37(2):233-236.

57. Schröder H, Morales-Molina JA, Bermejo S, et al. Relationship of abdominal obesity with alcohol consumption at population scale. *Euro J Nutr.* 2007;46(7):369-376.

58. Anderson BO, Berdzuli N, Ilbawi A, et al. Health and cancer risks associated with low levels of alcohol consumption. *Lancet Public Health.* 2023;8(1):e6-e7.

chapter 32

The Physician as a Nutrition Change Agent

Walter Willett, MD, MPH, Dr PH

Chapter Outline

CASE STUDY

A practicing physician is looking to have more of an impact on the "nutrition is medicine" movement. This physician has been seeing patients in her clinic practice for over 10 years and has seen the impact of fast food and processed food on the health and progression of disease in thousands of patients. She has gained education in nutrition through continuing medical education (CME) courses and has joined a national society with a focus on nutrition. This physician wants to do more and get involved in different ways.

1. In what ways can physicians serve to advance nutrition beyond the medical clinic visit?
2. How does a physician's own behavior impact their counseling behavior?
3. What can be done in worksites?

● INTRODUCTION

As physicians or other healthcare providers, most of our training is focused on counseling and treating patients on a one-on-one basis. This role of being trusted healers has deep traditions, developed over thousands of years. These highly personal interactions, however, are only one way by which physicians can enhance the diets and well-being of patients and society more broadly. To be most effective, an understanding of the broader determinants of diet and health can be helpful and are described here briefly.

Traditional Academic and Translational Pathways to Enhance Diets

One important path by which physicians can extend their contributions to improvements in nutrition is through an academic career. Until recently, this typically involved obtaining a PhD in biochemistry or physiology together with an MD degree and then conducting laboratory research in parallel with a clinical role. This path has a long and highly productive track record, providing the basis for our understanding of biochemical pathways and resulting in dozens of Nobel Prizes.

The resulting knowledge has had many practical applications, such as in fortification programs, the near-elimination of deficiency conditions such as rickets in high-income settings, and nutritional support for seriously ill patients. However, this work has had a surprisingly limited impact on our understanding of how foods and dietary patterns affect risks of the major chronic diseases such as cardiovascular disease, cancer, and neurodegenerative diseases. More recently, another academic path has emerged by combing an MD degree, often including specialty training, with a master in public health (MPH) degree emphasizing quantitative sciences. Research topics, rather than being laboratory-based, include development of methods for dietary assessment and monitoring, screening for nutritional inadequacies or excesses, and development and evaluation of interventions to improve diets for the prevention or management of illness. As with all academic pathways, publications are fundamentally important for disseminating knowledge and experiences. Academic physicians also help advance their research fields by presentations at meetings and by serving as peer reviewers of research proposals and papers submitted to journals. Another opportunity to have an impact is to serve on the editorial team for a nutrition or medical journal. Teaching and mentoring is also a central component of an academic career by which knowledge and experience are transmitted to new generations. All too often, even the most fundamental information on diets and health has not been included in the curricula of medical schools[1]; medical students and physicians can advocate for more nutrition content in medical school, residency, and continuing medical education programs.

Physicians can also pursue careers in many governmental and non-governmental organizations traditionally involved with diet and nutrition. These could include state, national, and international organizations such as the U.S. Centers for Disease Control and Prevention, the World Health Organization, or UNICEF, and typically involve development, implementation, and management of programs implementing knowledge. Existing public health positions at all levels of government also provide opportunities to creatively incorporate nutrition-enhancement programs where they do not already exist.

ACTING BEYOND TRADITIONAL PATHWAYS

Physicians and other healthcare providers have many opportunities to promote better diets and health beyond their practice with individual patients or an academic career involving teaching, mentoring, and research. The social-ecological model, described earlier in "Introduction to Behavior Change" (Chapter 26), was developed to convey the circles of factors that influence the actions or status of individuals,[2] and was adapted by Cheung to focus on diet and nutrition (see Figure 32-1). The diets of individuals are strongly influenced, both favorably and unfavorably, by our immediate social environment that includes family, friends, and peers. Our surrounding community further influences our diets; this includes schools, healthcare system, grocery stores, restaurants, worksites, and vending

machines. Broader societal factors such as media, marketing, food cultures, systemic racism, agricultural policies, and international trade policies also have strong effects on the availability, cost, and attractiveness of foods. This perspective helps to identify potential targets for policies and other actions to improve the nutritional status of individuals and populations.[3]

The degree to which physicians can become involved in non-traditional efforts to improve nutrition can range from occasional commitments of time to being the focus of a person's life's work. A matrix for thinking about such opportunities is shown in Figure 32-2 that considers different sectors (schools, health care, worksites, food environment, physical environment, mass media, and economic) and level of action (individual, family, community, state, national, and global). No person can be an actor at all of these intersections, but almost everyone can find one or more opportunities to have an important influence.

GETTING INVOLVED WITH SCHOOLS AND SCHOOL SYSTEMS

From preschool through university and professional education, schools should be places of learning about and experiencing good nutrition and well-being. Physicians can volunteer to give special lectures about diet and health for classes attended by their children, and they can advocate for high standards for foods and beverages available and serve on committees or boards at their child's school. These educational and advocacy roles can also extend to the larger community, state, and national level.

Examples might be as local as setting standards for bake sales as fundraisers (or sales of fruit and nuts rather than baked goods), or developing national standards for food served in schools. Such standards have largely eliminated sales of sugar-sweetened beverages at elementary schools nationally, but these changes were initiated and powered by local advocacy. Nationally, the implementation of standards for school lunch programs has dramatically improved these meals; in just several years, the quality score increased from 58 to 82 on a scale of 100.[4]

GETTING INVOLVED WITH HEALTHCARE SYSTEMS

Although the healthcare system should be the lead sector in promoting healthy nutrition, the unfortunate reality is that this sector has largely been missing in action. Incorporation of monitoring of patients' diets and providing motivation and education directed at enhancement of diets should be at the core of medical practice. Physicians can do much to integrate nutrition into our healthcare systems, whether working in solo practice, a small or large group, a community hospital, a large healthcare system, or the financial or regulatory aspects of state or national healthcare infrastructure. Waiting rooms in our healthcare facilities are an underutilized opportunity to provide nutritional education, such as with posters, handouts, and videos about healthy eating. Hospitals have unfortunately often been incubators of obesity and cardiometabolic disease by serving unhealthy foods to both patients and in their cafeterias

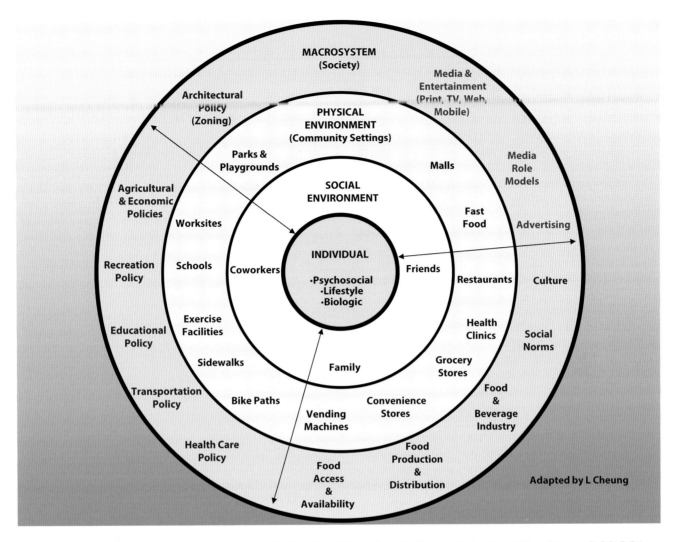

FIGURE 32-1 • Socio-ecological model as applied to diets. (Reproduced with permission from Lilian Cheung D.SC, R.D.)

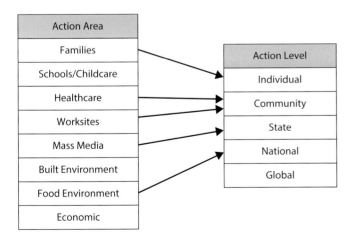

FIGURE 32-2 • Opportunities to promote healthier diets. As a hypothetical example, "X" could describe the activities of a primary care physician who does not keep soda at home, regularly counsels patients on healthy eating, has initiated a committee at his/her admitting hospital to improve the quality of foods for patients and staff, occasionally writes commentaries for a state-wide newspaper, and serves on a national committee of a professional organization to promote healthier diets.

where their staff and visitors dine. Not long ago, the only nutritional information in the cafeteria of one of Harvard's leading teaching hospitals was a sign at eye level in a large dessert section proclaiming "Try our fat-free chocolate brownie" (which was of course loaded with sugar and white flour). Until 2011, the Children's Hospital of Philadelphia had a McDonald's in the lobby. All too often, inpatients are by default served meals loaded with refined starch, sugar, and salt. Our healthcare institutions should be setting the best possible example of healthy and delicious meals. Fortunately, this is starting to change in some places, often led by institutional dietitians and physicians working together. At Massachusetts General Hospital, the cafeteria for staff and visitors has flagged foods with red, yellow, and green ratings, with suggestions for alternatives to red-flagged foods; this strategy has shifted purchases to healthier choices.[5] At the Brigham and Women's Hospital, patients receive menus with information on healthy eating and an array of healthy options. Also, adjusting prices of beverages combined with education reduced purchases of sugar-sweetened beverages, although this practice was abandoned for obscure reasons.[6] At the Harvard T. H. Chan School of Public Health cafeteria, subsidies for the salad bar increased sales,[7] and removal of red meat from the grill with replacement by other types of burgers led to a large increase in sales.[8] In many healthcare settings, physicians have worked with dietitians and others to establish teaching kitchens to provide hands-on facilities for patients to acquire skills in preparation of healthy meals (see Chapter 29, "Culinary Medicine"). Much more needs to be done to make our healthcare system a health-promoting system, and physicians are well positioned to effect this change.

Although we are not aware of systematic survey data on the prevalence of overweight/obesity data among healthcare workers, this is visibly a serious issue, including both the lowest paid and professional staff, consistent with national rates of approximately 70% of adults.[9] A contributing factor may be that the quality of foods available to hospital staff in cafeterias and dining facilities in hospitals has frequently been unhealthy and unappealing to many, yet there may be few other options. The prevalence of obesity/overweight in healthcare workers may be heightened because for many, healthy eating is challenging due to low incomes, systemic racism that has made healthy food options less accessible, irregular hours, and stressful work. The health consequences of the obesity epidemic for healthcare workers have been further magnified by COVID-19 because obesity and diabetes are major risk factors for severe outcomes, including death.[10] Also, many of these employees live in crowded conditions that promote transmission of infectious diseases, must commute using public transportation, and are directly exposed to infected patients. Diet quality itself appears to be a risk factor for severe COVID-19 independent of obesity.[11] For all of these reasons, the healthcare system has a special obligation to ensure, without stigmatization, that those who work in the system have access to healthy and affordable diets. Physicians can provide leadership to make better options readily available and affordable for all employees.

WORKING WITH WORKSITES

Beyond the healthcare system, many employers have developed programs to promote healthier diets as part of overall wellness programs for employees.[12] This is in part motivated by potential financial benefits due to reduction in absenteeism and greater "presence" at work, and by providing a benefit that is valued. The specific programs have varied widely, and can include education, provision of healthier options in cafeterias, and subsidies for healthier choices. In an umbrella review,[12] 19 meta-analyses of worksite dietary interventions were identified, with highly varied outcome evaluations. Evidence of benefit was found for increases in consumption of fruits and vegetables, reductions in dietary fat (many interventions were done when this was thought to be an appropriate goal), and reductions in body weight and blood cholesterol levels. Some evidence of reduction in absenteeism was seen and no adverse financial consequences were reported. Much work remains to optimize worksite dietary interventions and their evaluation; some physicians may have the opportunity to motivate such programs and participate in their implementation and reporting.

Although no formal surveys appear to have been conducted, our impression is that biomedical research laboratories appear to be poor examples of health promotion, as the primary offerings at seminars and research meetings are often pizza and soda. Physicians working in this environment have an opportunity to set a better example.

ADDRESSING THE FOOD ENVIRONMENT

The ubiquity of food in today's America, mostly of poor quality and sometimes described as "the toxic food environment," is thought to be one of the drivers of the ongoing obesity epidemic.[13] As noted, our healthcare facilities have often contributed to this poor environment, and physicians have a special voice in this setting. More broadly, physicians can lead or support efforts to improve diet quality or limit availability of unhealthy foods in other contexts; the possibilities are almost as endless as the number of unhealthy products being promoted. Actions can range from low-intensity actions such as education to labeling of contents of calories and other food constituents, setting standards for procurement of foods by institutions, limiting sales of unhealthy foods and beverages around schools or health care facilities, taxing soda or "junk food," to elimination of unhealthy foods such as has been done for trans-fatty acids. Because influences of industry groups are especially powerful at the national level in the United States, changes are more likely to be feasible at local and state levels. For example, soda taxes implemented in Berkely and Philadelphia have resulted in reduced consumption.[14,15] In Mexico, physicians have led successful efforts to tax soda and unhealthy snacks.[16]

ADDRESSING THE BUILT ENVIRONMENT

Although not directly related to diet, control of the obesity epidemic will need to incorporate greater adoption of regular physical activity than exists at present. Physical activity and nutrition are interconnected in many ways, as described in Chapter 31, "The Six Pillars of Lifestyle Medicine and Nutrition," and how nutrition interconnects with the others. Unfortunately, our physical environment has been built to minimize physical activity such as by making automobiles the primary mode of transportation, and constructing buildings that emphasize escalators and elevators rather than stairways. Although good health care includes assessment of a patient's pattern of physical activity and counseling about incorporation of physical activity into daily lives, this may be difficult for many patients if they do not live in an environment with safe places to walk, bicycle, or play. These facilities can have profoundly important impacts on health; for example, Denmark has an extensive bicycle system that is routinely used for transportation, and regular bicycle riding to work is associated with a 30% reduction in overall mortality.[16] Physicians can play an important advocacy role in development of these facilities, whether at the neighborhood, city, state, or national levels.

WORKING WITH MEDIA

The forms of communication beyond direct person-to-person exchanges have grown dramatically in recent years and can be used to promote both healthy and unhealthy diets. Unfortunately, these proportions are highly imbalanced because major corporations and powerful agricultural groups spend many billions of dollars per year on research to subvert human vulnerabilities and buy vast amounts of television time and print media. Their effectiveness in promoting unhealthy products has been augmented by artificial intelligence to deliver personalized messages based on analyses of purchases, clicks, and other data. Many institutions have been subverted; for example, the U.S. Department of Agriculture operates a "check-off" program that involves a small tax on beef, dairy, and other products, and uses this to promote cheese and beef while at the same time, their dietary guidelines (which have no funding for promotion) recommend that these foods be limited.[17] Also, the plethora of new digital media has created major financial challenges for traditional print and electronic media, so that all forms of media, including medical journals are competing for attention using sensationalism to attract readers and viewers[18]; physicians can play a role by writing letters or working with journalists to correct misinformation.

Despite the huge expenditures in media for promotion of foods that undermine health, physicians have access to "free" media space that is underutilized. As noted above, the walls, tables, and digital resources of our offices and worksites provide an opportunity to convey accurate, positive information about the benefits of healthy eating and other behaviors. Physicians can also write timely letters to the editors of local, regional, or national news media; author more extensive commentaries on nutrition-related topics; or give informed interviews for traditional newsprint, radio, or TV media. The "social media" is a morass of solid, scientifically based information as well as hyped news stories or purposeful disinformation motivated by many factors. As daunting as it may be, physicians can add credible and informed voices to this environment, sometimes specifically in response to egregiously misleading or false claims.

Perhaps the most egregious use of media is marketing directed at children to promote consumption of unhealthy foods and beverages that will increase risks of obesity and diabetes and thus cause suffering and premature death. Due to heavy lobbying efforts by industry, some members of Congress have blocked efforts to limit this exploitation, and voluntary rules have had minimal effects.[19] Despite limited success thus far, greater support from the medical community to protect our children could potentially make an important difference.

FOCUSING ON ECONOMICS

Economic factors strongly influence dietary choices, and on average healthier diets cost more than less healthy diets. However, at any cost, the healthfulness of diets can vary greatly, and it is possible to eat healthfully on a low budget.[20] For example, carrots, winter squash, and cabbage are inexpensive vegetables, and beans, peanuts, and peanut butter are inexpensive sources of protein. However, availability of these foods and the knowledge to prepare them in flavorful and enjoyable ways (which are central to the traditional diets of many cultures) is often limited. Physicians can support, or be directly involved

in, local programs to promote healthful nutrition on limited budgets. As mentioned in Chapters 29 and 30 on Culinary Medicine and Nutrition Counseling with Group Visits, teaching cooking skills and educating patients about eating on a budget can empower them to adopt and sustain healthy eating patterns.

Taxes and subsidies can also be used to tip the balance to support healthful eating. For example, the soda tax enacted by Philadelphia with the leadership of Tom Farley, MD, was created with the intent to use the income for health and nutrition programs for children.[21] This has the double benefit of reducing soda consumption and also providing funding for much-needed programs and infrastructure. Notably, taxes attract greater public support if the income is targeted to the needs of children, and physicians are in a position to advocate for these policies. Elsewhere, Farley has described the role of physicians in developing programs to improve nutrition in New York City.[22]

National economic policies related to food are highly contentious as this involves the titans of the food and agricultural sectors; these debates converge in the periodic renewal of the "Farm Bill" in Congress. Because each state has two senators regardless of population, the playing field is strongly tilted toward agricultural interests that are traditionally focused on production of beef, milk, and commodity crops, rather than fruits, vegetables, nuts, and legumes (except for soy, which is primarily fed to animals). By far, the largest part of the Farm Bill budget funds food assistance programs including SNAP (Supplemental Nutrition Assistance Program, formerly food stamps) and WIC (Special Nutritional Supplementation Program for Women, Infants, and Children). These are essential programs that have greatly reduced food insecurity, but the bargain struck in Congress has been that no limits should be placed on purchases with SNAP funds, even though soda and foods based on sugar and refined starch are fueling the epidemics of obesity and diabetes, and that these are driving health costs upward. Notably, even a majority of SNAP recipients recognize that limits on the use of SNAP funds for purchases of soda and "junk food" would be appropriate.[23] Moving national economic policies related to food is a daunting task, but physicians could work to improve SNAP by making it more supportive of healthy eating. In general, successes are more likely at local and state levels, where the power of agricultural and industry interests may be more limited.

LEADING BY EXAMPLE

Probably the most important action physicians can take to promote better diets for their patients and others is to lead by example. Adoption of healthy habits by physicians is important because of a natural hesitancy to promote a behavior that we do not practice ourselves. Smoking reduction provides a strong precedent; physicians who smoked (now very few in the United States) are less likely than nonsmokers to discuss smoking cessation with their patients,[24] and physician counseling does reduce patient smoking, although cessation typically takes many attempts.[25] Similar examples of physician personal behaviors being associated with likelihood of counseling patients have been documented for physical activity, wearing seatbelts, and using sunscreen.[26] Physicians publicly practicing healthy behaviors can also contribute to establishing social norms. As one example, in the 1950s America's best-known cardiologist, Paul Dudley White, regularly rode his bicycle to work at Massachusetts General Hospital, which helped make this normal behavior.

Practicing healthy diets also involves gaining practical experience in finding, preparing, and enjoying healthy foods, and this experience and dealing with the accompanying challenges can be shared with patients and others. Because few physicians have received training in nutrition, continuing education courses may be one way to develop knowledge and skills in this area.

SUMMARY

In addition to their central role in caring for individuals, physicians can be important change makers to improve nutrition and promote well-being. This has traditionally been done by engagement in research, teaching, mentoring, and participating in professional organizations.

Physicians can also be engaged in policy changes at many levels, from family to national and international. For both their own well-being and effectiveness as change makers, adoption of healthy dietary practices in their own lives is important.

TAKE-AWAY POINTS

1. Physicians play a central role in caring for individuals, and have traditionally extended their contributions by engaging in research, publication in professional journals, teaching, and mentoring.
2. A physician can also be a nutritional change agent by engaging with schools, healthcare systems, the food environment, the built environment, media messages, and development of economic policies.
3. Engagement can be at any level, beginning with personal behaviors to community, state, national, and global levels.
4. Important changes often begin locally, in part because positive changes can be contagious and also because powerful opposing economic actors may have less influence at that level.

CASE STUDY ANSWERS

1. This physician could engage in activities and policies related to nutrition within schools, the healthcare system, other worksites, the food and built environments, or media. This could be at levels from his/her own family and community to national or international; beginning locally can often make the most sense.
2. In many behavior-related areas, such as smoking avoidance, physicians who practiced healthy behaviors were more effective in counseling patients, and staying healthy oneself is important to be effective. Also, by adopting a healthy behavior, one gains understanding about barriers to overcome and practical ways to do so.

3. Worksites are potentially effective venues for improving dietary practices because many people consume a substantial part of their total food intake there, and some control of the food environment is possible. Physicians can be advocates for improving foods provided at worksites and be advisors where the leadership is already motivated to support healthy food offering. Specific actions can include helping to create health-promoting menus and educational material about diet and health, monitoring food availability and quality such as sodium audits, and working with food services to enhance procurement policies.

REFERENCES

1. Devries S, Willett W, Bonow RO. Nutrition education in medical school, residency training, and practice. *JAMA.* 2019;321(14):1351-1352.
2. Bronfenbrenner U. *The Ecology of Human Development: Experiments by Nature and Design.* Harvard University Press; 1979.
3. Willett WC, Wood M, Childs D. *Thinfluence.* Rodale; 2014.
4. *School Meals Are Healthier After Major Nutrition Reforms. Mathematica [Internet].* 2019. Available at: https://www.mathematica.org/news/school-meals-are-healthier-after-major-nutrition-reforms.
5. Thorndike AN, Gelsomin ED, McCurley JL, Levy DE. Calories purchased by hospital employees after implementation of a

cafeteria traffic light-labeling and choice architecture program. *JAMA Netw Open.* 2019;2(7):e196789.

6. Block JP, Chandra A, McManus KD, Willett WC. Point-of-purchase price and education intervention to reduce consumption of sugary soft drinks. *Am J Public Health.* 2010;100(8):1427-1433.

7. Michels KB, Bloom BR, Riccardi P, Rosner BA, Willett WC. A study of the importance of education and cost incentives on individual food choices at the Harvard School of Public Health cafeteria. *J Am Coll Nutr.* 2008;27(1):6-11.

8. Vadiveloo MK, Malik VS, Spiegelman D, Willett WC, Mattei J. Does a grill menu redesign influence sales, nutrients purchased, and consumer acceptance in a worksite cafeteria? *Prev Med Rep.* 2017;8:140-147.

9. Hales CM, Carroll MD, Fryar CD, Ogden CL. Prevalence of obesity and severe obesity among adults: United States, 2017–2018. *NCHS Data Brief.* 2020;(360):1-8.

10. Sawadogo W, Tsegaye M, Gizaw A, Adera T. Overweight and obesity as risk factors for COVID-19-associated hospitalisations and death: systematic review and meta-analysis. *BMJ Nutr Prev Health.* 2022;5(1):10-18.

11. Merino J, Joshi AD, Nguyen LH, et al. Diet quality and risk and severity of COVID-19: a prospective cohort study. *Gut.* 2021;70(11):2096-2104.

12. Schliemann D, Woodside JV. The effectiveness of dietary workplace interventions: a systematic review of systematic reviews. *Public Health Nutr.* 2019;22(5):942-955.

13. Godfrey JR. Toward optimal health: Dr. Kelly Brownell discusses the influence of the environment on obesity. *J Women's Health.* 2008;17(3):325-330.

14. Ng SW, Rivera JA, Popkin BM, Colchero MA. Did high sugar-sweetened beverage purchasers respond differently to the excise tax on sugar-sweetened beverages in Mexico? *Public Health Nutr.* 2019;22(4):750-756.

15. Bleich SN, Lawman HG, LeVasseur MT, et al. The association of a sweetened beverage tax with changes in beverage prices and purchases at independent stores. *Health Aff (Millwood).* 2020;39(7):1130-1139.

16. Colchero MA, Popkin BM, Rivera JA, Ng SW. Beverage purchases from stores in Mexico under the excise tax on sugar sweetened beverages: observational study. *BMJ.* 2016;352:h6704.

17. Wilde PE. Federal communication about obesity in the Dietary Guidelines and checkoff programs. *Obesity (Silver Spring).* 2006;14(6):967-973.

18. Oreskes N. Let Them eat meat? when journals behave irresponsibly, it can cause real harm. *Sci Am.* 2020;322(2):70.

19. Powell LM, Schermbeck RM, Chaloupka FJ. Nutritional content of food and beverage products in television advertisements seen on children's programming. *Child Obes.* 2013;9(6):524-531.

20. Bernstein AM, Bloom DE, Rosner BA, Franz M, Willett WC. Relation of food cost to healthfulness of diet among US women. *Am J Clin Nutr.* 2010;92(5):1197-1203.

21. Farley T. *E7: Thomas Farley on the Real Returns of the Philadelphia Soda Tax [Internet].* North Carolina; 2019. Podcast. Available at: https://wfpc.sanford.duke.edu/podcasts/thomas-farley-philadelphia-soda-tax/.

22. Farley T. *Saving Gotham: A Billionaire Mayor, Activist Doctors, and the Fight for Eight Million Lives.* W. W Norton & Company; 2015.

23. Leung CW, Wolfson JA. Perspectives from supplemental nutrition assistance program participants on improving SNAP policy. *Health Equity.* 2019;3(1):81-85.

24. Al-Hagabani MA, Khan MS, Al-Hazmi AM, Shaher BM, El-Fahel AO. Smoking behavior of primary care physicians and its effect on their smoking counseling practice. *J Family Med Prim Care.* 2020;9(2):1053-1057.

25. Stead LF, Buitrago D, Preciado N, Sanchez G, Hartmann-Boyce J, Lancaster T. Physician advice for smoking cessation. *Cochrane Database Syst Rev.* 2013;2013(5):CD000165.

26. Abramson S, Stein J, Schaufele M, Frates E, Rogan S. Personal exercise habits and counseling practices of primary care physicians: a national survey. *Clin J Sport Med.* 2000;10(1):40-48.

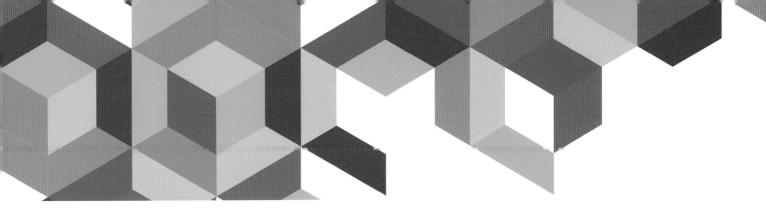

Index